Clinical Decision-Making Study Guide for

Medical-Surgical Nursing

Patient-Centered Collaborative Care

Sixth Edition

Donna D. Ignatavicius, MS, RN, ANEF

Speaker and Curriculum Consultant for
Academic Nursing Programs
Founder, Boot Camp for Nurse
Educators®
President, DI Associates, Inc.
Placitas, New Mexico

M. Linda Workman, PhD, RN, FAAN

Senior Volunteer Faculty
College of Nursing
University of Cincinnati
Cincinnati, Ohio;
Formerly Gertrude Perkins Oliva
Professor of Oncology
Frances Payne Bolton School of Nursing
Case Western Reserve University
Cleveland, Ohio

Clinical Decision-Making Study Guide prepared by

Candice K. Kumagai, RN, MSN

Clinical Instructor
University of Texas at Austin
Austin, Texas

Valerie O'Toole Baker, MSN, ACNS-BC

Assistant Professor
Villa Maria School of Nursing
Gannon University
Erie, Pennsylvania

Amy H. Lee, RN, MSN

Senior Lecturer
School of Nursing
Old Dominion University
Norfolk, Virginia

Tara McMillan-Queen, RN, ANP/GNP

Faculty II/Nurse Practitioner
Mercy School of Nursing
Carolinas Medical Center—Mercy
Charlotte, North Carolina

Linda L. Kerby, RN-C, BSN, MA, BA

Educational Consultant
Mastery Educational Consultations
Leawood, Kansas

Julie S. Snyder, MSN, RN, C

Adjunct Faculty, School of Nursing
Old Dominion University
Norfolk, Virginia

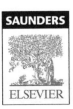

SAUNDERS

ELSEVIER

SAUNDERS

ELSEVIER

11830 Westline Industrial Drive
St. Louis, Missouri 63146

CLINICAL DECISION-MAKING STUDY GUIDE FOR
MEDICAL-SURGICAL NURSING:
PATIENT-CENTERED COLLABORATIVE CARE, SIXTH EDITION   ISBN: 978-1-4160-5479-5

Senior Editor: Lee Henderson
Senior Developmental Editor: Rae L. Robertson
Publishing Services Manager: Gayle May

Printed in the United States of America

Last digit is the print number: 9 8 7 6 5 4 3 2 1

Preface

The *Clinical Decision-Making Study Guide* is a companion publication for Ignatavicius & Workman's *Medical-Surgical Nursing: Patient-Centered Collaborative Care*, 6th Edition. This Study Guide, written by experts in the fields of adult medical-surgical nursing and nursing education, will help to ensure mastery of the textbook content and help you learn about collaborative practice in the care of the adult medical-surgical patient.

The 6th edition has been carefully revised and updated for an increased emphasis on clinical decision-making, and the use of Case Studies has been expanded.

The overall organization of the *Clinical Decision-Making Study Guide* directly corresponds to the unit/chapter name and number in the textbook so that you or your instructor can readily select the corresponding learning exercises in the Study Guide. Chapters are organized by the following sections:

- **Study/Review Questions** are designed to encourage prioritizing, clinical decision-making, and application of the steps of the nursing process. Questions have been thoroughly revised to focus on the question formats of the NCLEX Examination, and emphasize the NCLEX priorities of delegation, management of care, and pharmacology.
- Additional "real-world" **Case Studies** are included in this edition, allowing you to further develop your decision-making abilities in a variety of clinical situations.

Answers to the Study/Review Questions are now provided in the back of the Study Guide. Answer guidelines for the Case Studies are available on your Evolve website at http://evolve.elsevier.com/Iggy/ in the "Prepare for Class" folder.

The Evolve website also features an introductory "pre-chapter" that includes concrete study tips to help you make the most of your individual learning style.

The *Clinical Decision-Making Study Guide* is a practical tool to help you prepare for classroom examinations and standardized tests, as well as a review for clinical practice. This improved format will help you review and apply medical-surgical content and help you to prepare for the NCLEX Examination.

Contents

CHAPTER 1

Introduction to Medical-Surgical Nursing

STUDY/REVIEW QUESTIONS

1. The Institute of Medicine report *To Err Is Human* highlighted the need to improve patient safety. Which national organization requires its accredited agencies to meet specific national patient safety goals?
   a. National Hospital Council
   b. *Healthy People 2010*
   c. National Patient Safety Foundation
   d. The Joint Commission

2. What is the purpose of the Rapid Response Team (RRT)?
   a. Provide Code Blue teams in case of simultaneous emergencies
   b. Enable the nurse to recognize changes in patient status before an acute emergency
   c. Replace immediate consultation with the physician or medical resident
   d. Comprise teams of staff already familiar with the patient's medical diagnosis

3. In addition to skills in techniques and procedures, the medical-surgical nurse must also perform what other competencies?
   a. Teaching and patient advocacy
   b. Spiritual counseling and support
   c. Rehabilitation strategies and methods
   d. Administrative scheduling and budgeting

4. Which factor is likely to be one of the most common causes of medical errors?
   a. Lack of technical experience
   b. Overload of information
   c. Poor communication
   d. Maliciousness and criminal intent

5. Which nursing activity is the best practice in patient teaching of older adults?
   a. Speaking loudly and turning up the volume on any audio presentation
   b. Using soothing music in the background to promote relaxation
   c. Assessing the need for glasses and hearing aids as appropriate
   d. Giving instructions at bedtime, so information can be understood better

6. Which is the best way for the nurse to assess the patient's learning after teaching?
   a. Have the patient write a summary of the points covered.
   b. Ask the patient to repeat the information back.
   c. Quiz the patient on relevant points in the instruction.
   d. Repeat the important points to the patient.

7. Which type of evidence is rated highest on a Level of Evidence Scale?
   a. Well-designed case control with cohort studies
   b. Randomized trials of small descriptive studies
   c. Well-designed controlled trials without randomization
   d. Systematic review or meta-analysis of all randomized controlled trials

8. Which is the best use of information from electronic sources, such as websites or e-mail, in retrieving data for the evidence-based practice process?
   a. Being sure to include links to articles so the reader can follow up on subsequent results
   b. Evaluating the information for credibility and reliability before putting it into use
   c. Using only university-related sources to ensure the most current results
   d. Assessing the number of hits the sources have on a search engine to determine popularity

9. Which action exemplifies the goal of case management in an acute care setting?
   a. Making sure the patient's dietary choices meet prescribed nutritional needs
   b. Scheduling home visits after discharge and monitoring patient progress
   c. Monitoring the patient's vital signs and noting trends of elevations
   d. Reviewing the patient's hospital bill for accuracy and any excessive charges

10. Which action best demonstrates a collaborative nursing function?
    a. Requesting the assistance of another staff member to turn a patient
    b. Administering medications as prescribed by the health care provider
    c. Notifying the family members of a change in the patient's condition
    d. Making a referral to the case manager to assist with discharge planning

11. Which occurrence does the Joint Commission's National Patient Safety Goals designate as a high-risk issue?
    a. Health care workers' exposure to infectious diseases in the workplace
    b. Violating privacy considerations of patients' confidential information
    c. Administering medication that is not familiar to the nurse
    d. Failure to review patients' food allergies before serving meals

2 CHAPTER

Introduction to Complementary and Alternative Therapies

STUDY/REVIEW QUESTIONS

1. **Crossword Puzzle.** Complete each item by placing the correct answer in the appropriate number (across or down) in the puzzle.

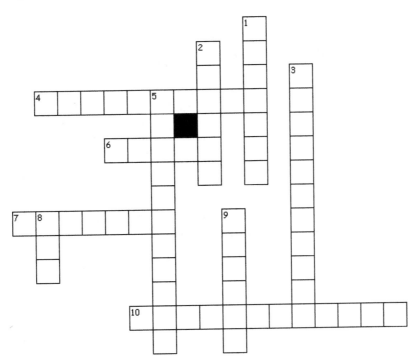

Across

4. A reflective therapy that is a tool for recording the process of one's life.
6. Therapeutic _____ is the use of the hands on or near the body with the purpose of healing.
7. Uses various strokes and pressure to manipulate soft tissues for therapeutic purposes.
10. Use of essential oils to promote relaxation and sleep.

Down

1. Uses the senses to form a mental representation of an object, place, event, or situation.
2. A mind-body exercise.
3. Uses needles on various acupoints throughout the body to treat certain conditions.
5. Uses fingers to press certain points on the body to treat certain conditions.
8. Abbreviation for a therapy that uses animal companionship to promote positive health outcomes.
9. _____ preparations, plants used for medicinal purposes.

2. What is one way that the National Center for Complementary and Alternative Medicine (NCCAM) advances scientific research?
   a. Promotes manipulative and body-based therapies
   b. Makes complementary therapies available to certain patients
   c. Provides patient handouts on the benefits of complementary medicine
   d. Investigates and evaluates efficacy of complementary therapies

3. For each category of complementary therapy listed below, name at least two examples.
   a. Systems of care _____
   _____
   b. Mind-body therapies _____
   _____
   c. Biologic-based therapies _____
   _____
   d. Manipulative and body-based therapies
   _____
   e. Energy therapies _____
   _____

Matching. *Match the herbal preparation with its intended use or effect.*

Herbal Preparation
a. Ginkgo biloba
b. Echinacea
c. Garlic
d. St. John's wort
e. Ginseng

Intended Use or Effect
_____ 4. Mild to moderate depression
_____ 5. Memory problems
_____ 6. Build immunity
_____ 7. Anti-aging
_____ 8. Lower cholesterol

Matching. *Match the herbal preparation with its caution or adverse effect. There may be more than one answer for each adverse effect, and answers may be used more than once.*

Herbal Preparation
a. Ginkgo biloba
b. Echinacea
c. Garlic
d. St. John's wort

Caution/Adverse Effect
_____ 9. Photosensitivity
_____ 10. May cause excessive bleeding if used with anticoagulant drugs
_____ 11. Should not be used for people with immune diseases

12. For what purposes might imagery be used? *(Select all that apply.)*
    a. Decrease pain
    b. Lessen fatigue
    c. Reduce nausea
    d. Promote arousal
    e. Decrease anxiety

13. Name three benefits of massage therapy.
    a. _____
    b. _____
    c. _____

14. The nurse prepares to give a massage to the older adult patient who has been bedridden for 3 days. When the patient's back is exposed, the nurse notes an area of redness on the sacrum that is about 6 cm in diameter. What is the best action for the nurse to take?
    a. Massage the area vigorously using long, flowing strokes.
    b. Massage the area with rhythmic stroking using light touch.
    c. Avoid massaging over an area of skin that is reddened or bruised.
    d. Use rapid, continuous strokes while massaging.

15. Which statements about aromatherapy are true? *(Select all that apply.)*
    a. Aromatherapy involves the use of essential oils to stimulate the sense of smell.
    b. Essential oils may be applied in compresses, used in baths, or applied to the skin.
    c. Because essential oils are natural, they do not need to be diluted before being applied topically.
    d. Lavender has been used for stimulation and to promote concentration.
    e. Rose oil has been used to promote relaxation and sleep.
    f. Allergies should be assessed before using essential oils.

16. Identify at least five considerations regarding the safety of herbal preparations that the nurse should keep in mind while considering herbal therapy for a patient.

    a. _____
    _____

    b. _____
    _____

    c. _____
    _____

    d. _____
    _____

    e. _____
    _____

17. The patient has been diagnosed with chronic pain. Before suggesting that the patient try meditation as a pain management method, what must the nurse consider?
    a. Patient's personal preference and medical condition
    b. Patient's ability to ambulate
    c. Possible negative outcomes such as grief
    d. Patient's willingness to commit to meditation three times per day

18. The nurse is teaching the patient about massage therapy. Which statement by the patient demonstrates a correct understanding of the nurse's instruction?
    a. "Firm finger pressure is applied to certain points on the body."
    b. "After 5 minutes, a gentle tingling sensation is felt."
    c. "Massage is sometimes painful."
    d. "Using various stroke techniques will produce relaxation."

19. The patient is taking garlic to lower cholesterol levels. What information does the nurse provide to the patient about this herbal supplement?
    a. Blood glucose levels should be monitored when taking garlic.
    b. Look for unusual bleeding or bruising.
    c. Garlic is not effective in the capsule form.
    d. Avoid taking garlic with coffee, tea, or cola.

3 CHAPTER

Common Health Problems of Older Adults

STUDY/REVIEW QUESTIONS

1. Which statements about the health of older adults in the United States are true? *(Select all that apply.)*
   a. The fastest growing group is between 85 and 90 years of age.
   b. Only 5% of older adults are in nursing homes, but most of the adults on acute care units are 65 or older.
   c. The incidence of chronic illness increases with advanced age.
   d. The lowest rate of suicide is in the older adult population.
   e. Men live longer than women.

2. Identify four interventions to reduce relocation stress in the older hospitalized patient.

   a. _____
   _____
   _____

   b. _____
   _____
   _____

   c. _____
   _____
   _____

   d. _____
   _____
   _____

3. Which statements would be included in an educational program on wellness behaviors for the older adult? *(Select all that apply.)*
   a. Allow at least 10 to 15 minutes of sun exposure 2 to 3 times weekly.
   b. Take one aspirin twice a day.
   c. Obtain a yearly influenza vaccination.
   d. Create a hazard-free environment to prevent falls.
   e. Increase calcium intake to between 1000 and 1500 mg daily.
   f. Reduce dietary intake of complex carbohydrates and fiber.
   g. Take time alone at home and relax.

4. Which statement regarding how nutrition is affected in older adults is true?
   a. Changes in smell and taste can result in decreased use of sugar.
   b. Older adults need increased calorie intake to maintain ideal body weight.
   c. Loneliness and boredom may impact the older adult's incentive to eat.
   d. Obesity is the most common nutritional problem in nursing homes.

5. What are direct benefits of exercise? *(Select all that apply.)*
   a. Decreases anxiety
   b. Reduces muscle strength
   c. Improves sleep apnea
   d. Increases mobility
   e. Decreases risk of heart disease
   f. Restricts caloric intake

6. Which assessment findings in the older adult patient indicate an increased risk for falls? *(Select all that apply.)*
    a. Increased mobility
    b. Macular degeneration
    c. Balance instability
    d. Full joint ROM
    e. Peripheral neuropathy

7. The nurse is caring for the confused older patient at risk for falls. Which intervention does the nurse avoid using with this patient?
    a. Remind the patient to use ambulatory devices as needed.
    b. Instruct the patient to limit activity as much as possible.
    c. Provide appropriate lighting in the patient's environment.
    d. Make sure the patient's eyeglasses are functional.

8. The patient requires physical restraints. Which interventions must the nurse perform for this patient? *(Select all that apply.)*
    a. Check the patient every 30 to 60 minutes.
    b. Release the restraints at least every 4 hours.
    c. Turn on the television to provide distraction.
    d. Place the patient in an area for careful observation.
    e. Decrease communication with the patient.

9. Which type of psychoactive drugs requires the most careful monitoring by the nurse due to the drug's potency?
    a. Antidepressants
    b. Antipsychotics
    c. Antianxiety agents
    d. Sedative-hypnotics

Matching. *Match the physiologic changes affecting drug use in older adults with their associated pharmacokinetic actions.*

Pharmacokinetic Actions
a. Absorption
b. Distribution
c. Metabolism
d. Excretion

Physiologic Changes

_____ 10. Increased gastric pH

_____ 11. Reduced glomerular filtration

_____ 12. Decreased cardiac output

_____ 13. Decreased liver enzyme activity

True or False? *Read each statement and write T for true or F for false in the blanks provided.*

_____ 14. Older adults have less reserve capacity in most organ systems.

_____ 15. Drug reactions are usually less severe in older adults due to reduced metabolism.

_____ 16. When prescribing medications for older adults, a policy of generalized "start high but taper quickly" is essential for safety.

_____ 17. All symptoms should be assessed for possible adverse reactions to medications in the older adult population.

18. Which intervention is effective in helping to reorient the patient suffering from delirium?
    a. Talk to the patient using a calm voice.
    b. Restrict visitors during periods of agitation.
    c. Remove personal items and store them safely.
    d. Apply wrist restraints to keep the patient from pulling at tubing.

19. Which symptoms of depression in older adults should be carefully evaluated by the health care provider? *(Select all that apply.)*
    a. Early morning insomnia
    b. Reluctance to participate in social activities
    c. Anger and aggressive behavior
    d. Increased appetite and overeating
    e. Excessive daytime sleeping

20. In planning care for the patient with dementia, the nurse identifies which intervention as the first priority goal of care?
    a. Prevent cognitive decline.
    b. Reorient on a regular basis.
    c. Prevent injury.
    d. Assist with ambulation.

21. Which statements regarding elder abuse are true? *(Select all that apply.)*
    a. The abuser is often a close family member or caregiver.
    b. Only physically dependent older adults are vulnerable to elder abuse.
    c. Elder neglect is categorized as a type of elder abuse.
    d. Approximately one-half of all cases involve physical force.
    e. There is a need for mandatory reporting laws for suspected elder abuse.

Matching. Match the type of elder abuse with its definition.

Type of Abuse
a. Neglect
b. Physical abuse
c. Financial abuse
d. Emotional abuse

Definitions

_____ 22. Mismanagement or misuse of an older patient's property or resources.

_____ 23. Intentional use of threats, humiliation, intimidation, and isolation.

_____ 24. Examples include hitting, burning, pushing, and molesting the patient.

_____ 25. Failure to provide for basic needs, such as food and clothing.

Matching. For each statement identify whether it describes dementia or delirium. Answers will be used more than once.

Types of Confusion
a. Dementia
b. Delirium

Descriptions

_____ 26. Temporary, acute confusional state that is a symptom of a variety of treatable conditions

_____ 27. Permanent, progressive loss of cognitive function

_____ 28. A common type includes Alzheimer's disease

_____ 29. Duration continues for hours to less than 1 month

_____ 30. Characterized by a rapid onset

Matching. Match the terms with their definitions.

Terms

a. Fallophobia
b. Presbyopia
c. Polypharmacy
d. Nocturia

Descriptions

_____ 31. Urination at night

_____ 32. The use of multiple drugs

_____ 33. Psychological fear of falling in older adults

_____ 34. Farsightedness that worsens with aging

CASE STUDY: MEDICATION USE IN OLDER ADULTS

Use a separate sheet of paper to answer the questions in this Case Study. Answer guidelines for this Case Study are available on your Evolve website at http://evolve. elsevier.com/Iggy/ in the "Prepare for Class" folder.

An 80-year-old patient is brought to the emergency department (ED) after fainting at home. His serum digoxin level is 2.3 ng/mL. He is transferred to a medical-telemetry nursing unit. The next day the nurse asks the patient to tell her about his routine for taking his daily digoxin tablets. He states that he was told to check his pulse every morning before taking a pill. He does this in his kitchen because the clock on the wall has big numbers and he can see the second hand go around. The nurse asks him how long he measures his pulse. He replies "I keep counting the beats until I get to 60. Sometimes it takes a long time. Then I take my heart pill." Later he tells you that he hates "having so many pills to take" and admits having trouble remembering to take his pills. He states that he sometimes can't remember which pills to take with breakfast and which to take at night.

1. Identify factors that may affect the patient's understanding of digoxin self-administration.

2. What specific pharmacokinetic factor should be considered when giving digoxin to an older adult?

3. What can the nurse suggest to assist this patient to take his multiple medications correctly?

4. Devise a teaching-learning plan to reteach this patient about taking digoxin at home.

5. Discuss how the nurse can validate whether the teaching plan has been effective.

4 CHAPTER

Cultural Aspects of Health and Illness

STUDY/REVIEW QUESTIONS

Matching. *Match the terms with the appropriate definitions.*

Terms

a. Culture
b. Subculture
c. Culture care preservation
d. Cultural competence
e. Culture care accommodation
f. Cultural assessment
g. Cultural restructuring
h. Transcultural nursing
i. Ethnocentrism
j. Cultural awareness

Definitions

_____ 1. A way to help people of a particular culture retain or preserve relevant care values so they can maintain and/or preserve their well-being, recover from illness, or face handicaps and/or death

_____ 2. The ability of health care providers and organizations to understand and respond effectively to the cultural and linguistic needs that patients bring to the health care setting

_____ 3. An integrated pattern of human behavior which is learned and transmitted to succeeding generations that includes thought, speech, action, and artifacts

_____ 4. The judging of others through the exclusive lens of one's own cultural beliefs

_____ 5. An area of study and practice that focuses on the care, health, and illness patterns of people with similarities and differences in their cultural beliefs, values, and practices

_____ 6. Data collected or research conducted to learn about the culture of patients

_____ 7. Interventions that help patients to reorder or greatly modify their lifeways; providing a lifeway more beneficial or healthier than that practiced before the changes were co-established with the patients

_____ 8. The process through which one becomes respectful, appreciative, and sensitive to the values, beliefs, lifeways, practices, and problem-solving strategies of a patient's culture

_____ 9. Part of a larger culture of the patient

_____ 10. Professional actions and decisions that help people of a designated culture adapt to or negotiate with others for a beneficial or satisfying health outcome with professional care providers

11. Purnell's model consists of 12 domains and their concepts to assess and understand an individual's cultural heritage. Which domain is *not* relevant for nursing care?
    a. Language and dialect
    b. Religious practices
    c. Dietary needs
    d. Cultural shock

True or False? *Write T for true or F for false in the blanks provided. If the statement is false, correct the statement to make it true.*

_____ 12. Cultural practices that should be included as part of a cultural assessment include nutrition, family roles, pregnancy and childbirth, death rituals, and spirituality.

_____ 13. Transcultural nursing focuses on the care, health, and illness patterns of people with various cultural beliefs, values, and practices.

_____ 14. In the 2000 census, minorities accounted for 43.8% of the total population in the United States.

_____ 15. One goal of *Healthy People 2010* is to eliminate disparities in health status experienced by racial and ethnic minorities.

_____ 16. All people within the same country have the same health care needs.

_____ 17. Garlic worn around the neck is thought to protect against cold and flu viruses in some cultures.

_____ 18. Pain is displayed the same way in all cultures.

19. How is "hypertension" referred to in some cultures?
    a. "High blood"
    b. "Low blood"
    c. "Hot blood"
    d. "Sour blood"

20. Which question or statement reflects the best way to consider a patient's religious or spiritual practice?
    a. "Do you have any dietary restrictions?"
    b. "Are you a Christian?"
    c. "Please tell me whether your religion allows you to accept blood products."
    d. "How can I help you in meeting any religious or spiritual needs you may have?"

21. You are the nurse for a patient who does not speak your language. In choosing an interpreter, rank the following choices from 1 to 3, with 1 being the most preferable arrangement and 3 being the least preferable.

    _____ a. Use a friend or family member of the patient.

    _____ b. Use a health care team member.

    _____ c. Use a person from the community or a local university.

22. The nurse is admitting an older adult who has cellulitis of her lower leg. The patient has been applying a homemade poultice to the leg for a week and refuses to remove it during the admission assessment. What does the nurse do?
    a. Remove the poultice in order to assess the lower leg.
    b. Inform the physician that the patient won't remove the poultice.
    c. Ask the patient about the poultice and how it has worked.
    d. Tell the patient that the leg won't heal until the doctor's orders are followed.

CASE STUDY: ASSESSMENT OF A CULTURE

Use a separate sheet of paper to answer the questions in this Case Study. Answer guidelines for this Case Study are available on your Evolve website at http://evolve. elsevier.com/Iggy/ in the "Prepare for Class" folder.

The hospital is opening an outreach clinic and has asked the nurse manager to help set it up. The clinic is located in a community with many recent immigrants from Guatemala.

1. What does the nurse need to know to be prepared to provide culturally appropriate care for the patients of this new clinic?
2. How will the nurse find that information?
3. How would the nurse address and work through issues related to spiritual beliefs that may be affecting a patient's condition?
4. What are some ways to ensure proper communication when working with the Guatemalan patients in this clinic?

5 CHAPTER

Pain: The Fifth Vital Sign

STUDY/REVIEW QUESTIONS

True or False? *Write T for true or F for false in the blanks provided. If the statement is false, correct the statement to make it true.*

_____ 1. "Pain is a universal experience" means that it is experienced by each patient in the same way.

_____ 2. Pain alters the quality of life more than any other single health-related problem.

_____ 3. Over the years, there have been major advances in how pain is managed.

_____ 4. Unrelieved and untreated pain is a major public health problem in the United States.

_____ 5. The nurse's primary role in managing pain is to administer analgesics as ordered.

6. Name three factors that affect a patient's perception of and response to pain.

   a. _____

   b. _____

   c. _____

7. Which description best describes the gate control theory?
   a. It is a complex phenomenon composed of sensory mechanisms located in the brain.
   b. Pain transmission is regulated by specialized cells located in the spinal column.
   c. Pain occurs because of increased sensitivity to painful stimuli.
   d. Perception of pain occurs by way of the stimulus transmitted directly to the brain.

8. Pain is a response caused by stimuli to the free nerve endings or receptors. What are these receptors called?
   a. Axons
   b. Fibers
   c. Nociceptors
   d. Endorphins

9. Briefly describe the four categories relating to the location of pain.

   a. Localized pain _____

   _____

   _____

   b. Projected pain _____

   _____

   _____

   c. Radiating pain _____

   _____

   _____

   d. Referred pain _____

   _____

   _____

10. The nurse is taking a health history of a patient who reports lower back pain for 10 months. How does the nurse categorize this pain?
    a. Acute pain
    b. Chronic cancer pain
    c. Non-cancer pain
    d. Somatic pain

11. Which characteristics pertain to somatic pain? *(Select all that apply.)*
    a. Sharp, burning or dull, aching, or cramping
    b. Diffuse, deep, and stabbing
    c. Painful numbness or shooting, burning, or fiery
    d. Poorly localized
    e. Skeletal muscle spasms
    f. Nerve compression
    g. Insertion site of wound drain
    h. Bladder spasms
    i. Pancreatitis
    j. Bony metastasis

12. Which characteristics pertain to neuropathic pain? *(Select all that apply.)*
    a. Sharp, burning or dull, aching, or cramping
    b. Diffuse, deep, and stabbing
    c. Painful numbness or shooting, burning, or fiery
    d. Poorly localized
    e. Skeletal muscle spasms
    f. Nerve compression
    g. Insertion site of wound drain
    h. Bladder spasms
    i. Pancreatitis
    j. Bony metastasis

13. Which characteristics pertain to visceral pain? *(Select all that apply.)*
    a. Sharp, burning or dull, aching, or cramping
    b. Diffuse, deep, and stabbing
    c. Painful numbness or shooting, burning, or fiery
    d. Poorly localized
    e. Skeletal muscle spasms
    f. Nerve compression
    g. Insertion site of wound drain
    h. Bladder spasms
    i. Pancreatitis
    j. Bony metastasis

14. Which statement is true about pain control barriers in the older adult patient?
    a. Older adults tend to underreport pain.
    b. Pain perception increases with age.
    c. The pain assessment scales are inaccurate.
    d. Cognitive impairment limits reliable pain assessment.

15. Identify the sources of these three types of pain:
    a. Somatic pain _____
    b. Visceral pain _____
    c. Neuropathic pain _____

16. The patient complains of a deep, localized, cramping type of pain. These assessment findings indicate which type of pain?
    a. Somatic
    b. Psychosomatic
    c. Neuropathic
    d. Visceral

17. The patient complains of a constant "achy" type of pain after abdominal surgery. This is an indication of which type of pain?
    a. Somatic
    b. Visceral
    c. Neuropathic
    d. Psychosomatic

Matching. For each of the characteristics listed, mark "AP" for acute pain, "CP" for chronic pain, or "B" for both.

Characteristics   Pain Description

AP = Acute pain
CP = Chronic pain
B = Both

_____ 18. Duration greater than 3 months

_____ 19. Intensity ranges from mild to severe

_____ 20. May be accompanied by anxiety and restlessness

_____ 21. May be accompanied by depression, fatigue, and decreased functional ability

_____ 22. Begins gradually and persists

_____ 23. Cause may be well-defined

_____ 24. Reversible

25. Which are physiologic responses that indicate the patient is experiencing pain? *(Select all that apply.)*
    a. Diaphoresis
    b. Restlessness
    c. Bradycardia
    d. Hypotension
    e. Bradypnea

26. What is the best type of pain scale to use for patients who have language barriers or reading problems, or for children?
    a. 0 to 10 numeric rating scale
    b. FACES (smile to frown)
    c. Verbal description scales
    d. No type of scale

27. Prioritize the drugs listed below, using the numbers 1 through 4, in the order that they might be prescribed for the relief of chronic pain.

    _____ a. Morphine

    _____ b. Ibuprofen

    _____ c. Amytriptyline

    _____ d. Oxycontin

28. The nurse monitors for gastric irritation, signs of bleeding, and bruising as side effects of which pain medications? *(Select all that apply.)*
    a. Aspirin (non-opioid analgesic, NSAID)
    b. Acetaminophen (non-opioid analgesic)
    c. Ibuprofen (non-opioid analgesic, NSAID)
    d. Morphine (opioid analgesic)
    e. Demerol (opioid analgesic)

29. The patient with chronic bone pain as a result of osteoarthritis or rheumatoid arthritis may be prescribed which agents? *(Select all that apply.)*
    a. Aspirin
    b. COX-2 inhibitor such as celecoxib (Celebrex)
    c. Opioid such as morphine
    d. Acetaminophen (Tylenol)
    e. NSAID such as ibuprofen (Motrin, Advil)

True or False? Write T for true or F for false in the blanks provided. If the statement is false, correct the statement to make it true.

_____ 30. The IM route is always the preferred route for most types of pain medication.

_____ 31. The oral route is always the preferred route for most types of pain medication.

_____ 32. The IV route is the most efficient route for pain management.

_____ 33. The transdermal route provides quick pain relief.

34. Which drugs can cause life-threatening seizures, particularly in the older adult, because of an accumulation of toxic metabolites? *(Select all that apply.)*
    a. Ibuprofen (Advil, Motrin)
    b. Morphine
    c. Meperidine (Demerol)
    d. Acetaminophen (Tylenol)
    e. Codeine

35. The patient is prescribed morphine sulfate, an opioid analgesic, for pain. Which nursing interventions decreases the risk of constipation? *(Select all that apply.)*
    a. Give foods low in bulk and roughage.
    b. Instruct the patient to increase water consumption.
    c. Administer a stool softener every morning.
    d. Change the dose of the opioid.
    e. Encourage activity.

36. Which statements are true regarding the side effects of respiratory depression as a result of administering an opioid analgesic? *(Select all that apply.)*
    a. Respiratory depression develops when opioid tolerance occurs.
    b. Monitor for respiratory depression in patients receiving opioids by IV administration, especially monitor opioid-naive adults.
    c. The pain, stress, and anxiety experienced by the patient are potent respiratory stimulants that may override or negate the respiratory depression resulting from the drugs.
    d. Respiratory depression is less of a problem in the older adult.
    e. The drug used to reverse the respiratory depression is known as naloxone (Narcan).
    f. A one-time dose of naloxone (Narcan) is all that is needed to reverse the effects of the opioid.
    g. Sedation will occur before opioid-induced respiratory depression.

37. Which statement about the adverse side effects of opioids is true?
    a. Bolus administration is less likely to produce central nervous system changes.
    b. Stimulants such as caffeine may counteract opioid-induced sedation.
    c. Opioid antagonists produce more respiratory depression than opioid agonists.
    d. Peripheral effects include vasoconstriction and elevated blood pressure.

Matching. *Match the definitions of physiologic sequelae associated with opioid use with their correct terms. Answers may be used more than once, and more than one term may apply to each sequela.*

Terms
a. Physical dependency
b. Tolerance
c. Addiction

Physiologic Sequelae

_____ 38. Persistent drug craving

_____ 39. Withdrawal symptoms upon abrupt cessation

_____ 40. Occurs in everyone who takes opioids over a period of time

_____ 41. Gradual resistance to effect of the opioid

_____ 42. Abuse for recreational purposes

_____ 43. Higher doses needed to achieve pain relief

_____ 44. A common fear in patients and health professionals

_____ 45. A psychological, not physical, phenomenon

_____ 46. Problem with amount of medication given to a patient with substance abuse

True or False? *Read the statements about patient-controlled analgesia (PCA) and write T for true or F for false in the blanks provided. If the statement is false, correct the statement to make it true.*

_____ 47. Meperidine (Demerol) is the drug most commonly used for PCA therapy.

_____ 48. The demand dose is ordered by the health care provider and is only available within specific intervals.

_____ 49. During the lockout interval, a dose will be delivered if the patient presses the button more than twice.

_____ 50. Two nurses should program the dosing parameters into the PCA delivery device.

_____ 51. Continuous or basal infusion of an opioid in addition to demand dosing causes overmedication.

_____ 52. Use of a PCA system may result in the patient needing less medication for pain than medication delivered by a nurse.

53. Which statements are true regarding the use of epidural catheters for pain management? *(Select all that apply.)*
    a. It is an external catheter located in the lumbar or thoracic region near the spinal cord.
    b. It is used for hospitalized patients with postoperative pain.
    c. Morphine and hydromorphone (Dilaudid) may be used, along with a local anesthetic such as bupivacaine.
    d. The nurse monitors for nausea and vomiting, pruritus, and infection at the insertion site.
    e. Catheters are usually in place for 12 to 24 hours.
    f. Urinary retention and weakness in the legs can occur.
    g. Pain assessments can be performed less frequently while receiving pain medications through epidural catheters.

54. Which nonpharmacologic therapies stimulate the skin and subcutaneous tissues to produce pain relief? *(Select all that apply.)*
    a. Massage
    b. Walking
    c. Passive ROM
    d. Heat application
    e. Therapeutic touch

55. The patient using a transcutaneous electrical nerve stimulation (TENS) unit asks the nurse how it works to decrease pain. What is the best response?
    a. "It delivers an electric shock to relieve muscle tension."
    b. "Low voltage currents block the pain you are having."
    c. "Endorphins are blocked which inhibit pain transmission."
    d. "The nerves causing pain will swell, raising the pain threshold."

56. Which statement about the strategy of distraction is true?
    a. Distraction is effective for acute and chronic pain relief.
    b. Distraction directly influences the cause of pain.
    c. Distraction should be used instead of other pain control measures.
    d. Distraction alters the perception of pain.

Matching. *Match the action or use with the corresponding adjuvant analgesic.*

Adjuvant Analgesics
a. Topical preparations such as Bio-Freeze gel
b. Oral local anesthetics such as mexiletine (Mexitil)
c. Antianxiety agents such as clonazepam (Klonopin)
d. Antiepileptic drugs such as gabapentin (Neurontin)
e. Antidepressants such as sertraline (Zoloft)

Actions/Uses

_____ 57. Used for neuropathy associated with diabetes mellitus

_____ 58. Used for its sedative effects at bedtime

_____ 59. Used for certain types of nerve injury pain

_____ 60. Used for electric, shocklike, continuous pain

_____ 61. Provides cryotherapy for muscle aches and pain

62. The nurse is teaching the patient about acupuncture as an alternative therapy for pain relief. Which statement by the patient indicates the nurse's teaching was effective?
    a. "Acupuncture is used for pain control and anesthetic purposes."
    b. "Acupuncture is commonly used to relieve pain and inflammation."
    c. "A local anesthetic is injected which decreases pain perception."
    d. "Needles are inserted into the body to temporarily deaden the nerve."

63. What is the drug category of choice for the treatment of mild-to-moderate bone pain?
    a. NSAIDs
    b. Opioids
    c. Anticonvulsants
    d. Antianxiety agents

Matching. Match the descriptions with their associated strategies for coping with pain. Answers may be used more than once.

Associated Strategies
a. Imagery
b. Relaxation
c. Hypnosis
d. Distraction

Descriptions

_____ 64. Massage

_____ 65. Deep-breathing exercises

_____ 66. Going for a walk

_____ 67. Mental experience of sensations or events

_____ 68. Altered state of consciousness

_____ 69. Focusing on pleasant or desirable feeling, sensation, or event

_____ 70. Losing an overall sense of reality

71. Which method would be the recommended route for controlling pain of a hospice patient with cancer who is unable to take oral medication?
    a. Intramuscular injection
    b. Continuous subcutaneous infusion
    c. Sublingual tablet
    d. Transdermal patch

True or False? Read the statements about fentanyl (Duragesic) patches and write T for true or F for false in the blanks provided. If the statement is false, correct the statement to make it true.

_____ 72. Duragesic is available in patch doses of 25 mcg/hr, 50 mcg/hr, 75 mcg/hr, and 100 mcg/hr.

_____ 73. It is reserved for those patients with continuous and relatively stable pain.

_____ 74. It is supplemented by intermittent doses of pain medication for episodic or breakthrough pain.

_____ 75. It is an easy-to-use method for anyone in chronic pain because it is easily titrated to control the pain.

_____ 76. When the patch is initially applied, it may take up to 24 hours before pain relief begins, so short-acting pain medication must be administered until the medication takes effect.

_____ 77. The patch is effective for 1 week; then a new patch is applied.

_____ 78. The patient's body temperature has no effect on absorption of the medication.

79. The nurse is preparing the patient for pain treatment that involves injecting a local anesthetic on or near a nerve root. Which term accurately describes this procedure?
   a. Cordotomy
   b. Rhizotomy
   c. Nerve block
   d. Ablation

CASE STUDY: THE PATIENT WITH PAIN

Use a separate sheet of paper to answer the questions in this Case Study. Answer guidelines for this Case Study are available on your Evolve website at http://evolve. elsevier.com/Iggy/ in the "Prepare for Class" folder.

The nurse is admitting the patient to a medical unit. She is 68 years of age and has a history of ovarian cancer. She had surgery 5 months ago and has had pain ever since the surgery. She reports that she has been taking Tylox tablets at home but that the pain is "never gone."

1. The patient describes her pain as a "10" on a scale of 1 to 10, deep, occasionally cramping, and sharp or stabbing. She waves her hand over her chest and abdomen when asked to pinpoint the location of the pain. What kind of pain is she experiencing?

2. During the pain assessment, the patient has difficulty identifying the location of her pain. She says, "It just hurts all over!" What can the nurse do to help her specify the exact location of pain?

3. During a discussion with the pain management nurse, it is suggested that the patient be given a Duragesic transdermal patch for pain management. She comments, "Oh, good! I know that will help make my pain go away quickly." What should the nurse say?

4. After consideration of her history and her pain, the pain management specialist recommends that the patient should receive patient-controlled analgesia (PCA). After discussing PCA therapy with her, an infusion is started with morphine as a basal infusion as well as interval self-dosing. The next morning while reviewing the infusion notes, the nurse sees that the patient dosed herself four times during the night. She is awake and states that her pain is now at a "5" and that she feels "a bit of relief now." Later that afternoon during rounds after lunch, the nurse sees that she is asleep and has not touched her meal. Her respiratory rate is 12, but she does not answer when the nurse calls her name. What should the nurse do at this point?

5. During evening rounds, the patient is found to be unresponsive, with respiratory rate of 7 breaths/min. Her son, who was staying with her, said that he "pushed the button a few times" while she was asleep because earlier she was complaining of hurting but wouldn't push it herself. What should the nurse do next?

6 CHAPTER

Genetic Concepts for Medical-Surgical Nursing

STUDY/REVIEW QUESTIONS

1. **Crossword Puzzle:** Complete each item by placing the correct answer in the appropriate number (across or down) in the puzzle.

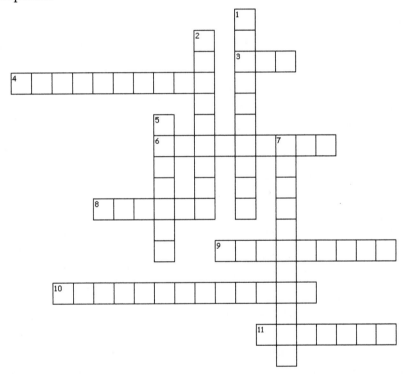

Across

3. Ribonucleic acid
4. The "pinched in" area of a chromosome where the two chromatids are joined
6. The 22 pairs of human chromosomes that do not code for the sexual differentiation of the individual
8. The complete set of genes for a species
9. _____ siblings; two siblings who share a womb and are born at the same time, but are the result of different fertilized eggs
10. The process of making a new strand of DNA
11. The complete set of chromosome pairs found in all of the individual's somatic cells

Down

1. Cellular DNA tightly condensed and coiled into a dense body
2. The observed expression of any given single gene trait (such as blood type, hair color)
5. A set of chromosomes consisting of half of each pair
7. _____ siblings; the product of one fertilized egg that split into two or more equal parts during embryogenesis

2. Humans have _____ chromosomes that are divided into _____ pairs.

3. What are autosomes?
   a. Chromosomes not involved in gender determination
   b. The organized arrangement of chromosomes in one cell
   c. The proteins needed to generate chromosome pairs
   d. Structures composed of two Xs as the sex chromosomes

4. When a person has homozygous alleles for a particular trait, the genotype and phenotype are the <u>same/different</u> *(circle one)*.

5. When a person has heterozygous alleles for a particular trait, the phenotype and the genotype are the <u>same/different</u> *(circle one)*.

6. For recessive traits, the phenotype and genotype are the <u>same/different</u> *(circle one)*.

7. Specify whether each characteristic is an autosomal dominant (AD) or autosomal recessive (AR) pattern of inheritance, or both (B).
   _____ a. In order for a trait to be expressed, both alleles must be present.
   _____ b. A trait is expressed even when only one allele of the pair is dominant.
   _____ c. The trait is found equally in males and females.
   _____ d. The trait is found in every generation with no skipping.
   _____ e. The trait may not appear in all generations of any one branch of a family.
   _____ f. The risk for an affected person to pass the trait to his or her children is 50% with each pregnancy.
   _____ g. The children of an affected mother and an affected father will always be affected (100% risk).
   _____ h. The trait can be transmitted to children if one parent is an unaffected carrier and the other parent is either a carrier or is affected.

True or False? *Reach each statement and write T for true or F for false in the blanks provided. If the statement is false, correct the statement to make it true.*

_____ 8. X-linked recessive genes have a dominant expressive pattern of inheritance in males and a recessive expressive pattern of inheritance in females.

_____ 9. The trait can be transmitted from father to son.

_____ 10. Transmission of the trait is from father to daughters, who will be carriers.

_____ 11. Female carriers have a 100% risk (with each pregnancy) of transmitting the gene to their children.

12. Which statement best reflects the correct actions of the health care professional who is providing genetic counseling?
    a. "This test will tell us everything about you!"
    b. "We are going to perform this testing because you asked for it and it won't affect your family in any way."
    c. "The results of this genetic testing will be sent to your health insurance carrier immediately."
    d. "I'm here to provide information so that you can make an informed decision about genetic testing."

13. When assessing for genetic risks, which factors indicate that a patient may have an increased genetic risk for a disease or disorder? *(Select all that apply.)*
    a. A close family member has an identified genetic problem.
    b. A patient tells you that he was exposed to a carcinogenic substance during a war.
    c. A patient has been diagnosed with two different types of cancer.
    d. A patient's sister had breast cancer at age 24.
    e. A patient's father was diagnosed with rheumatic fever at 10 years of age.

14. Which disorders have a genetic pattern of inheritance? *(Select all that apply.)*
    a. Malignant hyperthermia
    b. Gallstones
    c. Cystic fibrosis
    d. Acute lymphocytic leukemia
    e. Polycystic kidney disease
    f. Sickle cell disease

15. Write "SLR" for the disorders that have a sex-linked recessive pattern of inheritance, and write "FC" for those that have familial clustering.

    _____ a. Hemophilia

    _____ b. Hypertension

    _____ c. Alzheimer's disease

    _____ d. Red-green color blindness

    _____ e. G6PD deficiency

    _____ f. Schizophrenia

CHAPTER 7

Substance Abuse and Medical-Surgical Nursing

STUDY/REVIEW QUESTIONS

1. In the table below, identify the six categories of substances most commonly abused, describe the action and effect on the body, and give examples of the abused substance for each category.

Categories	Action of Substance and Overall Effects on the Body	Examples

True or False? *Read the statements about substance abuse and write T for true or F for false in the blanks provided. If the statement is false, correct the statement to make it true.*

_____ 2. Nurses and other health care professionals are not susceptible to substance abuse.

_____ 3. Nurses who need assistance in managing their own substance abuse must contact professional help on their own.

_____ 4. A plan of care for the patient with substance abuse should be based only on the type of chemical used.

_____ 5. Substance abuse only includes illicit or illegal drugs.

_____ 6. Substance abuse is only related to teenagers and young adults.

_____ 7. Any socioeconomic group is susceptible to substance abuse.

_____ 8. Knowledge of the patient's religious preference will influence the treatment modality.

_____ 9. Older adults are at risk for substance abuse because of normal body changes related to the aging process.

_____ 10. Women are generally susceptible to substance abuse because of biologic predisposition and stressors in the environment.

11. Which statements regarding substance abuse, stress, and addiction are true? *(Select all that apply.)*
    a. Stress is a contributing factor for substance abuse.
    b. When the body experiences stress, the brain reacts by decreasing the level of stress hormones.
    c. Stress responses that are frequently triggered can result in a more sensitive response to the substance.
    d. Addiction results in the continuous understimulation of the brain pleasure pathways.
    e. Metabolic imbalance is the primary factor associated with addiction.

12. Identify the two stimulants that are prescribed therapeutically for attention deficit disorders, obesity, and narcolepsy.
    a. _____
    b. _____

13. What assessment finding indicates to the nurse that the patient is a chronic user of cocaine, particularly "crack" cocaine?
    a. Increased blood pressure
    b. Perforation of nasal septum
    c. Irritation of eyes
    d. Rapid heart rate

14. Cardiopulmonary arrest can occur with the first use of which stimulant?
    a. Amphetamine
    b. Cocaine
    c. Inhalant
    d. Methamphetamine

15. Which sign/symptom should a patient who is withdrawing from stimulants be assessed for?
    a. Insomnia
    b. Chills
    c. Seizures
    d. Fever

16. Abusers of cocaine are most likely to develop which condition?
    a. Physical dependence
    b. Psychological dependence
    c. Psychological aversion
    d. Physical withdrawal

17. What is the optimum method for reducing fever in the patient with overdose or withdrawal symptoms from methamphetamine?
    a. Antipyretics such as aspirin or acetaminophen
    b. Evaporation methods such as cool, moist towels
    c. Cooling blanket with circulating water
    d. Hydration with cold beverages

18. Identify the stimulant that has both stimulant and sedative properties. Explain how this drug affects the body.
    _____
    _____
    _____
    _____
    _____
    _____

True or False? Read the statements about hallucinogens and related compounds and write T for true or F for false in the blanks provided.

_____ 19. Flashbacks are a common phenomenon when psychedelic drugs are used.

_____ 20. There are no therapeutic uses for hallucinogens that are acceptable for medical treatment.

_____ 21. Ketamine or "Special K" is also known as the "date rape drug."

_____ 22. The effects of LSD can last up to 12 hours.

_____ 23. Addiction to hallucinogens is physical in nature, not psychological.

24. Which drug affects the serotonin- and dopamine-producing neurons in the brain?
    a. Alcohol
    b. Nicotine
    c. PCP
    d. MDMA

25. In cases of ketamine overdose, the nurse is prepared to treat which life-threatening condition?
    a. Irregular heartbeat
    b. Loss of muscle control
    c. Shortness of breath
    d. Respiratory failure

26. The patient in the emergency department presents with coma of undetermined origin. This patient should be evaluated for the use of which drug?
    a. Marijuana
    b. GHB (gamma hydroxybutyrate)
    c. Rohypnol (flunitrazepam)
    d. MDMA (methylenedioxymethamphetamine)

27. Briefly describe assessment findings in a patient suspected of PCP abuse.

    _____

    _____

    _____

28. Which drug is used experimentally to control chronic pain?
    a. Heroin
    b. Marijuana
    c. Methadone
    d. Oxycodone

29. Which are effects of long-term or heavy use of marijuana? *(Select all that apply.)*
    a. Physical relaxation
    b. Slowed reaction time
    c. Respiratory changes
    d. Poor work performance
    e. Memory difficulties

30. As a result of action on the cerebral cortex and the reticular activating system, barbiturates produce which effect?
    a. Decrease of inhibitions
    b. Enhancement of cognitive processes
    c. Regulation of the sleep-wake cycle
    d. Production of hallucinations

True or False? Read the statements about depressants and write T for true or F for false in the blanks provided. If the statement is false, correct the statement to make it true.

_____ 31. Abuse is present when the patient continues to use benzodiazepines after clinical signs of need for the treatment have subsided.

_____ 32. Dependence on barbiturates takes a long time to occur.

_____ 33. Older adults can tolerate only small doses of the barbiturate group.

_____ 34. The safest method for withdrawing a patient from depressants is to gradually reduce the dosage.

_____ 35. Alcohol abuse occurs only when a person has a strong craving for alcohol.

36. Anxiety, restlessness, insomnia, irritability, and impaired attention are assessment findings for withdrawal from which drug?
    a. Barbiturates
    b. Benzodiazepines
    c. Opioids
    d. Alcohol

37. An assessment of a postoperative patient with a history of substance abuse documents diaphoresis, agitation, elevated blood pressure, and tremors. These assessment findings are symptoms of which kind of drug withdrawal?
    a. Benzodiazepine
    b. Barbiturate
    c. Alcohol
    d. Amphetamine

38. Alcohol withdrawal is evaluated by categories of severity. On a separate sheet of paper, briefly explain the assessment findings that would be monitored by the nurse for each of the three alcohol withdrawal categories:
    a. Minor
    b. Major
    c. Life-threatening

39. The hospitalized patient has a history of alcoholism. How soon after the patient's last drink does the nurse monitor the patient for withdrawal symptoms?
    a. 8 hours
    b. 24 hours
    c. 12 to 48 hours
    d. 36 to 72 hours

40. The patient is brought to the emergency department by a friend who states that they had been at a party with "lots of booze." The friend claims to be the designated driver, but is concerned because the patient passed out in the car and was unable to walk to his apartment. A blood alcohol level is drawn, and the results are 350 mg/dL. What does this level indicate?
    a. Mild to moderate intoxication
    b. Marked intoxication
    c. Severe intoxication
    d. Alcohol overdose

41. The patient is in the rehabilitation unit for treatment of alcohol withdrawal. Which drug is the nurse prepared to administer to prevent seizures and delirium tremens (DTs)?
    a. Thiamine
    b. Chlordiazepoxide (Librium)
    c. Disulfiram (Antabuse)
    d. Atenolol (Tenormin)

42. In the older adult, substance abuse commonly can be a problem related to alcohol and which kinds of drugs? *(Select all that apply.)*
    a. Stimulants
    b. Depressants
    c. Opioids
    d. Prescription drugs
    e. Over-the-counter drugs

43. Opioids and morphine are drugs of addiction because of which effects?
    a. Analgesic and euphoric
    b. General numbing
    c. Stimulating
    d. Hallucinogenic

44. Which opioid derivative has no medical use in the United States?
    a. Cocaine
    b. Heroin
    c. Methadone
    d. Oxycodone

45. The patient enters the emergency department and is diagnosed with opiate withdrawal grade 2. What do the assessment findings of this patient include?
    a. Increased vital signs, abdominal cramps, diarrhea, vomiting, and weakness
    b. Drug craving, anxiety, and drug-seeking behavior
    c. Dilated pupils, muscle twitching, and anorexia
    d. Sweating, lacrimation, yawning, and rhinorrhea

46. The patient is admitted to the emergency department with a possible opioid overdose. She is semiconscious, has dilated pupils, and her respiratory rate is 8 breaths/min. Which drug does the nurse prepare to administer?
    a. Meperidine (Demerol)
    b. Midazolam (Versed)
    c. Disulfiram (Antabuse)
    d. Naltrexone (ReVia)

47. Which age groups are most likely to use inhalants for psychoactive effects? *(Select all that apply.)*
    a. Children
    b. Young adults
    c. Middle-aged adults
    d. Older adults
    e. Adults older than 65 years

48. Which are examples of solvents?
    a. Butane lighters, whipping cream aerosols, and spray paints
    b. Cyclohexanol nitrite and amyl nitrite
    c. Paint thinners, gasoline, glues, and paper correction fluid
    d. Hair or deodorant sprays, ether, and chloroform

True or False? Read the statements about inhalants and write T for true or F for false in the blanks provided. If the statement is false, correct the statement to make it true.

_____ 49. A method to increase the effect of the inhalant is to dispense the substance from a paper bag to increase the concentration of the inhalant.

_____ 50. Inhalant toxicity treatment consists of administration of an antidote and supportive care.

51. Which condition is a reversible effect of inhalants?
    a. Liver and kidney damage
    b. Hearing loss
    c. Limb spasms
    d. Bone marrow suppression

52. Anabolic steroids are abused for which reason?
    a. Euphoric effects
    b. Increased physical strength and performance
    c. Reduced aggressive tendencies
    d. Improved fertility in males

Matching. Match each substance with its toxic effects.

Substances
a. Inhalants
b. Anabolic steroids
c. Methamphetamines
d. Lysergic acid (LSD)
e. GHB or "liquid ecstasy"
f. Cocaine

Toxic Effects

_____ 53. Respiratory depression, bradycardia, coma

_____ 54. Paranoid ideas, "hearing colors," brain damage, psychosis

_____ 55. Cardiopulmonary arrest, possibly with first use

_____ 56. Growth of facial hair, changes in menses, deepened voice

_____ 57. Chemical smell, red eyes, slurred speech, dazed appearance

_____ 58. Hyperthermia, convulsions, stroke

8 CHAPTER

Rehabilitation Concepts for Chronic and Disabling Health Problems

STUDY/REVIEW QUESTIONS

Matching. Match the interdisciplinary team member with the example of the type of work performed. *Answers may be used more than once, and there may be more than one answer for each example.*

Interdisciplinary Team Members

a. Physiatrist
b. Rehab nurse/case manager
c. Physical therapist
d. Occupational therapist
e. Speech-language pathologist
f. Recreational/activity therapist
g. Cognitive therapist
h. Social worker
i. Psychologist
j. Vocational counselor
k. Nursing or therapy assistant
l. Patient

Types of Work Performed

_____ 1. Screens, tests, and recommends feeding techniques for dysphagia

_____ 2. Assists in job placement and seeking work-related training

_____ 3. Works with patients in learning to feed, bathe, and dress themselves

_____ 4. Teaches patients skills related to coordination such as picking up coins from a table

_____ 5. Specializes in rehabilitation medicine

_____ 6. Involved in patient and family coping skills

_____ 7. Identifies community resources

_____ 8. Coordinates the team's plan of care

_____ 9. Teaches patient skills to achieve mobility

_____ 10. Assists with care such as bathing and feeding

_____ 11. Works directly with patients who have experienced head injuries and have difficulty with memory

_____ 12. Assists patients in learning new interests or hobbies

_____ 13. Involved in all aspects of restoration and maintenance of optimal health

_____ 14. Teaches patients how to talk again and works with swallowing problems

_____ 15. Performs comprehensive physical, psychosocial, and spiritual assessments

_____ 16. Discharge planning to determine adequacy of current situation and potential needs and how care will be provided to meet those needs

_____ 17. Has final authority regarding teaching plan

18. As a result of a car accident, the adult patient is unable to perform certain activities of daily living (ADLs) such as bathing without assistance. This is an example of which concept listed below?
    a. Rehabilitation
    b. Impairment
    c. Disability
    d. Handicap

19. Which problem is the leading cause of disabling conditions in young adults and the third leading cause of death in adults 45 to 54 years of age?
    a. Stroke
    b. Cancer
    c. Arthritis
    d. Accidents

20. What best describes the primary goal of the rehabilitation team?
    a. To rely on a specific plan of care standardized to the medical diagnosis
    b. To identify and use one conceptual framework to serve as the sole model for the practice of rehabilitation nursing
    c. To restore as much function as possible of the injured or diseased body part to facilitate the patient's independence
    d. To enable patients and their families identify strategies to successfully meet short-term goals

True or False? *Read each statement and write T for true or F for false in the blanks provided. If the statement is false, correct the statement to make it true.*

_____ 21. Fatigue and physical complications often affect the length of time of a given workout session.

_____ 22. Older adults are at increased risk for injury related to antihypertensive medications and orthostatic hypotension.

_____ 23. Diarrhea is a risk factor because increased intestinal motility.

_____ 24. Patients are at risk for ineffective coping related to a lack of family and significant other support systems.

_____ 25. Assess for urinary problems present before illness or rehabilitation to determine effectiveness of a bladder training program.

_____ 26. Turning the patient every 2 hours is adequate for the skin type of the older adult.

_____ 27. Encouraging ingestion of 2000 to 2500 mL of fluid per day is an important consideration in the prevention of complications from flaccid bladder and heart disease.

28. The patient with decreased cardiac output is entering a rehabilitation program. What will the nurse expect to find during the assessment of this patient?
    a. Shortness of breath on activity
    b. Ability to ambulate without angina
    c. Feeling rested upon awakening from sleep
    d. Ability to move from sitting to standing position easily

29. The paraplegic patient is entering a rehabilitation program. What does the nurse focus on first in assessing this patient?
    a. Family and cultural background
    b. Baseline hemoglobin and hematocrit measurements
    c. Habits of bowel elimination before illness
    d. Manual dexterity, muscle control, and mobility

30. The patient with a neurogenic bladder is to be taught how to perform intermittent self-catheterization. Before beginning the teaching-learning sessions, what will the nurse assess in this patient first?
    a. Motor function of both upper extremities
    b. Type of neurogenic bladder the patient has
    c. Patient's gender
    d. Age of the patient

31. To maintain skin integrity of the patient in a rehabilitation unit, what does the nurse assess? *(Select all that apply.)*
    a. Sensation of the skin
    b. Depth and diameter of an open lesion
    c. Ability to move extremities
    d. Presence or absence of exudate and odor
    e. Ability to change position as needed

32. Which statements correctly describe the Functional Independence Measure (FIM)? *(Select all that apply.)*
    a. It is a basic indicator of the severity of a disability.
    b. It tries to measure what a person should do, whatever the diagnosis or impairment.
    c. It tries to measure what a person actually does, whatever the diagnosis or impairment.
    d. The assessment may be performed by any health care discipline.
    e. Categories for assessment are self-care, sphincter control, mobility and locomotion, communication, and cognition.
    f. Evaluations may be done at specified times during therapy to determine patient progress.

Matching. For each of the activities listed, specify whether it is an activity of daily living or independent living skill.

Type
a.   Activity of daily living
b.   Independent living skill

Activity

_____   33.   Bathing

_____   34.   Using the telephone

_____   35.   Dressing

_____   36.   Ambulating

_____   37.   Shopping

_____   38.   Preparing food

_____   39.   Feeding self

_____   40.   Housekeeping

41. What best describes the purpose of a vocational assessment for the patient in rehabilitation?
    a. Assist the patient to find meaningful training, education, or employment after discharge from a rehabilitation setting.
    b. Evaluate and retrain patients with deficits that distort consonant and vowel sound production.
    c. Identify resources to assist with patient injuries that cause deficits in cognition.
    d. Demonstrate improvements in physical, social, cognitive, and emotional functions.

42. The nurse reviews with the patient the results of manual muscle testing performed by physical therapy. What ability of the patient does this procedure determine?
    a. Body flexibility and muscle strength
    b. Range of motion and resistance against gravity
    c. Muscle strength and amount of pain on movement
    d. Voluntary versus involuntary muscle movement

43. When assisting a patient with a hemiparesis to transfer or ambulate, what does the nurse instruct the patient to do?
    a. Lean the body weight backward.
    b. Use the weaker hand to assist.
    c. Lean the body weight toward the nurse.
    d. Use the strong hand to assist.

44. Which items would be helpful to use when transferring the quadriplegic patient to a bed or chair? *(Select all that apply.)*
    a. Gait belt
    b. Sliding board
    c. "Quad" cane
    d. Long-handled reacher
    e. Bedside table

45. The patient with impaired physical mobility must be monitored for which early potential complication?
    a. Pressure ulcers
    b. Renal calculi
    c. Osteoporosis
    d. Fractures

46. Which methods to prevent pressure ulcers resulting from immobility are best to teach patients and their significant others? *(Select all that apply.)*
    a. Change position often to relieve pressure on all bony prominences.
    b. Maintain good skin care by keeping the skin clean and dry.
    c. Inspect the skin at least once a day for problems such as reddened areas that do not fade readily.
    d. Use pressure-relieving devices as a substitute for changing position.
    e. Eat foods high in protein, carbohydrates, and vitamins for sufficient nutrition.

47. When assessing the patient who is to perform resistive exercises, what must be present in order for the exercises to be productive?
    a. Limited range of motion
    b. Full range of motion
    c. Full strength
    d. Ability to exercise to the point of pain

48. Which assistive-adaptive device would be recommended for the patient with a weak hand grasp?
    a. Gel pad
    b. Foam buildups
    c. Hook and loop fastener straps
    d. Buttonhook

49. When teaching the patient with hemiplegia about energy conservation techniques, which method does the nurse include?
    a. Using a walker instead of a cane
    b. Scheduling physical therapy immediately before eating
    c. Using a bedside commode
    d. Scheduling recreational activities in afternoon or evening

50. Which statement is true about the use of mechanical pressure-relieving devices?
    a. They effectively eliminate the need to turn patients.
    b. Patients still require regular repositioning.
    c. They prevent pressure ulcers in debilitated patients.
    d. They have been shown to be ineffective against pressure ulcers.

51. The patient has a lower motor neuron injury below T12. This injury results in which type of neurogenic bladder?
    a. Reflex or spastic
    b. Flaccid
    c. Uninhibited
    d. Inhibited

52. The patient with a flaccid bladder will have which urinary elimination problem?
    a. Incontinence and inability to empty the bladder completely
    b. Incontinence caused by inability to wait until on a commode or bedpan
    c. Urinary retention and dribbling because of overflow of urine
    d. Incontinence due to loss of sensation

Matching. Match the bladder training intervention with the type of neurogenic bladder problem. Answers may be used more than once.

Neurogenic Bladder Problem
a. Reflex or spastic
b. Flaccid
c. Uninhibited

Bladder Training Intervention

_____ 53. Credé maneuver

_____ 54. Facilitating/triggering

_____ 55. Intermittent catheterization

_____ 56. Medications

_____ 57. Consistent toileting schedule

_____ 58. Valsalva maneuvers

_____ 59. Regulation of fluid intake

_____ 60. Drinking fluids to promote an acidic urine

61. Which statements are correct principles for performing an intermittent catheterization? (*Select all that apply.*)
    a. A catheter is inserted every 2 to 4 hours.
    b. It is usually performed after the Valsalva or Credé maneuver.
    c. A residual of less than 150 mL increases the interval between catheterization.
    d. The maximum time interval between catheterizations is 6 hours.
    e. The patient uses sterile technique at home.

62. Which medication would the patient with a flaccid bladder most likely be given?
    a. Dantrolene sodium (Dantrium)
    b. Bethanechol chloride (Urecholine)
    c. Flavoxate hydrochloride (Urispas)
    d. Oxybutynin chloride (Ditropan)

63. The nurse is instructing the patient about which beverages to drink in order to create acidic urine. Which beverages does the nurse include in the teaching? (*Select all that apply.*)
    a. Orange juice
    b. Prune juice
    c. Apple juice
    d. Tomato juice
    e. Cranberry juice

64. Which patient is most likely to have a flaccid bowel dysfunction?
    a. 28-year-old man with a crushed pelvis
    b. 54-year-old man with Guillain-Barré syndrome
    c. 18-year-old woman with a displaced cervical fracture
    d. 48-year-old woman who has multiple sclerosis

65. Digital stimulation of the anus as a method of re-establishing bowel control is most successful in the patient who has had what problem?
    a. Myocardial infarction and is starting cardiac rehabilitation
    b. Chronic diarrhea resulting from radiation to the bowel
    c. Bowel incontinence resulting from a cerebrovascular accident
    d. Spinal cord injury resulting from a diving accident

66. What is the drug of choice for long-term management of bowel dysfunction?
    a. Milk of magnesia
    b. Senna concentrate (Senokot)
    c. Dulcolax or glycerin suppository
    d. Psyllium (Metamucil)

67. Which food is a part of breakfast for the patient with bowel dysfunction?
    a. Dried apricots or plums
    b. White bread
    c. Cheddar cheese
    d. Sausage links

68. Lower motor neuron disease or injury results in which bowel dysfunction?
    a. Flaccid bowel pattern
    b. Reflex (spastic) bowel pattern
    c. Uninhibited bowel pattern
    d. Inhibited bowel pattern

69. Which description characterizes the uninhibited bowel pattern dysfunction?
    a. Defecation occurring suddenly and without warning.
    b. Defecation occurring infrequently and in small amounts.
    c. Frequent defecation, urgency, and complaints of hard stool.
    d. Intermittent constipation and diarrhea.

Matching. *Match each intervention with the appropriate condition. The conditions may be used more than once.*

Conditions
a. Total urinary incontinence
b. Constipation
c. Risk for impaired skin integrity
d. Decreased cardiac output
e. Impaired physical mobility

Interventions
_____ 70. Perform major tasks in the morning
_____ 71. Complete the Braden Scale
_____ 72. Credé maneuver
_____ 73. Perform gait training
_____ 74. Wheelchair "push-ups"
_____ 75. Use a tilt table
_____ 76. Digital stimulation

CHAPTER 9

End-of-Life Care

STUDY/REVIEW QUESTIONS

Matching. Match each term related to loss with its correct definition.

Terms

a. Death
b. Dying
c. Grieving
d. Mourning

Definitions

_____ 1. Reaction to loss

_____ 2. Termination of life

_____ 3. The outward social expression of loss

_____ 4. A process leading to the end of life

5. Which statement regarding the approach to hospice/end-of-life care is correct?
   a. Hospice programs only include provision of care in the home.
   b. Admission to hospice is involuntary and directed by a physician's order.
   c. The focus is on facilitating quality of life just for the dying patient.
   d. An interdisciplinary team approach is used for the care of the patient and family.

6. The patient receiving nursing care in a home hospice program can expect which kind of care?
   a. The use of high-technology equipment such as ventilators until time of death.
   b. Around-the-clock skilled direct nursing patient care until time of death.
   c. Pain and symptom management that will achieve the best quality of life.
   d. Complete relief of only distressing physical symptoms.

7. To qualify for hospice benefits, a criterion for admission is that the patient's prognosis needs to be limited to what amount of time?
   a. 2 weeks or less
   b. 3 months or less
   c. 6 months or less
   d. 1 year or less

8. Which items are relevant to the concept of hospice? *(Select all that apply.)*
   a. Unit of care is the patient and family.
   b. Preferred location is in the hospital setting.
   c. Interdisciplinary team approach is used.
   d. Focus is on alleviating pain and suffering.
   e. Hospice care does not hasten death.

9. Place in correct sequence, using the numbers 1 through 3, the events that occur with multiple organ dysfunction syndrome (MODS).

   _____ a. Anaerobic metabolism, acidosis, hyperkalemia, and tissue ischemia

   _____ b. Release of toxic metabolites and destructive enzymes

   _____ c. Inadequate blood flow to body tissues and cells

10. Which statement is correct regarding the assessment of the terminally ill patient?
    a. Assess only the patient; do not include the family's perception of the patient's symptoms.
    b. When the patient is unable to communicate, there is no need to assess symptoms of distress any longer.
    c. Assess patients who are unable to communicate distress by observing for objective signs of discomfort.
    d. Assesses the patient for dyspnea, agitation, nausea, and vomiting only.

11. Which intervention should be done when performing postmortem care?
    a. Place the head of the bed at 30 degrees.
    b. Remove pillows from under the head.
    c. Leave a Foley (indwelling) catheter in place in the bladder.
    d. Place pads under the hips and around the perineum.

12. Which interventions after the patient's death are appropriate to perform? *(Select all that apply.)*
    a. Remove the body to the morgue or funeral home immediately after death.
    b. Follow agency policies to remove all tubes and lines from the body.
    c. A death certificate may accompany the body to the funeral home.
    d. Provide privacy for the family and significant others with the deceased.
    e. Allow family and/or significant other to perform religious and cultural customs.

Matching. *Match the term with its correct definition.*

Terms
a. Living will
b. Durable power of attorney for health care
c. Patient Self-Determination Act
d. Do not resuscitate (DNR)

Definitions

_____ 13. A legal document that appoints a person to make decisions regarding health care for someone else who becomes unable to make his or her own decisions

_____ 14. A physician's order that specifies that a patient has indicated that he or she does not want CPR

_____ 15. A legal document that instructs health care providers and family members of what life-sustaining treatment one wants or does not want if that person becomes unable to make these decisions

_____ 16. Requires that all patients admitted to health care agencies be asked if they have written advance directives

17. The hospice patient is deteriorating and the family is concerned about his restlessness and confusion. Which intervention is the nurse prepared to perform?
    a. Notify the primary health care provider and request orders for transfer to the hospital.
    b. Provide analgesics and oxygen as ordered, and make the patient as comfortable as possible.
    c. Initiate IV hydration to provide the patient with necessary fluids.
    d. Encourage the family to assist the patient to eat in order to gain energy.

True or False? Read each statement and write T for true or F for false in the blanks provided. If the statement is false, correct the statement to make it true.

_____ 18. Although anorexia is normal, patients should be forced to eat small, frequent meals.

_____ 19. Cessation of food ingestion is a natural process and hydration with IV fluids can cause distressing respiratory symptoms.

_____ 20. The patient's sense of hearing may be intact even though the patient is withdrawn from the external environment.

_____ 21. The symptom that a terminally ill patient most fears is dyspnea.

_____ 22. Pain is a not a universal problem, although it is common and has many causes.

_____ 23. The goals for a patient with dyspnea are to relieve the primary cause and the psychological distress and autonomic response.

_____ 24. *Dyspnea* is defined as a respiratory rate of fewer than 20 breaths/min with observed labored breathing.

_____ 25. Dyspnea is common in about 50% to 70% of dying patients and is considered by health care providers to be the worst symptom of distress when a patient is near death.

_____ 26. Nausea and vomiting occur in about 40% of terminally ill patients in the last week of life.

_____ 27. There are a variety of causes of nausea and vomiting, including constipation from opioid therapy.

_____ 28. Nausea and vomiting are prevalent only in individuals with certain types of cancer.

_____ 29. Agitation may be decreased with alternative therapies such as music or aromatherapy.

30. The most common treatment of pain in the terminally ill patient is administration of which kind of therapy?
    a. Opioids
    b. Steroids
    c. Nonsteroidal anti-inflammatory agents
    d. Radiation treatments

31. Which phrase correctly describes palliative care?
    a. Care for patients with a prognosis of 6 months or less
    b. Diagnoses and treatment for patients with a life-threatening illness
    c. Patient care with a focus on treatment of symptoms
    d. Patient education about relevant treatment alternatives

32. While caring for the Native American/American Indian patient who is dying, what cultural concept should the nurse keep in mind?
    a. Traditional Native American/American Indian families are male-dominated.
    b. Expression of grief is open, especially among women.
    c. Families will not allow the patient to die alone.
    d. Family members are likely to avoid visiting the terminally ill family member.

10 CHAPTER

Concepts of Emergency and Trauma Nursing

STUDY/REVIEW QUESTIONS

Matching. Match the job descriptions with the interdisciplinary team members.

Interdisciplinary Team Members
a. Forensic nurse examiner
b. Paramedic
c. Emergency medical technician
d. Psychiatric crisis nurse team
e. Emergency medicine physician

Job Descriptions

_____ 1. May work with patients involved with a sudden serious illness or the death of a loved one

_____ 2. Advanced life support provider who can perform advanced techniques, such as cardiac monitoring, advanced airway management and intubation, or giving intravenous drugs en route to the hospital

_____ 3. Offers basic life support interventions such as oxygen, basic wound care, splinting, spinal immobilization, and may carry automated external defibrillators (AEDs)

_____ 4. Obtains patient histories, collects abuse and domestic violence evidence, and offers counseling and follow-up for victims of rape and child abuse

_____ 5. Physician with specialized education and training in emergency patient management

6. The emergency department (ED) nurse is preparing a report on a patient being admitted for bacterial meningitis. Which points are included in the ED nurse's report to the medical-surgical nurse? *(Select all that apply.)*
   a. "Patient reports severe headache with high fever that started 4 days ago."
   b. "Patient currently alert and oriented x 2; speech clear, but rambling."
   c. "Patient is divorced and currently does not have any health insurance."
   d. "IV normal saline into left anterior forearm; received first dose of IV ceftriaxone (Rocephin) at 0700."
   e. "Past history of chronic obesity and fractured femur at age 5."
   f. "Lumbar puncture results are pending, but meningococcal meningitis is suspected."
   g. "Received 1000 mg acetaminophen for pain (9/10) and fever 103° F at 0400; pain continues (7/10), temperature now 100.9° F."

7. The ED nurse is attempting to transfer the patient to the medical-surgical unit. When the receiving nurse answers the phone, he says, "You people always dump these admissions on us during shift change." Which response by the ED nurse represents the best attempt at respectful negotiation?
   a. "I am sorry. I realize you are busy, but we are busy too."
   b. "When would you be willing to take our patients?"
   c. "If you could take the report, we could hold the patient until after shift change."
   d. "I apologize for the timing. We just received the bed assignment."

8. The nurse is interviewing a psychiatric patient who has been verbally aggressive for the past several hours according to the family. The family states, "He won't hurt anybody." However, the patient is pacing and appears suspicious and angry. Which strategy does the nurse use to conduct the interview?
   a. Sit at eye level with the patient in a quiet, secluded room.
   b. Conduct the interview standing near the door in a quiet room.
   c. Bring the entire family in and have everyone sit in comfortable chairs.
   d. Have the security guard stand by the patient during the interview.

9. The nurse is working alone in triage. It is a busy night and the waiting room is full of people who are restless and unhappy about having to wait. Which situation warrants the nurse to activate the panic button under the triage desk?
   a. The line for patients waiting to be triaged becomes overwhelmingly long.
   b. EMS calls to announce they are en route with a patient in full arrest.
   c. Several patients in the waiting room start to complain very loudly.
   d. A person walks in and starts threatening the registration staff with a weapon.

10. The ED nurse is caring for the patient who was found in an alley with no identification and no known family. The nurse must give medication to the patient. What is the correct procedure?
    a. Emergent conditions prevent identification, so the nurse gives the medication as ordered.
    b. The patient is designated as John Doe and the nurse uses two unique identifiers.
    c. The nurse validates the order with another nurse and both verify that the patient is unidentified.
    d. The nurse gives the medication and identification is made as soon as possible.

11. The nurse is working in the ED with an emergency physician, but the physician is currently involved in the care of several critical patients. The ED nurse must initiate care for patients under interdisciplinary and medical protocols. Which intervention is the *least* likely to be covered by a standing protocol?
    a. Give 50% dextrose IV push for low blood sugar.
    b. Obtain an arterial blood gas and start oxygen therapy.
    c. Ventilate per Ambu bag with 100% oxygen and intubate.
    d. Start a peripheral IV with normal saline at 125 mL/hour.

12. The older adult patient had been waiting in the ED for over 48 hours due to extremely high volume. Risk for Impaired Skin Integrity is identified and the charge nurse delegates turning the patient every 2 hours to the nursing assistants. Since the ED is busy, the patient is not turned and begins to develop a pressure ulcer. What does the charge nurse do to prevent a recurrence of this type of problem for future patients? *(Select all that apply.)*
    a. Nothing; in the overall priorities of the ED, the situation is inevitable.
    b. Make anecdotal notes and counsel all the involved nursing assistants.
    c. Delegate the duty of turning and repositioning to the primary nurses.
    d. File an incident report and seek resolution at the systems level.

13. An older couple on vacation comes to the ED. The man appears to be having a stroke and is unable to speak clearly or coherently. His wife is very distraught and states, "He has many allergies and takes many medications, but I can't remember anything right now!" What does the nurse do to quickly obtain accurate drug and allergy information?
    a. Call the patient's family physician for a phone report about his drugs and allergies.
    b. Call one of the patient's children and stress the urgency and importance for accurate information.
    c. Help the wife to calm down and tell her that she must remember the information.
    d. Check for a medical alert bracelet; help the wife to look in the patient's suitcase.

Matching. *Match the types of trauma with their descriptions.*

Trauma Types
a. Penetrating trauma
b. Blast effect
c. Rapid acceleration-deceleration forces
d. Blunt trauma

Descriptions
_____ 14. Impact forces such as with fists, kicks, or a baseball bat
_____ 15. Energy from an exploding bomb
_____ 16. High-speed crashes; produces tearing and shearing of anatomic structures
_____ 17. Injury from sharp objects and projectiles such as knives or icepicks

18. The patient is brought to the ED by friends who report "he probably overdosed on downers." The patient has a decreased level of consciousness and a decreased gag reflex; his face and chest are covered with emesis; he demonstrates spontaneous sonorous respirations; and pulse oximetry is 87% on room air. What type of airway management does the nurse expect this patient to receive?
    a. Supplemental oxygen per nasal cannula at 4-6 L/min
    b. Bag-valve-mask and 100% oxygen to assist with ventilatory effort
    c. Non-rebreather mask with high-flow oxygen
    d. Endotracheal intubation with initial high-concentration oxygen

19. The ED nurse is caring for several patients, all of whom are currently lying on stretchers either pending discharge or awaiting transfer to a hospital bed. Which patients are at risk for falls? *(Select all that apply.)*
    a. Patient with chronic pain who received 10 mg PO oxycodone for myalgia
    b. Opioid-naive teenager with a fracture who received 3 mg IV morphine for pain
    c. Middle-aged woman with severe vomiting and frequently watery stools
    d. Child with a fever of 102° F, crying, with an ear infection
    e. Older adult patient with acute dementia secondary to infection

20. The patient was involved in a high-speed motor vehicle accident. The physician instructs the nurse to prepare for several urgent procedures because of severe injury and physical compromise. Which procedure does the nurse prepare for first?
    a. Central line insertion
    b. Peritoneal lavage
    c. Chest tube insertion
    d. Endotracheal intubation

21. A child has sustained a closed fracture which requires reduction. The physician tells the nurse that the child will receive IV conscious sedation. What is the priority nursing diagnosis related to this procedure?
    a. Impaired Tissue Perfusion
    b. Risk for Ineffective Breathing Pattern
    c. Risk for Impaired mobility
    d. Acute Pain

22. For the each patient listed, indicate whether they should be triaged as emergent (E), urgent (U), or nonurgent (N).

    _____ a. 56-year-old man with severe unilateral back pain and previous history of kidney stones

    _____ b. 23-year-old woman with severe abdominal pain; positive home pregnancy test; BP 90/50 mm Hg

    _____ c. 35-year-old man with chest pain and diaphoresis

    _____ d. 10-year-old girl with vomiting, diarrhea, and abdominal pain onset 4 hours after eating fish

    _____ e. 6-year-old with a temperature of 101° F and flu-like symptoms

    _____ f. 44-year-old man with a dislocated elbow

    _____ g. 85-year-old man with new onset of confusion; BP elevated compared to his usual reading

    _____ h. 65-year-old woman with redness and swelling on the forearm associated with a bee sting

23. The patient is brought to the ED by the family because he has verbally threatened others and attempted to stab the neighbor's dog. What does the nurse do in order to ensure the safety of the patient and others? *(Select all that apply.)*
    a. Search the patient's belongings and secure personal effects.
    b. Instruct the patient's family to stay with him and call for help as necessary.
    c. Remove dangerous equipment from the room, such as sharps containers or portable instruments.
    d. Escort the patient to the waiting area where he can readily be observed by the triage nurse.
    e. Use a metal detector to search for objects that could be used as weapons.
    f. Instruct nursing students to avoid wearing a stethoscope around their necks.

24. Which patient has the greatest need for the nurse to advocate for a social services consult?
    a. Toddler who bumped her head on a table; observation for 24 hours is required
    b. Homeless woman who has a urinary tract infection and a vaginal yeast infection
    c. Woman who was punched and beaten by her husband and sustained a broken jaw
    d. Man who drove himself to the hospital and was treated with a long leg cast

25. Which function represents an appropriate referral to the case manager?
    a. Facilitate referral to a primary care provider who is taking new patients.
    b. Contact the peripherally inserted central catheter (PICC) line nurse to start an IV because the patient has bad veins.
    c. Investigate whether the patient is abusing and overusing ED services.
    d. Follow the patient into the community setting and evaluate the home environment.

26. The patient died in the ED after sustaining multiple injuries that occurred during an aggravated assault. The family arrives after the patient is pronounced dead and they ask to see the body. What does the nurse do?
    a. Explain that viewing the body would be too traumatic because all the tubes must remain in place for the forensic exam.
    b. Remove any tubes or debris that are near the patient's face and then cover the rest of the body with a blanket.
    c. Explain what they will see; dim the lights; leave the patient's face exposed, but cover the rest of the body with a blanket.
    d. Suggest that the family could spend time with their loved one at the mortuary after the medical examiner is finished.

27. The nurse is working in a Level III trauma community hospital. A motor vehicle accident occurs nearby and all the victims are brought to the facility. Which patient must be transferred immediately after stabilization to a Level I facility?
    a. Passenger with an obvious open fracture of the right tibia-fibula
    b. Child restrained in a car seat with a large forehead laceration
    c. Unrestrained driver who is unconscious, but has no apparent external injuries
    d. Passenger with abdominal pain, vaginal bleeding, and reports pregnancy

28. The nurse is evaluating the lower extremities of several patients. Which description represents the *least* serious physical presentation?
    a. Pain in calf; lower leg is swollen and red.
    b. Progressively increasing pain; distal portion is cool and bluish.
    c. Decreased sensation; lower leg has widespread brownish discoloration.
    d. Tight sensation in ankle; skin appears tight, shiny, and edematous.

Matching. Match the interventions with the primary survey categories. Answers may be used more than once.

Categories
a. Airway/cervical spine
b. Breathing
c. Circulation
d. Disability
e. Exposure

Interventions

_____ 29. Maintain alignment of cervical spine.

_____ 30. Re-evaluate level of consciousness frequently.

_____ 31. Use direct pressure for external bleeding.

_____ 32. Observe for chest wall trauma or other physical abnormalities.

_____ 33. Establish patent airway.

_____ 34. Remove all clothing to allow for thorough assessment.

_____ 35. Maintain vascular access with a large-bore catheter.

36. The ED trauma team is preparing to receive a motor vehicle accident victim with severe chest trauma with coughing of blood and a crush injury to the right leg. What type of personal protective equipment (PPE) does the nurse assigned to be the recorder put on?
   a. No PPE is necessary because the nurse is only recording and not giving direct care
   b. Gloves
   c. Gown, gloves, eye protection, face mask, a cap, and shoe covers
   d. The patient situation must first be assessed before determining what PPE to wear

37. A parent brings her 2-year-old child to the ED, stating, "She fell and bumped her head and forearm." Which behavior by the child causes the nurse the *least* concern during the initial triage interview?
   a. Crying and reaching for the parent as the nurse approaches
   b. Alert and still, quietly watching as the nurse approaches
   c. Asleep, limp, with even and unlabored respirations
   d. Crying loudly and inconsolably since she was brought in

38. What is the fastest way for the nurse to estimate the systolic blood pressure in the patient who is being resuscitated?
   a. Palpate for presence of a radial pulse.
   b. Use the automated blood pressure cuff.
   c. Place the patient on a cardiac monitor.
   d. Check for the presence of capillary refill.

39. The patient comes to the ED after falling off a roof. He displays absent breath sounds over the left chest, severe respiratory distress, hypotension, jugular vein distention, and tracheal deviation. Based on these assessment findings, for which condition does the nurse anticipate the patient must receive immediate treatment?
   a. Tension pneumothorax
   b. Cardiac arrest
   c. Airway obstruction
   d. Hemothorax

40. The nurse is helping the physician treat the patient with a tension pneumothorax. What type of equipment does the nurse obtain to immediately alleviate this life-threatening condition?
   a. Large adult endotracheal tube
   b. 14-gauge IV catheter 3-6 cm long
   c. Chest tube insertion tray
   d. Tracheostomy tray

41. The nurse's next-door neighbor has sustained a deep laceration to the right upper arm and there is active bright red bleeding. What does the nurse do to immediately control the bleeding?
   a. Apply a tourniquet just above the laceration.
   b. Have the neighbor lie flat and elevate the arm.
   c. Apply direct pressure with a thick, dry towel.
   d. Apply a sterile gauze and wrap the wound with an Ace bandage.

42. The patient who sustained multiple injuries in a job site accident has a BP of 100/60 and pulse of 120/min. Two large-bore IVs are established and IV fluid resuscitation is initiated. After receiving IV fluid, repeat vital signs are BP 94/56, pulse 135/min; then BP 80/50, pulse 150/min. With these vital signs, the patient is likely to require blood products after how many liters of IV fluid?
   a. 1
   b. 2
   c. 4
   d. 5

43. The nurse is caring for the patient with a head injury whose Glasgow Coma Scale score is 3. This score indicates the patient is most likely to do what?
   a. Withdraw from painful stimuli
   b. Open eyes spontaneously
   c. Moan with incoherent speech
   d. Be totally unresponsive

44. The patient involved in a boating accident has extensive injuries and comes to the ED in wet clothes. The nurse identifies a risk for hypothermia. Which interventions does the nurse implement? *(Select all that apply.)*
   a. Remove wet clothing
   b. Infuse warm IV solutions
   c. Set the room temperature at 90° F
   d. Give sips of warm fluid
   e. Use a heat lamp

45. Each patient listed below has entered the ED's waiting area. Place them in order of priority, with 1 being the highest priority and 4 being the lowest priority.

   _____ a. 3-year-old child with inconsolable high-pitched crying, high fever, headache, and nuchal rigidity

   _____ b. 65-year-old man having diaphoresis with left anterior crushing chest pain

   _____ c. 32-year-old woman reporting upper abdominal pain and vomiting green bile emesis

   _____ d. 16-year-old boy with a broken arm from skateboarding, pulse and sensation intact

46. The patient comes to the ED with severe respiratory distress. He has a long history of chronic respiratory disease and now requires endotracheal intubation. How does the nurse assess this patient's lung compliance?
   a. Auscultate the lung fields, especially for coarse crackles
   b. Sense the degree of difficulty in ventilating with a bag-valve-mask
   c. Monitor the pulse oximeter for decreasing saturation levels
   d. Count the respiratory rate and observe the respiratory effort

True or False? *Write T for true or F for false in the blanks provided. If the statement is false, correct the statement to make it true.*

_____ 47. The Emergency Severity Index is the universally accepted triage system recognized in the United States.

_____ 48. The vast majority of people who come to the ED do not need resuscitation.

_____ 49. After the physician has evaluated the patient, the nurse is responsible for providing follow-up care, but does not need to reassess the patient.

_____ 50. It is illegal to search a patient and his or her belongings even if the nurse believes that the patient may be seriously mentally ill.

_____ 51. Educational materials and discharge instructions should be available at the 6th grade reading level or lower.

_____ 52. The patient comes to the ED for an exacerbation of chronic back pain. This would be a good time to perform education about weight loss.

_____ 53. Intentional injury is the leading cause of death for Americans under the age of 35 and is one of today's most significant public health problems.

_____ 54. The overall goal of the trauma system is to save lives.

CASE STUDY: THE TRAUMA PATIENT

Use a separate sheet of paper to answer the questions in this Case Study. Answer guidelines for this Case Study are available on your Evolve website at http://evolve. elsevier.com/Iggy/ in the "Prepare for Class" folder.

The patient is a 37-year-old man who was the driver in a high-speed motor vehicle accident. EMS reports that his vehicle was struck on the driver's side by a truck and the victim had to be extracted using the "jaws of life." The patient was wearing a seatbelt and he was unconscious when EMS arrived, but he has intermittently aroused reporting extreme pain in the chest and pelvis area. He arrives secured to a backboard with a C-collar in place. His breathing is uneven and becomes increasingly more labored as he is transferred to the ED stretcher. Vital signs are respirations 35/min; pulse 125/min; blood pressure 86/40 mm Hg; cardiac monitor shows sinus tachycardia. The resuscitation team includes an ED physician, primary nurse, secondary nurse, respiratory therapist, and a nursing assistant.

1. During the primary survey, what is the *highest* priority intervention?
2. When assessing breathing during the primary survey, what is included in this assessment?
3. Discuss interventions that accompany the ABCDE of the primary survey.
4. Discuss with a classmate several ways that assessment, interventions, and responsibilities could be divided between the primary and secondary nurse. (Use your critical thinking skills and discuss your answer with your instructor.)
5. What duties would be appropriate to delegate to the nursing assistant?
6. What is the purpose of the secondary survey?
7. Why is the mechanism of injury (MOI) important in trauma cases? In the scenario above, speculate about the relationship of the mechanism of injury and the EMS report on the patient's complaints and injuries.
8. Explain why the patient is likely to have a nasogastric tube and a Foley catheter inserted.

11

CHAPTER

Care of Patients with Common Environmental Emergencies

STUDY/REVIEW QUESTIONS

1. Which of the following are predisposing factors associated with heat-related illness? *(Select all that apply.)*
   a. High humidity
   b. Low humidity
   c. Obesity
   d. Anemia
   e. Seizures
   f. Dehydration
   g. Beta-adrenergic blockers

2. The nurse is providing patient education about the prevention of heat-related illness. Which statement is correct?
   a. "Wear lightweight, dark-colored clothing when working outside."
   b. "Plan to limit activities at the hottest time of day."
   c. "Avoid fluids with electrolytes before, during, and after exercise."
   d. "Use a sunscreen with an SPF of at least 45."

3. A television meteorologist has been doing a photo shoot during a day when temperatures reached 110° F. Later in the day, he reports that he feels weak, has a headache, and feels nauseated and dizzy. He states that he had water with him but often forgot to drink it. His body temperature is 98.9° F. What is this patient suffering from?
   a. Classic heat stroke
   b. Exertional heat stroke
   c. Heat exhaustion
   d. Fluid overload

4. During a summer marathon at a beach resort city, a runner suddenly collapses after running in the race for 1 hour. The weather has been extremely hot during the race day, with temperatures of almost 100° F and high humidity. The runner's body temperature is 105.2° F, she is confused and sweating. What is this patient suffering from?
   a. Classic heat stroke
   b. Exertional heat stroke
   c. Heat exhaustion
   d. Dehydration

5. For the runner in question number 4, what first aid interventions would be performed while waiting for an ambulance to arrive? *(Select all that apply.)*
   a. Placing ice packs on the neck, axillae, chest, and groin
   b. Immersion in ice
   c. Removal of clothing
   d. Wetting the body with tepid water, then fanning rapidly to cool by evaporation
   e. Oral antipyretics, such as acetaminophen or aspirin

6. The nurse is participating in a local community sports day. The day is hot and humid and children are running around excitedly. Prevention of heat-related injuries would include which interventions? *(Select all that apply.)*
   a. Encouraging children to eat high-energy snacks, such as sports bars
   b. Advising parents that children with disabilities should not participate
   c. Setting up a shade tent with areas for rest and relaxed play
   d. Limiting direct sun exposure to 2 hours during the hottest time of the day
   e. Using a sunscreen with an SPF factor of at least 15 and reapplying frequently
   f. Wearing lightweight, light-colored, loose-fitting clothing and a hat

7. The nurse is volunteering at the first-aid station at a local community fair. The weather is predicted to be hot and humid. In planning care for people who may experience heat-related illness in this setting, what should the nurse obtain?
   a. Supply of salt tablets and bottles of water
   b. Bags of IV normal saline and IV insertion equipment
   c. Several water spray bottles and a portable fan
   d. Supply of educational pamphlets and sunscreen samples

8. It is the middle of summer and the weather has been hot and humid for several weeks. Which patient has the highest risk for severe heat-related illness?
   a. Older adult woman who lives alone in an apartment with no air conditioning
   b. Well-conditioned athlete who is participating in a marathon
   c. Experienced construction worker who is working on an outdoor structure
   d. Young child who is participating in an organized team sport

9. The nurse has received reports on several patients who were admitted for heat-related illnesses. The patient who has the most severe case of heat-related illness exhibits which signs/symptoms?
   a. Headache; heavy perspiration; temperature of 101° F
   b. Feeling of illness; nausea and vomiting
   c. Significant sunburn to extremities, face, and neck; temperature of 102° F
   d. Hot and dry skin; alert and oriented to person; pulse of 110

10. A homeless man is found lying in a vacant lot in the middle of July. He is lethargic and confused and he has sustained severe sunburns on the exposed areas of his skin. His core temperature is 106° F. What do prehospital emergency cooling measures include for this patient? *(Select all that apply.)*
    a. Administering cold IV fluid
    b. Stripping off all clothing
    c. Packing the axilla and groin with ice
    d. Encouraging sips of cool water
    e. Sponging with tepid water and fanning

11. A young migrant worker who has been living in a garden shed for several months is brought to the ED. He is alert and conversant, but appears fearful and somewhat confused. His skin is hot and dry and his lips are cracked and bleeding. His skin turgor is poor and he appears malnourished. His blood pressure is 96/60 mm Hg, pulse is 120, respirations 30, temperature is 105° F. In addition to high-flow oxygen, what does the nurse anticipate the ED physician will initially order?
    a. IV normal saline and a Foley catheter
    b. IV Ringer's lactate and an NG tube
    c. IV 5% dextrose and acetaminophen (Tylenol)
    d. IV 45% saline and chlorpromazine (Thorazine)

12. An older adult man with a history of chronic dementia is brought to the ED by his son. The son states that his father sustained a snakebite. What is a key question that the nurse should ask the son to gauge the potential risk for envenomation?
    a. "Do you think he sustained a 'dry' bite?"
    b. "What kind of first-aid did you try?"
    c. "Did the snake have a triangular head?"
    d. "Does your father seem unusually anxious?"

13. The patient sustained a bite from a pit viper and is admitted for observation. Which potential complications does the nurse observe for? *(Select all that apply.)*
    a. Local tissue necrosis
    b. Pulmonary hypertension
    c. Massive tissue swelling
    d. Renal failure
    e. Hypovolemic shock
    f. Increased intracranial pressure

14. The nurse is participating in a summer hike with a group of children. Suddenly the children start screaming, "Snake! Snake!" One little girl is sitting in a tall grassy area, clutching her ankle and crying. What is the first priority in the field care of this child?
    a. Remove any constricting clothing.
    b. Maintain the extremity below the level of the heart.
    c. Move the child to a safe area and encourage rest.
    d. Keep the child warm and provide calm reassurance.

15. The nurse is on a backpacking trip. One of the hikers sustains a pit viper bite to the lower leg. Transportation to the hospital will be delayed by several hours while others go for help. The nurse decides that the circumstances warrant which first-aid measure?
    a. Elevating the leg and applying cool packs
    b. Incising the fang marks with a pocket knife
    c. Checking the puncture site for swelling and pain
    d. Applying a constricting band proximal to the fang marks

16. The patient arrives in the ED after sustaining a cottonmouth snakebite. What are the immediate interventions for this patient?
    a. Establishing a central line with normal saline
    b. Applying a pressure bandage
    c. Monitoring blood pressure and cardiac function
    d. Administering antivenin

17. The patient is admitted for a poisonous snakebite. The nurse observes that the patient has hematuria, hemoptysis, petechiae, and extensive bruising. These clinical observations indicate to the nurse that the patient may be experiencing which hemorrhagic complication associated with snakebite?
    a. Disseminated intravascular coagulation
    b. Agranulocytosis
    c. Thrombocytopenia
    d. Aplastic anemia

18. The patient sustained a snakebite and the physician has determined that the patient should receive antivenin (*Crotalidae*) polyvalent (ACP), which is horse (equine) serum that contains antibodies against the venom. Prior to administering the antivenin, which action does the nurse perform that is specifically related to this treatment?
    a. Cleanse the skin with chlorhexidine.
    b. Perform skin testing for allergy.
    c. Assess the location of the fang marks.
    d. Inject a topical anesthetic into the skin.

19. The patient is to receive antivenin (*Crotalidae*) polyvalent (ACP) for treatment of a rattlesnake bite 10 days ago. Which symptoms indicate that the patient may have the beginning of serum sickness?
    a. Skin rash with pruritus
    b. Nausea and vomiting
    c. Dizziness and lightheadedness
    d. Malaise and excessive fatigue

20. The patient is transported to the ED by a family member after sustaining a snakebite on a hiking trip. The patient may be a potential candidate for *Crotalidae* Polyvalent Immune Fab (CroFab). In order to safely administer therapy, which question would the nurse ask?
    a. "What type of snake inflicted the bite?"
    b. "How much time has passed since the snakebite occurred?"
    c. "Do you have a history of DVT or do you take Coumadin?"
    d. "Do you have allergies to papaya or pineapple?"

21. The patient sustained a snakebite 2 hours ago and the physician orders *Crotalidae* Polyvalent Immune Fab (CroFab). What is the priority nursing intervention in administering this medication to the patient?
    a. Monitor for symptom control after the first dose.
    b. Monitor the patient closely for hives, rash, or difficulty breathing.
    c. Give the bolus dose slowly over 10 minutes.
    d. Give the medication within 3 hours of the snakebite.

22. The patient sustained a coral snakebite on the forearm approximately 12 hours ago and he has been admitted for observation. He reported a mild transient pain, but was otherwise asymptomatic on admission. Which clinical manifestations are early signs of envenomation?
    a. Nausea, vomiting, and pallor
    b. Difficulty speaking and swallowing
    c. Total flaccid paralysis
    d. Severe pain and swelling at the site

23. The patient sustained a coral snakebite and developed severe complications. Which two diagnostic test results reveal the physiologic insufficiency and/or damage that occurs with envenomation?
    a. Arterial blood gas (ABG) and creatinine kinase (CK)
    b. Complete blood count (CBC) and partial thromboplastin time (PTT)
    c. Blood urea nitrogen (BUN) and serum creatinine
    d. Electrocardiogram (ECG) and Troponin I

24. The patient is admitted for a coral snakebite and is to receive antivenin *Micrurus fulvius*. While waiting for the arrival of the antivenin, which equipment does the nurse prepare in case the most significant risk associated with the administration of the antivenin should occur?
    a. Resuscitation equipment, epinephrine, and antihistamines
    b. Cooling blanket, cool mist humidifier, and antipyretics
    c. Padding for siderails, oral suction equipment, and anticonvulsants
    d. Oral suction equipment, emesis basin, and antiemetics

25. The patient is receiving an infusion of antivenin *Micrurus fulvius*. He reports subjective itching at the infusion site that radiates up the arm, and the nurse notes a raised red welt in the axillary area of the same arm. What is the priority nursing action for this patient?
    a. Slow the infusion and reassess the site.
    b. Stop the infusion and give epinephrine or antihistamine.
    c. Flush the line with saline and call the physician.
    d. Discontinue the IV and reestablish the IV at another site.

26. The nurse's next-door neighbor calls because he has just killed a snake that has bitten him on the arm while he was gardening. He does not know how to identify the snake. What features lead the nurse to believe that this snake is poisonous? *(Select all that apply.)*
    a. Triangular head
    b. Two fangs that are curved
    c. The snake hissed before biting
    d. Depression in the skin between each eye and nostril
    e. Diamond pattern on its back
    f. Black, red, and yellow bands of color on the snake (red bands next to black bands)
    g. Black, red, and yellow bands of color on the snake (red bands next to yellow bands)

27. The patient sustained a snake bite and calls the ED for instructions. Besides calling for an ambulance, what does the nurse instruct the patient to do?
    a. Apply ice to the wound.
    b. Incise the wound to allow the blood to flow freely.
    c. Place a constricting band proximal to the wound that does not impair venous drainage or arterial flow.
    d. Place a constricting band proximal to the wound that is tight enough to reduce arterial flow of the venom.

Matching. *Match the type of envenomation with its physical manifestations.*

Type of Envenomation
a. Pit viper envenomation
b. Coral snake envenomation
c. Both types

Manifestation

_____ 28. Mild and transient pain at the bite site

_____ 29. Severe pain, swelling, and bruising at the bite site

_____ 30. Formation of vesicles or hemorrhagic bullae

_____ 31. Cranial and peripheral nerve deficits

_____ 32. Nausea and vomiting

_____ 33. Coagulopathy

_____ 34. Total flaccid paralysis

_____ 35. Minty, rubbery, or metallic taste in the mouth

36. When administering antivenin, the nurse needs to monitor closely for which common complication?
    a. Hemorrhage
    b. Neurologic impairment
    c. Anaphylactic shock
    d. Seizures

37. **Crossword Puzzle.** Complete the crossword puzzle using the clues listed below.

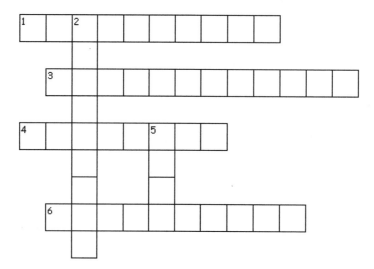

Across

1. The type of hairs launched by the spiders in 2 down that may induce a severe inflammatory reaction if they penetrate the eyes or skin.
3. This type of spider hides in areas that are dark and secluded, and are also known as fiddle-backs or violin spiders *(two words)*.
4. The type of bee that cannot sting repeatedly when disturbed.
6. This type of spider is often found in cool, damp areas such as outdoor log piles, under rocks, or in sheds or garages. The female has a red hourglass pattern on her ventral abdomen *(two words.)*

Down

2. The largest spiders in the arachnid class.
5. The venom of this type of scorpion is neuro-toxic.

Matching. Match the first aid and hospital interventions with the appropriate spider bite. Some interventions may be appropriate for both types of spider bites.

Spider Bites

a. Brown recluse spider
b. Black widow spider

Interventions

_____ 38. Apply cold compresses.

_____ 39. Elevate extremity.

_____ 40. Administer opioid pain medications.

_____ 41. Administer muscle relaxants.

_____ 42. Administer oral dapsone.

_____ 43. Administer tetanus prophylaxis.

_____ 44. Monitor for seizures and rapidly rising BP.

_____ 45. Antivenin is available for use.

_____ 46. Débridement and skin grafting may be needed later for severe wounds to heal.

47. The patient calls the physician's office after sustaining a spider bite on the arm 3 hours ago asking for advice about whether to come into the office or hospital for evaluation. She denies any allergic reactions or shortness of breath. Which question would be the most relevant in helping the patient to make the decision?
    a. "Do you have Benadryl at the house?"
    b. "Is your arm painful or swollen?"
    c. "Were you able to capture or identify the spider?"
    d. "Was the spider hiding in a dark secluded area?"

48. The patient calls the ED for advice on immediate first aid for a brown recluse spider bite on his hand. He denies allergic response or shortness of breath and states that he plans to see his physician, but is currently about 2 to 3 hours away. What does the nurse advise the patient to do?
    a. Apply a warm pack and elevate the extremity.
    b. Wash the bite area several times with soap and water.
    c. Apply ice and rest as much as possible.
    d. Apply a snug constricting band at the wrist level.

49. The patient sustained a brown recluse bite and has been admitted for IV antibiotics and wound management. Which laboratory value indicates that the patient may be developing a serious complication from the bite?
    a. Increased red blood count
    b. Increased platelet count
    c. Decreased white blood count
    d. Decreased blood urea nitrogen

50. The patient was bitten by a brown recluse spider 4 days ago. The nurse observes petechiae, reddish bruising, ecchymoses, and prolonged bleeding after venipunctures. The patient also has a platelet count of 10,000/μL. What do these findings indicate?
    a. Thrombocytopenia
    b. Hemolytic anemia
    c. Aplastic anemia
    d. Agranulocytosis

51. Which patient is most likely to develop complications related to a black widow spider bite?
    a. Older adult woman with heart disease who denies pain at the site
    b. Small asymptomatic child who was bitten 6 hours ago
    c. Teenager reporting intense pain at the site
    d. Man who initially applied an ice pack to the site

52. The nurse is assessing a patient who reports being bitten by a black widow spider. The patient may have clinical signs and symptoms that mimic which disorder?
    a. Myocardial infarction
    b. Peritonitis
    c. Small bowel obstruction
    d. Deep vein thrombosis

53. Although antivenin for black widow spider bites is rarely used because of the high risk for anaphylaxis and serum sickness, the nurse must be prepared to administer antivenin to patients exhibiting which signs/symptoms or conditions? *(Select all that apply.)*
    a. Pregnancy
    b. Uncontrolled hypertension
    c. Respiratory arrest
    d. Severe muscle spasms and pain
    e. Uncontrolled seizures
    f. Priapism

54. The patient reports severe skin inflammation after sustaining a tarantula bite. On close inspection, the nurse observes that the skin area is covered with fine hairs. What is the first intervention for this skin irritation?
    a. Flush the skin with sterile normal saline
    b. Wash the area thoroughly with soap and water
    c. Apply sticky tape to the skin and pull off to remove hairs
    d. Gently scrape the skin with a rigid plastic card

55. The patient reports a scorpion sting to the back of the hand. There is no obvious redness or inflammation at the suspected sting site. Which assessment technique does the nurse use to confirm a bark scorpion sting?
    a. Raise the arm and observe for blanching.
    b. Observe for the stinger embedded in the skin.
    c. Look for puncture marks surrounded by fine hairs.
    d. Gently tap at the suspected area to elicit pain.

56. The patient is admitted for observation following a bark scorpion sting. The nurse monitors the patient for which type of systemic complications?
    a. Hyperglycemia, hyperkalemia, and dyspnea
    b. Hypoglycemia, hypotension, and subnormal temperature
    c. Bradycardia, respiratory distress, and decreased urine output
    d. High fever, hypertension, and tachycardia

57. The patient is being treated for a bark scorpion sting. He is currently alert, but somewhat confused. He complains of localized pain (5/10) at the site and requires frequent oral suction. Vital signs are temperature 102° F, pulse 95, respirations 12, and BP 140/ 85. Which medication order does the nurse question?
    a. Acetaminophen 650 mg PRN for fever
    b. Tetanus toxoid 0.5 mL intramuscularly x 1 dose
    c. Morphine 20 mg intravenous push for severe pain
    d. Atropine 0.4 mg subcutaneously for hypersalivation

58. The patient sustained a bark scorpion sting and the physician considers the administration of *Centruroides exilicauda* antivenin if the patient's condition worsens. Which chronic health condition does the nurse assess for that could potentiate a hypersensitivity reaction?
    a. Hypertension
    b. Asthma
    c. Diabetes mellitus
    d. Cardiac disease

59. A person is stung by a wasp at a picnic. The person has no difficulty breathing and no history of allergic reaction to bee or wasp stings. What is the priority first-aid action for this person?
    a. Remove the stinger with a pair of tweezers.
    b. Gently scrape the stinger off with the edge of a credit card.
    c. Apply an ice pack to the area and elevate.
    d. Observe the area for signs of inflammation prior to taking any action.

60. A teenager is brought to the ED with a reported bee sting. The nurse observes facial swelling, an audible wheeze, and labored rapid breathing. The teen's girlfriend reports he has been vomiting and having trouble speaking and breathing. What does the nurse anticipate the priority medication order will be?
    a. IV normal saline bolus of 400 mL
    b. 50 mg diphenhydramine (Benadryl) PO
    c. 0.5 mL of 1:1000 epinephrine IM
    d. 100 mg methylprednisolone sodium succinate (Solu-Medrol) IV infusion

61. The physician orders IV infusion of epinephrine for an older adult patient who is not responding to the IM epinephrine that was administered for an allergic reaction to a bee sting. In conjunction with the epinephrine administration, which action does the nurse take?
    a. Place the patient on a cardiac monitor.
    b. Place the patient on continuous pulse oximetry.
    c. Obtain an order for an ECG.
    d. Obtain an order for an arterial blood gas.

62. The patient calls the physician's office asking for advice about whether to seek immediate medical attention for a bee sting. She has no shortness of breath or swelling to the face, throat, or lips. Which question will elicit information to assist the patient in making the decision?
    a. "Were you stung by an African 'killer bee'?"
    b. "Is the affected area red, painful, or swollen?"
    c. "Did you receive multiple stings?"
    d. "Were you able to remove the stinger?"

True or False? *Read the statements regarding bee and wasp stings and write T for true or F for false in the blanks provided.*

_____ 63. First aid for bee and wasp stings includes quick removal of the stinger and application of warm compresses.

_____ 64. Systemic effects develop if the individual is sensitive to the venom.

_____ 65. An anaphylactic reaction results in respiratory distress, laryngeal edema, and hypotension.

_____ 66. An "EpiPen" should be administered any time a bee or wasp sting occurs.

_____ 67. Subcutaneous epinephrine is recommended over the intramuscular (IM) route.

_____ 68. An oral antihistamine should also be administered if an allergic reaction is suspected.

_____ 69. People with a history of allergic reactions to bee or wasp stings should wear a medical alert tag.

70. The patient treated for a severe allergic reaction to a bee sting tells the nurse, "The doctor told me that I had to be careful about getting bee stings in the future, because I could have another allergic reaction." Based on the patient's statement, what is the nurse's first action?
    a. Repeat the information that the physician gave her.
    b. Assess the patient's understanding of allergic reactions and first aid.
    c. Advise the patient to obtain a medical alert bracelet.
    d. Ensure that the patient has a prescription for an EpiPen.

71. Which person has the greatest risk for injury from lightning strike?
    a. Jogger in the park at mid-morning in December
    b. Deer hunter walking through the woods in the evening in October
    c. Golfer out on the green in the late afternoon in June
    d. Camper walking on the beach during the early morning in April

72. Which lightening-strike victim should receive attention first?
    a. Teenager who is motionless except for shallow respirations; he has a weak pulse
    b. Middle-aged man, unconscious, with no palpable pulse
    c. Confused older adult woman with apparent paralysis in lower extremities
    d. Child crying, bleeding from ears, mottled skin, and decreased pulses in left leg

73. A construction worker who was struck by lightning is brought to the ED. He was reported to be unconscious, but CPR was started immediately and he awoke just before the arrival of EMS personnel. In the ED, he is alert and confused, and reports pain to his right hand and foot with fernlike marks. Which assessment tool is the priority for this patient?
    a. Glasgow Coma Scale
    b. Pulse oximeter
    c. Cardiac monitor
    d. Rule of Nines chart

74. The nurse receives a phone call from a child who says, "Mommy was hit by lightning! She's outside. I'm afraid to touch her! I'll get shocked too!" How does the nurse advise the child?
    a. "There is no danger in touching your mom. You won't get hurt."
    b. "It will be okay, just quickly run outside and see if she is breathing."
    c. "Is there anybody at home with you? Let me speak to an adult."
    d. "You stay in the house and someone will come to help very soon."

75. The patient reports that several weeks ago she and a friend were at the beach. The friend was struck by lightning and had cardiac arrest and now has severe cognitive impairment. The patient now reports headache, chronic pain, and extreme fatigue. What are these symptoms and this situation consistent with?
    a. Generalized anxiety disorder
    b. Delayed response lightning strike injury
    c. Post-traumatic stress disorder
    d. Occult lightning strike injury

76. The nurse is caring for a patient who had cardiac and respiratory arrest after being struck by lightning. The patient was resuscitated, and he is now alert and appears to be progressing toward recovery. The nurse observes tea-colored urine in the Foley drainage bag. What does the nurse suspect?
    a. This is a normal finding associated with trauma and resuscitation
    b. Dehydration
    c. Urinary tract infection
    d. Excessive muscle damage affecting the kidneys

77. The nurse is advising parents who are trying to organize a winter cross-country skiing trip. In assisting the parents to develop an appropriate winter clothing list, which articles should be taken on the trip? *(Select all that apply.)*
    a. Synthetic socks
    b. Cotton underwear
    c. Polyester fleece shirt
    d. Windproof outer jacket
    e. Hat made from Gore-Tex
    f. Sunglasses

78. The day camp nurse is with a group of children who have been participating in hiking, swimming, and crafts. The nurse sees a child who is soaking wet, stumbling, and taking off all of her clothes. What does the nurse suspect is wrong with this child?
    a. Snakebite
    b. High-altitude sickness
    c. Hypothermia
    d. Cold diuresis

79. The nurse is conducting a community presentation on cold weather safety. Which point is the nurse sure to include in the presentation?
    a. Hydration and water intake are not an issue, so pack extra clothes, not extra water.
    b. Wear multiple layers of socks when participating in winter sports.
    c. When driving in cold winter weather, carry extra clothes, food, and fluids.
    d. Hypothermia occurs only in the winter months in the United States.

80. Which signs/symptoms indicate the most severe case of hypothermia?
    a. Dysarthria, mental slowness, and increased urine output
    b. Shivering, tachypnea, and increased respiratory rate
    c. Confusion, inability to walk without stumbling and falling
    d. Bradycardia, hypotension, and decreased responsiveness

81. Which person is at highest risk for developing hypothermia?
    a. Teenager swimming with friends in a lake in September
    b. Trained athlete running in wet weather in December
    c. Infant being treated for upper respiratory infection in January
    d. Homeless alcoholic who depends on a city shelter year-round

82. The nurse is caring for a patient who suffered prolonged cold exposure during a hunting trip. The physician instructs the nurse to observe for "cold diuresis" and to administer a 400 mL fluid bolus if symptoms occur. What does the nurse monitor for?
    a. Increased urine output and tachycardia
    b. Diaphoresis and restlessness
    c. Generalized fluid loss with pale, cool skin
    d. Fluid retention with peripheral edema

83. Several people on a cross-country ski trip experience mild hypothermia. Which items does the nurse offer or obtain for the hypothermia victims? *(Select all that apply.)*
    a. Synthetic-fiber hat
    b. Bottle of water
    c. Caffeinated beverage
    d. Polyester fleece shirt
    e. Dry socks and gloves

84. The patient arrives at the ED after a prolonged cold exposure. The nursing assistant handles the patient with rough and vigorous movements during the transfer from stretcher to bed. Which complication has the nursing assistant's actions placed the patient at risk for?
    a. Ventricular fibrillation related to rough handling
    b. Third-degree heart block related to cold autotransfusion
    c. Tissue damage related to frostbite of the extremities
    d. Pulmonary emboli related to dislodgment of a clot

85. The physician orders core warming methods for a patient who has moderate hypothermia. What equipment would the nurse obtain in order to provide this therapy?
    a. Three-way Foley with warmed lavage fluid
    b. Axillary thermometer to monitor core temperature
    c. Ambu bag with warmed humidified oxygen
    d. Several warm blankets and warming pads

86. A man is found lying in an alley in cold weather for an unknown length of time. His hands, toes, and face show evidence of frostbite; otherwise there are no obvious injuries. He is severely obtunded with a pulse of 43 beats/min, respirations of 9/min, and a core temperature of 27° C. What is this patient's most immediate physiologic risk?
    a. Acute respiratory distress syndrome
    b. Pulmonary edema
    c. Cardiac arrest
    d. Acute renal failure

87. The nurse has volunteered at a storm shelter to identify potential problems related to cold-related injuries. Which person is at greatest risk for cold injury?
    a. Construction worker who is working outside to restore power.
    b. Homeless woman who has diabetes mellitus.
    c. Teenager who frequently smokes cigarettes.
    d. Obese middle-aged man with high blood pressure.

88. The nurse is working in a mountain clinic where there is a high incidence of cold-related injuries. Which signs/symptoms indicate the most severe case of frostbite?
    a. Large fluid-filled blisters with partial thickness skin necrosis
    b. Numbness, coldness, and bloodlessness of affected area
    c. Small blisters that contain dark fluid; skin is cool
    d. Pain, numbness, and pallor of the affected area

89. Which measures are *correct* when rewarming a victim of deep frostbite? *(Select all that apply.)*
    a. Rubbing the area helps speed the warming process.
    b. Rapid rewarming in a 38° C to 41° C water bath will be required.
    c. Rapid rewarming is avoided due to the possibility of seizures.
    d. Rewarming does not cause pain due to damage to the peripheral nerves.
    e. An opioid analgesic may be given because of the pain associated with rewarming.
    f. Dry heat may be applied as needed to assist in the rewarming process.
    g. After rewarming, the extremity should be elevated above the heart level.
    h. Immunization for tetanus prophylaxis will be needed.

90. The nurse is conducting a class about cold-weather hiking. To recognize early signs of frostbite, what should hiking partners observe each other frequently for?
    a. White, waxy appearance to exposed skin on the ears, nose, and cheeks
    b. Edema and redness over the exposed skin
    c. Mottled coloring of the skin
    d. Small blisters that contain dark fluid and areas that do not blanch

91. The ED nurse receives a phone call from someone stating that he and his friend have been out in the cold weather and his friend's fingers 3 through 5 appear white and waxy. What does the nurse direct the caller to do?
    a. Seek shelter immediately and massage and briskly rub the fingers.
    b. Seek shelter immediately and place the hands under the armpits.
    c. Seek medical attention immediately and intermittently apply dry heat while en route.
    d. Seek medical attention immediately and place fingers in cool water while en route.

92. The patient has sustained severe frostbite to the toes and lower legs. He received rewarming therapy in the ED and arrives to the medical-surgical unit with a splint on both legs. IV normal saline is infusing at 125 mL/hr. He reports severe pain in the lower extremities. Which physician order does the nurse question?
    a. Morphine 1-2 mg IV push PRN for pain in extremities
    b. Elevate bilateral lower extremities above the level of the heart
    c. Neurologic and circulation checks every 1 hour to bilateral lower extremities
    d. Apply compression bandage to bilateral lower extremities

93. The nurse is reviewing the CBC results for a patient who lives in a high mountain town. The patient's RBC is 6.8 million/mm^3. What does this lab value indicate?
    a. Anemia related to a decreased production of erythropoietin
    b. Polycythemia related to chronic hypoxia
    c. Pernicious anemia related to a regional dietary deficiency
    d. Cold antibody anemia related to cold temperature

94. The patient reports having a throbbing headache with nausea and vomiting "like the worst hangover of my life" after recently returning from a hiking trip to the mountains. The nurse suspects that the patient could be suffering from a high-altitude illness. Which question helps the nurse gather relevant information about this condition?
    a. "Did you experience any episodes of hypothermia during your trip?"
    b. "How quickly did you ascend to the top of the mountain range?"
    c. "Did you go skiing or hiking in a high-altitude area?"
    d. "Did you have trouble sleeping while you were in the mountains?"

95. The patient is admitted to the ED for high-altitude sickness. In the morning, he appears apathetic and declines to perform basic ADLs. Later in the shift, the patient is unable to move himself in bed or to independently sit upright. What condition does the nurse suspect?
    a. High-altitude cerebral edema (HACE)
    b. Severe hypoxemia
    c. Acute mountain sickness (AMS)
    d. Severe hypothermia

96. Which initial signs/symptoms indicate high-altitude pulmonary edema (HAPE)?
    a. Loss of appetite and dizziness when standing up too quickly
    b. Irritability, fatigue, and apathy
    c. Persistent cough and blue-tinged nail beds
    d. Headache with nausea and vomiting

97. A foreign service employee must take an emergency trip to a high mountain area. He normally lives in a coastal area and there is no time for him to acclimate. He asks the nurse if there is anything he can do to prevent acute mountain sickness (AMS). What does the nurse advise the patient to do?
    a. Ascend about 1000 feet at a time with intermittent periods of rest and to sleep at lower elevations if possible.
    b. Obtain gingko biloba from a herbalist; take just before ascending and every 8 hours during the trip.
    c. Obtain a prescription for acetazolamide; take 24 hours before ascent and for the first 2 days of the trip.
    d. See a physician as soon as the trip is completed for evaluation of possible respiratory or cerebral edema complications.

98. Which occurrence in the patient treated for AMS indicates that treatment with acetazolamide (Diamox) was effective?
    a. Decreased pulse rate and decreased urine output
    b. Increased urine output and an increased respiratory rate
    c. Periodic respirations during sleep and decreased pulse
    d. Decreased sleep disturbance and decreased respiratory rate

99. A rescue team is attempting to take the patient to the hospital for symptoms of HAPE. The descent to the hospital is delayed due to severe weather conditions. What is the most important treatment for this patient during the delay?
    a. Dexamethasone (Decadron)
    b. Furosemide (Lasix)
    c. Oxygen administration
    d. Avoidance of cold stress

100. Two teenagers bring their friend to the ED because "he was drowning." The patient is unconscious but shows spontaneous breathing, and he is immediately taken to the resuscitation area. Which question is most important for the nurse to ask the patient's friends in determining the outcomes for the patient?
    a. "Was this a fresh water or salt water drowning?"
    b. "Does he have any medical conditions, such as seizures?"
    c. "Was the water contaminated with chemicals or algae?"
    d. "How long was he under the water and not breathing?"

101. What response does the "diving reflex" cause in the body?
    a. Tachycardia with increased blood flow to the brain
    b. Vasoconstriction of vessels and increased cardiac output
    c. Increased myocardial oxygen use
    d. Enhanced blood flow to the brain and heart

102. At the lake, several people are looking out across the water and pointing to a swimmer in the distance who appears to be struggling to stay afloat and is shouting for help. What is the priority action in this situation?
    a. Safe rescue of the victim
    b. Removal of the victim from the water
    c. Gentle handling to prevent ventricular fibrillation
    d. Removal of excess fluid from the lungs

12 CHAPTER

Concepts of Emergency and Disaster Preparedness

STUDY/REVIEW QUESTIONS

Matching. *Match the abbreviations with the correct terms.*

Abbreviations

a. NNRT
b. NDMS
c. HAZMAT
d. ED
e. HICS
f. FEMA
g. WMD
h. EMS
i. PPE
j. DMAT
k. MRC
l. DMORT
m. MSRT

Terms

_____ 1. Emergency department

_____ 2. Federal Emergency Management Agency

_____ 3. Medical Reserve Corps

_____ 4. National Disaster Medical System

_____ 5. Disaster Mortuary Team

_____ 6. International Medical Surgical Response Team

_____ 7. Emergency medical services

_____ 8. Hazardous materials training

_____ 9. Personal protective equipment

_____ 10. Disaster Medical Assistance Team

_____ 11. Weapons of mass destruction

_____ 12. National Nurse Response Team

_____ 13. Hospital Incident Command System

14. For which event would the hospital's disaster plan typically be activated?
    a. Three-car collision on the freeway
    b. Fight between two local street gangs
    c. School bus involved in an accident
    d. Explosion at a chemical factory

15. The hospital in a small mountain town is updating their disaster plan to incorporate the "all hazards approach" and to address all credible threats to the area. Which disaster events are the likely priorities in this community's disaster plan? *(Select all that apply.)*
    a. Avalanches
    b. Floods
    c. Burns
    d. Car accidents
    e. Tornados
    f. Bioterrorism
    g. Blizzards

16. The hospital committee is reviewing the disaster plan of their small community hospital in a suburban area of a large city. What is a priority to include in this hospital's disaster plan?
   a. Plan for evacuation routes out of the city
   b. Plan for transporting patients to other hospitals
   c. Method to contact the National Disaster Medical System
   d. Stockpiling postexposure prophylactic antibiotics

17. The hospital staff is participating in a disaster drill and the nurse is assigned to organize personnel who are called in from home. Which task would be appropriate to delegate to a nursing assistant who usually works in the labor and delivery area?
   a. Stay with "black tag" patients in the holding area.
   b. Talk to the families of the "red tag" patients.
   c. Care for and support the "green tag" patients.
   d. Obtain vital signs of the "yellow tag" patients.

18. The nurse manager is evaluating the human resources on her unit that could be mobilized during a mass casualty event. What is a controllable factor in estimating the total number of available personnel?
   a. Worker illness
   b. Lack of qualified personnel
   c. Absenteeism
   d. Personal choice of quarantine

Matching. *Several individuals have been injured in a major explosion at an assembly plant. Classify the triage priority according to the color-coded disaster triage tag system (green, yellow, red, or black tag).*

Triage Tags
a. Black tag
b. Green tag
c. Red tag
d. Yellow tag

Triage Priorities

_____ 19. Patient who has died of his injuries

_____ 20. Patient with a fractured ankle

_____ 21. Patient who is short of breath and has broken ribs and a hemothorax

_____ 22. Patient with an open fracture of the femur

_____ 23. Patient who has a weak pulse and is bleeding profusely from a severe arm laceration

_____ 24. Patient who has a 4-inch leg laceration that is oozing blood slowly

_____ 25. Patient who has fallen and sprained her shoulder

26. The nurse based in Iowa is a volunteer member of the Medical Reserve Corps (MRC) and has been called to serve in Ohio where he does not hold an active nursing license. What should the nurse do?
    a. Determine if Ohio has reciprocity with Iowa before accepting deployment.
    b. Decline deployment because his nursing license will not allow him to practice in Ohio.
    c. Prepare for deployment because he will be considered a federal employee with valid licensure.
    d. Delay deployment until he has reviewed the nurse practice act that is specific to Ohio.

27. The nursing director of a long-term care facility is designated as the "incident commander" for the facility's disaster plan. What is the priority action for the incident commander?
    a. Call all the off-duty staff and ask them to come into work.
    b. Take inventory of available supplies according to the disaster plan.
    c. Activate the disaster management process according to the plan.
    d. Call the National Guard to move all the patients to other facilities.

28. The nurse is assigned to assist the "hospital incident commander" during a disaster drill. Which responsibility is appropriate for the nurse in this capacity?
    a. Call all nursing units to determine the number of patients who could potentially be discharged.
    b. Call the physical therapy department and direct therapists to assist in the operating room or the ICU.
    c. Go to the emergency department (ED) and assist with the triage of disaster victims to appropriate clinical areas.
    d. Contact the security department and instruct them to control the number of people who attempt to enter the hospital.

29. The nurse serves on a committee that is tasked to develop tools and aids that the "medical command physician" could use during a disaster event. What is an appropriate project for this purpose?
    a. Make a current list, including contact information, of trauma and orthopedic surgeons.
    b. Make a telephone tree for contacting the nursing and ancillary staff.
    c. Design a triage algorithm that addresses different types of disaster events.
    d. Design an algorithm for contacting the Federal Emergency Management Agency.

30. At 3:00 AM, the ED charge nurse of a large suburban hospital receives notification that a commercial plane has just crashed outside the city limits. What does the nurse do?
    a. Activate the hospital's disaster plan and initiate the staff telephone tree.
    b. Alert the ED unit manager at home and determine who can be discharged.
    c. Inform the medical director of the hospital and consult the hospital's disaster plan.
    d. Notify the night nursing supervisor and alert the ED physician(s).

31. A local news station calls the hospital seeking permission to verify the number of victims and details of a local disaster. What is the nurse's best response?
    a. "Please don't bother us now. We are swamped with victims."
    b. "We have a lot of stable victims and two people have died."
    c. "Please hold and I will connect you to the public relations officer."
    d. "I will connect you with the Emergency Command Center."

32. An experienced ED nurse is acting as the triage officer during a mass casualty event in a small rural hospital. Which task is part of this role?
    a. Direct patients who are tagged in the field to the designated areas.
    b. Triage all incoming patients for appropriate care and disposition.
    c. Identify the need for specialty care such as plastic or orthopedic surgery.
    d. Provide comprehensive nursing care to victims as they arrive.

33. During a disaster event, several nurses from the quality assurance department are reassigned to clinical roles. Which area is the most appropriate assignment for these nurses?
    a. Operating room to scrub in for emergency surgeries
    b. ED to take vital signs and transport patients
    c. ED to assist in the triage of incoming patients
    d. Clinic area to provide care for "green tag" patients

34. A city committee reviews possible scenarios related to a disaster event. Which is an example of the "greatest good for the greatest number of people?"
    a. The city's supply of antibiotics is sent to one hospital that has 25 victims with exposure to a bioterrorism agent.
    b. Twenty victims infected by a bioterrorism agent are placed on life support and mechanical ventilation.
    c. Thirty people with possible exposure to a bioterrorism agent are quarantined including five children who are asymptomatic.
    d. Elderly community members are treated with prophylactic antibiotics for a bioterrorism agent.

35. The nurse is making a personal emergency preparedness plan. What is the nurse sure to include in the plan?
    a. Make a disaster supply kit with clothing and basic survival supplies.
    b. Resolve the ethical conflicts of family and professional obligations.
    c. Stockpile antibiotics, first aid supplies, and resuscitation equipment.
    d. Teach family members about radiation and HAZMAT safety issues.

36. The patient comes to the ED worried that he has been exposed to anthrax after opening an envelope that contained a white powder. What is the first thing the emergency department nurse does?
    a. Have the patient wait in the ED waiting area until the decontamination team arrives.
    b. Separate the patient from others in the ED.
    c. Tell the patient to go outside to wait until the decontamination team arrives.
    d. Ask the patient for the envelope that contained the white powder.

37. The nurse is assigned to assist the incident commander who is evaluating the feasibility of deactivating the emergency response plan. The commander directs the nurse to accomplish certain tasks. Which task is the priority?
    a. Contact all hospital departments and determine if needs have been met.
    b. Go to the ED and supervise the inventory and restocking of supplies.
    c. Arrange for temporary sleeping quarters for exhausted staff members.
    d. Assist in the preparations of the critical incident stress debriefing.

38. The patient comes to the ED worried about possible exposure to a hazardous substance. He presents with periorbital swelling and redness on exposed skin areas (i.e., face and hands). The triage nurse elects to activate the hazardous materials decontamination plan. What precautions does this plan entail? (Select all that apply.)
    a. Staff wear protective gowns, gloves, masks, and protective eyewear.
    b. Patient is taken immediately to the closest available shower room.
    c. Patient is directed to remove all of his own clothing.
    d. Patient is directed to wash with soap and water and rinse liberally.
    e. Patient is instructed to wear gown, mask, gloves, and eyewear.
    f. Staff confiscate the patient's clothes and place them in a hazardous waste bag.

39. The nurse is working in the ED where several local gang members are being treated for gunshot and knife wounds. The nurse hears gunshots in the waiting room, followed by screaming and cries for help. What does the nurse do?
    a. Grab the resuscitation box and run to the waiting room.
    b. Assist all the ambulatory patients to leave through a back entrance.
    c. Alert the ED physician that additional trauma victims need care.
    d. Assess the level of threat to self and others and call for help.

Matching. Following a mass casualty event, the hospital is conducting an administrative debriefing and critical incident stress debriefing. Match the type of debriefing with the corresponding description of the two types.

Debriefing Types
a. Administrative debriefing
b. Critical incident stress debriefing

Purposes/Descriptions

_____ 40. Promotes effective coping strategies

_____ 41. Determines if there are opportunities to improve the disaster plan

_____ 42. Prevents the development of post-traumatic stress disorder (PTSD)

_____ 43. Provides for specially trained individuals to deal with the emotional needs of staff

_____ 44. Employs "ground rules" for the debriefing sessions

_____ 45. Allows feedback provided by participants to be used to modify or revise the plan

_____ 46. Keeps the media away from the debriefing with the use of a "doorkeeper"

_____ 47. Reviews activation and implementation of the emergency preparedness plan

CASE STUDY: DISASTER PREPAREDNESS

Use a separate sheet of paper to answer the questions in this Case Study. Answer guidelines for this Case Study are available on your Evolve website at http://evolve. elsevier.com/Iggy/ in the "Prepare for Class" folder.

The nurse is working in a small rural community hospital when the town is hit by a tornado. The nurse cares for several patients who are also neighbors or members of her church, one of whom dies from injuries sustained during the event. The nurse works several extra shifts immediately after the event and continues to help out in the community and cover shifts for other nurses whose homes and families were directly affected by the tornado. Several months later, the nurse notices that she has trouble sleeping and experiences generalized depression.

1. What are signs and symptoms of PTSD that health care personnel and victims of disasters might experience?

2. What is the purpose of the critical incident stress debriefing (CISD)?

3. What are the roles of the CISD team?

4. Discuss the general principles of CISD that are used to support health care personnel who are at risk for PTSD.

5. What are the best practices for preventing future episodes of PTSD?

13 CHAPTER

Assessment and Care of Patients with Fluid and Electrolyte Imbalances

STUDY/REVIEW QUESTIONS

Matching. *Match the physiologic influences on fluids and electrolytes in the body with their descriptions.*

Physiologic Influences

a. Diffusion
b. Filtration
c. Hydrostatic pressure
d. Osmolality
e. Osmolarity
f. Osmosis

Descriptions

_____ 1. "Water-pushing" pressure

_____ 2. The movement of electrolytes into or out of a cell

_____ 3. The movement of water only (the solvent) through a selectively permeable membrane

_____ 4. The unit of measure in a liter of solution that reflects the concentration of solutes

_____ 5. The unit of measure in a kilogram of solution that reflects the concentration of solutes

_____ 6. The movement of fluid through a membrane; usually occurs from capillaries to the interstitial space

7. The nurse is assessing the patient at risk for fluid volume excess. Which findings indicate that the patient has fluid volume excess? *(Select all that apply.)*
   a. Increased, bounding pulse
   b. Jugular venous distention
   c. Diminished peripheral pulses
   d. Presence of crackles
   e. Excessive thirst
   f. Elevated blood pressure
   g. Orthostatic hypotension
   h. Skin pale and cool to touch

8. Which analogy best approximates the principles of diffusion and concentration gradient?
   a. Game with four players on one side and eight on the other; two move over to create six per side
   b. Community fun run where 2000 participants move across the line in a mass start
   c. Basketball game of five players per side; all players move across the court
   d. Concert where 1000 people are trying to enter through a single gate

9. The patient's blood osmolality is 302 mOsm/L. What manifestation does the nurse expect to see in the patient?
   a. Increased urine output
   b. Thirst
   c. Peripheral edema
   d. Nausea

10. The patient is at risk for fluid volume excess. For self-management at home, what does the nurse teach the patient to do?
    a. Increase diuretic dose if swelling occurs.
    b. Limit the amount of free water in relation to sodium intake.
    c. Monitor his or her skin turgor.
    d. Weigh self each day on the same scale.

11. The older adult patient at risk for fluid and electrolyte problems is vigilantly monitored by the nurse for the first indication of a fluid balance problem. What is this indication?
    a. Fever
    b. Mental status changes
    c. Poor skin turgor
    d. Dry mucous membranes

12. Which person is most likely to have symptoms related to poor lymph circulation?
    a. Person with carpal tunnel syndrome
    b. Marathon runner
    c. Person with a history of myocardial infarction
    d. Frequent overseas flyer

13. Based on the factors of age, gender, and body type, which patient has the smallest percentage of total body water?
    a. Thin 78-year-old adult man
    b. Obese 35-year-old man
    c. Thin 25-year-old woman
    d. Obese 68-year-old woman

14. Which intake-output record represents the norm for the average adult?
    a. 500 mL of fluid per day, ingesting an additional 200 mL of fluid from food
    b. 1500 mL of fluid per day, ingesting an additional 800 mL of fluid from food
    c. 3000 mL of fluid per day, ingesting an additional 500 mL of fluid from food
    d. 5000 mL of fluid per day, ingesting an additional 100 mL of fluid from food

15. What is the consequence and clinical manifestation for the patient who does not meet the obligatory urine output?
    a. Increased salivation and alkalosis
    b. Increased thirst with dry mucous membranes
    c. Lethal electrolyte imbalance and acidosis
    d. Bradycardia and decreased nitrogen level

16. What is the minimum amount of urine per day needed to excrete toxic waste products?
    a. 200 to 300 mL
    b. 400 to 600 mL
    c. 500 to 1000 mL
    d. 1000 to 1500 mL

17. Which patient in the medical-surgical unit is most likely to have increased aldosterone secretion?
    a. Patient who has excessive salt ingestion
    b. Patient who drinks a lot of water
    c. Patient who loses a lot of fluid and sodium
    d. Patient who loses potassium and water

18. The patients with which conditions are at great risk for deficient fluid volume? (Select all that apply.)
    a. Fever of 103° F
    b. Extensive burns
    c. Thyroid crisis
    d. Water intoxication
    e. Continuous fistula drainage
    f. Diabetes insipidus

19. The nurse is working in a long-term care facility where there are numerous patients who are immobile and at risk for dehydration. Which task is best to delegate to the unlicensed assistive personnel (UAP)?
    a. Offer patients a choice of fluids every 1 to 2 hours.
    b. Check patients at the beginning of the shift to see who is thirsty.
    c. Give patients extra fluids around medication times.
    d. Evaluate oral intake and urinary output.

20. The nurse is assisting a community group to plan a family sports day. In order to prevent dehydration, what beverage does the nurse suggest be supplied?
    a. Iced tea
    b. Light beer
    c. Diet soda
    d. Bottled water

21. The nurse is assessing the weight of the patient with chronic renal failure. The patient shows a 2 kg weight gain since the last clinic appointment. This is equivalent to how many liters of fluid?
    a. 0.5
    b. 1
    c. 2
    d. 3

22. The nurse is evaluating the hydration status of the older adult patient. If the patient is dehydrated, the nurse expects to observe which type of cardiovascular change?
    a. Hypertension with bounding peripheral pulses
    b. Tachycardia with weak peripheral pulses
    c. Bradycardia and distended neck veins
    d. Increase in pulse pressure and systolic pressure

23. The nurse is caring for the patient with hypovolemia secondary to severe diarrhea and vomiting. In evaluating the respiratory system for this patient, what does the nurse expect to assess?
    a. No changes, because the respiratory system is not involved
    b. Hypoventilation, because the respiratory system is trying to compensate for low pH
    c. Increased respiratory rate, because the body perceives hypovolemia as hypoxia
    d. Normal respiratory rate, but a decreased oxygen saturation

24. The nurse is assessing skin turgor in the 65-year-old patient. What is the correct technique to use with this patient?
    a. Pinch the skin over the sternum and observe for tenting and resumption of skin to its normal position after release.
    b. Observe the skin for a dry, scaly appearance and compare it to a previous assessment.
    c. Pinch the skin over the back of the hand and observe for tenting; count the number of seconds for the skin to recover position.
    d. Observe the mucous membranes and tongue for cracks, fissures, or a pasty coating.

25. The emergency department (ED) nurse is caring for the patient who was brought in for significant alcohol intoxication and minor trauma to the wrist. What will serial hematocrits for this patient likely show?
    a. Hemoconcentration
    b. Normal and stable hematocrits
    c. Progressively lower hematocrits
    d. Decreasing osmolality

26. The nurse is caring for the child at risk for dehydration secondary to diarrhea, vomiting, and fever. The child is alert, quiet, and clinging to the parent. What is the best nursing intervention to rehydrate this patient?
    a. Give an oral rehydration solution such as Oralyte or Rehydralyte.
    b. Have the parent give small sips of preferred diluted fluids every 5 to 10 minutes.
    c. Obtain an order for IV access and an isotonic solution such as normal saline.
    d. Encourage the child to take as much water as possible and offer popsicles.

27. Which statements about the function of the lymphatic system are true? *(Select all that apply.)*
    a. Lymph fluid contains more protein than plasma.
    b. Lymph flow is slower than blood flow.
    c. Lymph flow is enhanced by a pump system.
    d. Lymphatic vessels carry lymph fluid toward the heart.
    e. Lymph fluid is filtered by lymph nodes.
    f. The lymphatic system takes lymph to the kidneys for excretion.

28. The nurse is caring for several older adult patients who are at risk for dehydration. Which task can be delegated to the UAP?
    a. Withhold fluids if patients are incontinent of bowels or bladder.
    b. Assess for and report any difficulties that patients are having in swallowing.
    c. Stay with patients while they drink and note the exact amount ingested.
    d. Divide the total amount of fluids needed over a 24-hour period and post a note.

29. The nurse assessing the patient notes a bounding pulse quality, neck vein distention when supine, presence of crackles in the lungs, and increasing peripheral edema. What condition does the nurse suspect?
    a. Fluid excess
    b. Fluid deficit
    c. Electrolyte imbalance
    d. Serum protein increase

30. The patient is at risk for fluid volume excess and dependent edema. Which task does the nurse delegate to the UAP?
    a. Massage the legs and heels to stimulate circulation.
    b. Evaluate the effectiveness of a pressure-reducing mattress.
    c. Assess the coccyx, elbows, and hips daily for signs of redness.
    d. Assist the patient to change position every 2 hours.

31. The nurse is reviewing orders for several patients who have risk for fluid volume excess. For which patient condition does the nurse question an order for diuretics?
    a. Pulmonary edema
    b. Congestive heart failure
    c. End-stage renal disease
    d. Ascites

32. The UAP reports to the nurse that the patient being evaluated for kidney problems has produced a large amount of pale yellow urine. What does the nurse do next?
    a. Instruct the UAP to measure the amount carefully and then discard the urine.
    b. Instruct the UAP to save the urine in a large bottle for a 24-hour urine specimen.
    c. Assess the patient for signs of fluid imbalance and check the specific gravity of the urine.
    d. Compare the amount of urine output to the fluid intake for the previous 8 hours.

33. On admission, the patient with pulmonary edema weighed 151 lbs; now the patient's weight is 149 lbs. Assuming the patient was weighed both times with the same clothing, same scale, and same time of day, how many milliliters of fluid does the nurse estimate the patient has lost?
    a. 500
    b. 1000
    c. 2000
    d. 2500

34. The nurse is giving discharge instructions to the patient with advanced congestive heart failure who is at continued risk for fluid volume excess. For which physical change does the nurse instruct the patient to call the health care provider?
    a. Greater than 3 lbs gained in a week or greater than 1 to 2 lbs gained in a 24-hour period
    b. Greater than 5 lbs gained in a week or greater than 1 to 2 lbs gained in a 24-hour period
    c. Greater than 15 lbs gained in a month or greater than 5 lbs gained in a week
    d. Greater than 20 lbs gained in a month or greater than 5 lbs gained in a week

35. The nurse is caring for several patients at risk for falls because of fluid and electrolyte imbalances. Which task related to patient safety and fall prevention does the nurse delegate to the UAP?
    a. Assess for orthostatic hypotension.
    b. Orient the patient to the environment.
    c. Help the incontinent patient to toilet every 1 to 2 hours.
    d. Encourage family members or significant other to stay with the patient.

36. The nurse is assessing the patient's urine specific gravity. The value is 1.035. How does the nurse interpret this result?
    a. Overhydration
    b. Dehydration
    c. Normal value for an adult
    d. Renal disease

Matching. *Match each electrolyte with its corresponding lab value and description. Answers can be used more than once.*

Electrolytes
a. Sodium
b. Potassium
c. Calcium
d. Phosphorus
e. Magnesium
f. Chloride

Normal Lab Values and Descriptions

_____ 37. Normal plasma value is 3.5 to 5.0 mEq/L

_____ 38. Major anion of extracellular fluid (ECF)

_____ 39. Normal value is 98 to 106 mEq/L

_____ 40. Main cation in ECF of the cell that maintains ECF osmolarity

_____ 41. Works in balance with calcium

_____ 42. Normal plasma value is 136 to 145 mEq

_____ 43. Has more activity in the cell than in the blood

_____ 44. Major cation of intracellular fluid (ICF) in the cell

_____ 45. Maintains action potentials in excitable membranes

_____ 46. Functions include contraction of skeletal and cardiac muscle

_____ 47. Normal value is 3.0 to 4.5 mg/dL

_____ 48. Major intracellular anion

_____ 49. Free form is physiologically active in the body

_____ 50. Normal value is 1.3 to 2.1 mg/dL

51. The patient is talking to the nurse about sodium intake. Which statement by the patient indicates an understanding of high sodium food sources?
    a. "I have bacon and eggs every morning for breakfast."
    b. "We never eat seafood because of the salt water."
    c. "I love Chinese food, but I gave it up because of the soy sauce."
    d. "Pickled herring is a fish and my doctor told me to eat a lot of fish."

52. Which statement best explains how antidiuretic hormone (ADH) affects urine output?
    a. It increases permeability to water in the tubules causing a decrease in urine output.
    b. It increases urine output as a result of water being absorbed by the tubules.
    c. Urine output is reduced as the posterior pituitary decreases ADH production.
    d. Increased urine output results from increased osmolarity and fluid in the extracellular space.

53. The nurse is assessing the patient's neuromuscular status to obtain a baseline because the patient is at risk for electrolyte imbalances. What technique does the nurse use to assess muscle strength in the legs?
    a. Ask the patient to push the feet against a flat surface and apply resistance to the opposite side of the flat surface.
    b. Ask the patient to walk around the room and observe for stride, gait, balance, and endurance.
    c. Instruct the patient to stand at the side of the bed and abduct each leg as high as possible.
    d. Support the patient's lower leg with the palm and move the knee through flexion and extension.

54. During shift report, the nurse discovers that the patient has low sodium. What gastrointestinal change does the nurse expect to find during the physical assessment?
    a. Minimal bowel sounds with frequent episodes of vomiting
    b. Absent bowel sounds with pronounced abdominal distention
    c. Hypoactive bowel sounds and complaints of constipation
    d. Hyperactive bowel sounds and abdominal cramps

55. Which patients are at risk for developing hyponatremia? *(Select all that apply.)*
    a. Postoperative patient who has been NPO for 24 hours
    b. Patient with decreased fluid intake for several days
    c. Patient with excessive intake of 5% dextrose solution
    d. Diabetic patient with blood glucose of 250 mg/dL
    e. Patient with overactive adrenal glands
    f. Tennis player in 100° F weather

Matching. *Match the clinical situations with the resulting effect leading to hypernatremia. Answers may be used more than once.*

Effects Leading to Hypernatremia

a.   Inadequate water intake
b.   Excess fluid loss
c.   Excess sodium intake
d.   Decreased sodium excretion

Clinical Situations

_____ 56.   Severe diarrhea

_____ 57.   Presence of fever

_____ 58.   Profound diaphoresis

_____ 59.   Primary hyperaldosteronism

_____ 60.   Kidney disease of the proximal tubule

_____ 61.   Confused and disoriented

_____ 62.   Multiple sodium bicarbonate injections

_____ 63.   Severe vomiting

_____ 64.   Restraints

65.   The physician has ordered therapy for the patient with low sodium and signs of fluid volume excess. Which diuretic is best for this patient?
a.   Conivaptan (Vaprisol)
b.   Furosemide (Lasix)
c.   Hydrochlorothiazide (HydroDiuril)
d.   Bumetanide (Bumex).

66.   The nurse is assessing the patient with a mild increase in sodium level. What early manifestation does the nurse observe in this patient?
a.   Muscle twitching and irregular muscle contractions
b.   Inability of muscles and nerves to respond to a stimulus
c.   Muscle weakness occurring bilaterally with no specific pattern
d.   Reduced or absent deep tendon reflexes

67.   The nurse is caring for the patient with hypernatremia caused by fluid and sodium losses. What type of IV solution is best for treating this patient?
a.   Hypotonic 0.225% sodium chloride
b.   Small-volume infusions of hypertonic (2% to 3%) saline
c.   Isotonic sodium chloride (NaCl)
d.   Isotonic Ringer's lactate

68.   Which serum value does the nurse expect to see in the patient with hyponatremia?
a.   Sodium less than 136 mEq/L
b.   Chloride less than 95 mEq/L
c.   Sodium less than 145 mEq/L
d.   Chloride less than 103 mEq/L

69.   The patient has a serum sodium level of 126 mEq/L. What assessment findings does the nurse expect to see in this patient?
a.   Constipation and paralytic ileus
b.   Watery diarrhea with abdominal cramping
c.   Muscle cramping and spasticity
d.   Tachypnea and diminished breath sounds

70.   The nurse is caring for the psychiatric patient who is continuously drinking water. The nurse monitors for which complication related to potential hyponatremia?
a.   Proteinuria/prerenal failure
b.   Change in mental status/increased intracranial pressure
c.   Pitting edema/circulatory failure
d.   Possible stool for occult blood/gastrointestinal bleeding

71. What is the intervention of choice for the patient with mild hypernatremia caused by excessive fluid loss?
    a. IV infusion of 10 units of insulin in 50 mL of 10% dextrose
    b. Replacement of table salt with salt substitute
    c. Furosemide (Lasix) 20 mg IV
    d. Increased oral water intake

72. The nurse is caring for several patients at risk for fluid and electrolyte imbalances. Which patient problem or condition can result in a relative hypernatremia?
    a. Use of a salt substitute
    b. Diarrhea
    c. Drinking too much water
    d. NPO status for a prolonged period

73. The nurse is caring for the older adult patient whose serum sodium level is 150 mEq/L. The nurse assesses the patient for which common manifestation associated with this sodium result?
    a. Gastrointestinal disorders
    b. Altered urinary elimination
    c. Impaired skin integrity
    d. Altered cerebral functioning

74. Which conditions cause the patient to be at risk for hypernatremia? (Select all that apply.)
    a. Renal failure
    b. Immobility
    c. Use of corticosteroids
    d. Watery diarrhea
    e. Cushing's syndrome

75. Which patient is most at risk for developing hypernatremia?
    a. Patient who dislikes drinking milk and lacks calcium in the diet
    b. Patient who is receiving total parenteral nutrition related to gastrointestinal surgery
    c. Patient with excessive diarrhea and vomiting from food poisoning
    d. Older adult patient with decreased sensitivity to thirst

76. Which precaution or intervention does the nurse teach the patient at continued risk for hypernatremia?
    a. Avoid salt substitutes
    b. Avoid aspirin and aspirin-containing products
    c. Read labels on canned or packaged foods to determine sodium content
    d. Increase daily intake of caffeine-containing foods and beverages

77. The nurse identifies the nursing diagnosis of Risk for Injury for the patient with hyponatremia. What is the etiology of this diagnosis?
    a. Altered mental capabilities
    b. Fragility of bones
    c. Immobility
    d. Altered senses

78. Which serum laboratory value indicates the patient has hypernatremia?
    a. Chloride greater than 95 mEq/L
    b. Sodium greater than 135 mEq/L
    c. Chloride greater than 103 mEq/L
    d. Sodium greater than 145 mEq/L

79. The nurse is teaching the patient to recognize foods that are high in sodium. Which food items does the nurse use as examples? (Select all that apply.)
    a. Egg roll with soy sauce
    b. White rice
    c. Salad with oil and vinegar dressing
    d. Bacon and eggs
    e. Cottage cheese and tomato
    f. Steak
    g. Soup with saltine crackers
    h. Steamed vegetables

Matching. *Identify which patient conditions cause the patient to be at risk for developing hyperkalemia or hypokalemia.*

Disorder

a. Hyperkalemia
b. Hypokalemia

Patient Conditions

_____ 80. Severe malnutrition in an older adult man

_____ 81. Chronic obstructive pulmonary disease (COPD) managed with prednisone

_____ 82. Short bowel syndrome with use of total parenteral nutrition

_____ 83. Multiple transfusions of packed red cells

_____ 84. End-stage renal disease

_____ 85. Hypertension managed with Aldactone

_____ 86. Metabolic alkalosis

_____ 87. Ileostomy

_____ 88. Early stage of severe burns

_____ 89. Respiratory acidosis

_____ 90. Diabetes insipidus

_____ 91. Uncontrolled diabetes mellitus

_____ 92. Trauma patient with crushed extremities

_____ 93. Congestive heart failure managed with loop diuretics

94. Which serum laboratory value does the nurse expect to see in the patient with hypokalemia?
   a. Calcium less than 8.0 mg/dL
   b. Potassium less than 5.0 mEq/L
   c. Calcium less than 11.0 mg/dL
   d. Potassium less than 3.5 mEq/L

95. The patient's potassium level is 2.5 mEq/L. Which clinical findings does the nurse expect to see when assessing this patient?
   a. Hypertension, bounding pulses, and bradycardia
   b. Moist crackles, tachypnea, and diminished breath sounds
   c. General skeletal muscle weakness, lethargy, and weak hand grasps
   d. Increased specific gravity and decreased urine output

96. The nurse administering potassium to the patient carefully monitors the infusion because of the risk for which condition?
   a. Pulmonary edema
   b. Cardiac dysrhythmia
   c. Postural hypotension
   d. Renal failure

97. Which changes on the patient's electrocardiogram (ECG) reflect hyperkalemia?
   a. Tall peaked T waves
   b. Narrow QRS complex
   c. Tall P waves
   d. Normal P-R interval

98. The nurse is teaching the patient about hypokalemia. Which statement by the patient indicates a correct understanding of the treatment of hypokalemia?
    a. "My wife does all the cooking. She shops for food high in calcium."
    b. "When I take the liquid potassium in the evening, I'll eat a snack beforehand."
    c. "I will avoid bananas, orange juice, and salt substitutes."
    d. "I hate being stuck with needles all the time to monitor how much sugar I can eat."

99. The nurse is caring for the patient who takes potassium and digoxin. For what reason does the nurse monitor both laboratory results?
    a. Digoxin increases potassium loss through the kidneys.
    b. Digoxin toxicity can result if hypokalemia is present.
    c. Digoxin may cause potassium levels to rise to toxic levels.
    d. Hypokalemia causes the cardiac muscle to be less sensitive to digoxin.

100. Which serum laboratory value does the nurse expect to see in the patient with hyperkalemia?
    a. Calcium greater than 8.0 mg/dL
    b. Potassium greater than 3.5 mEq/L
    c. Calcium greater than 11.0 mg/dL
    d. Potassium greater than 5.0 mEq/L

101. The patient has an elevated potassium level. Which assessment findings are associated with hyperkalemia? *(Select all that apply.)*
    a. Wheezing on exhalation
    b. Numbness in hands, feet, and around the mouth
    c. Frequent, explosive diarrhea stools
    d. Irregular heart rate and hypotension
    e. Circumoral cyanosis

102. The nurse is teaching the patient about foods high in potassium. Which food item does the nurse use as the best example?
    a. Bread
    b. Eggs
    c. Cereal grains
    d. Meat

103. The patient's serum potassium value is below 2.8 mEq/L. The patient is also on digoxin. The nurse quickly assesses the patient for which cardiac problem before notifying the physician?
    a. Cardiac murmur
    b. Cardiac dysrhythmia
    c. Congestive heart failure
    d. Cardiac tamponade

104. Which potassium levels are within normal limits? *(Select all that apply.)*
    a. 2.0 mmol/L.
    b. 3.5 mmol/L.
    c. 4.5 mmol/L.
    d. 5.0 mmol/L.
    e. 6.0 mmol/L.

105. The patient has hyperkalemia resulting from dehydration. Which additional laboratory findings does the nurse anticipate for this patient?
    a. Increased hematocrit and hemoglobin levels
    b. Decreased serum electrolyte levels
    c. Increased urine potassium levels
    d. Decreased serum creatinine

106. The 65-year-old patient has a potassium laboratory value of 5.0 mEq/L. How does the nurse interpret this value?
    a. High for the patient's age
    b. Low for the patient's age
    c. Normal for the patient's age
    d. Dependent upon the medical diagnosis

107. The patient's potassium level is low. What change in the cardiovascular system does the nurse expect to see related to hypokalemia?
    a. Tall, peaked T waves
    b. Weak, thready pulse
    c. Malignant hypertension
    d. Distended neck veins

Matching. *Match the following cellular compartments with their characteristics. Answers can be used more than once.*

Compartments

a. Extracellular compartment
b. Intracellular compartment

Characteristics

_____ 108. Contains the largest amount of body fluid

_____ 109. Contains plasma

_____ 110. Contains interstitial fluid

_____ 111. High in sodium and chloride content

_____ 112. High in potassium and phosphorous content

_____ 113. High in magnesium content

114. The patient with low potassium must have an IV potassium infusion. The pharmacy sends a 250 mL IV bag of dextrose in water with 40 mEq of potassium. The label is marked "to infuse over 1 hour." What does the nurse do?
    a. Obtain a pump and administer the solution.
    b. Double-check the physician's order and call the pharmacy.
    c. Hold the infusion because there is an error in labeling.
    d. Recalculate the rate so that it is safe for the patient.

115. The older adult patient needs an oral potassium solution, but is refusing it because it has a strong and unpleasant taste. What is the best strategy the nurse uses to administer the drug?
    a. Tell the patient that failure to take the drug could result in serious heart problems.
    b. Ask the patient's preference of juice and mix the drug with a small amount.
    c. Mix the solution into food on the patient's meal tray and encourage the patient to eat everything.
    d. Offer the drug to the patient several times and then document the patient's refusal.

116. The patient has a low potassium level and the physician has ordered an IV infusion. Before starting an IV potassium infusion, what does the nurse assess?
    a. Adequate urine output
    b. Oxygen saturation level
    c. Baseline mental status
    d. Apical pulse

117. Hyperkalemia can cause severe problems in which body system?
    a. Neuromuscular
    b. Cardiovascular
    c. Intestinal
    d. Respiratory

118. Which assessment findings are related to hypercalcemia? *(Select all that apply.)*
    a. Bradycardia
    b. Paresthesia
    c. Leg cramping
    d. Hyperactive bowel sounds
    e. Ineffective respiratory movements
    f. Shortened QT interval
    g. Impaired blood flow
    h. Profound muscle weakness

119. Which nursing interventions apply to patients with hypercalcemia? *(Select all that apply.)*
    a. Administer IV normal saline (0.9% sodium chloride).
    b. Assess the patient for a positive Homan's sign.
    c. Measure the abdominal girth.
    d. Massage calves to encourage blood return to the heart.
    e. Monitor for ECG changes.
    f. Provide adequate intake of vitamin D.
    g. During treatment, monitor for tetany.

120. The nurse is reviewing the laboratory calcium level results for the patient. Which value indicates mild hypocalcemia?
    a. 5.0 mg/dL
    b. 8.0 mg/dL
    c. 10.0 mg/dL
    d. 12.0 mg/dL

121. The patient with a recent history of anterior neck injury reports muscle twitching and spasms with tingling in the lips, nose, and ears. The nurse suspects these symptoms may be caused by which condition?
    a. Hypocalcemia
    b. Hypokalemia
    c. Hyponatremia
    d. Hypomagnesemia

122. Which patient conditions cause the patient to be at risk for hypocalcemia? *(Select all that apply.)*
    a. Crohn's disease
    b. Acute pancreatitis
    c. Removal or destruction of parathyroid glands
    d. Immobility
    e. Use of digitalis

123. The advanced practice nurse is assessing the patient with a risk for hypocalcemia. What is the correct technique to test for Chvostek's sign?
    a. Patient flexes arms against the chest and examiner attempts to pull the arms away from the chest.
    b. Place a blood pressure cuff around the upper arm and inflate the cuff to greater than the patient's systolic pressure.
    c. Tap the face just below and in front of the ear to trigger facial twitching of one side of the mouth, nose, and cheek.
    d. Lightly tap the patellar and Achilles tendons with a reflex hammer and measure the movement.

124. The nurse is caring for several patients with electrolyte imbalances. Which condition may require the patient to be put on seizure precautions?
    a. Hypercalcemia
    b. Hyperphosphatemia
    c. Hypocalcemia
    d. Hypokalemia

125. Which clinical condition can result from hypocalcemia?
    a. Stimulated cardiac muscle contraction
    b. Increased intestinal and gastric motility
    c. Decreased peripheral nerve excitability
    d. Increased bone density

126. Which patient is at greatest risk of developing hypocalcemia?
    a. 30-year-old Asian woman with breast cancer
    b. 45-year-old Caucasian man with hypertension and diuretic therapy
    c. 60-year-old African-American woman with a recent ileostomy
    d. 70-year-old Caucasian man on long-term lithium therapy

127. Which is a preventive measure for patients at risk for developing hypocalcemia?
    a. Increase daily dietary calcium intake to 1000 mg.
    b. Increase intake of phosphorus.
    c. Apply sunblock and wear protective clothing whenever outdoors.
    d. Administer calcium-containing IV fluids to patients receiving multiple blood transfusions.

128. The patient who has undergone which surgical procedure is at risk for hypocalcemia?
    a. Thyroidectomy
    b. Adrenalectomy
    c. Pancreatectomy
    d. Gastrectomy

129. Which medication order does the nurse clarify before administering the drug to the patient with hypocalcemia?
    a. Magnesium sulfate 1 g IM every 6 hours for four doses
    b. Aluminum hydroxide (AlternaGEL) 15 mL orally three times a day and at bedtime
    c. Calcium carbonate 1000 mg orally after meals and at bedtime
    d. Calcium gluconate 5 mEq IV PRN for tetany

130. What is a typical nursing assessment finding for the patient with hypocalcemia?
    a. Paresthesias and tingling followed by numbness
    b. Shortened ST segment, tachycardia, and hypertension
    c. Constipation and hypoactive bowel sounds
    d. Severe muscle weakness

131. Which intervention does the nurse implement for the patient with hypocalcemia?
    a. Encourage activity by the patient as tolerated, including weight-lifting.
    b. Encourage socialization and active participation in stimulating activities.
    c. Include a tracheostomy tray at the bedside for emergency use.
    d. Provide adequate intake of vitamin D and calcium-rich foods.

132. The patient has chronic renal failure (CRF). Which electrolyte imbalance often associated with hypocalcemia and CRF does the nurse monitor for?
    a. Hypophosphatemia
    b. Hyperphosphatemia
    c. Hyperkalemia
    d. Hyponatremia

133. Which food provides both calcium and vitamin D for the patient in need of supplemental diet therapy for hypocalcemia?
    a. Eggs
    b. Broccoli
    c. Milk
    d. Tofu

134. The patient shows a positive Trousseau's or Chvostek's sign. The nurse prepares to give the patient which urgent treatment?
    a. IV calcium
    b. Calcitonin (Calcimar)
    c. IV potassium chloride
    d. Large doses of oral calcium

135. Which is a preventive nursing intervention for patients at risk for developing hypercalcemia?
    a. Ensure adequate hydration.
    b. Discourage weight-bearing activity such as walking.
    c. Monitor the patient for fluid volume excess.
    d. Administer multivitamin tablets twice per day.

136. The nurse caring for the patient with hypercalcemia anticipates orders for which medications? *(Select all that apply.)*
    a. Magnesium sulfate
    b. Calcitonin (Calcimar)
    c. Furosemide (Lasix)
    d. Plicamycin (Mithracin)
    e. Calcium gluconate
    f. Aluminum hydroxide

137. The nurse instructs the UAP to use precautions with moving and use of a lifting sheet for which patient with an electrolyte imbalance?
    a. Young diabetic woman with hyperkalemia
    b. Psychiatric patient with hyponatremia
    c. Older woman with hypocalcemia
    d. Child with severe diarrhea and hypomagnesemia

138. The patient's laboratory results show a decrease in serum phosphorus level. The nurse expects to see a reciprocal increased change in which serum level?
    a. Calcium
    b. Potassium
    c. Sodium
    d. Magnesium

139. The patient has hyperphosphatemia. Which accompanying and potentially life-threatening electrolyte imbalance does the nurse monitor for?
    a. Hypercalcemia
    b. Hypocalcemia
    c. Hyponatremia
    d. Hyperkalemia

140. Which nursing interventions does the nurse include for the patient with hypophosphatemia?
    a. Aggressive treatment with parenteral phosphorous
    b. Administration of oral vitamin D and phosphorus supplements
    c. Concurrent administration of calcium supplements
    d. Elimination of beef, pork, and legumes from the diet

141. Which serum level of phosphorus represents hypophosphatemia?
    a. 2.5 mg/dL
    b. 3.5 mg/dL
    c. 4.5 mg/dL
    d. 5.5 mg/dL

Matching. *Match the clinical conditions with their effects on serum phosphorus levels. Answers are used more than once.*

Serum Phosphorus Levels
a. Hyperphosphatemia
b. Hypophosphatemia

Clinical Conditions
_____ 142. Tumor lysis syndrome
_____ 143. Malnutrition
_____ 144. Alcoholism
_____ 145. Hypoparathyroidism
_____ 146. Aluminum hydroxide-based antacids
_____ 147. Renal insufficiency
_____ 148. Respiratory alkalosis
_____ 149. Increased intake of phosphorus
_____ 150. Hyperparathyroidism

151. The physician orders magnesium sulfate ($MgSO_4$) for the patient with severe hypomagnesemia. What is the preferred route of administration for this drug?
    a. Oral
    b. Subcutaneous
    c. Intramuscular
    d. Intravenous

152. The nurse is assessing the patient with severe hypermagnesemia. Which assessment findings are associated with this electrolyte imbalance?
    a. Bradycardia and hypotension
    b. Tachycardia and weak palpable pulse
    c. Hypertension and irritability
    d. Irregular pulse and deep respirations

153. The patient on the medical-surgical unit suddenly has a severely elevated magnesium level. What does the nurse anticipate will happen next with this patient's care?
    a. Immediate transfer to the intensive care unit
    b. Discontinuation of magnesium sources so the patient can recover
    c. Administration of diuretics such as furosemide
    d. Administration of IV magnesium binder

154. The patient has a magnesium level of 0.8 mg/dL. Which treatment does the nurse expect to be ordered for this patient?
    a. Intramuscular magnesium sulfate
    b. Increased intake of fruits and vegetables
    c. Oral preparations of magnesium sulfate
    d. IV magnesium sulfate and discontinuation of diuretic therapy

155. The nurse monitors the effectiveness of magnesium sulfate by assessing which factor every hour?
    a. Deep tendon reflexes
    b. Vital signs
    c. Serum laboratory values
    d. Urine output

156. Which patient condition places the patient at risk for hypocalcemia, hyperkalemia, and hypernatremia?
    a. Hypothyroidism
    b. Diabetes mellitus
    c. Chronic renal failure
    d. Adrenal insufficiency

157. The patient with congestive heart failure is receiving a loop diuretic. The nurse monitors for which electrolyte imbalances? *(Select all that apply.)*
    a. Hypocalcemia
    b. Hypokalemia
    c. Hyponatremia
    d. Hypercalcemia
    e. Hyperkalemia
    f. Hypernatremia

158. Complete the chart below by indicating the reference range values for each electrolyte.

Major Serum Electrolyte

Electrolyte	Reference Range
Sodium (Na$^+$)	
Potassium (K$^+$)	
Calcium (Ca^{2+})	
Chloride (Cl$^-$)	
Magnesium (Mg^{2+})	
Phosphorus (Pi)	

CASE STUDY: THE PATIENT WITH A FLUID IMBALANCE

Use a separate sheet of paper to answer the questions in this Case Study. Answer guidelines for this Case Study are available on your Evolve website at http://evolve. elsevier.com/Iggy/ in the "Prepare for Class" folder.

The patient is a 45-year-old man who had GI surgery 4 days ago. He is NPO, has a nasogastric tube, and IV fluids of D_5 1/2 normal saline at 100 mL/hr. The nursing physical assessment includes the following: alert and oriented; fine crackles; capillary refill within normal limits (WNL); moving all extremities; complaining of abdominal pain, muscle aches, and "cottony" mouth; dry mucous membranes; bowel sounds hypoactive, last BM was 4 days ago; skin turgor is poor; 200 mL of dark green substance has drained from NG tube in last 3 hours. Voiding dark amber urine without difficulty. Intake for last 24 hours is 2500 mL. Output is 2000 mL including urine and NG drainage. Febrile and diaphoretic; BP 130/80; pulse 88; urine specific gravity 1.035; serum potassium 3.0 mEq/L; serum sodium 140 mEq/L; Cl 92 mEq/L; Mg 1.4 mg/dL.

1. Analyze the data in the case study. Do the findings indicate a fluid deficit or fluid excess problem? Support your answer with data from this patient.

2. What factors could be contributing to this problem?

3. Evaluate the patient's electrolyte values and give a rationale for the answer.

CASE STUDY: THE PATIENT WITH OVERHYDRATION

Use a separate sheet of paper to answer the questions in this Case Study. Answer guidelines for this Case Study are available on your Evolve website at http://evolve. elsevier.com/Iggy/ in the "Prepare for Class" folder.

A patient is admitted to the hospital with a decreased serum osmolality and a serum sodium of 126 mEq/L. The nurse recognizes that dehydration or overhydration may accompany hypotonic conditions.

1. Using Gordon's Functional Health Patterns, what questions would the nurse ask to assess the patient?

2. Which of the following assessments would indicate that the patient has fluid volume excess?
    a. Increased, bounding pulse
    b. Jugular venous distention
    c. Presence of crackles
    d. Elevated blood pressure
    e. Skin pale and cool to touch

3. After determining by an in-depth clinical assessment that the patient is not dehydrated, which intervention is best to correct this hypotonic overhydration?
    a. Administration of 0.9% NS
    b. Restriction of free water
    c. Administration of antihypertensives
    d. Restriction of potassium

4. What does the nurse monitor for as evidence of a worsening hypotonic condition?
    a. Mental status
    b. Urine output
    c. Skin changes
    d. Bowel sounds

CASE STUDY: THE PATIENT WITH DEHYDRATION

Use a separate sheet of paper to answer the questions in this Case Study. Answer guidelines for this Case Study are available on your Evolve website at http://evolve. elsevier.com/Iggy/ in the "Prepare for Class" folder.

The patient with a history of vomiting and diarrhea from the flu presents with a rapid pulse, orthostatic hypotension, urine output of 20 mL/hr, skin turgor poor with tenting, and increased respiratory rate.

1. Which type of dehydration does this patient have? Explain your answer.

2. In evaluating the patient's laboratory values, indicate whether the following values are likely to be normal, elevated, or decreased.
   a. Urine specific gravity
   b. Urine volume
   c. Serum sodium
   d. Serum hematocrit and hemoglobin
   e. Blood urea nitrogen (BUN)
   f. Serum osmolality

3. The compensatory mechanism responsible for the patient's rapid pulse is increased:
   a. circulation of angiotensin.
   b. sympathetic discharge.
   c. aldosterone production.
   d. renal reabsorption of sodium and water.

4. Immediate interventions to correct this patient's fluid volume imbalance include:
   a. rapid hydration with D_5W.
   b. administration of a loop diuretic.
   c. administration of an osmotic diuretic.
   d. rapid hydration with D_5/0.45% NS.

5. What is the most important thing to monitor to determine the patient's response to corrective interventions?
   a. Respiratory rate and depth
   b. Skin turgor
   c. Urinary output
   d. Weight

6. What indicates that the patient is having a negative response to fluid resuscitation?
   a. Increased blood pressure
   b. Urinary output of 40 mL/hr
   c. Presence of crackles
   d. Widening of pulse pressure

CASE STUDY: THE PATIENT WITH A POTASSIUM IMBALANCE

Use a separate sheet of paper to answer the questions in this Case Study. Answer guidelines for this Case Study are available on your Evolve website at http://evolve. elsevier.com/Iggy/ in the "Prepare for Class" folder.

A male adult patient is admitted for palpitations. His serum potassium level on admission is 5.4 mEq/L. Yesterday he ate two eggs, bacon, and toast for breakfast. For lunch he had a fresh fruit salad, and for dinner he ate baked halibut, baked potatoes, a salad, and spinach. He usually has a cola drink and dried fruit for a snack. He uses a salt substitute regularly. He tells the nurse that he has been taking spironolactone 50 mg once daily for hypertension for 2 months, but missed his 1-month follow-up appointment.

1. Identify the foods in his diet that may be contributing to his hyperkalemia.

2. Which ECG changes would be typical for a patient such as this?

3. Formulate relevant nursing diagnoses for this patient based on the above data.

4. This patient states that he has had abdominal cramping and several very loose diarrhea stools since yesterday. The physician orders a sodium polystyrene sulfonate (Kayexalate) retention enema to be given stat. Discuss the etiology of the patient's symptoms.

5. Explain whether the nurse should clarify the physician's order before administering the enema.

6. Will the patient continue to take the spironolactone? Explain.

7. Eventually the patient recovers and is scheduled for discharge. Develop a teaching-learning plan for him including information about his diet.

CASE STUDY: THE PATIENT WITH A SODIUM IMBALANCE

Use a separate sheet of paper to answer the questions in this Case Study. Answer guidelines for this Case Study are available on your Evolve website at http://evolve. elsevier.com/Iggy/ in the "Prepare for Class" folder.

The nurse is caring for a 77-year-old woman who was admitted after gardening on a hot summer day. Her daughter found her lying on the couch, slightly confused, and unable to get up to the bathroom. She is weak, anxious, and slightly confused to time and place. Her pulse is 110 beats/min; blood pressure is 108/58. Her skin is dry and urine specific gravity is 1.028. The nurse notes that the patient's deep tendon reflexes are slightly reduced.

1. Discuss whether this patient's serum sodium would be elevated, decreased, or normal.

2. What are the signs and symptoms that will occur in hypernatremia?

3. What treatment does the nurse expect this patient to receive at this time?

4. This patient will be discharged to home care. Develop a teaching plan for her.

14 CHAPTER

Assessment and Care of Patients with Acid-Base Imbalances

STUDY/REVIEW QUESTIONS

True or False? *Read the statements and write T for true or F for false in the blanks provided. If the statement is false, correct the statement to make it true*

_____ 1. Acid-base balance is mainly a function of cellular metabolism.

_____ 2. The immediate binding of excess hydrogen ions occurs primarily in the renal tubule.

_____ 3. Renal mechanisms are stronger for regulating acid-base balance and respond more rapidly than chemical and respiratory mechanisms.

_____ 4. The serum pH value is directly related to the concentration of hydrogen ion.

_____ 5. A main cause of increased bicarbonate levels is respiratory elimination of acid.

_____ 6. Ammonium is a major extracellular fluid (ECF) buffer.

_____ 7. The component released by the lungs to regulate pH is hydrogen.

_____ 8. The cause of respiratory acidosis is underelimination of carbon dioxide from the lungs.

_____ 9. Interference with alveolar-capillary diffusion results in hydrogen ion elimination and acidemia.

_____ 10. Combined acidosis is less severe than either metabolic acidosis or respiratory acidosis alone.

Fill in the blank.

11. An increase in the CO_2 level causes the free hydrogen ion level to increase and the pH to decrease, or become more _____.

12. The ratio between carbonic acid and bicarbonate should remain at _____.

13. In the healthy person, the kidneys control _____ levels and the lungs control _____ levels.

Matching. *Match the terms with their associated functions and substances. Answers may be used more than once.*

Terms

a. Acid
b. Base
c. Buffer
d. pH

Associated Statements

_____ 14. Accepts hydrogen ion

_____ 15. Donates hydrogen ion

_____ 16. Formed in the body as a result of metabolism

_____ 17. Releases or binds hydrogen ions into/from a fluid

_____ 18. Measure of the body's free hydrogen ion level

_____ 19. H_2CO_3

_____ 20. Increases as the amount of base increases

_____ 21. HCO_3^-

_____ 22. Hemoglobin

23. Use arrows to indicate the direction the carbonic anhydrase equation shifts when excess carbon dioxide is produced.

$$CO_2 + H_2O \qquad H_2CO_3 \qquad H^+ + HCO_3^-$$

24. For the conditions listed below, indicate whether plasma pH will increase (I) or decrease (D).

_____ a. Increase in CO_2

_____ b. Decrease in HCO_3^-

_____ c. Increase in lactic acid

_____ d. Increase in HCO_3^-

_____ e. Decrease in CO_2

Matching. *Match the buffer systems with their descriptive statements. Answers may be used more than once.*

Buffer Systems

a. Chemical
b. Respiratory
c. Renal
d. Protein

Statements

_____ 25. Chemoreceptor response to increase in CO_2

_____ 26. Binding of hydrogen ions to phosphate ions to form H_2PO_4

_____ 27. Reabsorbs HCO_3^-

_____ 28. Binds H^+ with HCO_3^-

_____ 29. Binds H^+ with hemoglobin

_____ 30. Response occurs within minutes

31. Which blood pH value is within normal limits?
    a. 7.27
    b. 7.37
    c. 7.47
    d. 7.5

32. Incomplete breakdown of glucose occurs whenever cells metabolize under anaerobic conditions to form lactic acid. Based on this knowledge of pathophysiology, which patient conditions could cause the patient to develop acidosis? *(Select all that apply.)*
    a. Sepsis
    b. Hypovolemic shock
    c. Use of a mechanical ventilator
    d. Prolonged nasogastric suctioning
    e. Respiratory depression

33. Which patient has the highest risk for acidosis because of excess production of hydrogen ions?
    a. Patient with a kidney stone
    b. Patient with chronic obstructive pulmonary disease
    c. Patient who is having a seizure
    d. Patient with continuous diarrhea

34. The patient's ABG results show an increase in pH. Which condition is most likely to contribute to this laboratory value?
    a. Mechanical ventilation
    b. Ketoacidosis
    c. Nasogastric suction
    d. Diarrhea

35. Which patient is most likely to have a decrease in bicarbonate?
    a. Patient with pancreatitis
    b. Patient with hypoventilation
    c. Patient who is vomiting
    d. Patient with emphysema

36. The patient has a new onset of shallow and slow respirations. While the patient's body attempts to compensate, what happens to the patient's pH level?
    a. Increases
    b. Decreases
    c. Stabilizes
    d. Fluctuates

37. The patient is at risk for acid-base imbalance. Which laboratory value indicates that the patient is acidotic?
    a. $Paco_2$ = 55 mm Hg
    b. CO_3^- = 25 mEq/L
    c. Lactate = 2.5 mmol/L
    d. pH = 7.30

38. Which type of medication increases the older adult patient's risk for acid-base imbalances?
    a. Antilipemics
    b. Hormonal therapy
    c. Diuretics
    d. Antidysrhythmics

Matching. *Match the etiologies of metabolic acidosis to their resulting states of pathophysiology. Answers may be used more than once.*

Etiology of Metabolic Acidosis
a. Hydrogen ion production
b. Hydrogen ion elimination
c. Base elimination
d. Base production

Pathophysiology State
_____ 39. Diabetic ketoacidosis
_____ 40. Renal failure
_____ 41. Dehydration
_____ 42. Seizures
_____ 43. Pancreatic insufficiency
_____ 44. Diarrhea

Matching. Match the pathophysiologic causes of respiratory failure with their associated conditions. Answers may be used more than once.

Associated Conditions

a.   Respiratory depression
b.   Inadequate chest expansion
c.   Airway obstruction
d.   Altered alveolar capillary diffusion

Pathophysiology

_____ 45.   Asthma

_____ 46.   Muscular dystrophy

_____ 47.   Morphine infusion

_____ 48.   Pulmonary embolus

_____ 49.   Bronchiolitis

_____ 50.   Ascites

_____ 51.   Stroke

_____ 52.   Flail chest

_____ 53.   Hemothorax

_____ 54.   Hyperkalemia

_____ 55.   Pneumonia

56.   Which medication usage could cause metabolic acidosis?
a.   Aspirin overdose
b.   Overuse of antacids
c.   Prolonged use of antihistamines
d.   Vitamin overdose

57.   Which nursing assessment finding indicates a worsening of respiratory acidosis?
a.   Decreased respiratory rate
b.   Decreased blood pressure
c.   Use of accessory respiratory muscles
d.   Pale nail beds

58.   Which patient is most likely to have respiratory acidosis?
a.   Patient who is anxious and breathing rapidly
b.   Patient with multiple rib fractures
c.   Patient with IV normal saline bolus
d.   Patient with increased urinary output

59.   Which patient requires assessment related to inadequate chest expansion, which places the patient at risk for respiratory acidosis?
a.   Patient with lordosis
b.   Patient with emphysema
c.   Patient on prolonged bedrest
d.   Patient in the first trimester of pregnancy

60.   The nurse reviews the ECG and cardiovascular status of the patient. Which findings are early changes associated with mild acidosis?
a.   Decreased heart rate with hypertension
b.   Hypotension and faint peripheral pulses
c.   Increased heart rate and increased cardiac output
d.   Peaked T waves and wide QRS complexes

61.   The nurse is assessing the patient with an acid-base imbalance by using Gordon's Functional Health Patterns. What primary areas are affected? *(Select all that apply.)*
a.   Values/Beliefs
b.   Activity-Exercise
c.   Health Perception–Health Management
d.   Elimination
e.   Sleep–Rest
f.   Cognitive–Perceptual
g.   Coping–Stress Tolerance

62. The nurse is testing the muscle strength of the patient at risk for acid-base imbalance. Which technique does the nurse use to test arm strength?
    a. Asks the patient to hold the arms straight out in front and the nurse observes for drift.
    b. The patient flexes the arms against the chest; the nurse tries to pull the arms from the chest.
    c. Asks the patient to pick up an object that weighs at least 10 lbs.
    d. The patient clasps the hands together and pushes as hard as possible.

63. The nurse assesses the acidotic patient's lower extremities for strength as part of the shift assessment. What finding does the nurse expect to see?
    a. There is bilateral weakness.
    b. There is weakness on the dominant side.
    c. There is no change from baseline.
    d. There is cramping, but no weakness.

64. The nurse observes tall peaked T waves on an ECG of the patient with metabolic acidosis. Before notifying the health care provider, the nurse also assesses the results of which laboratory test?
    a. Serum calcium
    b. Serum glucose
    c. Serum potassium
    d. Serum magnesium

Matching. Match the signs and symptoms to either metabolic acidosis or respiratory acidosis. Answers may be used more than once.

Acid-Base Condition
a. Metabolic acidosis
b. Respiratory acidosis

Signs and Symptoms

_____ 65. Kussmaul respirations

_____ 66. Shallow, rapid respirations

_____ 67. Warm, flushed skin

_____ 68. Skin pale to cyanotic

_____ 69. Elevated $Paco_2$

_____ 70. Decreased bicarbonate

71. What interventions are included in the plan of care for the patient with metabolic ketoacidosis? *(Select all that apply.)*
    a. Monitor ABG levels for decreasing pH level, as appropriate.
    b. Maintain patent IV access.
    c. Administer fluids as prescribed.
    d. Monitor for irritability and muscle tetany.
    e. Monitor determinants of tissue oxygen delivery, such as hemoglobin.
    f. Monitor loss of bicarbonate through the GI tract such as diarrhea.

72. What is the priority intervention for the patient with diabetic ketoacidosis?
    a. Administer bicarbonate.
    b. Give furosemide.
    c. Administer insulin.
    d. Administer potassium.

73. Which statement made by the patient indicates that he or she may have an alkaline condition?
    a. "I am more and more tired and can't concentrate."
    b. "I have tingling in my fingers and toes."
    c. "My feet and ankles are swollen."
    d. "I am short of breath all of the time."

74. Which patient is most likely to have respiratory alkalosis?
    a. Hypoxic patient
    b. Patient with a body cast
    c. Patient with a panic attack
    d. Morbidly obese patient

75. Which type of electrolyte imbalance does the nurse expect to see in the patient with metabolic alkalosis?
    a. Hyperkalemia
    b. Hypophosphatemia
    c. Hyperchloremia
    d. Hypocalcemia

76. Which patient is most likely to develop metabolic alkalosis as a result of base excess?
    a. Patient taking thiazide diuretics
    b. Patient who is having nasogastric suction
    c. Patient with severe vomiting
    d. Patient who had a massive blood transfusion

77. The nurse is assessing the patient with metabolic alkalosis. Which neuromuscular finding is the most ominous and warrants immediate notification of the health care provider?
    a. Muscle cramps
    b. Muscle twitching
    c. Hyperactive deep tendon reflexes
    d. Tetany

78. The nurse is caring for the patient with metabolic alkalosis secondary to diuretic medication. Which equipment does the nurse obtain to administer the correct therapy to this patient?
    a. Oxygen tubing and cannula or mask
    b. IV catheter and IV start kit
    c. Foley catheter and drainage bag
    d. Antiemetic drug and emesis basin

Matching. *Match each characteristic with its associated acid-base imbalance. Answers may be used more than once, and more than one answer may apply.*

Acid-Base Imbalance
a. Respiratory acidosis
b. Metabolic acidosis
c. Respiratory alkalosis
d. Metabolic alkalosis

Characteristics

_____ 79. May occur as a result of anxiety

_____ 80. Results from bicarbonate loss

_____ 81. Caused by hypoventilation

_____ 82. May be a result of blood transfusions

_____ 83. May be caused by diarrhea

_____ 84. Associated with Kussmaul respiration

_____ 85. Associated with ingestion of antacids

_____ 86. Results in hypocalcemia

_____ 87. Compensation occurs through renal reabsorption of bicarbonate

_____ 88. Compensation occurs through hyperventilation

_____ 89. Compensation occurs through hypoventilation

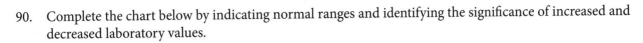

90. Complete the chart below by indicating normal ranges and identifying the significance of increased and decreased laboratory values.

Acid-Base Assessment

Test	Normal Range for Adults		Significance of Abnormal Findings
	Arterial	**Venous**	

pH
  Adult <90 yr
 	
  >90 yr
			Increased:
			
			Decreased:

Pao$_2$
  Adult <90 yr
 	
  >90 yr
	mm Hg
	
	mm Hg
			Increased:
			
			Decreased:

Paco$_2$	mm Hg	mm Hg	Increased: Decreased:
Bicarbonate	mEq/L	mEq/L	Increased: Decreased:
Lactate	mg/dL mmol/L	mg/dL mmol/L	Increased: Decreased:

Matching. *Match the arterial blood gas value to the corresponding acid-base imbalance. Answers may be used more than once.*

Acid-Base Imbalance
a. Metabolic acidosis
b. Respiratory acidosis
c. Metabolic alkalosis
d. Respiratory alkalosis
e. Normal values

ABG Values

_____ 91. pH 7.30, Paco$_2$ 66, bicarbonate 38, Pao$_2$ 70

_____ 92. pH 7.52, Paco$_2$ 45, bicarbonate 36, Pao$_2$ 95

_____ 93. pH 7.55, Paco$_2$ 24, bicarbonate 20, Pao$_2$ 95

_____ 94. pH 7.28, Paco$_2$ 24, bicarbonate 15, Pao$_2$ 95

_____ 95. pH 7.35, Paco$_2$ 24, bicarbonate 15, Pao$_2$ 95

_____ 96. pH 7.45, Paco$_2$ 50, bicarbonate 42, Pao$_2$ 80

_____ 97. pH 7.45, Paco$_2$ 41, bicarbonate 25, Pao$_2$ 97

98. The patient has a low pH level. Which other concurrent change does the nurse expect to see in this patient?
    a. Elevated serum sodium level
    b. Elevated serum potassium
    c. Decreased serum chloride level
    d. Decreased serum calcium level

99. What is the safest way to administer oxygen to the patient with chronic respiratory acidosis?
    a. High-volume intermittent positive pressure
    b. Low-flow oxygen (2 L/min) via nasal cannula
    c. High-flow 40% oxygen via face mask
    d. Positive end-expiratory pressure (PEEP)

100. Which assessment finding indicates that the patient with chronic respiratory acidosis is responding favorably to treatment?
    a. Nail beds pale, extremities cool
    b. Respiratory stridor with inspiration
    c. Expectorating clear, thin mucus
    d. Diffuse crackles auscultated bilaterally

101. In order to ensure the safety of the patient with metabolic alkalosis, which task is best to delegate to the unlicensed assistive personnel (UAP)?
    a. Watch the patient when he or she eats or drinks anything.
    b. Sit with the patient to prevent wandering.
    c. Keep the siderails in the "up" position.
    d. Remove all sharp objects from the bedside table.

102. Determine whether the arterial blood values indicate an acid or alkaline condition.
    a. $Paco_2$ = 66 mm Hg _____
    b. Bicarbonate = 16 mEq/L _____
    c. pH = 7.55 _____
    d. pH = 7.32 _____

CASE STUDY: THE PATIENT WITH RESPIRATORY ACIDOSIS

Use a separate sheet of paper to answer the questions in this Case Study. Answer guidelines for this Case Study are available on your Evolve website at http://evolve. elsevier.com/Iggy/ in the "Prepare for Class" folder.

The patient is a 75-year-old man with a history of emphysema. He comes to the emergency department (ED) reporting a productive cough that causes chest pain and fatigue. "I am having more problems breathing than usual."

1. What should the nurse include in the initial history when a patient is suspected of having an acid-base imbalance?

2. Which assessment indicates that this patient has impaired gas exchange?
   a. Decreased urine output
   b. Bradycardia
   c. Decreased chest expansion
   d. Hypotension

3. Which ABG value indicates that this patient is retaining carbon dioxide?
   a. $Paco_2$ = 40 mm Hg
   b. $Paco_2$ = 60 mm Hg
   c. Bicarbonate = 42
   d. Pao_2 = 60 mm Hg

4. The patient's baseline ABG values are: pH 7.36; $Paco_2$ 60 mm Hg, Pao_2 52 mm Hg, bicarbonate 42 mEq/L. Which ABG result would most likely indicate that he is having a negative response to the administration of oxygen?
   a. pH 7.35; $Paco_2$ 64, Pao_2 60, bicarbonate 42 mEq/L
   b. pH 7.36, $Paco_2$ 60, Pao_2 60, bicarbonate 42 mEq/L
   c. pH 7.36, $Paco_2$ 60, Pao_2 58, bicarbonate 38 mEq/L
   d. pH 7.33, $Paco_2$ 66, Pao_2 66, bicarbonate 42 mEq/L

5. Based on the answer for question 4, is the patient's respiratory acidosis compensated or uncompensated? Explain your answer.

6. The patient is admitted with a diagnosis of pneumonia. What immediate interventions are needed for this patient?

7. Later in the shift, the nurse notes that his oxygen is set at 5 L/minute. The patient says that he asked the UAP to turn up his oxygen because he was having trouble breathing. What actions, if any, should the nurse take at this time?

CASE STUDY: THE PATIENT WITH METABOLIC ACID-BASE IMBALANCE

Use a separate sheet of paper to answer the questions in this Case Study. Answer guidelines for this Case Study are available on your Evolve website at http://evolve. elsevier.com/Iggy/ in the "Prepare for Class" folder.

A 65-year-old woman with a recent history of cellulitis is admitted to the hospital with fever, shortness of breath, and hypotension. She has had a 2-day history of diarrhea. Her ABG reveals a pH of 7.30, $Paco_2$ of 28, Pao_2 of 88, and bicarbonate of 17 mEq/L.

1. What additional information could the nurse collect using Gordon's Functional Health Patterns?

2. This patient's symptoms are most likely a result of which condition?
   a. Metabolic acidosis
   b. Metabolic alkalosis

3. The bicarbonate level of 17 mEq/L is the result of which factor?
   a. Respiratory hypoventilation
   b. Overelimination of bicarbonate
   c. Respiratory compensation
   d. Underelimination of hydrogen ions

4. Which finding indicates a worsening acidotic condition?
   a. Increased blood pressure
   b. Anxiety
   c. Decreasing pH
   d. Increased urinary output

5. What does this patient critically need to reverse the condition?
   a. Fluids
   b. Oxygen
   c. Calcium
   d. Potassium

6. Explain whether or not bicarbonate would be given to this patient to correct her condition.

7. What other laboratory values would be important to monitor at this time? Explain your answer.

15 CHAPTER

Infusion Therapy

STUDY/REVIEW QUESTIONS

1. The nurse is caring for several patients in need of IV therapy. Which task is best to assign to the licensed practical nurse (LPN) or licensed vocational nurse (LVN)?
    a. Draw blood from a central line.
    b. Insert a peripheral IV with saline lock.
    c. Hang a hyperosmolar solution.
    d. Change a central line dressing.

2. The nurse is preparing to start an infusion of 10% de1xtrose. Why does the nurse infuse the solution through a central line?
    a. Osmolarity of the solution could cause phlebitis or thrombosis.
    b. The patient could be at risk for fluid overload.
    c. Viscosity of the solution would slow the infusion.
    d. The solution should not be mixed with other drugs or solutions.

3. The nurse is preparing to give the patient IV drug therapy. What information does the nurse need before administering the drug? *(Select all that apply.)*
    a. Indications, contraindications, and precautions for IV therapy
    b. Appropriate dilution, pH, and osmolarity of solution
    c. Rate of infusion and dosage of drugs
    d. Generic, chemical, and brand name of the drug
    e. Compatibility with other IV medications
    f. Percentage of adverse events for the drug
    g. Specifics of monitoring because of immediate effect

4. The charge nurse is reviewing IV therapy orders. What information is included in each order? *(Select all that apply.)*
    a. Specific type of solution
    b. Rate of administration
    c. Specific drug dose to be added to the solution
    d. Method for diluting drugs for the solution
    e. Specific type of administration equipment

5. The nurse must insert a short peripheral IV catheter. In order to decrease the risk of deep vein thrombosis or phlebitis, which vein does the nurse choose for the infusion site?
    a. Hand
    b. Foot
    c. Forearm
    d. Antecubital

6. The patient requires IV therapy via a peripheral line. What considerations does the nurse use when inserting the peripheral IV? *(Select all that apply.)*
    a. Use either an upper or lower extremity for the insertion site.
    b. Start with more distal sites, such as the hand veins.
    c. Start with more proximal sites, such as the forearm.
    d. Choose the patient's nondominant arm.
    e. Do not use the arm if the patient had a mastectomy on that side.
    f. If the vein is hard and cordlike, use an indirect approach.
    g. Avoid placing an IV over the palm side of the wrist.

7. The nurse is assessing the patient's IV site and identifies signs and symptoms of infiltration. What does the nurse do next?
   a. Discontinue the IV.
   b. Apply a sterile dressing.
   c. Elevate the extremity.
   d. Apply cold compresses.

8. The nurse is selecting a site for peripheral IV insertion. Which patient condition influences the choice of left versus right upper extremity?
   a. Pneumothorax with a chest tube on the right side
   b. Myocardial infarction with pain radiating down the left arm
   c. Right hip fracture with immobilization and traction in place
   d. Regular renal dialysis with a shunt in the left upper forearm

9. The nurse is attempting to insert a peripheral IV when the patient reports tingling and a feeling like "pins and needles." What does the nurse do next?
   a. Change to a short-winged butterfly needle.
   b. Stop immediately, remove the catheter, and chose a new site.
   c. Ask the patient to wiggle the fingers to stimulate circulation.
   d. Pause the procedure and gently massage the fingers.

10. The patient has been on prolonged steroid therapy. In assessing the patient for IV insertion, what finding does the nurse expect to see?
    a. Skin and vein fragility that makes repeated venipuncture difficult
    b. Skin that is thick, tough, dry, and difficult to puncture
    c. Edema or puffiness making visualization of veins difficult
    d. Rash with excoriation from scratching which limits site selection

11. Under what circumstances does the nurse elect to use only one secondary set rather than a secondary set for each medication?
    a. When multiple intermittent medications are required
    b. To eliminate the cost of using multiple secondary sets
    c. When the nurse is using the backpriming method
    d. When the medications are compatible

12. When using an intermittent administration set to deliver medications, how often does the Infusion Nurse's Society recommend that the set be changed?
    a. Every 24 hours
    b. Every shift
    c. Every morning
    d. After every dose

13. The nurse is supervising a student nurse who is preparing an IV bag with IV administration tubing. Which action by the student nurse causes the nurse to intervene?
    a. The student touches the drip chamber.
    b. The sterile cap from the distal end of the set is removed.
    c. The distal end is attached to a needleless connector.
    d. The student touches the tubing spike.

14. Complete the chart below by describing the criteria for grades of phlebitis.

Phlebitis Scale from INS Standards of Practice

Grade	Criteria
0	
1	
2	
3	
4	

15. The nurse is caring for the patient with a Groshong catheter. According to the manufacturer's recommendations, which technique does the nurse use in maintaining this type of catheter?
    a. Flush the catheter with heparin.
    b. Flush the catheter with saline.
    c. Avoid flushing the catheter.
    d. Aspirate the catheter to remove clots.

16. The patient has a peripherally inserted central catheter (PICC) line placed by an advanced practice nurse at the bedside. Before using the catheter, how is its placement verified?
    a. The physician who ordered the procedure verifies placement.
    b. The line is aspirated gently and the nurse watches for blood return.
    c. A chest x-ray is taken which shows the catheter tip in the lower superior vena cava.
    d. The line is slowly flushed with 10 mL of saline while the nurse notes the ease of flow.

17. The patient requires a nontunneled percutaneous central catheter. What is the nurse's role in this procedure?
    a. Insert the catheter using sterile technique.
    b. Place the patient in Trendelenberg position.
    c. Read the chest x-ray to validate placement.
    d. Select and prepare the insertion site.

18. The patient requires an infusion of packed red blood cells (PRBCs). Which factor allows the nurse to infuse the PRBCs through the patient's PICC line?
    a. Length of the PICC allows infusion within 6 hours.
    b. The nurse is unable to obtain an infusion pump.
    c. Lumen size of the PICC is 4F or larger.
    d. PRBCs can be warmed before infusion.

19. Which patient is the most likely candidate for a tunneled central venous catheter?
    a. Patient with trauma from a motor vehicle accident
    b. Patient in need of IV antibiotics for several weeks
    c. Patient in need of permanent parental nutrition
    d. Patient in need of intermittent chemotherapy

20. Which central venous access device requires piercing of the skin each time the device is accessed?
    a. Broviac catheter
    b. Groshong catheter
    c. Hickman catheter
    d. Implanted port

21. Which nursing interventions are implemented when caring for the patient with an implanted port? *(Select all that apply.)*
    a. A noncoring needle is used to access the port before an infusion.
    b. The port must be flushed daily with saline when not in use.
    c. The external catheter requires dressing changes every other day.
    d. A topical anesthetic cream may be used before accessing the port.
    e. Careful palpation is required before accessing the septum.

22. A 65-year-old patient has been receiving IV fluids at 100 mL/hr of $D_51/2\%$ NS for the past 3 days, along with IV antibiotic therapy. After receiving the new antibiotic, the patient reports general itching and difficulty catching his breath. The nurse notes audible wheezing and rhonchi over the lung fields bilaterally and a rash over his back and chest. What complication do these assessment findings indicate?
    a. Infection in the blood
    b. Allergic reaction
    c. Speed shock
    d. Circulatory overload

23. The patient has a central line inserted in the vena cava. The nurse assesses the patient for which potential complication related to the procedure?
    a. Pneumothorax
    b. Air embolism
    c. Circulatory overload
    d. Cardiac dysrhythmias

24. The nurse is helping the physician insert a central line when the patient develops chest pain and shortness of breath with decreased breath sounds and restlessness. What does the nurse do next?
    a. Tell the patient "Relax, the procedure will soon be over."
    b. Administer pain medication to minimize the pain of insertion.
    c. Administer oxygen and plan to assist with insertion of a chest tube.
    d. Monitor ongoing pulse oximetry and respiratory changes.

25. A triple lumen catheter central line is inserted in the patient. What does the nurse do immediately after the procedure?
    a. Start IV fluids but at a slower rate to prevent any fluid overload.
    b. Watch and wait for any complications before using the site.
    c. Get a portable chest x-ray immediately and hold IV fluids until results are obtained.
    d. Assess vital signs and assess the patient; if patient is stable, start IV fluids.

26. After a tubing change to the patient's central line, the line is later found to be disconnected from the catheter. The patient develops chest pain and restlessness, heart rate of 120 beats/min, blood pressure drops to 90/40, and pulse oximetry is 89%. What does the nurse do next?
    a. Place the patient in Trendelenburg position on the left side, clamp the catheter, and notify the physician.
    b. Assess for patency of the catheter, change the tubing, and resume IV fluids.
    c. Notify the physician, remove the central line, apply pressure, and place the patient in a semi-Fowler's position.
    d. Notify the physician and administer urokinase to declot the catheter.

27. Which nursing intervention is key in preventing an infection in the patient with a central line?
    a. Administer antibiotics for at least a week in a timely manner.
    b. Use aseptic technique when administering medications and changing tubing.
    c. Change the catheter every 72 hours and tubing every 24 hours.
    d. Monitor the patient's temperature for any elevation and give acetaminophen as needed.

28. The patient with an implanted port is discharged to home and will receive long-term therapy on an outpatient basis. How frequently must the port be flushed between courses of therapy?
    a. Daily
    b. Weekly
    c. Monthly
    d. When therapy resumes

29. The nurse is preparing to deliver IV infusion therapy through an implanted port. What technique does the nurse use to access the port?
    a. Palpate the port to locate the septum, scrub, and access with a Huber needle.
    b. Scrub the port with alcohol and access with a needleless device.
    c. Scrub the port with Betadine and flush using a 10 mL syringe.
    d. Palpate the port, scrub, and access with a winged butterfly needle.

30. The patient is discharged to home with an implanted port. Which discharge instruction does the nurse give the patient?
    a. Clean the port every day with an alcohol pad.
    b. An external dressing is not required.
    c. Flush the port daily using a heparin flush syringe.
    d. Apply a topical anesthetic cream daily.

31. The nurse is preparing to give IV infusion therapy to the patient. When is the choice of using a glass container appropriate?
    a. When the patient needs a rapid infusion of fluids
    b. When the patient needs emergency transportation
    c. When the nurse must accurately read the container
    d. When the drug is incompatible with a plastic container

32. The patient requires a 2-month course of antibiotics to treat a resistant infection. Which device is chosen for this therapy?
    a. Short peripheral catheter
    b. Midline catheter
    c. Nontunneled percutaneous central catheter
    d. PICC

33. The nurse is attaching an administration set to a central venous catheter. Which type of equipment decreases the risk of accidental disconnection or leakage?
    a. Slip lock connector
    b. Luer-Lok connector
    c. Extension set
    d. Needleless connector

34. The nurse is adding a filter to an IV administration setup. Where is the best place to add the filter to the IV line?
    a. As close to the solution container as possible
    b. Immediately below the infusion pump
    c. At any convenient connection point
    d. As close as possible to the catheter hub

35. Which safety measures does the nurse apply to decrease the risk of catheter-related bloodstream infection (CR-BSI) related to needleless systems? *(Select all that apply.)*
    a. Clean needleless system connections vigorously every 24 hours.
    b. Do not tape connections between tubing sets.
    c. Use evidence-based hand hygiene guidelines from the Centers for Disease Control and Prevention (CDC) and the Occupational Safety and Health Administration (OSHA).
    d. Attend educational offerings to prevent or minimize CR-BSI.
    e. Use needleless systems only when necessary.
    f. Discard needleless equipment in a biohazard container.

36. The patient is receiving IV therapy via an infusion pump. What is a nursing responsibility related to the therapy and equipment?
    a. Count the number of drops per minute.
    b. Monitor the patient's infusion site and rate.
    c. Check the equipment at the end of the infusion.
    d. Position the container for gravity flow.

37. The patient's IV site is very edematous, the pump continues to infuse fluids, and the patient reports burning at the site. The nurse notices a clear fluid leaking from the insertion site. The nurse interprets these findings as an indication of which condition?
    a. Hematoma
    b. Phlebitis
    c. Infiltration
    d. Infection

38. Identify whether each characteristic relates to a pump (P) or a controller infusion device (CID).

    _____ a. Delivers fluids under pressure

    _____ b. Relies on gravity to create fluid flow

    _____ c. Is pole-mounted or ambulatory and portable

    _____ d. Is best for accurate infusion

    _____ e. Counts drops to regulate flow

39. The nurse is assessing the patient's IV insertion site. What features does the nurse look for in the assessment? (Select all that apply.)
    a. Observe for redness and swelling.
    b. Check that the dressing is clean and dry.
    c. Ensure that the dressing is adherent to the skin.
    d. Observe for yellow discoloration.
    e. Observe for hardness or drainage.

40. The patient's central venous IV site is covered with a transparent membrane dressing. How often does the nurse change this dressing?
    a. Every 24 hours
    b. Every 48 hours
    c. At least every 7 days
    d. The dressing does not need changing

41. The nurse is changing the dressing on the patient's peripheral IV site. In which direction does the nurse remove the dressing?
    a. From proximal to distal
    b. Toward the nurse
    c. Laterally from side to side
    d. Away from the insertion site

42. The nurse has removed the dressing from the patient's central venous catheter site. In order to monitor the catheter position, what does the nurse do?
    a. Gently push the catheter into the insertion site.
    b. Slightly retract the catheter and observe the position.
    c. Mark the catheter with a pen to monitor the length.
    d. Note the length of the catheter which is external to the insertion site.

43. The nurse is caring for the patient with a central venous catheter. What measures does the nurse use to prevent air emboli when changing the administration set or connectors? (Select all that apply.)
    a. The patient lies flat so the catheter site is below the heart.
    b. Use the pinch clamp that can be closed during the procedure.
    c. Use sterile technique when handling the equipment.
    d. Have an assistant apply pressure at the insertion site.
    e. Ask the patient to perform the Valsalva maneuver by holding the breath and bearing down.

44. After assessing the patency of the patient's IV catheter, the nurse attempts to flush the catheter and meets resistance. What does the nurse do next?
    a. Get a larger-sized syringe and repeat the flush attempt.
    b. Use a heparinized solution and repeat the flush attempt.
    c. Gently force-flush the catheter using the push-pause method.
    d. Stop the flush attempt and discontinue the IV.

45. The nurse is preparing to draw blood from the patient who has a central line. The patient's spouse asks, "Why can't you just take the blood out of that big IV line?" What information does the nurse use to explain why the central line is not used for blood draws? *(Select all that apply.)*
    a. Additional hub manipulation is a major cause of CR-BSI.
    b. Heparin used in flushing can interfere with coagulation studies.
    c. Electrolytes in the IV fluid may alter the results of serum electrolytes.
    d. Infusion of antibiotics can interfere with peak serum levels of the drug.
    e. The blood vacutainer may cause the catheter to temporarily collapse.

46. The nurse is flushing the patient's short peripheral IV catheter. What does the nurse typically use for this procedure?
    a. 3 mL of normal saline
    b. 5 mL of heparin
    c. 10 mL of normal saline
    d. 30 mL of bacteriostatic saline

47. Place the steps of removing a peripheral catheter in the proper order using the numbers 1 through 7.

    _____ a. Hold pressure on the site until hemostasis is achieved.

    _____ b. Immediately cover the puncture site with dry gauze.

    _____ c. Assess the catheter tip to make sure it is intact and completely removed.

    _____ d. Slowly withdraw the catheter from the skin.

    _____ e. Lift opposite sides of the transparent dressing.

    _____ f. Document catheter removal and the appearance of the IV site.

    _____ g. Pull laterally to remove the dressing from the site while stabilizing the catheter.

48. The nurse is attempting to remove a PICC line and feels resistance. What technique does the nurse use first to attempt to resolve this problem?
    a. Gently pull on the catheter while the patient holds his or her breath.
    b. Place a cold pack on the extremity and give the patient a cold drink.
    c. Use simple distraction techniques and deep breathing.
    d. Place the patient in Trendelenberg position.

49. The nurse is assessing the short peripheral catheter after removal and it appears that the catheter tip is missing. What does the nurse do next?
    a. Notify the health care provider.
    b. Assess the patient for symptoms of emboli.
    c. Apply firm pressure to the insertion site.
    d. Assess the extremity for coldness, cyanosis, or numbness.

50. The nurse is assessing the veins of the older adult patient before inserting a peripheral IV. Which technique does the nurse use to distend the veins?
    a. Tie the tourniquet very loosely and far from the vein.
    b. Elevate the extremity above the heart on a small pillow.
    c. Ask the patient to flex and extend the arm at the elbow.
    d. Inflate a blood pressure cuff to slightly below diastolic pressure.

51. The nurse is caring for the patient receiving arterial therapy via the carotid artery. What important nursing action is specific to this therapy?
    a. Assess the extremities for sensation and pulses.
    b. Monitor respirations for rate and regularity.
    c. Perform frequent neurologic assessments.
    d. Place antiembolic stockings on the patient's lower extremities.

52. Which patient is a candidate for intraperitoneal therapy?
    a. Patient receiving total parental nutrition
    b. Patient receiving blood and blood products
    c. Chemotherapy patient
    d. Patient receiving medications for diagnostic tests

53. During intraperitoneal therapy, the patient reports nausea and vomiting. What does the nurse do next?
    a. Help the patient move from side to side.
    b. Flush the catheter with normal saline.
    c. Reduce the flow rate and give antiemetics.
    d. Obtain an order for an abdominal x-ray.

54. In what position does the nurse place the patient before starting intraperitoneal therapy?
    a. Semi-Fowler's
    b. Prone
    c. Supine
    d. Side-lying

55. Which patient is a candidate for hypodermoclysis?
    a. Patient requiring long-term antibiotic therapy
    b. Patient with a bleeding disorder
    c. Patient requiring rapid large-volume infusion
    d. Patient requiring palliative care

56. The nurse is preparing to start a hypodermoclysis treatment on the patient. What is the preferred insertion site?
    a. Anterior forearm
    b. Anterior tibial area
    c. Lateral aspect of the upper arm
    d. Area under the clavicle

57. The home health nurse is adjusting the rate for a hypodermoclysis treatment. What is the usual maximum rate for this therapy?
    a. 2 mL/hr
    b. 30 mL/hr
    c. 80 mL/hr
    d. 125 mL/hr

58. The home health nurse is caring for the patient receiving hypodermoclysis therapy. How often are the subcutaneous sites rotated?
    a. Every 4 hours
    b. Every 24 hours
    c. At least every 3 days
    d. At least once a week

59. The nurse is caring for the patient receiving intrathecal pain medication. Which agent is preferred for cleaning the access site?
    a. Alcohol
    b. Soap and water
    c. Povidone iodine
    d. Chlorhexidine gluconate

60. The patient is receiving epidural medication therapy. The nurse assesses for which potential problem specific to this type of therapy?
    a. Meningitis
    b. Loss of bowel function
    c. Respiratory distress
    d. Cardiac dysrhythmias

61. The patient is brought to the emergency department (ED) after a serious motor vehicle accident. Which factor makes the patient a candidate for intraosseous (IO) therapy?
    a. Patient has a history of chronic renal failure.
    b. Endotracheal intubation is difficult to accomplish.
    c. Patient is an older adult and very thin.
    d. IV access cannot be achieved within a few minutes.

62. The patient has an IO needle in place. Why does the nurse advocate for removal of the device within 24 hours after insertion?
    a. There is an increased risk for osteomyelitis.
    b. There is an increased risk for arterial insufficiency.
    c. The device hinders patient mobility.
    d. The device is unstable and easily dislodged.

63. **Crossword Puzzle.** Complete the crossword puzzle below by answering the questions about complications of IV therapy.

Across

1. During a central line dressing change, the nurse notes redness and swelling at the catheter insertion site, and a small amount of purulent drainage. The nurse suspects _____ at the insertion site.

3. During rounds, the nurse notes that the patient's IV site is swollen, cool, and that the IV has stopped infusing. The patient reports tenderness at the IV site. The nurse suspects _____.

4. The patient is receiving an infusion of chemotherapy, and the nurse monitors the IV infusion and site closely because the medication may cause tissue damage if it escapes into the subcutaneous tissue. The medication is known as a(n) _____.

8. After multiple IV start attempts, the nurse finally starts a peripheral IV infusion. However, that evening, the area is swollen, tender, red at the site, and the vein looks engorged. The infusion has stopped. The nurse suspects a(n) _____ at the IV site.

Down

2. Medication infuses into the subcutaneous tissue and may result in tissue sloughing. This is known as _____.

5. Two days after a peripheral IV infusion has been discontinued, the patient calls the clinic because he noticed a red, cordlike vein on his forearm above the old IV site. The nurse suspects _____.

6. The patient receiving heparin has accidentally dislodged his IV catheter. A new IV has been started, but the old site is slightly swollen, bruised, and very tender. The skin condition would be documented as _____.

7. After a dose of IV penicillin, the patient reports itching and has a rash across his back. Slight wheezes are audible. This is a(n) _____ reaction.

9. After hanging an IVPB antibiotic, the nurse steps out when called by another patient. The nurse returns after a few minutes to find that the IV antibiotic has completely infused. The patient reports dizziness, chest tightness, and has an irregular pulse and a flushed face. The nurse suspects _____.

CASE STUDY: THE PATIENT RECEIVING INTRAVENOUS THERAPY

Use a separate sheet of paper to answer the questions in this Case Study. Answer guidelines for this Case Study are available on your Evolve website at http://evolve. elsevier.com/Iggy/ in the "Prepare for Class" folder.

The patient is an older adult resident at a skilled nursing facility. She needs to receive IV antibiotics and fluids for pneumonia via a peripheral catheter. She is alert and cooperative and understands the need for therapy.

1. What considerations does the nurse have in establishing a peripheral IV site in an older patient?

2. What should be included in the documentation for initiating IV therapy for this patient?

3. The patient reports that her arm hurts where she is receiving the IV, especially when the antibiotic is given. What is the nurse's best action at this time?

4. What possible complications may explain her discomfort?

5. After examining the site, the nurse decides to discontinue the IV. It is restarted in her other arm, and the infusion set at 50 mL/hr as ordered. When the nurse rechecks her in an hour, the entire 1000 mL bag of normal saline has infused. The patient reports shortness of breath and she has puffiness around her eyes and engorged neck veins. Assessment of breath sounds reveals crackles over both lower lobes, and her blood pressure is 154/96. Another nurse says that the patient is experiencing speed shock because the saline went in too fast. Is the nurse correct? Explain your answer.

6. What should the nurse do at this time?

16 CHAPTER

Care of Preoperative Patients

STUDY/REVIEW QUESTIONS

1. Which statement best describes the preoperative period?
   a. It begins when the patient makes the appointment with the surgeon to discuss the need for surgery.
   b. It is the time during which the patient receives education and testing related to the impending surgery.
   c. It is a time during which the patient's need for surgery and willingness to have it is established.
   d. It begins when the patient is scheduled for surgery and ends at the time of transfer to the surgical suite.

Matching. Match each category of surgery with its description.

Categories of Surgery
a. Palliative
b. Diagnostic
c. Restorative
d. Cosmetic
e. Curative

Definitions

_____ 2. Alters or enhances personal appearance

_____ 3. Improves the patient's functional ability

_____ 4. Resolves a health problem by repairing or removing the cause

_____ 5. Determines the origin or cause of a disorder

_____ 6. Relieves symptoms of a disease process, but does not cure

7. The patient is scheduled for resection of nerve roots. What type of surgery is this?
   a. Palliative
   b. Restorative
   c. Diagnostic
   d. Ablative

8. Specify whether the urgency of the surgery is elective (EL), urgent (U), or emergent (EM).

   _____ a. A 22-year-old nursing student is scheduled for an appendectomy.

   _____ b. A 77-year-old woman is scheduled for a total knee replacement.

   _____ c. A 55-year-old man is scheduled for a colon resection due to a small bowel obstruction.

9. The nurse screens the preoperative patient for conditions that may increase the risk for complications during the perioperative period. Which condition is a possible risk factor?
   a. The patient is 70 years old and obese.
   b. The procedure planned is a bunionectomy.
   c. The patient is 5 feet tall and weighs 100 pounds.
   d. The surgery is planned as an ambulatory/same-day surgical procedure.

True or False? Read each statement and write T for true or F for false in the blanks provided. If the statement is false, correct the statement to make it true.

_____ 10. The nurse functions as the patient advocate by reporting to the surgeon and anesthesiology personnel any abnormalities found on the physical assessment.

_____ 11. Throughout the physical assessment, the nurse focuses on the problem areas identified from the patient's history that are limited to body systems affected directly by the surgical procedure.

_____ 12. In the preoperative setting, the nurse is functioning as a patient advocate when the patient's home environment, self-care capabilities, and support systems are assessed and used in the discharge planning process.

_____ 13. As a patient advocate, the nurse can provide the patient with educational materials appropriate to the patient's ability to learn.

_____ 14. When the nurse evaluates preoperative laboratory test values, only abnormal values related to the surgery need to be reported to the surgeon and anesthesiology personnel.

_____ 15. Patients who have had minor outpatient surgery do not usually require discharge planning.

16. The nurse is preparing the patient for surgery. Which common laboratory tests does the nurse anticipate to be ordered? *(Select all that apply.)*
   a. Total cholesterol
   b. Electrolyte levels
   c. Uric acid
   d. Clotting studies
   e. Serum creatinine

17. Which statement is true regarding the patient who has given consent for a surgical procedure?
   a. Information necessary to understand the nature of and reason for the surgery has been provided.
   b. The length of stay in the hospital has been preapproved by the managed care provider.
   c. Information about the surgeon's experience has been provided.
   d. The nurse has provided detailed information about the surgical procedure.

18. Which statement best describes the collaborative roles of the nurse and surgeon when obtaining the informed consent?
    a. The nurse is responsible for having the informed consent form on the chart for the physician to witness.
    b. The nurse may serve as a witness that the patient has been informed by the physician before surgery is performed.
    c. The nurse may serve as witness to the patient's signature after the physician has the consent form signed before preoperative sedation is given and before surgery is performed.
    d. The nurse has no duties regarding the consent form if the patient has signed the informed consent form for the physician, even if the patient then asks additional questions about the surgery.

19. The nurse has received the patient in the holding area who is scheduled for a left breast biopsy. What is the priority safety measure for this patient before surgery?
    a. Ensure the patient knows who will be performing the surgery.
    b. Ask the patient to mark the site with a marker.
    c. Instruct the patient to perform leg exercises to prevent a deep vein thrombosis.
    d. Determine who the support persons are for the patient.

20. The diabetic patient is scheduled for surgery in the morning. Which procedure does the nurse expect on the morning of surgery?
    a. Usual dose of insulin will be given to maintain the patient's blood glucose level.
    b. Increased dose of insulin will be given to offset the physical stress caused by the procedure.
    c. Modified dose of insulin will be given, based on the patient's blood glucose.
    d. No insulin will be given because the patient is NPO.

21. Complete the chart below about the aspects of preoperative teaching about postoperative procedures and exercises.

Procedure/Exercise	Purpose
Breathing exercises and incentive spirometry	
	Performed along with deep breathing. Help to expel secretions, keep the lungs clear, promote full aeration of the lungs, and prevent pneumonia and atelectasis
Antiembolism stockings and elastic wraps	
	Devices that provide intermittent periods of compression to the lower leg, thus preventing venous stasis and enhancing venous flow
Early ambulation	
	Passive or active, these help prevent joint rigidity and muscle contracture

CASE STUDY: THE PREOPERATIVE PATIENT

Use a separate sheet of paper to answer the questions in this Case Study. Answer guidelines for this Case Study are available on your Evolve website at http://evolve. elsevier.com/Iggy/ in the "Prepare for Class" folder.

The patient is a 42-year-old woman who is scheduled for a total hysterectomy under general anesthesia this morning. She is admitted to the preoperative area in the same-day surgery admitting area. During the admission assessment, the patient mentions to the nurse that her last menses was 2 months ago and that the bleeding was heavier than usual, which she assumes is why her surgeon is recommending the surgery. When asking her about medications that she takes, the patient denies taking any prescription medicines but does mention taking a baby aspirin a day and assorted herbal medicines for the bleeding.

1. What assessment should the nurse make to determine this patient's nutritional status and potential risk from the preoperative preparation and surgery?

2. Which laboratory results should the nurse review? State the rationales for doing so.

3. Prioritize teaching needs for this patient before surgery.

4. Develop a teaching-learning plan for this patient's postoperative care.

5. Identify any patient conditions or information that is to be shared with the surgeon or anesthesiologist.

6. The patient states that she doesn't know whether her hysterectomy will be done vaginally or abdominally. Recognizing that the patient is in need of more information, what would the nurse do?

7. The patient asks if she will lose a lot of blood in surgery and, if so, can her daughter donate blood that she can receive if needed. What teaching would you give the patient concerning blood donations?

8. Identify which category of surgery is related to each aspect of this patient's impending surgery.
    a. Reason:
    b. Urgency:
    c. Degree of risk of surgery:
    d. Extent of surgery:

9. While this patient is waiting in the preoperative area, she begins to cry, saying she is fearful of the surgery and "going under." What interventions could be used to reduce the patient's anxiety?

10. The patient is about to be sent to the operating room. What items on a final checklist should be evaluated before leaving the preoperative area?

17 CHAPTER

Care of Intraoperative Patients

STUDY/REVIEW QUESTIONS

1. Which nursing intervention can reduce the preoperative patient's anxiety?
   a. Provide a climate of privacy, comfort, and confidentiality when caring for the patient.
   b. Instruct the patient that after the preoperative medication has taken effect, the anxiety will go away.
   c. Avoid discussing the activities taking place around the patient while in the holding area.
   d. Assist members of the surgical team readying the operating room suite.

Matching. *Match the perioperative personnel with the descriptions of duties in the perioperative area.*

Personnel

a. Surgeon
b. Holding area nurse
c. Anesthesiologist
d. Circulating nurse
e. Scrub nurse
f. Specialty nurse

Duties

_____ 2. Coordinates, oversees, and participates in the patient's nursing care while the patient is in the operating room

_____ 3. Assumes responsibility for the surgical procedure and any surgical judgments about the patient

_____ 4. Manages the patient's care while the patient is in this area and initiates documentation on a perioperative nursing record

_____ 5. Educated in a particular type of surgery and responsible for intraoperative nursing care specific to patients needing that type of surgery

_____ 6. Sets up the sterile field, assists with the draping of the patient, and hands sterile supplies, sterile equipment, and instruments to the surgeon

_____ 7. Physician who specializes in the administration of anesthetic agents

8. During surgery, what things do anesthesia personnel monitor, measure, and assess? *(Select all that apply.)*
    a. Intake and output
    b. Vital signs
    c. Cardiopulmonary function
    d. Level of anesthesia
    e. Family concerns
    f. Room temperature

Matching. Match the nursing interventions with their stages of general anesthesia.

Stages of Anesthesia
a. Stage 1
b. Stage 2
c. Stage 3
d. Stage 4

Nursing Interventions

_____ 9. Prepare for and assist in treatment of cardiovascular and/or pulmonary arrest. Document in record.

_____ 10. Shield patient from extra noise and physical stimuli. Protect the patient's extremities. Assist anesthesia personnel as needed. Stay with patient.

_____ 11. Close operating room doors and control traffic in and out of room. Position patient securely with safety belts. Maintain minimal discussion in operating room.

_____ 12. Assist anesthesia personnel with intubation of patient. Place the patient in position for surgery. Prep the patient's skin in area of operative site.

13. The acute, life-threatening complication of malignant hyperthermia (MH) results from the use of which agents?
    a. Hypnotics and neuromuscular blocking agents
    b. Succinylcholine and inhalation agents
    c. Nitrous oxide and pancuronium for muscle relaxation
    d. Fentanyl and regional anesthesia for spinal block

14. Which clinical features are found in an MH crisis? *(Select all that apply.)*
    a. Sinus tachycardia
    b. Tightness and rigidity of the patient's jaw area
    c. Lowering of the blood pressure
    d. A decrease in the end-tidal carbon dioxide level
    e. Skin mottling and cyanosis
    f. An extremely elevated temperature at onset
    g. Tachypnea

15. The surgical team understands that time is crucial in recognizing and treating an MH crisis. Once recognized, what is the treatment of choice?
    a. Danazol gluconate
    b. Dilantin sodium
    c. Diazepam sulfate
    d. Dantrolene sodium

16. Which factor may lead to an anesthetic overdose in the patient?
    a. Amount of anesthesia retained by fat cells
    b. Limited muscle relaxant effects in the patient
    c. Slowed metabolism and drug elimination
    d. An uncooperative patient

17. The patient experiences MH immediately after induction of anesthesia. What are the priority nursing interventions? *(Select all that apply.)*
    a. Identifying the triggering allergy
    b. Wrapping the extremities with cold towels
    c. Assessing ABGs and serum chemistries
    d. Applying a cooling blanket over the torso
    e. Administering lower doses of the inhalation agents

Matching. Match the nursing interventions with the potential complications, which can be prevented with appropriate patient positioning and monitoring.

Anatomic Area/Complications
a. Brachial plexus/paralysis; loss of sensation
b. Radial nerve/wrist drop
c. Medial or ulnar nerves (hand deformities)/peroneal nerve (foot drop)
d. Tibial nerve/loss of sensation on the plantar surface of the foot
e. Joints/stiffness, pain, inflammation

Interventions

_____ 18. Support the wrist with padding; do not overtighten wrist straps.

_____ 19. Place pillow or foam padding under bony prominences; maintain good body alignment; slightly flex joints and support with pillows, trochanter rolls, and pads.

_____ 20. Place a safety strap above the ankle; do not place equipment on lower extremities.

_____ 21. Pad the elbow, avoid excessive abduction, secure the arm firmly on an arm board positioned at shoulder level.

_____ 22. Place a safety strap above or below the area. Place a pillow or padding under the knees.

23. In which situation is regional anesthesia useful?
    a. For procedures performed by robotics
    b. When the patient has experienced a previous reaction to blood transfusions
    c. For an endoscopy or cardiac catheterization
    d. In patients with serious medical problems

Matching. Match the anesthetic agent with its characteristic.

Agents

a. Halothane
b. Nitrous oxide
c. Desflurane
d. Thiopental sodium
e. Ketamine HCl
f. Propofol
g. Fentanyl
h. Tetracaine

Characteristics

_____ 24. Used for local or regional anesthesia.

_____ 25. A barbiturate; low incidence of post-operative nausea and vomiting.

_____ 26. Emergence reactions such as halluci-nations, unpleasant dreams, and rest-lessness are common.

_____ 27. Excellent postoperative analgesia, but may cause significant respiratory de-pression.

_____ 28. Short-acting; patient becomes respon-sive quickly postoperatively.

_____ 29. Sweet smell makes it easy to use in children.

_____ 30. May cause coughing and excitement during induction.

_____ 31. Needs addition of other agents for lon-ger procedures.

32. To avoid electrical safety problems during sur-gery, what does the nurse do?
    a. Observes for breaks in sterile technique
    b. Continuously assists the anesthesia pro-vider
    c. Ensures proper placement of the ground-ing pads
    d. Monitors the operating room with avail-able cameras

33. Which medical condition increases the pa-tient's risk for surgical wound infection?
    a. Anxiety
    b. Hiatal hernia
    c. Diabetes mellitus
    d. Amnesia

Matching. *Match the type of anesthesia with its appropriate definition.*

Type of Anesthesia

a. Topical anesthesia
b. Local infiltration
c. Nerve block
d. Spinal anesthesia
e. Epidural anesthesia

Definitions

_____ 34. Injection of the anesthetic agent into the epidural space; the spinal cord areas are never entered. Used for lower extremity surgeries, as well as anorectal, vaginal, perineal, and hip surgeries.

_____ 35. Injection of anesthetic agent into or around a nerve or group of nerves, resulting in blocked sensation and motor impulse transmission. Used to prevent pain during a procedure or to identify the cause of pain. A type of regional anesthesia.

_____ 36. Agents applied directly to the area of skin or mucous membrane to be anesthetized. Onset is within 1 minute; duration is up to 30 minutes.

_____ 37. Injection of an anesthetic agent directly into the tissue around an incision, wound, or lesion. Blocks peripheral nerve function at its origin.

_____ 38. Also called *intrathecal block*; injection of anesthetic agent into the cerebrospinal fluid in the subarachnoid space. Used for lower abdominal and pelvic surgery.

39. Which patient would be a candidate for conscious sedation? *(Select all that apply.)*
    a. Endoscopy
    b. Caesarean section delivery
    c. Closed fracture reduction
    d. Cardiac catheterization
    e. Suturing a laceration
    f. Abdominal surgery
    g. Cardioversion

CASE STUDY: THE INTRAOPERATIVE PATIENT

Use a separate sheet of paper to answer the questions in this Case Study. Answer guidelines for this Case Study are available on your Evolve website at http://evolve. elsevier.com/Iggy/ in the "Prepare for Class" folder.

A 71-year-old man is scheduled to receive orthopedic surgery in 3 hours. The nurse in the holding area has assessed the patient and begins to prepare him for the surgical procedure.

1. This patient has his intravenous catheter inserted and had a surgical shave performed before surgery. The patient is expected to be free from injury during surgery. Identify nursing diagnoses that would be appropriate for this patient.

2. While this patient is in the holding area, members of the surgical team are preparing the surgical suite. Identify factors related to physical safety in the surgical suite and give the rationale for each.

3. Identify three factors related to what the surgical team does to minimize risk of surgical infection for the patient; also identify the rationale for each.

4. The patient sees the surgical team scrubbing their hands and arms and states "Oh, it makes me feel good to know that their hands are going to be sterile for my surgery." Evaluate this statement.

5. The surgeon, nurse, and anesthesiologist have discussed anesthesia options with the patient, who agrees that an epidural anesthetic will be a good choice for him. What are potential complications the surgical team should be aware of with this choice? What are the symptoms of these potential complications?

6. Identify the circulating nurse's responsibilities for this patient during the intraoperative period.

7. As the surgical team closes the operative wound, what type of skin closures would you expect to see?

18 CHAPTER

Care of Postoperative Patients

STUDY/REVIEW QUESTIONS

1. Which description illustrates the beginning of the postoperative period?
   a. Completion of the surgical procedure and arousal of the patient from anesthesia
   b. Discharge planning initiated in the preoperative setting
   c. Closure of the patient's surgical incision
   d. Completion of the surgical procedure and transfer of the patient to the postanesthesia care unit (PACU) or intensive care unit

2. What is the primary purpose of a PACU?
   a. Follow-through on the surgeon's postoperative orders
   b. Ongoing critical evaluation and stabilization of the patient
   c. Prevention of lengthened hospital stay
   d. Arousal of patient following the use of conscious sedation

3. Which signs/symptoms are considered postoperative complications? *(Select all that apply.)*
   a. Sedation
   b. Pain at the surgical site
   c. Pulmonary embolism
   d. Hypothermia
   e. Wound evisceration

4. If a patient experiences a wound dehiscence, which description illustrates what is happening with the wound?
   a. Purulent drainage is present at incision site because of infection.
   b. Extreme pain is present at incision site.
   c. A partial or complete separation of outer layers is present at incision site.
   d. The inner and outer layers of the incision are separated.

5. When the patient describes being able to see "internal organs" at the incision site, what is the patient describing?
   a. An infection
   b. Evisceration
   c. Poor wound healing
   d. Split skin sutures

6. During PACU care, part of the nursing assessment includes the dressing. What characteristics does the nurse note?
   a. The amount of adhesive in place on the dressing
   b. The size and output of the drains used
   c. Amount, color, odor, and consistency of drainage on the dressing
   d. The appearance of the wound under the dressing

7. The nurse transfers the patient to the PACU. What is included in the standard hand-off report for the patient?
   a. Signed and dated informed consent form
   b. Record of performing preoperative teaching related to postoperative care
   c. Notation to call the health care provider for specific PACU orders
   d. Type and extent of the patient's surgical procedure

Matching. *Match the assessment findings that may be noted for patients in the PACU with their corresponding body systems. Answers may be used more than once. More than one body system may be involved in an assessment finding.*

Body Systems
a. Respiratory
b. Cardiovascular
c. Fluid and electrolyte balance
d. Neurologic
e. Renal/urinary
f. Gastrointestinal
g. Integumentary

Assessment Findings

_____ 8. Eyes open on command

_____ 9. Symmetrical chest wall expansion

_____ 10. Foley catheter to facilitate drainage

_____ 11. Absent dorsalis pedis pulsations

_____ 12. Use of accessory muscles

_____ 13. Large amount of sanguineous drainage

_____ 14. Negative Homans' sign

_____ 15. IV infusion of dextrose 5% Ringer's lactate

_____ 16. States name when asked

_____ 17. Rounded, firm abdomen

_____ 18. Exhalation felt from nose or mouth

_____ 19. Decreased blood pressure

_____ 20. Wound edges approximated

_____ 21. Dry mucous membranes

_____ 22. Vomiting

_____ 23. Pupils constrict equally

_____ 24. Sternal retraction

_____ 25. Nasogastric tube in place

_____ 26. Evisceration

_____ 27. Dullness over symphysis pubis

_____ 28. Tenting

_____ 29. Faint heart sounds

_____ 30. Wound dressing dry

_____ 31. Absent bowel sounds

_____ 32. Vesicular crackles

_____ 33. Hand grips equal

_____ 34. Simultaneous apical and radial pulsations

_____ 35. Dehiscence

_____ 36. Snoring

37. The patient arrives in the PACU. Which action does the nurse perform first?
    a. Assess for a patent airway and adequate gas exchange.
    b. Rate the patient's pain using the 0-10 pain assessment scale.
    c. Position the patient in a supine position to prevent aspiration.
    d. Calculate the PCA pump maximum dose per hour to avoid an overdose.

38. The patient arrives at the PACU and the nurse notes a respiratory rate of 10 with sternal retractions. The report from anesthesia personnel indicates that the patient had received fentanyl during surgery. Place in sequential order, using the numbers 1 to 7, the nursing interventions to be performed.

    _____ a. Monitor the patient for effects of anesthetic for at least 1 hour.

    _____ b. Have suction available appropriate to the patient's available airway.

    _____ c. Closely monitor vital signs and pulse oximetry readings until the patient responds.

    _____ d. Do not leave the patient unattended until he or she is able to respond fully.

    _____ e. Observe for significant reversal of anesthesia.

    _____ f. Administer oxygen as ordered, monitoring pulse oximetry.

    _____ g. Maintain an open airway through positioning and suction as needed.

39. The nurse is teaching incisional care to the patient who has been discharged after abdominal surgery. Which instructions does the nurse include?
    a. Do not rub or touch the incision site.
    b. Practice proper handwashing.
    c. Clean the incision site two times a day with soap and water.
    d. Splint the incisional site as often as needed for comfort.

40. The health care team determines the patient's readiness for discharge from the PACU by noting a postanesthesia recovery score of at least 10. After determining that all criteria have been met, the patient is discharged to the hospital unit or home. Review the patient profiles after 1 hour in the PACU listed below. Number the patients in order of anticipated discharge from the PACU area.

    _____ a. 10-year-old girl, tonsillectomy, general anesthesia. Duration of surgery 30 minutes. Immediate response to voice. Alert to place and person. Able to move all extremities. Respirations even, deep, rate of 20. VS are within normal limits. IV solution is D_5RL. Has voided on bedpan. Eating ice chips. Complaining of sore throat.

    _____ b. 35-year-old woman, cesarean section, epidural anesthesia. Duration of surgery 27 minutes. Awake and alert. Able to bend knees and lift lower extremities. Respirations 16 breaths/min and unlabored. Foley draining 300 mL urine. IV of RL infusing. VS are within normal limits.

    _____ c. 55-year-old man, repair of fractured lower left leg. General anesthesia. Duration of surgery 1 hour, 30 minutes. Drowsy, but responds to voice. Nausea and vomiting twice in PACU. No urge to void at this time. IV infusing D_5NS. Pedal pulses noted in both lower extremities. VS: T 98.6° F; P 130; R 24; BP 124/76.

    _____ d. 24-year-old man, reconstruction of facial scar. General anesthesia. Duration of surgery 2 hours. Sleeping, groans to voice command. VS are within normal limits. Respirations 10 breaths/min. No urge to void. IV of D_5RL infusing. Complains of pain in surgical area.

    _____ e. 42-year-old woman, colonoscopy. IV conscious sedation. Awake and alert. Up to bathroom to void. IV discontinued. Resting quietly in chair. VS are within normal limits.

41. The nurse is caring for the patient who has had abdominal surgery. After a hard sneeze, the patient reports pain in the surgical area, and the nurse immediately sees that the patient has a wound evisceration. What should the nurse do? Include in your answer the timing of the interventions.

42. Which intervention for postsurgical care of the patient is correct?
    a. When positioning the patient, use the knee gatch of the bed to bend the knees and relieve pressure.
    b. Gentle massage on the lower legs and calves helps promote venous blood return to the heart.
    c. Encourage bedrest for 3 days after surgery to prevent complications.
    d. The patient should splint the surgical wound for support and comfort when getting out of bed.

43. The morning after the patient's lower leg surgery, the nurse notes that the dressing is wet from drainage. The surgeon has not yet been in to see the patient on rounds. What does the nurse do about the dressing?
    a. Removes the dressing and puts on a dry, sterile dressing
    b. Reinforces the dressing by adding dry, sterile dressing material on top of the existing dressing
    c. Applies dry, sterile dressing material directly to the wound, then retapes the original dressing
    d. Does nothing to the dressing but calls the surgeon to evaluate the patient immediately

44. The health care provider removed the patient's original surgical dressing 2 days after surgery. Which characteristic describes normal drainage?
    a. Thick and yellow
    b. Cream-colored
    c. Serosanguineous
    d. Coffee ground-like

CASE STUDY: THE POSTOPERATIVE PATIENT

Use a separate sheet of paper to answer the questions in this Case Study. Answer guidelines for this Case Study are available on your Evolve website at http://evolve. elsevier.com/Iggy/ in the "Prepare for Class" folder.

A 30-year-old woman is admitted to the recovery area following a laparoscopy for an ovarian cyst removal. She is a small woman: 5 feet 1 inch and 103 pounds. Her surgery lasted 1 hour and 45 minutes, and the circulating nurse reported that she had a severe hemorrhage from the surgical site during that time. Upon admission to the PACU, the patient's blood pressure is 112/62, pulse range is 84 to 92, and respirations are 20 and shallow. She is groggy but answers when asked questions. An IV infusion of 1000 mL of D_5 Ringer's lactate is infusing at a rate of 200 mL per hour, and 800 mL remains in the bottle. During surgery, 100 mL of D_5 Ringer's lactate and 500 mL of normal saline were infused. An endotracheal tube (ET) is in place.

1. What assessments should the nurse perform before removing the ET?
2. How often should the nurse monitor the patient's vital signs?

A very slight amount of drainage is present on her dressing. Her blood pressure has been rising slowly and is now 20 mm Hg higher than the time recorded during surgery. She is restless and her respirations are 24 per minute.

3. After reviewing the above data, the nurse performs further assessment. What additional parameters should be assessed and why?
4. The nurse contacts the surgeon who orders the IV rate be reduced to 100 mL per hour. What is the reason for this order?
5. The patient's condition stabilizes and she is transferred to the postsurgical nursing unit. Discuss the information that the PACU nurse should report to the unit nurse.

19
CHAPTER

Inflammation and the Immune Response

STUDY/REVIEW QUESTIONS

1. Which statements about the purpose of the immune system are true? *(Select all that apply.)*
   a. The immune system provides protection from and eliminates or destroys microorganisms.
   b. The immune system is able to identify non-self proteins and cells.
   c. The immune system removes foreign proteins and other substances.
   d. The immune system protects against allergic/anaphylactic reactions.
   e. The immune system is able to prevent healthy body cells from being destroyed.

2. Which factors may affect the function of the immune system? *(Select all that apply.)*
   a. Nutritional status
   b. Environmental conditions
   c. Drugs
   d. Previous/current disease
   e. Age

True or False? *Write T for true or F for false in the blanks provided.*

_____ 3. The ability of the immune system to recognize self versus non-self cells is called *self-tolerance*.

_____ 4. Most immune cells originate in the bone marrow and are released in the blood at maturity.

_____ 5. The immune system cells are the only body cells capable of determining self from non-self.

_____ 6. The presence of inflammation always indicates that an infection is present.

_____ 7. Immunocompetence refers to the function and interaction of four immunity processes.

8. The actions of leukocytes provide the body protection against invading organisms. Which is *not* one of those actions?
   a. Phagocytic destruction of foreign invaders and unhealthy or abnormal self cells
   b. Lytic destruction of foreign invaders and unhealthy self cells
   c. Production of antibodies directed against invaders
   d. Production of cytokines that decrease specific leukocyte growth and activity

9. Which statement about the inflammatory response is true?
   a. Response is different with each incident.
   b. Response is the same whether the insult to the body is a burn or otitis media.
   c. Response depends on the location in the body.
   d. Response is specific to the cell type invaded or injured.

10. The inflammatory response is present in which conditions? *(Select all that apply.)*
    a. Sprain injuries to joints
    b. Surgical wounds
    c. Poison ivy
    d. Scalding burn injury
    e. Appendicitis

11. Which cell types associated with the inflammatory response participate in phagocytosis?
    a. Neutrophils and eosinophils
    b. Macrophages and neutrophils
    c. Macrophages and eosinophils
    d. Eosinophils and basophils

12. The body produces the most of which type of white blood cell?
   a. Macrophages
   b. Eosinophils
   c. Neutrophils
   d. Band neutrophils

Matching. Match the cell characteristics with the types of cells. Answers may be used more than once.

Cell Types
a. Neutrophil
b. Macrophage
c. Basophil
d. Eosinophil

Characteristics

_____ 13. 12- to 18-hour life span

_____ 14. 1% to 2% of total WBCs

_____ 15. Contains chemicals such as histamine

_____ 16. Can participate in multiple episodes of phagocytosis

_____ 17. When mature, capable of phagocytosis

_____ 18. Clinical sign of left shift indicates not enough mature cells being produced

_____ 19. Liver and spleen have greatest concentration

_____ 20. Vascular leak syndrome

_____ 21. The number in circulation increases during an allergic response

22. Which statements about phagocytosis are true? *(Select all that apply.)*
   a. It is a process that engulfs invaders and destroys them by enzymatic degradation.
   b. It rids the body of debris and destroys foreign invaders.
   c. It is done in a predictable manner.
   d. It is a function of all leukocytes.
   e. Phagocytosis involves six very important steps.

23. When an injury or invasion occurs, which functions will the phagocytic cell perform? *(Select all that apply.)*
   a. Release chemotaxins or leukotaxins
   b. Initiate repair of damaged tissue
   c. Generate specific antibodies
   d. Gain direct contact with the antigen or invader
   e. Recognize "non-self"

24. Complement activation and fixation is a mechanism of opsonization. When stimulated, phagocytic adherence includes 20 different inactive protein components that will:
   a. Cause individual complement proteins to activate, join together, surround the antigen, and adhere.
   b. Join together, cause individual complement proteins to activate, surround the antigen, and adhere.
   c. Cause individual phagocytic cells to clump together, forming a barrier to an invader.
   d. Stimulate the bone marrow to increase production of macrophages.

25. What are phagocytes capable of doing?
   a. Making antibodies
   b. Ingesting cells
   c. Secreting complement
   d. Producing insulin

26. Which are cardinal signs of inflammation that should be assessed by the nurse? *(Select all that apply.)*
    a. Warmth
    b. Redness
    c. Swelling
    d. Pain
    e. Decreased function

27. In which stage are all the signs of inflammation present?
    a. I
    b. II
    c. III
    d. IV

28. At the time of inflammation, a colony-stimulating factor stimulates bone marrow to perform which action?
    a. Produce leukocytes in less time
    b. Produce immature leukocytes
    c. Release immature leukocytes
    d. Synthesize immunoglobulins

29. The substance commonly called "pus" is produced by exudate in which stage of inflammation?
    a. I
    b. II
    c. III
    d. IV

30. Neutrophils attack and destroy foreign material and remove dead tissue through which process?
    a. Phagocytosis
    b. Adherence
    c. Cytokines
    d. Fixation

31. When B-lymphocytes, part of the antibody-mediated immunity (AMI) response, become sensitized to an antigen, what do they do next?
    a. Release colony-stimulating factors
    b. Cause leukocytes to aggregate
    c. Generate specific antibodies
    d. Suppress phagocytosis

32. When a person is exposed to an antigen, seven special actions take place in sequence. In which step do antibodies bind to the antigen and form an immune complex?
    a. 2
    b. 4
    c. 5
    d. 7

33. Which cells interact in the presence of an antigen to start antibody production? *(Select all that apply.)*
    a. B-lymphocytes
    b. Macrophages
    c. Neutrophils
    d. T-helper/inducer cells
    e. T-suppressor cells

34. Which statement about B-lymphocytes sensitizing to one antigen is true?
    a. Once sensitized, B-lymphocytes are always sensitized to that antigen.
    b. Plasma cells produce the antigen.
    c. The plasma cell lies dormant until the next exposure.
    d. Memory cells prevent plasma cells from oversecreting antibodies.

35. In what way is AMI different from cell-mediated immunity (CMI)?
    a. AMI is more powerful than CMI.
    b. AMI can be transferred from one person to another; CMI cannot.
    c. CMI requires constant re-exposure for "boosting"; AMI does not.
    d. CMI requires inflammatory actions for best function; AMI function is independent of inflammatory actions.

Matching. Match the actions with the antibody-binding reactions.

Antibody-Binding Reactions
a. Agglutination
b. Lysis
c. Precipitation
d. Inactivation (neutralization)
e. Complement fixation

Actions
_____ 36. Cell membrane destruction
_____ 37. Large, insoluble antibody molecules
_____ 38. Clumping-like antibody action
_____ 39. Activated by IgG and IgM
_____ 40. Covers antigen's active site

41. Which statement is true about innate-native immunity? *(Select all that apply.)*
   a. It is genetically determined, nonspecific, and cannot be transferred.
   b. It adapts to individual exposure and invasion.
   c. It cannot be altered by environmental or physiologic changes.
   d. It requires a special interaction with antibody-mediated immunity for activation.

Matching. Match the type of immunity with its correct definition.

Immunity Types
a. Natural active
b. Artificial active
c. Innate-native
d. Passive
e. Active

Definitions
_____ 42. Immunity that occurs when antibodies are created in another person or animal.
_____ 43. Immunity which is a naturally occurring feature of a person.
_____ 44. Protections developed by vaccination or immunization.
_____ 45. Antigens enter the body and the body makes antibodies against the antigen.
_____ 46. Antigen enters the body without human assistance; antibodies are made against the antigen.

47. Which cells are the T-lymphocyte subsets that are critically important to CMI? *(Select all that apply.)*
   a. Helper/inducer T-cell
   b. Suppressor T-cell
   c. Cytotoxic/cytolytic T-cell
   d. Natural killer cells
   e. Cytokines

48. Which statement best describes the function of CD4+ (cluster of differentiation 4, or T4+) cells?
   a. They participate in specialized episodes of phagocytosis directed against cancer cells.
   b. They provide a frame or lattice for tissue repair and regeneration after inflammatory events.
   c. They secrete lymphokines that can enhance the activity of other WBCs.
   d. They deliver a "lethal hit" of lytic substance to a target cell in response to antibody-dependent lysis.

Matching. Match each type of cell with its function. Answers may be used more than once.

Cell Type
a. Suppressor cell
b. Natural killer cell
c. Helper/inducer T-cell
d. Cytotoxic/cytolytic T-cell

Function
_____ 49. Prevents overreaction
_____ 50. Binds with infected cell's antigen that results in death of affected cell
_____ 51. Secretes lymphokines that stimulate activities of other cells of the immune system
_____ 52. Exerts cytotoxic effect without first undergoing period of sensitization
_____ 53. Regulates variety of inflammatory and immune responses

True or False? Write T for true or F for false in the blank provided.

_____ 54. Cancer prevention is assisted by CMI through its surveillance system.

55. The action of which cell types must be suppressed to prevent acute rejection of transplanted organs? *(Select all that apply.)*
a. Eosinophils
b. Suppressor T-cells
c. Natural killer cells
d. Cytotoxic/cytolytic T-cells
e. Helper/inducer T-cells

Matching. Match the types of rejection with their descriptors. Answers may be used more than once.

Types of Rejection
a. Hyperacute
b. Acute graft
c. Chronic

Descriptors
_____ 56. Immediate
_____ 57. Includes both cellular and antibody-mediated mechanisms
_____ 58. Rejection cannot be stopped
_____ 59. Occurs within 1 week to 3 months
_____ 60. Leads to organ destruction
_____ 61. Does not mean loss of transplant
_____ 62. Accelerated graft atherosclerosis
_____ 63. Triggers blood clotting cascade
_____ 64. Fibrotic and scarlike tissue
_____ 65. Major cause of death in heart transplant patients
_____ 66. Is antibody-mediated

67. What precaution or intervention has the highest priority for the patient going home on maintenance drugs after receiving a kidney transplant?
a. Monitoring for bacterial and fungal infections
b. Avoiding the use of table salt
c. Measuring abdominal girth daily
d. Avoiding blood donation

Matching. Match each antibody characteristic with its correct antibody type.

Antibody Types
a. IgA
b. IgE
c. IgG
d. IgM

Characteristics

_____ 68. Mediates ABO incompatibility reactions in blood transfusions

_____ 69. Mediates many types of allergic reactions

_____ 70. Present in body secretions such as tears, mucus, saliva

_____ 71. Has the highest percentage in the blood

72. Complete the table below.

Drug	Use
Cyclosporine	
Tacrolimus FK506 (Prograf)	
Corticosteroids	
Daclizumab (Zenapax)	
Muromonab-CD3 (Orthoclone OKT3)	

Matching. Match the drugs listed to their related problems, precautions, or uses in transplant rejection.

Drugs
a. Cyclosporine
b. Tacrolimus FK506
c. Corticosteroids
d. Daclizumab
e. Muromonab-CD3

Descriptions

_____ 73. Induction of capillary leak syndrome is common; may require premedication with corticosteroids.

_____ 74. Immunosuppression is more profound than what occurs with other agents.

_____ 75. There is a high incidence of flu-like symptoms.

_____ 76. May also be used as a rescue agent in kidney rejection.

_____ 77. May stimulate hyperglycemia, increase body and facial hair, and cause gingival hyperplasia.

78. Which drug should *not* be given with grapefruit juice?
a. Sirolimus (Rapamune)
b. Mycophenolate sodium (Myfortic)
c. Basiliximab (Simulect)
d. Antithymocyte globulin (Atgam)

20
CHAPTER

Care of Patients with Arthritis and Other Connective Tissue Diseases

STUDY/REVIEW QUESTIONS

1. Identify these abbreviations commonly used in relation to connective tissue disease.

   a. CTD _____

   b. DJD _____

   c. OA _____

   d. HRT _____

   e. ESR _____

   f. TJR _____

   g. TJA _____

   h. DVT _____

   i. CPM _____

   j. RA _____

   k. TMJ _____

   l. PSS _____

   m. SLE _____

2. A rheumatic disease is any condition or disease of which body system?
   a. Cardiovascular
   b. Hematopoeitic
   c. Integumentary
   d. Musculoskeletal

3. Connective tissue diseases are characterized by which features? *(Select all that apply.)*
   a. Chronic pain
   b. Dry skin
   c. Decreased function
   d. Joint deterioration
   e. Autoimmune disorder

4. What are the most common sites for osteoarthritis?
   a. Hands, back, hips, and knees
   b. Hands, elbows, and pelvis
   c. Hands, back, and pelvis
   d. Knees, hips, and back

5. During erosion of the cartilage associated with osteoarthritis, which event also occurs?
   a. Excessive formation of scar tissue
   b. Widening of the joint space and "filling in" with osteoclasts
   c. Nerve degeneration resulting in joint paresthesias
   d. Bone cyst formation and joint subluxation

6. In what way does obesity influence the development of osteoarthritis?
   a. The obese person has a reduced inflammatory response with less joint swelling.
   b. The high body fat levels of the obese patient lubricate joints and improve mobility.
   c. The extra weight of obesity increases the degeneration rate of hip and knee joints.
   d. Obesity has no positive or negative influence on development of osteoarthritis.

7. Which patient is most likely to develop osteoarthritis?
   a. Obese older woman living alone
   b. Slender, nonsmoking, middle-aged man
   c. Muscular, young construction worker
   d. Young woman with family history of rheumatoid arthritis

8. How would the patient describe crepitus?
   a. Spasms of surrounding muscles
   b. Pain with motion
   c. A continuous grating sensation
   d. Protruding bony lumps

133

9. Which characteristic is associated with Heberden's nodes?
   a. Found at the distal interphalangeal joints
   b. Found at the proximal interphalangeal joints
   c. Usually appear unilaterally
   d. Found primarily in lower-extremity joints

10. The presence of fluid in the knees may be diagnosed as which condition?
   a. Subcutaneous swelling
   b. Joint nodules
   c. Joint effusions
   d. Joint deformities

11. Osteoarthritis affecting the spine may present as what kind of pain?
   a. Localized pain at L3-4, bone spurs, stiffness, and muscle spasm
   b. Radiating pain at L3-4, C4-6, stiffness, muscle spasms, and bone spurs
   c. Localized pain at T6 to T12, stiffness, and muscle atrophy
   d. Radiating pain throughout the spine, stiffness, and muscle spasms

12. Which response from the patient with advanced osteoarthritis alerts the nurse to a problem coping with the image and role changes necessitated by disease progression?
   a. "I used to be a playground assistant; now I work with children who need help with reading."
   b. "I must be getting younger. I used to tie my shoes; now I am using Velcro closures just like my kids."
   c. "I find it easier to do my ironing sitting down rather than standing up."
   d. "I try to avoid public places so no one will see my ugly hands."

13. To determine an alteration in the patient's body image and self-esteem, what does the nurse assess as priorities? *(Select all that apply.)*
   a. Church affiliation
   b. Personal care of self
   c. Demeanor as happy or sad
   d. Expression of feeling of reacting to change
   e. Number of years the patient has been married

14. The patient is admitted with osteoarthritis. On assessment, the nurse notes that the patient walks with a limp. What is the priority nursing diagnosis?
   a. Activity Intolerance
   b. Impaired Physical Mobility
   c. Ineffective Health Maintenance
   d. Chronic Osteoarthritis

15. The nurse is teaching the patient with osteoarthritis about taking prescribed ibuprofen (Motrin). Which statement by the patient indicates a correct understanding of the medication?
   a. "I'll take the medication between meals."
   b. "The medication will affect my appetite."
   c. "The medication will help my pain and swelling."
   d. "I should stop the medication if my joints swell."

16. The teaching plan for the patient with arthritis includes complementary and alternative therapies. Which therapies does the nurse include? *(Select all that apply.)*
   a. Imagery
   b. Gene therapy
   c. Acupuncture
   d. Music therapy
   e. Thermal modalities

17. When educating the patient regarding total joint replacement (TJR), what does the nurse do first?
   a. Ask whether the patient has insurance.
   b. Review instructions and ask the patient to repeat them back.
   c. Assess the patient's knowledge and begin education if needed.
   d. Ask if the doctor has explained the procedure.

18. During the surgery for TJR, the nurse expects the patient to receive which procedure? *(Select all that apply.)*
   a. An intravenous antibiotic
   b. Blood transfusion
   c. An antibiotic in the cement
   d. Local anesthetic
   e. Immunosuppressant drug therapy

True or False? Read each statement and write T for true or F for false in the blanks provided.

_____ 19.   Polymethyl methacrylate is a fixer that holds new prostheses in place but will most likely need replacement in several years.

_____ 20.   After a total hip replacement, subluxation or total dislocation can occur if the legs are in the abducted position.

21.   Which items are contraindications for total joint arthroplasty? *(Select all that apply.)*
    a.   Infection
    b.   Severe pain
    c.   Advanced osteoporosis
    d.   Severe inflammation
    e.   Open wound

22.   After total hip replacement, what are the signs of dislocation?
    a.   Hip pain, shortening of leg, and leg rotation
    b.   Swelling in hip, hip pain, and leg rotation
    c.   Swelling of leg, shortening of leg, and leg rotation
    d.   Swelling of hip, shortening of leg, and leg rotation

23.   What is the treatment for dislocation of a total hip replacement?
    a.   Manipulation and bedrest
    b.   Bedrest and pain medication
    c.   Manipulation and immobilization
    d.   Manipulation and continuation of previous care

24.   Which symptom should be reported to the physician as a possible sign of infection following a total hip replacement?
    a.   Confusion and excessive or malodorous drainage
    b.   Swelling of the foot and bruising
    c.   Diaphoresis and lowered blood pressure
    d.   Pain in surgical area

True or False? Read each statement and write T for true or F for false in the blanks provided.

_____ 25.   The most potentially life-threatening complication following TJR is venous thromboembolism.

_____ 26.   The TJR patient's erythrocyte sedimentation rate (ESR) is elevated, which may indicate infection at the site.

_____ 27.   Initial drainage from the surgical site of the TJR is most likely to be about 250 mL.

28.   After TJR, how are the drains removed that were placed during surgery?
    a.   By the surgeon
    b.   They are allowed to fall out
    c.   At the first dressing change
    d.   By the physical therapist when weight-bearing has started

29.   After TJR, when is hemoglobin and hematocrit monitored?
    a.   First postoperative day only
    b.   Only after a transfusion
    c.   Only if there is drainage on the dressings
    d.   Two to three days postoperatively

30.   Which precautions are used to reduce the chance of having a blood transfusion reaction? *(Select all that apply.)*
    a.   Autologous transfusions
    b.   Nonsteroidal anti-inflammatory drugs (NSAIDs)
    c.   Epoietin alfa administration
    d.   Neuroaxial anesthesia
    e.   Blood salvage

31.   How does a continuous peripheral nerve blockade (CPNB) device work?
    a.   Infuses intravenous opioids.
    b.   Infuses a local anesthetic into the surgical site.
    c.   Circulates cold liquids within a wrap around the incision site.
    d.   Stimulates vibration-sensitive receptors in the incision area to "close the gate" on pain.

32. Adlea is a refined capsaicin product. If infused directly into the surgical joint, how is its mechanism of action described?
    a. Numbness results from calcium flooding the nerve cells, which then shut down.
    b. Capsaicin shuts down C fiber receptors.
    c. Depletes calcium stores in nerve cells and blocks pain transmission.
    d. Local anesthetic numbs nerves in the operative region.

33. Postoperative total hip replacement patients can develop numerous complications. Which intervention is the priority in preventing complications?
    a. Bedrest with pillow between the legs
    b. Adequate diet and fluid intake
    c. Getting out of bed on the first postoperative day
    d. Sitting on the side of the bed

34. Which postoperative complication occurs more frequently among patients who have total hip replacements than among patients who have total knee replacements?
    a. Deep vein thrombosis
    b. Joint dislocation
    c. Acute pain
    d. Infection

35. For patients who have TJRs, the risk of deep vein thrombosis (DVT) is high. Which statements are true? *(Select all that apply.)*
    a. Older adults are at high risk for DVT and compromised circulation.
    b. Thinner patients are more at risk than obese patients.
    c. Patients with a history of DVT are at high risk for recurrence.
    d. Leg exercises must be started in the immediate postoperative period.
    e. Use of an abduction splint will decrease the risk of DVT.

36. The patient had a total hip arthroplasty. Which interventions does the nurse perform to prevent a DVT from occurring? *(Select all that apply.)*
    a. Instruct to delay ambulation postoperatively.
    b. Apply thigh-high stockings.
    c. Administer an anticoagulant such as aspirin.
    d. Use the foot sole pumps as needed.
    e. Apply sequential compression devices (SCDs).

37. To prevent a DVT, several types of anticoagulant medications can be ordered. Which is the most commonly used drug during hospitalization?
    a. Oral or parenteral aspirin
    b. Warfarin
    c. Intravenous tPA
    d. Subcutaneous low–molecular weight (LMW) heparin

38. It is important to monitor which laboratory test for patients on anticoagulant therapy with LMW heparin after total joint arthroplasty? *(Select all that apply.)*
    a. Prothrombin time and international normalized ratio (INR)
    b. Oxygen saturation
    c. Complete blood count
    d. Activated partial thromboplastin time
    e. Platelet count

39. Postoperative care for total knee replacement may include which techniques? *(Select all that apply.)*
    a. Hot compresses to the incisional area
    b. Continuous passive motion (CPM) used immediately or several days postoperatively
    c. Ice packs or cold packs to the incisional area
    d. The use of a CPM machine in the daytime and an immobilizer at night
    e. Maintaining abduction

40. Postoperative care following finger and wrist replacements includes which techniques? *(Select all that apply.)*
    a. Traction
    b. Joint wrapped in a bulky dressing
    c. Splint, brace, or cast
    d. Abduction pillow
    e. Elevation of the arm to prevent edema
    f. CPM machine

41. Impaired Physical Mobility is an appropriate nursing diagnosis for a total hip replacement patient. What is the priority intervention for this patient?
    a. Encourage use of assistive devices such as a walker when ambulating.
    b. Recommend to quickly decrease rest periods between activities.
    c. Instruct to flex the hips 90 degrees or greater.
    d. Instruct to sit on a soft chair with a raised back.

42. What is an important health teaching point for the patient with TJR?
    a. "Do as much as you can as often as you can."
    b. "Reach beyond the physical therapist's instructions."
    c. "Protect the joint."
    d. "No pain, no gain."

43. Although arthritis is not curable, many "cures" are marketed to patients with the disease. What does the nurse encourage the patient to do?
    a. Take advantage of clinical trials or experimental therapy.
    b. Check with the Arthritis Foundation for appropriate modalities.
    c. Buy special liniments and creams.
    d. Take herbals and vitamins.

44. When evaluating the patient with arthritis and TJR, the nurse assesses for which expected outcome?
    a. Perform ADLs with one person assisting.
    b. Verbally express comfort and pain relief.
    c. Ambulate with crutches or a walker.
    d. Perform passive range of motion (ROM) exercises three times a shift.

45. Which statements regarding rheumatoid arthritis (RA) are true? *(Select all that apply.)*
    a. It is a chronic, progressive, systemic inflammatory process.
    b. It primarily affects the synovial joints.
    c. It is known to have periods of remission.
    d. It occurs most often in older men and women.
    e. It often involves an inflamed, red rash.

46. Because of the inflammatory process in RA, a pannus forms in the joint. What is a pannus?
    a. Scar tissue restricting the joint
    b. Vascular granulation tissue in the joint
    c. Necrotic tissue sloughing into the joint
    d. Fluid encapsulated in the joint

47. What common musculoskeletal health problem is often associated with RA?
    a. Paget's disease
    b. Fibromyalgia
    c. Marfan syndrome
    d. Osteoporosis

48. Although the etiology of RA is unknown for certain, it is considered to be what type of disorder?
    a. An autoimmune disease
    b. Associated with aging
    c. Genetic
    d. The result of joint misuse

49. For the following manifestations of RA, specify whether they are early (E) or late (L) manifestations.
    _____ a. Joint deformities
    _____ b. Joint inflammation
    _____ c. Osteoporosis
    _____ d. Vasculitis
    _____ e. Subcutaneous nodules
    _____ f. Paresthesias
    _____ g. Low-grade fever
    _____ h. Anemia

50. Which patient-reported symptoms are typical of RA?
    a. "My hands are stiff, swollen, and tender."
    b. "My right hand is weak."
    c. "My left hand is stiff and swollen."
    d. "My knees are swollen and stiff."

51. When the patient has RA of the temporomandibular joint, what is the major complaint?
    a. Pain on chewing and opening the mouth
    b. Headache at the temple
    c. Toothache
    d. Earache

52. What is the most common area of involvement of RA in the spine?
    a. Lumbar spine
    b. Sacral spine
    c. Cervical spine
    d. Thoracic spine

53. Complications of spinal involvement in RA may be seen as which signs/symptoms? *(Select all that apply.)*
    a. Compression of the phrenic nerve that controls the diaphragm
    b. Resulting subluxation of the first and second vertebrae
    c. Becoming quadriplegic or quadriparetic
    d. Bilateral sciatic pain in the legs
    e. Numbness of the hands and feet

54. In patients with RA, where might Baker's cysts be located?
    a. Ankles
    b. Wrists
    c. Popliteal bursae
    d. Achilles tendon

55. In late RA, the patient may have systemic involvement called "flares." How are these described?
    a. Moderate to severe weight loss
    b. Fever and fatigue
    c. Muscle atrophy
    d. Joint contractures

56. Which condition is *not* consistent with the patient with RA?
    a. Ischemia
    b. Deformed joints
    c. Weight loss
    d. Subcutaneous nodules

57. What are the manifestations of Sjögren's syndrome in patients with advanced RA?
    a. Dry eyes, dry mouth, and dry vagina
    b. Obstruction of secretory glands and ducts
    c. Nodules in the lungs
    d. Enlarged spleen and liver

58. What might a psychosocial examination of the patient with advanced RA reveal? *(Select all that apply.)*
    a. Role changes
    b. Poor self-esteem and body image
    c. Grieving and depression
    d. Loss of control and independence
    e. Inability to perform relaxation techniques

59. In RA, autoantibodies (rheumatoid factors [RFs]) are formed that attack healthy tissue, especially synovium, causing which condition?
    a. Nerve pain
    b. Bone porosity
    c. Ischemia
    d. Inflammation

60. Which conditions may be present in the patient with an elevated ESR? *(Select all that apply.)*
    a. Inflammation or infection in the body
    b. Pregnancy
    c. Vasculitis and organ damage
    d. Anemia
    e. Muscular dystrophy

61. What CBC laboratory values does the nurse expect for the patient with RA? *(Circle "high" or "low" for each value.)*

    a. Hemoglobin: High   Low

    b. Hematocrit: High   Low

    c. RBC: High   Low

    d. WBC: High   Low

    e. Platelets: High   Low

62. Arthrocentesis done on the patient with RA may reveal which element(s) in the synovial fluid of the joint?
    a. Glucose and glycogen
    b. Inflammatory cells and immune complexes
    c. Protein, such as albumin
    d. Platelet aggregation

63. The nurse is teaching the patient about the common side effects of chronic salicylate and NSAID therapy. Which body system side effects does the nurse focus on in the teaching plan?
    a. Central nervous system
    b. Skin
    c. Gastrointestinal
    d. Cardiovascular

Matching. Match each drug with the possible side effect of which the nurse should be aware in patients with RA. Side effects may be used more than once.

Drugs
a. Salicylates
b. NSAIDs
c. Steroids
d. Plaquenil (Antimalarial)
e. Methotrexate (Rheumatrex)
f. Minocycline
g. Analgesics
h. Etanercept (Enbrel)
i. Gold salts
j. Leufonamide (Arava)

Side Effects
_____ 64. Headache, dizziness, drowsiness
_____ 65. Diabetes, infection, hypertension
_____ 66. Gastrointestinal problems
_____ 67. Bone marrow suppression, mouth sores
_____ 68. Rash, blood dyscrasias, renal involvement
_____ 69. Red, itchy rash at injection site
_____ 70. Retinal toxicity
_____ 71. Low incidence of adverse effects and resistance
_____ 72. Hair loss, diarrhea, decreased WBCs and platelets

73. The nurse is performing an assessment of the patient with RA. Which findings does the nurse expect?
    a. Head and neck pain
    b. Early morning joint pain
    c. Increased ROM in the hands
    d. Absence of joint swelling

74. The nurse's plan of care for the patient with RA includes which interventions? *(Select all that apply.)*
    a. Ensure optimal pain relief.
    b. Utilize the prone position.
    c. Encourage frequent rest periods.
    d. Decrease exercise to every other day.
    e. Recommend liberal use of arthritic creams.

Matching. Match the drugs to their correct descriptions.

Drugs

a. NSAIDs
b. Methotrexate
c. Biologic response modifiers
d. Gold therapy

Descriptions

_____ 75. The first choice for the treatment of mild RA

_____ 76. The first choice for the treatment of moderate to severe RA

_____ 77. Used less commonly now and requires a test dose before the first injection

_____ 78. Requires a purified protein derivative (PPD) test be performed to rule out the presence of tuberculosis

79. Which statement best describes discoid lupus?
    a. It is the most frequently diagnosed type of lupus.
    b. It results in an increase in immune complexes within the joint cavity.
    c. It is not a systemic condition and is limited to involvement of the skin.
    d. It is a lupus-like syndrome that occurs in patients taking certain medications.

80. What can be expected for the patient with recently diagnosed systemic lupus erythematosus (SLE)?
    a. An acute inflammatory disorder
    b. Spontaneous remission and exacerbations
    c. Symptoms limited to arthritis
    d. Symptoms limited to skin lesions

81. What is the most common cause of death in patients with SLE?
    a. Cardiac failure
    b. Skin involvement
    c. Central nervous system involvement
    d. Renal failure

82. Which laboratory test is the only significant test for diagnosing the patient with discoid lupus?
    a. Antinuclear antibody
    b. Serum complement
    c. Complete blood count
    d. Skin biopsy

83. What is the priority diagnosis for the patient with progressive systemic disease (PSS) or scleroderma?
    a. Disturbed Body Image
    b. Impaired Skin Integrity
    c. Activity Intolerance
    d. Impaired Physical Mobility

84. Which finding does the nurse expect to see in the patient admitted with systemic sclerosis?
    a. Multiple joint deformities
    b. Chronic use of immunosuppressant therapy
    c. Rash and discoid lesions
    d. CREST syndrome

85. The patient with scleroderma may have which problems? *(Select all that apply.)*
    a. Dysphagia, esophageal reflux
    b. Smooth tongue
    c. Malabsorption problems causing malodorous diarrhea stools
    d. Butterfly lesions on the face and nose
    e. Spiderlike hemangiomas

86. Raynaud's phenomenon in the patient with scleroderma may present as which signs/symptoms? *(Select all that apply.)*
    a. Digit necrosis
    b. Excruciating pain
    c. Autoamputations of digits
    d. Periungual lesions
    e. Peripheral neuropathy

87. What are characteristics of primary gout? (Select all that apply.)
    a. Results from medications such as diuretics
    b. Sodium urate deposited in the synovium
    c. Affects large joints most commonly
    d. Affects middle-aged and older men
    e. Peak time of onset after age 50

88. What part of the body is first affected by gout?
    a. Fingers
    b. Knees
    c. Great toe
    d. Shoulder

True or False? *Read each statement and write T for true or F for false in the blanks provided. If the statement is false, correct the statement to make it true.*

_____ 89. The patient with acute gout cannot tolerate having the joint touched or moved.

_____ 90. The patient with chronic gout may have tophi on the outer ear.

91. The patient who was prescribed colchicine for gout reports abdominal pain associated with nausea, vomiting, and diarrhea for 48 hours. To what does the nurse attribute these signs/symptoms?
    a. Common side effects of colchicine
    b. Signs of drug toxicity
    c. Not taking colchicine 30 minutes before a meal
    d. Not administering the drug via IV route

92. Polymyalgia rheumatica and temporal arteritis present with which symptoms? (Select all that apply.)
    a. Stiffness
    b. Low-grade fever
    c. Arthralgias
    d. Decreased ESR
    e. Polycythemia

93. Patients with ankylosing spondylitis have the threat of which condition?
    a. Compromised respiratory function
    b. Cardiac involvement
    c. Hip pain
    d. Dysphagia

94. Which are common findings in the patient with Reiter's syndrome?
    a. Conjunctivitis and urethritis
    b. Erythema and psoriasis
    c. Arthritis and weight loss
    d. Paresthesias and fatigue

95. Which manifestation is expected in the patient with Marfan syndrome?
    a. Obesity
    b. Shortened hands and feet
    c. Short, swollen fingers
    d. Excessive height

96. Lyme disease is identified early by which signs/symptoms? (Select all that apply.)
    a. Known bite from deer tick
    b. Bull's-eye rash at onset
    c. Facial paralysis
    d. Dysphagia
    e. Generalized erythema

True or False? *Read the statements below and write T for true or F for false in the blanks provided. If the statement is false, correct the statement to make it true.*

_____ 97. Lyme disease is treated with antibiotics over an extended period of time (10 to 21 days).

_____ 98. Pseudogout is a mimic of gout depositing uric acid crystals in the joints.

99. The nursing assessing the patient with fibromyalgia identifies the trigger points by palpation. In which specific areas does the nurse expect to elicit pain and tenderness? *(Select all that apply.)*
    a. Neck
    b. Feet
    c. Trunk
    d. Lower back
    e. Hands

100. The patient is prescribed amitriptyline (Elavil) for the diagnosis of fibromyalgia. What kind of drug is this medication?
    a. Anti-inflammatory
    b. Antirheumatic
    c. Antidepressant
    d. Antipsychotic

Matching. *Match the disease or condition with its definition.*

Diseases/Conditions
a. Polyarthralgia
b. Polymyositis
c. Polymyalgia rheumatica
d. Giant cell arteritis
e. Ankylosing spondylitis
f. Sjögren's syndrome
g. Lyme disease

Definitions

_____ 101. Systemic infectious disease that is caused by the spirochete *Borrelia burgdorferi*

_____ 102. Affects the vertebral column and causes spinal deformities

_____ 103. Diffuse, inflammatory disease of skeletal (striated) muscle

_____ 104. Systemic vasculitis that affects large and midsized arteries

_____ 105. Aching around multiple joints

_____ 106. Clinical syndrome characterized by stiffness, weakness, and aching of the proximal musculature

_____ 107. Inflammatory condition in which secretory ducts and glands are obstructed

CASE STUDY: THE PATIENT WITH RHEUMATOID ARTHRITIS

Use a separate sheet of paper to answer the questions in this Case Study. Answer guidelines for this Case Study are available on your Evolve website at http://evolve. elsevier.com/Iggy/ in the "Prepare for Class" folder.

The patient comes to the clinic with symptoms of fatigue and hand and wrist pain for 3 months. The patient reports the fatigue has started to interfere with sleep, and NSAIDs have provided minimal pain relief. The nurse assesses that the proximal interphalangeal (PCP) and metacarpophalangeal (MCP) joints of both hands are warm, swollen, and painful to touch with limited ROM. Diagnostic tests reveal a positive rheumatoid factor, elevated antinuclear antibody (ANA), and ESR of 32 mm/hr. The patient is diagnosed with RA, and the health care provider prescribes a regimen of prednisone 10 mg orally daily, methotrexate (Rheumatrex) 15 mg orally weekly, and folate once per day.

1. What clinical manifestations of RA did the patient exhibit? Explain the pathophysiologic basis for these clinical manifestations.

2. What discharge teaching instructions should the nurse provide for prednisone, methotrexate (Rheumatrex), and folate therapy?

3. What are four minimum interventions the nurse can suggest to manage the patient's fatigue?

21 CHAPTER

Care of Patients with HIV Disease and Other Immune Deficiencies

STUDY/REVIEW QUESTIONS

1. Which statement about immunodeficiency is true?
   a. It causes a decrease in the patient's risk for infection.
   b. It is always acquired.
   c. It occurs when a person's body cannot recognize antigens.
   d. It is the same as autoimmunity.

Matching. Match the descriptions with the types of immunodeficiencies.

Immunodeficiencies

a. Primary
b. Secondary
c. Human immunodeficiency virus (HIV)
d. Acquired immunodeficiency syndrome (AIDS)
e. Immunodeficiency

Descriptions

_____ 2. Last and most serious stage of HIV infection

_____ 3. Disease/deficiency present since birth

_____ 4. Chronic infection with immunodeficiency virus

_____ 5. Disease/deficiency acquired as a result of viral infection, contact with a toxin, or medical therapy

_____ 6. Deficient immune response as a result of impaired or missing immune components

True or False? Write T for true or F for false in the blank provided.

_____ 7. Everyone who has AIDS has HIV infection, and everyone who has HIV infection has AIDS.

8. Using Table 21-1 in the textbook, identify the HIV/AIDS clinical classification (A, B, or C) for these symptoms and diagnoses:

_____ a. Bacterial endocarditis

_____ b. Toxoplasmosis

_____ c. Kaposi's sarcoma

_____ d. Persistent generalized lymphadenopathy

_____ e. Herpes zoster

_____ f. Idiopathic thrombocytopenic purpura

_____ g. Fever and diarrhea lasting over a month

_____ h. Cytomegalovirus retinitis

_____ i. Severe cervical dysplasia

9. Which statement best describes a retrovirus?
   a. It is a fungus that infects other cells in order to replicate.
   b. It carries its genetic material on a single-stranded RNA.
   c. It is any infection that results from a deficient immune system.
   d. It carries its genetic material on a double-stranded RNA.

10. Which immune function abnormality is a result of HIV infection?
    a. Lymphocytosis
    b. CD4+ cell depletion
    c. Increased CD8+ cell activity
    d. Long macrophage life span

11. Which group is experiencing the highest increase in the number of HIV infections?
    a. Men having sex with other men
    b. Intravenous drug users
    c. Women having sex with men
    d. Asian immigrants

12. Which descriptions are characteristic of a nonprogressor? *(Select all that apply.)*
    a. Has been infected for 10 years
    b. Is asymptomatic
    c. Has no CD4+ or T-lymphocytes
    d. Is immunocompetent
    e. Are functional antibodies

13. Which conditions may be the first signs of HIV in women? *(Select all that apply.)*
    a. Vaginal candidiasis
    b. Bladder infections
    c. Cervical neoplasia
    d. Pelvic inflammatory disease (PID)
    e. Mononucleosis

14. Which statement regarding HIV/AIDS among older adults is true?
    a. The risk for HIV infection after exposure is minimal for older adults.
    b. Older men are more susceptible to HIV infection than are older women.
    c. It is not necessary to assess an older adult for a history of drug abuse.
    d. Older adults who participate in high-risk behaviors are susceptible to HIV infection.

15. What is the most important means of preventing HIV spread or transmission?
    a. Engineering
    b. Education
    c. Isolation
    d. Counseling

16. HIV can be transmitted by which routes? *(Select all that apply.)*
    a. Viral
    b. Sexual
    c. Parenteral
    d. Airborne
    e. Perinatal

17. Highly activated antiretroviral therapy (HAART) causes what effect?
    a. Reversal of a patient's antibody status
    b. Decrease of the viral load
    c. Increase of the viral load
    d. More detectable HIV

18. The patient is an IV drug user who regularly shares needles and syringes with friends. What information does the nurse provide to decrease the patient's risk of HIV through shared needles and syringes after each use?
    a. Fill and flush the syringe with clear water, then fill the syringe with bleach, shake approximately 1 minute, and rinse with clear water.
    b. Fill and flush the syringe with water, then fill the syringe with soap and hot water, shake 2 minutes, and rinse with cold water.
    c. Rinse needles after each use with a bleach and water solution, then allow to air dry.
    d. Rinse needles after each use with rubbing alcohol and water solution, then rinse with water.

19. Which practice is recommended by the CDC to prevent sexual transmission of HIV?
    a. Use of latex condoms
    b. Use of natural membrane condoms
    c. Use of topical contraceptives
    d. Use of antiviral medications

20. Which symptoms does the nurse assess in the patient diagnosed with HIV? (*Select all that apply.*)
    a. Shortness of breath
    b. Weakness and numbness
    c. Skin lesions
    d. Visual changes
    e. Night sweats

21. Which opportunistic infections can be observed in AIDS? (*Select all that apply.*)
    a. Protozoan
    b. Viral
    c. Bacterial
    d. Fungal
    e. Gastroenteritis

22. The patient with *Pneumocystis carinii* pneumonia (PCP) usually presents with which symptoms?
    a. Dyspnea, tachypnea, persistent dry cough, and fever
    b. Cough with copious thick sputum, fever, and dyspnea
    c. Low-grade fever, cough, and shortness of breath
    d. Fever, persistent cough, and vomiting

23. The patient presenting with toxoplasmosis may have which signs and symptoms? (*Select all that apply.*)
    a. Speech difficulty
    b. Shortness of breath
    c. Visual changes
    d. Impaired gait
    e. Mental status changes

24. Cryptosporidiosis is a form of gastroenteritis in which diarrhea can amount to a loss of how many liters of fluid per day?
    a. 1 to 2
    b. 3 to 5
    c. 5 to 8
    d. 15 to 20

25. Where can candidiasis occur in the body? (*Select all that apply.*)
    a. Mouth
    b. Esophagus
    c. Vagina
    d. Nose
    e. Ears

True or False? *Write T for true or F for false in the blanks provided.*

_____ 26. Cryptococcosis is a type of meningitis.

_____ 27. Histoplasmosis is a localized respiratory infection.

_____ 28. *Mycobacterium avium-intracellulare* complex (MAC) is the most common bacterial infection among people with HIV/AIDS.

29. Where in the body can cytomegalovirus (CMV) present with symptoms? (*Select all that apply.*)
    a. Eyes, causing visual impairment
    b. The kidneys as glomerulonephritis
    c. Respiratory tract, causing pneumonitis
    d. Gastrointestinal tract, causing colitis
    e. The heart as cardiomyopathy

30. How does the herpes simplex virus (HSV) manifest itself in patients with HIV and AIDS? *(Select all that apply.)*
    a. Maculopapular lesions that can spread
    b. A chronic ulceration after vesicles rupture
    c. Vesicles located in the perirectal, oral, and genital areas
    d. Numbness and tingling occurring before the vesicle forms
    e. Itching localized in the perianal area

31. Shingles results from varicella zoster virus (VZV) leaving the nerve ganglia and entering the body by which route?
    a. Mucous membranes
    b. Pulmonary spaces
    c. Body fluids and other tissue areas
    d. Bone marrow

32. Lymphomas associated with AIDS include which types? *(Select all that apply.)*
    a. Non-Hodgkin's B-cell
    b. Immunoblastic
    c. Hodgkin's
    d. Burkitt's
    e. Primary brain

33. The patient diagnosed with AIDS reports a nonproductive cough, loss of appetite, intermittent bouts of diarrhea, and weight loss during the past several months. What is the priority nursing diagnosis for this patient?
    a. Impaired Gas Exchange
    b. Diarrhea
    c. Risk of Infection
    d. Imbalanced Nutrition

34. Which treatments are intended to boost the immune system? *(Select all that apply.)*
    a. Radiation therapy
    b. Bone marrow transplantation
    c. Lymphocyte transfusion
    d. Administration of interleukin-2
    e. Infusion of lymphokines

35. Pentamidine isethionate can be administered to the patient with PCP by which routes? *(Select all that apply.)*
    a. Orally
    b. Intravenously
    c. Intramuscularly
    d. Inhalation (by aerosol)
    e. Topically

36. Which conditions cause severe pain in HIV disease and AIDS? *(Select all that apply.)*
    a. Enlarged organs
    b. Peripheral neuropathy
    c. Tumors
    d. High fevers
    e. Dry skin

37. What methods or agents are used to treat Kaposi's sarcoma? *(Select all that apply.)*
    a. Radiotherapy
    b. Chemotherapy
    c. Antibiotics
    d. Cryotherapy
    e. Surgery

38. Which actions are useful in helping orient the patient? *(Select all that apply.)*
    a. Repeating person, place, and time
    b. Using clocks and calendars
    c. Giving the mini mental state examination (MMSE) screening test
    d. Having familiar items present
    e. Providing uninterrupted time

39. The nurse assesses the patient diagnosed with advanced AIDS for malnutrition. Which findings does the nurse most likely assess? *(Select all that apply.)*
    a. Pain
    b. Anorexia
    c. Incontinence
    d. Diarrhea
    e. Vomiting

40. Corticosteroids perform which actions? *(Select all that apply.)*
    a. Block the movement of neutrophils and monocytes through cell membranes.
    b. Increase cell production in the bone marrow.
    c. Reduce the number of circulating T-cells, resulting in suppressed cell-mediated immunity.
    d. Decrease intracranial pressure.
    e. Constrict blood vessels.

True or False? *Read each statement and write T for true or F for false in the blanks provided. If the statement is false, correct the statement to make it true.*

_____ 41. The higher the degree of blood concentration of HIV, the greater the risk of sexual transmission.

_____ 42. The person with HIV infection can transmit the virus to others at all stages of disease.

_____ 43. Lesions resulting from Kaposi's sarcoma are painful and have purulent drainage.

_____ 44. Opportunistic infections are usually prevented by a properly functioning immune system of the HIV patient.

_____ 45. AIDS dementia complex (ADC) is caused by infection of the cells in the central nervous system by HIV.

_____ 46. Patients with HIV should know that as CD4+ counts lower, clinical manifestations decrease.

_____ 47. A patient is leukopenic if the WBC is less than 3500 /mm³ and lymphopenic if lymphocytes are fewer than 1500 /mm³.

_____ 48. The viral load test measures the presence of HIV genetic material in the patient's blood and helps with monitoring the disease progression.

_____ 49. Antiretroviral drug therapy kills the virus before it is able to replicate.

_____ 50. HIV is more easily transmitted from infected female to uninfected male than from infected male to uninfected female.

51. Which methods or items are means of transmitting HIV? *(Select all that apply.)*
    a. Sexual intercourse
    b. Household utensils
    c. Breast milk
    d. Toilet facilities
    e. Mosquitoes

52. The nurse is teaching the patient about preventing HIV infection through sexual contact. Which statement made by the patient indicates effective teaching?
    a. "A latex condom with spermicide provides the best protection against getting infected with HIV."
    b. "Mutually monogamous sex with a noninfected partner will best prevent HIV infection."
    c. "Contraceptive methods like implants and injections are recommended to prevent HIV transmission."
    d. "If my partner and I are both HIV-positive, unprotected sex is permitted."

53. Rank each risk for transmission of HIV from highest to lowest risk using the numbers 1 through 4.

_____ a. Intravenous drug use

_____ b. Blood and blood product transfusions

_____ c. Sexual exposure

_____ d. Perinatal transmission from mothers with AIDS

54. For each laboratory test, indicate whether the presence of HIV will increase (I), decrease (D), or cause no change (NC) in the levels.

_____ a. CD4+

_____ b. CD8+

_____ c. WBC

_____ d. Lymphocytes

55. Complete the chart below regarding drug therapy for HIV.

Drug	Classification	Therapeutic Use	Nursing Intervention
Pentamidine isethionate			
Metronidazole (Flagyl)			
Zidovudine (Retrovir)			
Ritonavir (Norvir)			
Enfuvirtide (Fuzeon)			
Nevirapine (Viramune)			
Fluconazole (Diflucan)			

56. The patient diagnosed with HIV is receiving medications to reduce the viral load and improve CD4+ lymphocyte counts. Which term accurately describes this HIV/AIDS drug regimen?
    a. Interferon treatment
    b. Antiviremia
    c. ELISA administration
    d. HAART therapy

CASE STUDY: THE PATIENT WITH HIV

Use a separate sheet of paper to answer the questions in this Case Study. Answer guidelines for this Case Study are available on your Evolve website at http://evolve. elsevier.com/Iggy/ in the "Prepare for Class" folder.

A 42-year-old man who was diagnosed as HIV-positive 10 years ago is admitted to the hospital with AIDS. He has been on antiretroviral therapy since his diagnosis, and his CD4+ count has consistently been above 500 for the past 10 years. He now reports increased dyspnea for 3 days and "being very cold." The nurse assesses a dry nonproductive cough and crackles in the right and lower lung bases. Vital signs are BP 156/90 mm Hg, HR 110 BPM, RR 28-30 breaths/min and regular, and an oral temperature of 102.4° F. Diagnostic tests reveal a WBC count of 4000 /μL, lymphocytes 13%, CD4+ T-cell count of 300 /mm^3, CD4+ count of 160 mm^3, and decreased RBC and thrombocyte levels. The patient's current drug regimen includes stavudine (Zerit) 40 mg twice daily, zidovudine (Retrovir) 300 mg twice daily, and indinavir (Crixivan) 800 mg every 8 hours.

1. What is the significance of the patient's CD4+ cell count?

2. What nursing interventions will be most helpful for this patient?

3. What nursing considerations are necessary to ensure the patient is compliant with his antiretroviral medication therapy?

22
CHAPTER

Care of Patients with Immune Function Excess: Hypersensitivity (Allergy) and Autoimmunity

STUDY/REVIEW QUESTIONS

1. Which type I hypersensitivity reaction requires immediate intervention by the nurse?
   a. PPD test result of 10 mm
   b. Anaphylaxis
   c. Vasculitis
   d. Fever

2. "Overreactions" to invaders or foreign antigens can be the result of what? *(Select all that apply.)*
   a. Hypersensitivity
   b. Allergic response
   c. Autoimmune response
   d. Phagocytosis
   e. Increased cardiac output

3. Which statement best describes allergy or hypersensitivity?
   a. Excessive response to the presence of an antigen
   b. Excessive response against self-cells and cell products
   c. Failure of the immune system to recognize self cells as normal
   d. Failure of the immune system to recognize foreign cells and microbial invaders

Matching. *Match the type of hypersensitivity to a clinical example. Types may be used more than once.*

Hypersensitivities
a. Type I: immediate
b. Type II: cytotoxic
c. Type III: immune complex-mediated
d. Type IV: delayed
e. Type V: stimulated

Clinical Examples

_____ 4. Autoimmune hemolytic anemia

_____ 5. Poison ivy

_____ 6. Hay fever

_____ 7. Graves' disease

_____ 8. Serum sickness

_____ 9. Anaphylaxis

_____ 10. Myasthenia gravis

_____ 11. Graft rejection

_____ 12. Allergic asthma

_____ 13. Vasculitis

14. Which type of therapy for allergy management administers small increasing amounts of identified allergens subcutaneously?
    a. Alternative
    b. Progressive
    c. Symptomatic
    d. Desensitization

Matching. *Match the terms with their corresponding descriptions.*

Causes
a. Allergen
b. Leukotriene
c. Histamine
d. Rhinorrhea

Reactions

_____ 15. Increases capillary permeability, nasal and conjunctival mucous secretions, and itching

_____ 16. Promotes allergic responses mediated by IgE

_____ 17. Runny nose, clear drainage, and pink mucosa

_____ 18. Responsible for secondary phase of type I hypersensitivity reactions

19. Which techniques are used for allergy management? *(Select all that apply.)*
    a. Avoidance
    b. Desensitization
    c. Conization
    d. Antibiotics
    e. Injections

20. Which methods are used for testing for allergies? *(Select all that apply.)*
    a. Topical serums
    b. Scratch test
    c. Intravenous
    d. Intradermal
    e. Skin biopsy

Matching. *Match the drug types with their corresponding actions.*

Drug Types
a. Decongestant
b. Antihistamine
c. Corticosteroids
d. Mast cell stabilizers
e. Leukotriene antagonist

Actions

_____ 21. Competes for histamine at histamine receptor sites

_____ 22. Causes vasoconstriction, reducing edema; may be combined with anticholinergics

_____ 23. Decreases inflammation and immune response in a short time

_____ 24. Prevents mast cells from opening when allergen binds with IgE

_____ 25. Prevents leukotriene synthesis and blocks leukotriene receptors

26. Which common symptoms will the patient manifest almost immediately after being exposed to an allergen? *(Select all that apply.)*
    a. Angioedema
    b. Apprehension
    c. Chills
    d. Fever
    e. Urticaria

27. The patient in anaphylaxis who is going into respiratory failure will demonstrate which symptoms? *(Select all that apply.)*
    a. Laryngeal edema
    b. Hypoxemia
    c. Hypocapnia
    d. Dehydration
    e. Crackles
    f. Wheezing
    g. Dry mouth

28. For the patient with anaphylaxis described above, what would the nurse expect to find?
    a. Hypertension and rapid, weak pulse
    b. Hypotension and rapid, weak pulse
    c. Hypertension and rapid, bounding pulse
    d. Hypotension and rapid, bounding pulse

True or False? Reach each statement and write T for true or F for false in the blanks provided. If the statement is false, correct the statement to make it true.

_____ 29. Rhinitis may or may not be an allergic response.

_____ 30. Desensitization therapy can last 5 years.

_____ 31. After the proper dose of epinephrine is administered to a patient having an anaphylactic reaction, the nurse must wait 60 minutes before repeating the dose.

_____ 32. The body's response to epinephrine is constriction of the blood vessels, increased myocardial contractions, and dilation of bronchioles.

_____ 33. The anaphylactic patient should be observed for fluid overload.

_____ 34. Latex allergies are manifested only in dermatitis, so latex-free gloves are the only necessary precaution for those with a latex allergy.

_____ 35. A person who is allergic to bananas must be aware of the possibility that he or she could develop a latex allergy.

_____ 36. In a type III immune complex reaction, the deposited immune complex activates complement, and tissue and vessel damage results.

_____ 37. Benadryl is the oral drug of choice for type IV delayed hypersensitivity reactions.

_____ 38. Patients with a history of allergy to bee stings should carry a prescription for injectable epinephrine at all times.

39. The nurse is assessing the patient experiencing a cytotoxic reaction to IV drugs. What does the nurse do first?
    a. Discontinue drug administration.
    b. Decrease the infusion rate.
    c. Call the health care provider.
    d. Increase the IV fluid rate.

40. What are the clinical manifestations of systemic lupus erythematosus that are caused by immune complex reaction?
    a. Vasculitis, nephritis, arthritis
    b. Hypertension, anemia
    c. Destruction of mucus-producing glands
    d. Increased urinary output

41. Serum sickness occurs less frequently than in the past for what reason?
    a. Vaccines are no longer made from horse and rabbit serum.
    b. Patients have become less sensitive to allergens.
    c. Penicillin and related drugs and some animal serums are antitoxins.
    d. Manufacturing techniques produce vaccines that contain fewer impurities.

42. Which responses are characterized as type IV delayed hypersensitivity reactions? *(Select all that apply.)*
    a. Positive PPD test for tuberculosis
    b. Anaphylaxis after insect sting
    c. Thrombocytopenic purpura
    d. Contact dermatitis
    e. Graft rejection

43. What is the most important aspect of treating type V stimulating reactions?
    a. Medication management and observation for adverse effects
    b. Removing stimulated tissue to return the organ to normal functioning
    c. Monitoring for other organ involvement
    d. Surgical removal of secondary immune tissue

44. Which description best characterizes autoimmunity?
    a. Cell-mediated immune response that does not cause an antibody-mediated response
    b. The synthetic substances used to stimulate or suppress the response of the immune system
    c. Inappropriate immune response to one's own healthy cells and tissues
    d. An altered immune response that results in an immediate hypersensitivity reaction

45. Which disorders are types of autoimmune diseases? *(Select all that apply.)*
    a. Polyarteritis nodosa
    b. Systemic lupus erythematosus
    c. Hypothyroidism
    d. Rheumatic fever
    e. Hashimoto's thyroiditis

46. Autoimmune diseases occur mostly in which group of women?
    a. African American
    b. Asian American
    c. White
    d. Hispanic

47. In whom does Sjögren's syndrome mostly appear?
    a. Men 35 to 40 years of age
    b. Women younger than 25 years of age
    c. Women 35 to 40 years of age
    d. Men and women 35 to 40 years of age

48. What is the most common cause of Sjögren's syndrome thought to be?
    a. A bacterial infection
    b. A viral infection
    c. Inflammation
    d. An allergic reaction

49. The nurse suspects Sjögren's syndrome because the patient reports which common symptoms? *(Select all that apply.)*
    a. Increased tooth decay
    b. Burning and itching of the eyes
    c. Painful intercourse
    d. Nosebleeds
    e. Shortness of breath

50. The nurse expects the lab values on the patient with Sjögren's syndrome to include which results? *(Select all that apply.)*
    a. Increased presence of general antinuclear antibodies
    b. Elevated levels of IgM rheumatoid factor
    c. Decreased presence of anti-SS-A or anti-SS-B antibodies
    d. Decreased erythrocyte sedimentation rate
    e. Increased circulating platelets

Matching. Match each symptom with the appropriate intervention/treatment. Some treatments are used for more than one symptom.

Symptoms

a. Dry eyes
b. Dry mouth
c. Vaginal dryness
d. Pain control

Treatments

_____ 51. Water-soluble lubricants

_____ 52. Artificial tears

_____ 53. Systemic pilocarpine

_____ 54. Room humidifiers

_____ 55. Artificial saliva

_____ 56. Blocking tear outflow duct

_____ 57. Nonsteroidal anti-inflammatory drugs (NSAIDs)

58. Goodpasture's syndrome is a disorder of auto-antibodies against which body components?
   a. Skin cells and vascular tissue
   b. Hepatic support cells and RBCs
   c. Glomerular basement membrane and neutrophils
   d. Capillary walls and intima

59. What do the symptoms of Goodpasture's syndrome include? *(Select all that apply.)*
   a. Hemoptysis
   b. Increased urine output
   c. Bradycardia
   d. Shortness of breath
   e. Weight loss
   f. Generalized edema

60. Which organ is often damaged which can cause death in Goodpasture's syndrome?
   a. Heart
   b. Liver
   c. Thyroid
   d. Kidney

61. The patient has been diagnosed with Goodpasture's syndrome. Which drug therapy does the nurse expect to administer?
   a. Corticosteroids
   b. Vasopressors
   c. Antibiotics
   d. Muscle relaxants

62. Plasmapheresis may be used to treat immune complex responses such as Goodpasture's syndrome. Which statement best describes this treatment?
   a. Blood is circulated through a machine that removes excess fluids.
   b. 300 to 500 mL of blood is intermittently removed to decrease immune complexes.
   c. Autoantibodies are removed from blood plasma.
   d. IV immunoglobulins (IVIGs) are infused.

63. Which nursing intervention is most important for the nurse to do before administering any drug or therapeutic agent to the patient?
   a. Ask the patient about allergies to drugs or other substances.
   b. Compare the wristband name with the drug administration record.
   c. Verify the order with the prescriber.
   d. Calculate the prescribed drug dosage twice.

64. The patient who had a PPD test has redness and a 9 mm induration at the injection site. The nurse suspects which type of hypersensitivity reaction?
   a. Type I, immediate
   b. Type II, cytotoxic
   c. Type III, immune complex-mediated
   d. Type IV, delayed

65. The patient reports a runny nose with clear drainage, watery eyes, and a scratchy throat. The nurse determines the patient has been in close contact with several cats. Which hypersensitivity reaction does the nurse suspect the patient is experiencing?
    a. Type I, immediate
    b. Type II, cytotoxic
    c. Type III, immune complex-mediated
    d. Type IV, delayed

66. The nurse is assessing the patient with shortness of breath, hemoptysis, tachycardia, and generalized edema. Which autoimmune disorder does the nurse suspect this patient is experiencing?
    a. Goodpasture's syndrome
    b. Transplant reaction
    c. Glomerulonephritis
    d. Hemolytic reaction

CASE STUDY: THE PATIENT WITH HYPERSENSITIVITY

Use a separate sheet of paper to answer the questions in this Case Study. Answer guidelines for this Case Study are available on your Evolve website at http://evolve. elsevier.com/Iggy/ in the "Prepare for Class" folder.

A 62-year-old woman is admitted for total knee replacement surgery. Following surgery, cefazolin sodium (Ancef), 2 g, was ordered to be given intravenous piggyback (IVPB) every 8 hours for 24 hours. She received her first dose when she arrived at the orthopedic unit after surgery. Vital signs upon arrival: BP 136/84, P 88, R 12, T 98.8° F.

1. The patient has a history of allergy to penicillins. With this history, what type of hypersensitivity reaction is this patient most likely to experience?

Thirty minutes after the medication was started, the patient calls the nurse and reports "itching all over" and difficulty breathing. The nurse notes facial edema and audible wheezing. The patient's skin is red with large, swollen blotches over her arms, trunk, and back. Her systolic blood pressure is 118/78, pulse 108, and respirations 24. The IVPB antibiotic bag has infused about three-fourths of the dose.

2. What should the nurse's *first* action be?

3. The nurse stays with the patient to monitor her condition. What must the nurse observe for during this time?

4. What medications and by what route should the nurse expect the physician to prescribe? Explain the rationale for the medications used in this situation. What other interventions should follow?

5. What precautions should have been taken by the health care provider to prevent this problem?

23 CHAPTER

Cancer Development

STUDY/REVIEW QUESTIONS

1. Nurses have an important role in which components of cancer care? *(Select all that apply.)*
   a. Diagnosis of cancer
   b. Education of the public regarding cancer prevention
   c. Education of the public regarding early detection
   d. Education of the public regarding cancer treatment
   e. Treatment modalities for cancer

2. Which statement is true about hypertrophy and hyperplasia?
   a. Hypertrophy and hyperplasia are the same, except that one is in an organ and the other is in tissue.
   b. Hypertrophy is the expansion of cells; hyperplasia is an increased number of cells.
   c. Hypertrophy is an increase in the number of cells; hyperplasia is the expansion of cells.
   d. Hypertrophy is a decrease in the number of cells; hyperplasia is the shrinkage of cells.

3. Which are characteristics of neoplasia? *(Select all that apply.)*
   a. New or continued cell growth that is not needed for tissue replacement
   b. Is always malignant
   c. Has a parent cell that was normal
   d. Typically leads to death
   e. Is always abnormal
   f. Some cause no harm

4. Which statements about cell mitosis are true? *(Select all that apply.)*
   a. It is a term for cell division.
   b. Mitosis occurs to develop normal tissue.
   c. Mitosis occurs to replace damaged or lost tissue.
   d. Mitosis occurs randomly throughout the life cycle.
   e. *Apoptosis* is another term for mitosis.
   f. Mitosis occurs only when body conditions and nutrition are appropriate.

True or False? Write T for true or F for false in the blanks provided. If the statement is false, correct the statement to make it true.

_____ 5. Normal body cells are recognized by their appearance, size, and shape.

_____ 6. Each cell in the body performs one special function that contributes to homeostasis.

_____ 7. All cells produce fibronectin, which binds them closely together so they do not migrate.

_____ 8. All cells capable of mitosis have a specific pattern or cycle they follow.

_____ 9. Most cells in the body spend their existence in a reproductive resting state, or M phase, of the cell cycle.

_____ 10. Embryonic cells are aneuploid.

_____ 11. Cell division (mitosis) happens throughout our lives at a well-controlled rate to maintain the tissues and organs.

_____ 12. *Pluripotency* is a term referring to the flexibility of embryonic cells to mature into any cell.

_____ 13. Anaplasia is a term which refers to the cell's distinct shape and differentiation, causing the cell to closely resemble the parent cell.

14. How is a gene that is "turned on" described?
    a. Repressed
    b. Suppressed
    c. Expressed
    d. Depressed

15. Benign cells have which characteristics? *(Select all that apply.)*
    a. Tissue unnecessary for normal function
    b. Resemble the parent tissue
    c. Have a small nucleus
    d. Perform their differentiated function
    e. Invade other tissues
    f. Nonmigratory
    g. Aneuploid

16. Which statements are true of cancer cells? *(Select all that apply.)*
    a. They are slow-growing.
    b. Cancer cells divide nearly continuously.
    c. They are harmful to the body.
    d. They are abnormal.
    e. Cancer cells contain a small nucleus.
    f. They have an unlimited life span.

17. Why do cancer cells spread throughout the body? *(Select all that apply.)*
    a. They make little fibronectin.
    b. They are able to metastasize.
    c. They are persistent in their growth.
    d. Cell division occurs under adverse conditions.
    e. They have only one enzyme on their surface.

18. Which are actions of carcinogens? *(Select all that apply.)*
    a. Damage the DNA
    b. Change the activity of a cell
    c. Turn off proto-oncogenes
    d. Create allergic reactions
    e. Begin the initiation step of carcinogenesis

True or False? *Write T for true or F for false in the blanks provided. If the statement is false, correct the statement to make it true.*

_____ 19. If growth conditions are right, widespread metastatic disease can develop from just one cancer cell.

_____ 20. In carcinogenesis and oncogenesis, a normal cell undergoes malignant transformation.

_____ 21. Initiators start irreversible mutations in a normal cell.

_____ 22. Once a cell has been initiated, it is a recognizable tumor.

_____ 23. As the tumor cells grow, there are changes within the tumor cells themselves allowing for "selection advantages."

24. Which characteristics describe the initiated cell's responses to the promoter? *(Select all that apply.)*
    a. Promoted or enhanced cell growth
    b. Shortened latency period
    c. Lengthened latency period
    d. Metastasis
    e. Irreversible changes in the cell

25. Promoters may include which factors? *(Select all that apply.)*
    a. Chemicals
    b. Hormones
    c. Drugs
    d. Antibodies
    e. Viruses

26. If a primary tumor is located in a vital organ, what happens?
    a. The organ's rate of cell division is increased.
    b. The organ's response to injury is decreased.
    c. There is interference with the organ's functioning.
    d. Function of the organ is initially increased.

27. Which statement correctly describes metastatic tumors?
    a. They are caused by cells breaking off from the primary tumor.
    b. They become less malignant over time.
    c. They are usually less harmful than a primary tumor.
    d. They become the tissue of the organ where they spread.

28. During metastasis, which actions take place? *(Select all that apply.)*
    a. Tumor vascularization results in blood supply to the tumor.
    b. Enzymes open up pores in the patient's blood vessels.
    c. Clumps of the cells break off for transport.
    d. Cells stop circulating and then invade.
    e. Increased tumor size causes invasion of surrounding tissues.

True or False? Write T for true or F for false in the blanks provided.

_____ 29. Brain tumors usually metastasize only within the central nervous system.

_____ 30. During metastasis, local seeding takes place near the primary site.

_____ 31. Lymphatic spread is usually to primary sites with few lymph nodes.

32. Which characteristics describe a "high-grade" tumor? *(Select all that apply.)*
    a. Barely resembles the parent cell
    b. Slow-growing
    c. Rapidly metastasizes
    d. Easiest to cure
    e. Very aggressive

33. Which information can be obtained from grading a tumor?
    a. Cause of the cancer
    b. Location of metastasis
    c. Cell differentiation
    d. How long the cancer has been present

34. What is performed during clinical staging of suspected cancer?
    a. Clinical tests
    b. Biopsy
    c. Major surgery
    d. Radiation therapy

35. What are the primary factors influencing the development of cancer? *(Select all that apply.)*
    a. Environmental exposure to carcinogens
    b. Gender of the patient
    c. Genetic predisposition
    d. Immune function
    e. Health history

36. Indicate whether cancer arises commonly (C) or rarely (R) from each of the following tissues or organs in adults.
    _____ a. Heart muscle
    _____ b. Bone marrow
    _____ c. Skin
    _____ d. Nerve tissue
    _____ e. Lining of the gastrointestinal tract
    _____ f. Lining of the lungs
    _____ g. Skeletal muscle

37. Which statements are true about tobacco and cancer risk? *(Select all that apply.)*
    a. Tobacco is considered an initiator of cancer.
    b. Tobacco is considered a promoter of cancer.
    c. A person's risk for cancer depends on the amount of tobacco use.
    d. A person's risk for cancer depends on the type of tobacco use.
    e. Those who receive secondhand tobacco smoke have the same risk for cancer as those in direct contact with tobacco smoke.

38. Ionizing radiation is found in which elements? *(Select all that apply.)*
    a. Radon
    b. Uranium
    c. Soil
    d. Water
    e. Medical x-rays

39. Which factors are forms of UV radiation? *(Select all that apply.)*
    a. Sun (solar)
    b. Tanning beds
    c. Medical x-rays
    d. Radon
    e. Germicidal lights

40. A few viruses are known as *oncoviruses* because they perform which actions? *(Select all that apply.)*
    a. Infect the cell
    b. Break the DNA chain
    c. Insert their own genetic material
    d. Mutate the cell's DNA
    e. Grow slowly

41. How does the immune system protect the body from cancer? *(Select all that apply.)*
    a. By using cell-mediated immunity
    b. By using natural killer cells
    c. By using antibody-mediated immunity
    d. By using helper T-cells
    e. Identifying cancer cells as "non-self" cells

42. Which people are considered to be at greater risk for developing cancer? *(Select all that apply.)*
    a. Organ transplant recipients
    b. Adults over the age of 60
    c. People with AIDS
    d. African Americans
    e. People who are immunocompromised

43. For which types of cancer is risk modifiable? *(Select all that apply.)*
    a. Breast
    b. Colon
    c. Ovarian
    d. Prostate
    e. Cervical
    f. Lymphatic

44. Which are cancers that have genetic predisposition? *(Select all that apply.)*
    a. Breast
    b. Colorectal
    c. Melanoma
    d. Bladder
    e. Lung

45. Which group has the highest rate of incidence, death rate, and largest increase in incidence of cancer?
    a. Whites
    b. Hispanics
    c. African Americans
    d. Asian Americans

46. Which patient would have the best prognosis for survival based on the TNM staging classification listed?
    a. $T_{IS}N_0M_0$
    b. $T_xN_xM_x$
    c. $T_2N_1M_0$
    d. $T_2N_3M_1$

47. The American Cancer Society reports that the cancer incidence and survival rate are related to which factors? *(Select all that apply.)*
    a. Gender
    b. Availability of health care services
    c. Early health care
    d. Age
    e. Race

48. Which are included in the seven warning signs of cancer? *(Select all that apply.)*
    a. Hoarseness
    b. A thickening lump
    c. Obvious change in a mole
    d. Inability of a sore to heal
    e. Difficulty swallowing

49. Which are dietary practices that may help reduce the risk of cancer? *(Select all that apply.)*
    a. Low-fat diet
    b. Avoidance of nitrates
    c. Eating foods high in vitamins A and C
    d. Maximize intake of red meat
    e. Increase fiber intake

50. Which measures are considered secondary prevention for cancer? *(Select all that apply.)*
    a. Yearly mammography for women over age 40
    b. Avoidance of tobacco
    c. Yearly fecal occult blood testing in adults
    d. Removing colon polyps
    e. Using sunscreen when outdoors
    f. Colonoscopy at age 50 and then every 10 years
    g. Chemoprevention with vitamin therapy

24 CHAPTER

Care of Patients with Cancer

STUDY/REVIEW QUESTIONS

1. Which type of cancer puts patients at greatest risk for infection?
   a. Breast cancer
   b. Leukemia
   c. Lung cancer
   d. Prostate cancer

2. Cancer invading the bone marrow can cause which effects? *(Select all that apply.)*
   a. Hypokalemia
   b. Decreased RBCs
   c. Pathologic fractures
   d. Degenerative joint disease
   e. Thrombocytopenia

3. How is cachexia described?
   a. Electrolyte imbalance in the patient with cancer
   b. Decreased cognition and confusion
   c. Extreme body wasting and malnutrition
   d. Chemotherapy-induced nausea and vomiting

4. Which statement about gastrointestinal function and cancer is true?
   a. Only cancers within the gastrointestinal system alter gastrointestinal function.
   b. Gaining weight during cancer therapy indicates successful treatment.
   c. A low-fat diet improves survival rates for people with cancer.
   d. The liver is a common site of cancer metastasis.

5. Which common hematologic conditions result from cancer invading the bone marrow? *(Select all that apply.)*
   a. Cachexia
   b. Anemia
   c. Bruising
   d. Thrombocytopenia
   e. Bleeding

True or False? Write T for true or F for false in the blanks provided. If the statement is false, correct the statement to make it true.

_____ 6. Pain is present with all cancers.

_____ 7. Patients with lung cancer can develop pulmonary edema and dyspnea.

_____ 8. The primary goal of cancer treatment is to cure the patient.

_____ 9. Surgery for a cancer patient may be a part of diagnosis or treatment.

10. The patient asks the nurse why untreated cancers cause gastrointestinal problems. What is the nurse's best response?
    a. "A tumor in the bowel can decrease your ability to absorb necessary nutrients."
    b. "The tumor makes you not feel hungry or thirsty and affects your urinary output."
    c. "It stops the absorption of necessary fat and protein enzymes."
    d. "Cancers in the GI tract are known to cause related bowel problems."

11. Which factors determine the type of therapy for cancer? *(Select all that apply.)*
    a. Type and location of cancer
    b. Overall health of the patient
    c. Whether the cancer has metastasized
    d. Family history and genetics
    e. Previous lymph node biopsy

12. Which example illustrates appropriate prophylactic cancer surgery?
    a. Excision of lesions shown on biopsy to be "precancerous"
    b. Removing part of a tumor to provide pain relief
    c. Removal of a mole that is often irritated by the patient's waistband
    d. Breast reconstruction after a mastectomy

13. What is the purpose of cytoreductive surgery for cancer?
    a. Cancer prevention by removal of "at-risk" tissue
    b. Cancer control by reducing the size of the tumor
    c. Cancer cure by removing all gross and microscopic tumor tissue
    d. Improving the function or appearance of a previously treated body area

14. Palliative surgery may be performed for which reasons? *(Select all that apply.)*
    a. Relieving pain
    b. Relieving an obstruction
    c. Curing the cancer
    d. Diagnostic staging
    e. Destroying the tumor

15. For what purposes may cancer survivors need reconstructive surgery? *(Select all that apply.)*
    a. Breast reconstruction
    b. Revision of scars and release of contractures
    c. Bowel reconstruction
    d. Pain relief
    e. Increase organ function

16. What is an appropriate nursing diagnosis for the postsurgical patient who has lost a body part?
    a. Dysfunctional Grieving
    b. Disturbed Body Image
    c. Anxiety
    d. Chronic Sorrow

True or False? *Read the statements about radiation therapy and write T for true or F for false in the blanks provided. If the statement is false, correct the statement to make it true.*

_____ 17. Cell damage occurs with any exposure to radiation, which may cause the cell to die or lose the ability to divide.

_____ 18. The dosage of radiation is commonly determined by cell cycle.

_____ 19. Normal cells are not damaged during radiation therapy.

_____ 20. Each cell has its own response to radiation, such as dying, becoming sterile, or repairing itself.

_____ 21. The goal of radiation therapy is to administer enough treatment to kill all of the cancer cells.

_____ 22. Brachytherapy involves the use of isotopes placed on or near the cancer tissue, making the patient hazardous to others.

_____ 23. Unsealed radiation sources can be given orally, intravenously, or as an instillation in a body cavity, making patients and their excrement radioactive for 48 hours.

_____ 24. Needles and seeds for sealed radiation sources make the patient and his or her excrement radioactive.

_____ 25. Teletherapy is also called *beam therapy*.

26. What is the meaning of the "inverse square law" for radiation exposure?
    a. The further away a person is from a radiation source, the less radiation is absorbed.
    b. When chemotherapy is added to the treatment regimen, less radiation is needed.
    c. As the distance from the radiation source increases, more tumor cells are killed.
    d. Less radiation is needed if natural sources are used.

27. Which factors are used to determine the cancer patient's absorbed radiation dose? *(Select all that apply.)*
    a. Intensity of radiation exposure
    b. Proximity of radiation source to the cells
    c. Duration of exposure
    d. Age of the patient
    e. Previous radiation therapy

28. Why is the therapeutic dose of radiation fractionated for cancer treatment?
    a. To reduce total treatment cost
    b. To ensure a higher cancer cell kill with less damage to normal cells
    c. To prevent profound bone marrow suppression with resulting anemia
    d. To allow time for chemotherapy to first reduce the tumor size

29. At what point is the patient radioactive when receiving radiation treatment by teletherapy and therefore a potential danger to other people?
    a. The patient is never radioactive
    b. When the linear accelerator is turned on
    c. For the first 24 to 48 hours after treatment
    d. Until the radiation source has decayed by at least one half-life

30. What are the systemic side effects of radiation?
    a. Altered taste sensation and fatigue
    b. Skin changes and permanent local hair loss
    c. Diarrhea and tooth loss
    d. Immunosuppression and weight gain

31. For the patient undergoing external radiation therapy, what do the nurse's instructions include? *(Select all that apply.)*
    a. Do not remove the markings.
    b. Do not use lotions or ointments.
    c. Avoid direct skin exposure to sunlight for up to a year.
    d. Use soap and water on the affected skin.
    e. Do not rub treated areas.

32. Why does the nurse wear a dosimeter when providing care to the patient receiving brachytherapy?
    a. Indicate special expertise in radiation therapy
    b. Protect the nurse from absorbing radiation
    c. Determine the amount of radiation exposure experienced
    d. Ensure that the radiation source remains active

33. What is the rationale for chemotherapy as a cancer treatment?
    a. Less expensive and safer than radiation therapy
    b. Decreases the patient's risk for life-threatening complications
    c. Systemic treatment for cancer cells that may have escaped from the primary tumor
    d. Concentrates in secondary lymphoid tissues and prevents widespread metastasis

Matching. Match each type of chemotherapy with the corresponding action.

Chemotherapy

a. Antimitotic agents
b. Topoisomerase inhibitor
c. Antimetabolites
d. Alkylating agent

Type of Action

_____ 34. "Counterfeit" chemicals that fool cancer cells into using them, but prevent cell division

_____ 35. Causes major damage to DNA and RNA synthesis

_____ 36. Cross-links DNA; prevents RNA synthesis

_____ 37. A plant source that interferes with formation of microtubules

38. What is the lowest level of bone marrow activity and WBCs called?
    a. Anemia
    b. Nadir
    c. Leukopenia
    d. Immunosuppression

39. Each chemotherapeutic agent has a specific nadir. What is important to do when giving combination therapy?
    a. Give two agents with like nadirs.
    b. Avoid giving agents with like nadirs at the same time.
    c. Allow for one agent's nadir to recover before giving another agent.
    d. Give two agents from the same drug class.

40. Chemotherapy drug dosage is based on total body surface area (TBSA); therefore, what is it important for the nurse to do?
    a. Ask the patient's height and weight.
    b. Weigh and measure the patient.
    c. Assess body mass index.
    d. Measure abdominal girth.

41. What does a course of chemotherapy normally include? *(Select all that apply.)*
    a. Rounds every week for a total of 6 weeks
    b. Variance with patient's responses to therapy
    c. Timed dosing of the therapy to minimize normal cell damage
    d. A concurrent dose of radiation
    e. The administration of one specific anticancer drug

42. Most chemotherapy is administered intravenously. What is the major potential complication?
    a. Electrolyte imbalance
    b. Bruising
    c. Extravasation
    d. Thrombus formation

43. Which side effect of chemotherapy is most serious?
    a. Nausea and vomiting
    b. Peripheral neuropathy
    c. Bone marrow suppression
    d. Dry desquamation of the skin

44. The nurse administering a vesicant must be prepared for complications and must have knowledge of which information?
    a. The antidote
    b. The pH of the vesicant
    c. How to use hot or cold packs
    d. Type of available dressings

45. Indicate which chemotherapeutic agents are vesicants (V) and which are irritants (I).

    _____ a. Daunorubicin
    _____ b. Mitomycin C
    _____ c. Bleomycin
    _____ d. Vincristine
    _____ e. Paclitaxel

46. When thinning or loss of hair is a known side effect of a drug being administered, what does the nurse do? *(Select all that apply.)*
    a. Have the patient use gentle hair shampoo.
    b. Help the patient select wigs, turbans, or scarves.
    c. Instruct the patient that hair loss is permanent.
    d. Remind the patient to avoid washing the hair.
    e. Suggest complementary and alternative therapies to the patient.

47. Which statements are true regarding nausea and vomiting related to chemotherapy administration? *(Select all that apply.)*
    a. It is a common side effect of emetogenic agents.
    b. It usually lasts for 1 to 2 days after administration.
    c. It lasts as long as 3 weeks after administration.
    d. It is purely psychosomatic.
    e. Most chemotherapy drugs do not induce vomiting.

48. Which phrase best describes stomatitis?
    a. Lesions located in the GI tract
    b. An infection within the stomach lining
    c. A generalized infection within the bowel lining
    d. Sores located in the mouth

49. Because of the rapid cell division in the gastrointestinal tract, what is the effect of chemotherapy?
    a. Kills off the cells immediately
    b. Prevents the body from replacing cells
    c. Causes cells to be killed more rapidly than they can be produced
    d. Helps to increase cell division

50. What techniques are included in oral care for the patient with stomatitis? *(Select all that apply.)*
    a. Observation
    b. Hard-bristled tooth brush
    c. Saline mouthwash
    d. Glycerin swabs
    e. Commercial mouthwashes
    f. Petrolatum jelly to lips after each mouth care

51. Bone marrow suppression causes a decrease in which bodily components to occur? *(Select all that apply.)*
    a. Leukocytes
    b. Parenchyma
    c. Erythrocytes
    d. Platelets
    e. Blood

52. What clinical manifestations does the nurse expect in the patient who has chemotherapy-induced bone marrow suppression? *(Select all that apply.)*
    a. Alopecia
    b. Fatigue
    c. Bleeding gums
    d. Dry skin
    e. Diarrhea
    f. Pallor

True or False? *Read each statement about biological response modifiers and write T for true or F for false in the blanks provided.*

_____ 53. Biological response modifier drugs stimulate the immune system to produce cells.

_____ 54. The most important role of biological response modifiers is the prevention of cancer development.

55. The nurse is responsible for teaching both the immunosuppressed patient and the family about health promoting activities. Which is the most important activity to teach?
    a. Handwashing
    b. Isolation
    c. Boiling dishes
    d. Wearing masks

Matching. *Match each biological response modifier to its action.*

Modifiers

a. Interleukins
b. Interferons
c. Monoclonal antibodies

Actions

_____ 56. Bind with cell and prevent cell division

_____ 57. Help immune system recognize and destroy cancer cells

_____ 58. Help cancer cells revert to original characteristics

59. The biological response modifiers have which positive effect on the patient receiving chemotherapy?
    a. Less risk of life-threatening infections
    b. Reduced incidence of alopecia
    c. Reduced severity of nausea
    d. Euphoria and increased libido

60. Side effects of interleukin therapy can be dramatic. The patient may need to be treated in a critical care unit for which side effects? *(Select all that apply.)*
    a. Fluid shifts
    b. Severe inflammatory reaction
    c. Capillary leak
    d. Nausea and vomiting
    e. Tissue swelling

61. What are common immediate reactions to biological response modifier therapy?
    a. Fever, chills, nausea and vomiting, malaise
    b. Fever, chills, rigor, malaise
    c. Hypertension, constipation
    d. Hives, diarrhea, low back pain

62. The patient with cancer tells the nurse she has numbness and weakness in her legs. What is the nurse's best response?
    a. "Are you having any back pain?"
    b. "Have you been exercising vigorously?"
    c. "When was your last dose of pain medication?"
    d. "Don't worry. This is a normal response to chemotherapy."

63. Which manifestation and/or piece of laboratory data alerts the nurse to the possibility of syndrome of inappropriate antidiuretic hormone (SIADH) in the patient who has cancer?
    a. Tall T-waves on ECG and hyperkalemia
    b. Positive Chvostek's sign and hypocalcemia
    c. Kussmaul respirations and hypochloremia
    d. Weight gain of 6 lbs. and hyponatremia

Matching. *Match the colony stimulating factor (CSF) agent with the type of cell affected.*

CSF Agents

a. Sargramostim (Leukine)
b. Epoietin alfa (Epogen, Procrit)
c. Filgrastim (Neupogen)
d. Oprelvekin (Neumega)

Cell Types

_____ 64. Erythrocytes

_____ 65. Neutrophils

_____ 66. Platelets

_____ 67. Monocytes and macrophages

68. The patient with lymphoma reports severe facial swelling, tightness of the gown collar, and epistaxis. Which complication does the nurse suspect?
    a. Tumor lysis syndrome
    b. Cancer-induced hypercalcemia
    c. Superior vena cava syndrome
    d. Congestive heart failure

69. Which condition is a common cause of death in patients with cancer?
    a. Myeloid leukemia
    b. Sepsis
    c. Allergic reactions
    d. Blood transfusions

70. The patient has a diagnosis of cancer with a gram-negative infection. The nurse assesses bleeding from many sites throughout the body. For which condition does the nurse expect to perform nursing interventions?
    a. Sepsis
    b. Anemia
    c. Disseminated intravascular coagulation
    d. SIADH

71. The patient diagnosed with bone cancer reports fatigue, loss of appetite, and constipation. Which laboratory result does the nurse report immediately?
    a. Potassium level of 4.2 mEq/L
    b. Magnesium level of 2.0 mg/dL
    c. Sodium level of 14 mEq/L
    d. Calcium level of 10.5 mEq/dL

72. The patient with advanced breast cancer reports severe back pain and leg weakness. Based on these symptoms, what does the nurse suspect?
    a. Isolated limb perfusion
    b. Lower back cancer
    c. Spinal cord compression
    d. Bladder tumor

CASE STUDY: THE PATIENT RECEIVING CHEMOTHERAPY

Use a separate sheet of paper to answer the questions in this Case Study. Answer guidelines for this Case Study are available on your Evolve website at http://evolve. elsevier.com/Iggy/ in the "Prepare for Class" folder.

A 63-year-old woman is seen in the cancer therapy unit for her first round of chemotherapy for breast cancer. She had a lumpectomy 2 months ago and a double-lumen peripherally inserted central catheter (PICC) line inserted at that time. Her medications include 5-fluorouracil (Adrucil), ifosfamide (Ifex), and mesna (Mesnex). Ondansetron (Zofran) is ordered for nausea.

1. How does the nurse explain to the patient what the drug mesna is for and why it is being administered?

2. Before giving chemotherapy, the nurse prepares to give the ondansetron. The patient asks why she is getting that medication "when I'm not even nauseated." How should the nurse answer the patient?

3. After 10 days, the patient comes to the office for follow-up laboratory work. The results are as follows:
   - Sodium: 135 mEq/L
   - Potassium: 3.7 mEq/L
   - Hemoglobin: 8.5 g/dL
   - Hematocrit: 25%
   - Red blood cells: 2.3 million/mm^3
   - White blood cells: 2.8 mm^3
   - Platelets: 45,000 mm^3/mL

   Which laboratory values are expected at this time? What is the cause of these altered laboratory values?

4. What, if anything, can be done to protect this patient during this period? What other drugs may be ordered at this time?

25 CHAPTER

Care of Patients with Infection

STUDY/REVIEW QUESTIONS

Matching. *Match the terms related to infection to their correct definitions.*

Terms
a. Communicable
b. Reservoirs
c. Pathogen
d. Pathogenicity
e. Colonization
f. Susceptible host
g. Virulence
h. Normal flora

Definitions

_____ 1. Cause agent

_____ 2. Infection recipient

_____ 3. Ability to cause disease

_____ 4. Degree of communicability

_____ 5. Characteristic bacteria

_____ 6. Pathogenic microbes present but no symptoms

_____ 7. Sources of infectious agents

_____ 8. Transmitted from person to person

9. Transmissions of infection require a reservoir. Which is an example of an animate reservoir?
   a. People
   b. Water
   c. Soil
   d. IV solution

Matching. *Match each type of pathogen with its description.*

Pathogens
a. Toxin
b. Exotoxin
c. Endotoxin

Descriptions

_____ 10. Substances produced and released by certain bacteria, such as tetanus and diphtheria, into the surrounding environment

_____ 11. Substances produced in cell walls of certain bacteria, such as typhoid, and released by cell lysis

_____ 12. Protein molecules released by bacteria to affect host cells at distant sites

13. Which factors increase the patient's susceptibility to infection? *(Select all that apply.)*
    a. Alcohol consumption
    b. Steroid use
    c. Diabetes mellitus
    d. Nicotine use
    e. Oral contraceptives
    f. High-protein diet
    g. Advanced age

14. Which nursing intervention best decreases the patient's susceptibility to infection?
    a. Using standard precautions
    b. Removing soiled linens
    c. Restricting all visitors
    d. Avoiding direct contact

Matching. *Match the portal of entry with its method of transmission. Answers may be used more than once.*

Portals of Entry
a. Bloodstream
b. Skin/mucous membrane
c. Genitourinary tract
d. Gastrointestinal tract
e. Respiratory tract

Methods of Transmission

_____ 15. Droplet

_____ 16. Ingestion

_____ 17. Intravascular device

_____ 18. Insect bite

_____ 19. Catheterization

_____ 20. Laceration

Matching. *Match the contact site for infection to its mode of transmission. Answers may be used more than once.*

Modes of Transmission
a. Airborne
b. Vehicle
c. Vector
d. Direct
e. Indirect

Contact Sites

_____ 21. Skin-to-skin

_____ 22. Contaminated needle

_____ 23. Sneezing

_____ 24. Contaminated food

_____ 25. Lyme disease

True or False? *Read the statements about infection and write T for true or F for false in the blanks provided. If the statement is false, correct the statement to make it true.*

_____ 26. The portal of exit for an infection may be the same as the portal of entry.

_____ 27. The body's skin is the best barrier or defense against infection.

_____ 28. Phagocytosis decreases a patient's risk for infection.

_____ 29. The use of gloves eliminates the need to wash your hands.

_____ 30. Artificial nails have a low risk of spreading infection.

_____ 31. Nosocomial infection means that the infection was caused by health care staff.

32. Effective handwashing is vital in preventing the spread of infection. Place the steps of proper handwashing technique in the correct order using the numbers 1 through 4.

    _____ a. Apply friction under water for 15 seconds.

    _____ b. Wet, soap, and lather hands.

    _____ c. Rinse hands thoroughly.

    _____ d. Dry hands adequately.

33. Which situation requires using soap and water for handwashing?
    a. Before a sterile dressing change
    b. After removing sterile gloves
    c. Dry skin
    d. Hands feeling sticky

Matching. Match each precaution with the example of its use.

Precautions
a. Contact precautions
b. Droplet precautions
c. Standard precautions
d. Airborne precautions

Uses

_____ 34. All body secretions and excretions, most membranes and tissue, excluding perspiration, are potentially infectious.

_____ 35. Uses negative airflow rooms, high-efficiency particulate air (HEPA) filters, or ultraviolet (UV) lights.

_____ 36. Infection transmitted by droplet; an example is meningitis.

_____ 37. Transmission by touch of patient or environment; examples are methicillin-resistant *Staphylococcus aureus* (MRSA) and vancomycin-resistant *Enterococcus* (VRE).

38. How are complications of infection usually caused? *(Select all that apply.)*
    a. Incorrect choice of antibiotic
    b. Poor patient compliance
    c. Patient unable to afford medication
    d. The patient's overall health condition
    e. The patient taking too much of the prescribed medication

39. A localized infection may include which symptoms? *(Select all that apply.)*
    a. Chills
    b. Cool and clammy skin
    c. Fever
    d. Pain
    e. Pus
    f. Redness
    g. Swelling

Matching. *Match each diagnostic test with its description.*

Tests

a. Biopsy
b. Scanning
c. Ultrasonography
d. Radiographic studies
e. Erythrocyte sedimentation rate
f. Complete blood count
g. Culture
h. Sensitivity

Descriptions

_____ 40. Pathogen is isolated for identification.

_____ 41. Pathogen is tested for antibiotic reactions.

_____ 42. Checks WBC, neutrophils, lymphocytes, monocytes, eosinophils, and basophils.

_____ 43. Measures rate of RBC fall through plasma; increased rate indicates infection or inflammation.

_____ 44. X-ray films used to monitor infection.

_____ 45. Noninvasive procedure: used particularly for diagnosing heart valve problems.

_____ 46. Use of radioactive agents to determine presence of inflammation.

_____ 47. Tissue specimen obtained for tissue culture.

48. The patient has had a bacterial infection for 3 days and laboratory results show the percentage of immature neutrophils has increased at a greater rate than mature neutrophils. How does the nurse interpret these findings?
    a. The patient is very sick and immunocompromised.
    b. There is a unilateral shift to the right in the differential.
    c. The infection was caused by antimicrobial agents.
    d. There is a shift to the left in the differential.

True or False? *Read the statements about infection and write T for true or F for false in the blanks provided. If the statement is false, correct the statement to make it true.*

_____ 49. Antibiotic therapy should not begin until after the culture specimen is obtained.

_____ 50. Patients with a temperature greater than 100° F are considered to have a systemic infection.

_____ 51. Older adult patients may have a severe infection with no fever.

_____ 52. A superinfection is an infection with an extremely resistant microbe.

53. In the patient with an infection, which common interventions may be used to reduce fever? *(Select all that apply.)*
    a. Antipyretic drugs such as aspirin or acetaminophen
    b. External cooling, cooling blankets, cool compresses
    c. Fluid administration, oral and IV
    d. Antimicrobial therapy with antibiotic, antiviral, or antifungal agents
    e. Opening the windows and door to the patient's room

54. Name the antimicrobials that correspond to each drug action listed below.

   a. Inhibits reproduction_____

    _____

   b. Injures the cytoplasmic membrane _____

    _____

   c. Inhibits nucleic acid synthesis _____

    _____

   d. Inhibits cell wall synthesis _____

    _____

55. The patient has been prescribed gentamicin drug therapy. Which nursing intervention ensures effective antimicrobial therapy?
   a. Avoid the use of acetaminophen while on this medication.
   b. Deliver a sufficient dosage and duration of therapy.
   c. Take the medication with food.
   d. Closely monitor the patient's temperature.

Matching. Match the organism to its disease manifestation.

Organisms
a. *Escherichia coli*
b. *Plasmodium* sp.
c. Pinworm
d. *Streptococcus sp.*
e. *Pneumocystis carinii*
f. *Entamoeba histolytica*
g. Rickettsiae
h. Rhinovirus
i. *Candida albicans*

Disease Manifestations
_____ 56. Rocky Mountain spotted fever
_____ 57. Thrush
_____ 58. Diarrhea
_____ 59. Common cold
_____ 60. Malaria
_____ 61. Urinary tract infection
_____ 62. Anal pruritus
_____ 63. Pharyngitis
_____ 64. Pneumonia

65. The patient is diagnosed with mycobacterium tuberculosis. Which nursing intervention does the nurse implement for this patient?
   a. Wash hands before and after entering the room.
   b. Ensure the patient has a private room with negative airflow.
   c. Use contact and droplet precautions.
   d. Place contaminated gloves outside the room.

66. Which body fluids are *likely* to transmit blood-borne diseases? *(Select all that apply.)*
   a. Feces
   b. Blood
   c. Semen
   d. Sputum
   e. Breast milk

67. The patient reports fever, chills, headache, and swollen glands in the groin and axillary areas. When the nurse assesses multiple reddened areas on both lower extremities, the patient states, "Those are flea bites from the refugee camp mission that I went to." What does the nurse suspect?
   a. Plague (*Yersinia pestis*)
   b. Erythema multiforme (Stevens-Johnson syndrome)
   c. Smallpox (variola virus)
   d. Measles (rubeola)

68. The patient who had previously reported flu-like symptoms which seemed to be improving woke up today with severe dyspnea, tachycardia, fever, and diaphoresis. What does the nurse suspect?
   a. Meningitis
   b. Influenza
   c. Inhalation anthrax (*Bacillus anthracis*)
   d. Respiratory syncytial virus

69. The patient who has returned from a camping trip reports severe vomiting and diarrhea and is experiencing symmetrical flaccid paralysis. The patient reports eating mostly canned foods during the trip. What does the nurse suspect?
   a. Meningitis
   b. Botulism
   c. Variola virus
   d. Inhalation anthrax

70. The nurse is caring for multiple patients in a temporary hospital after severe flooding in the area. Several patients have high fever, headache, and a papular rash over the face and extremities, including the palms of the hands. Some of the skin lesions are vesicular and pustular. What does the nurse suspect?
   a. Pandemic infection
   b. Superinfection
   c. Plague (*Yersinia pestis*)
   d. Smallpox (variola virus)

26 CHAPTER

Assessment of the Skin, Hair, and Nails

STUDY/REVIEW QUESTIONS

Matching. Match each property with its appropriate layer of skin.

Layer of Skin
a. Fat
b. Dermis
c. Epidermis

Property

_____ 1.   Contains elastin

_____ 2.   Serves as insulator

_____ 3.   Contains no cells

_____ 4.   Collagen is main component

_____ 5.   Does not have a separate blood supply

_____ 6.   Provides padding

_____ 7.   Innermost layer of skin

_____ 8.   Rich in sensory nerves

_____ 9.   Synthesis of vitamin D

_____ 10. Melanin production

11.   The dark-skinned patient is admitted for pneumonia. During shift report, the nurse learns that the patient is at risk for Ineffective Tissue Perfusion, Peripheral. How does the nurse assess for cyanosis?
a. Observe for shallow and rapid respirations.
b. Check the tongue and lips for a gray color.
c. Auscultate for decreased breath sounds throughout lung fields.
d. Inspect the palms and soles for a yellow-tinged color.

12.   The patient is at risk for fluid volume deficit. The nurse assesses this patient's skin using which assessment technique?
a. Brush the skin surface and observe for flaking.
b. Push on the skin and observe for blanching.
c. Gently pinch the skin on the chest and observe for tenting.
d. Push on the skin over the tibia and observe for depth of indentation.

13. The patient with a history of congestive heart failure goes to the outpatient clinic for a follow-up appointment. How does the nurse assess for dependent edema in this patient?
    a. Palpate the dorsum of the foot or the medial ankle.
    b. Weigh the patient and compare to the baseline weight.
    c. Check the patient's buttocks or lower back.
    d. Ask the patient about intake and output.

14. The nurse is assessing the skin of the older adult patient who is at risk for dehydration due to excessive vomiting. The skin appears dry and loose. Where is the best site for the nurse to check skin turgor on this patient?
    a. Facial cheek
    b. Upper arm
    c. Anterior chest
    d. Mid-thigh

15. The nurse is preparing patient education material about healthy skin. What is the single most important preventive health behavior the nurse promotes?
    a. Limit continuous sun exposure.
    b. Drink plenty of water.
    c. Practice good skin hygiene.
    d. Eat a well-balanced diet.

16. The thin and malnourished patient requires emergency abdominal surgery. After the operation, in order to promote wound healing, what does the nurse encourage?
    a. High-calorie diet
    b. Low-sodium and low-carbohydrate diet
    c. High-quality protein diet
    d. Low-fat diet with vitamin supplements

Matching. *Match the definition or characteristic of the integumentary system with the correct term.*

Terms
a. Elastin
b. Sebum
c. Lichenified
d. Pruritus
e. Petechiae
f. Ecchymoses
g. Macular
h. Papular
i. Turgor
j. Hirsutism

Defining Characteristics

_____ 17. Itching

_____ 18. Small, reddish-purple lesions that do not fade or blanch when pressure is applied

_____ 19. Raised rash

_____ 20. Skin becomes thickened

_____ 21. Lubricates the skin and reduces water loss from the skin surface

_____ 22. Indicates amount of skin elasticity

_____ 23. Excessive growth of body hair or hair growth in abnormal body areas

_____ 24. Large bruised areas of hemorrhage; vary in size

_____ 25. Fine, flat rash

_____ 26. Major component of the elastic fiber

27. The nursing student must perform a skin assessment on an older adult patient and observe for signs of skin breakdown. What does the student do to meet the clinical objective and demonstrate good time-management skills?
    a. Examine the skin while bathing or assist the patient with hygiene.
    b. Complete the assessment before the end of the clinical experience.
    c. Check to see if the primary nurse has already completed the assessment.
    d. Perform the examination when the patient willingly consents and agrees.

28. The nurse is caring for the patient who sustained trauma and blood loss. The patient is alert and anxious, blood pressure is low, and the heart rate is high. Which skin characteristics are most likely to manifest during impending shock?
    a. Dry, flushed appearance
    b. Cool, pale, moist skin
    c. Bluish color that blanches with pressure
    d. Poor turgor with a rough texture

29. The patient is being referred to a dermatologist for evaluation of a rash of unknown origin. The patient has trouble articulating specific information because of "nervousness." Which questions does the nurse use to help the patient practice for the specialist appointment? *(Select all that apply.)*
    a. "Why do you have the rash?"
    b. "When did you first notice the rash?"
    c. "Where on the body did the rash first start?"
    d. "How do you feel about the skin rash?"
    e. "Are you having an itching or burning sensation?"
    f. "What makes the problem better or worse?"
    g. "Have you been having fever or sore throat?"

30. In regulating body temperature, how much evaporative water loss can occur during hot weather or exercise?
    a. 600 mL/day
    b. 900 mL/day
    c. 2 L/day
    d. 10 to 12 L/day

31. The nurse is caring for the very dark-skinned patient who has high risk for thrombocytopenia. Which area of the patient's body is the best place to check for petechiae?
    a. Anterior chest
    b. Oral mucosa
    c. Palmar surface
    d. Periorbital area

32. The nurse is performing a skin assessment on the patient and notes an area on the forearm that feels hard or "woody." What does the nurse interpret this physical finding as?
    a. Inflammation
    b. Subcutaneous fat
    c. Psoriasis
    d. Skin cancer

True or False? Questions 33 through 40 pertain to integumentary changes in older adults. Write Y for yes if the described change occurs as a result of aging, or N for no if the change does not occur as a result of aging.

_____ 33. Decreased thickness in the epidermal layer results in increased skin transparency and fragility replacement.

_____ 34. Thinning of the fat layer decreases the susceptibility to hypothermia.

_____ 35. Increased active melanocytes result in decreased sensitivity to sun exposure.

_____ 36. Increased susceptibility to shearing forces results in blisters, purpura, skin tears, and pressure-related skin problems.

_____ 37. Decreased vitamin D production increases susceptibility to osteomalacia.

_____ 38. Decreased epidermal mitotic activity results in delayed wound healing.

_____ 39. Increased epidermal permeability decreases susceptibility to irritants.

_____ 40. Increased thermoregulatory alterations predispose to heat stroke.

41. The patient reports a rash that itches, but denies fever, shortness of breath, or other symptoms. Which questions does the nurse ask to help determine if the patient is having an allergic reaction? *(Select all that apply.)*
    a. "Are you taking any new medications?"
    b. "Have you been using any different soaps or lotions?"
    c. "Is your skin unusually dry or flaky?"
    d. "Have you been exposed to any new cleaning solutions?"
    e. "Have you noticed any new bruises or brownish discolorations?"
    f. "Have you had any changes in your diet?"

42. The nurse is performing a physical exam on the patient and observes a dark asymmetrical lesion on the patient's back. The patient states, "I can't see back there and I don't know how long it has been there." What is the most important intervention for this patient?
    a. Encourage the patient to make an appointment with a dermatologist.
    b. Teach the patient how to do a total skin self-evaluation.
    c. Instruct the patient on self-care measures, such as use of sunscreen.
    d. Obtain an order for a fungal culture and take a fungal specimen.

43. To differentiate between color changes in the nail bed related to vascular supply and those from pigment disposition, what does the nurse do?
    a. Examine the nail plate under a Wood's light.
    b. Assess for thickness.
    c. Blanch the nail bed.
    d. Evaluate for lesions.

44. The nurse is taking a medication history of the patient and performing a physical assessment on the skin. During the assessment the nurse notes that the skin is thin, fragile, and papery. The nurse specifically asks if the patient takes which type of medication?
    a. Anticoagulants
    b. Oral hypoglycemics
    c. Steroids
    d. Herbal preparations

45. The young female patient reports an unusual increase in facial hair. Which question helps the nurse to identify the need for a genital examination?
    a. "Have you noticed any bruising or unusual bleeding?"
    b. "Have you noticed any deepening of your voice quality?"
    c. "Are you having any trouble urinating?"
    d. "Does your skin seem unusually dry and flaky?"

46. Which statement about dandruff is true?
    a. Dandruff flakes are caused by a dry scalp.
    b. Dandruff is merely a cosmetic problem.
    c. Severe dandruff could cause hair loss.
    d. Brushing your hair every day prevents dandruff.

47. The nurse is caring for several older adult patients in a long-term care facility. The patient with which disorder has the greatest risk to develop a staphylococcal infection secondary to an ingrown toenail?
    a. Chronic obstructive pulmonary disease
    b. Hypertension
    c. Osteoarthritis
    d. Diabetes mellitus

Matching. Match each alteration in color to its underlying cause or condition.

Alteration in Color
a. Blue
b. Yellow-orange
c. Red (erythema)
d. Brown
e. White (pallor)

Underlying Cause or Condition

_____ 48. Pregnancy (melasma), Addison's disease

_____ 49. Bleeding from vessels into tissue

_____ 50. Liver disorders, chronic renal failure, or increased hemolysis of red blood cells

_____ 51. Vasoconstriction, sudden emotional upset

_____ 52. Fever, cellulitis

53. The nurse is assessing the patient who is African American with very dark skin. Which technique does the nurse use to assess the health of the nail?
    a. Gently squeeze the end of the finger, exert downward pressure, then release the pressure.
    b. Obtain a color chart to identify the normal color of nails for the dark-skinned patient.
    c. Observe the nail bed for a pale pink color and a shiny, smooth surface.
    d. Soak the fingertips in warm water, then gently push back the cuticle.

54. The patient reports a subjective sensation of pain and tenderness "because my arthritis is flaring up." In order to assess for inflammation, what does the nurse do?
    a. Place the hand just above the area and feel for radiant warmth.
    b. Use fingertips to gently depress tissue area and then release and observe.
    c. Use the back of the hand to palpate the area for warmth.
    d. Using the palmar surface of the hand, make a circular motion over the area.

55. The patient has a history of mild congestive heart failure. The nurse is assessing the patient's lower extremities; the skin is tight and shiny, but the patient currently denies pain or distress, saying "Oh, my legs just get like that." How does the nurse interpret these findings?
    a. Fluid retention and edema
    b. Early signs of poor circulation
    c. Early stage of infection
    d. Normal for this patient

56. The nurse is caring for the patient who is several days postoperative. The nursing assistant reports that the patient's linens were changed, but are wet again. The nurse notes that the patient's skin is excessively warm and moist. What is the nurse's priority action?
    a. Initiate intake and output
    b. Take the patient's temperature
    c. Direct the nursing assistant to change the linens
    d. Help the patient with hygiene

Matching. Identify the probable causes for each skin manifestation identified below.

Causes

a. Dehydration, sudden severe weight loss, or normal aging
b. Fungal infection
c. Hormone imbalance
d. Prolonged hypoxia or lung cancer

Manifestations

_____ 57. Increased body hair growth on the face in the female patient

_____ 58. Drumstick appearance of nail shape

_____ 59. Decreased skin turgor

_____ 60. "Heaped up" appearance of the older adult's toenail

61. The nurse is assessing the patient with a chronic skin condition. During the interview, the nurse observes that the patient has poor eye contact and tries to keep the affected skin area covered with a scarf. The nurse identifies which nursing diagnosis based on this first interaction?
    a. Social Isolation
    b. Disturbed Body Image
    c. Anxiety
    d. Powerlessness

62. The nurse is assessing the patient's skin and notes a slightly darkened area over the left ankle. The patient denies pain, but reports a recent problem with the area. Based on the skin appearance and the patient's report, what does the nurse do next?
    a. Ask the patient if there was a serious and deep burn to the area.
    b. Observe the area for scar tissue.
    c. Ask the patient if there was an inflammation to the area.
    d. Take a scraping of the skin for culture.

63. The nurse is caring for the older adult patient with very dark skin. The patient has a low hemoglobin and hematocrit. How does the nurse assess for pallor in this patient?
    a. Observe the mucous membranes for an ash-gray color.
    b. Use indirect and low fluorescent lighting.
    c. Gently push on the skin and watch for blanching.
    d. Inspect the conjunctivae for a yellowish color.

64. The nurse is interviewing the patient who has come to the walk-in clinic and observes the patient has matted hair, body odor, and soiled clothes. Which conditions does the nurse assess for that could be contributing to the patient's overall hygiene? *(Select all that apply.)*
    a. Range of motion and strength to perform self-care
    b. Access to shower facilities and a laundry
    c. Financial ability to pay water and heating bills
    d. Patient's perception of how he or she appears to others
    e. Diabetes mellitus or hypertension
    f. Intactness of sensory functions (i.e., sight, smell)
    g. Patient's knowledge (or memory) of how to perform hygiene care

65. The physician has ordered diagnostic testing to determine whether the patient has a fungal infection of the skin. Which test does the nurse prepare the patient for?
    a. Shave biopsy
    b. Punch biopsy
    c. Wood's light examination
    d. KOH test

66. The patient reports a history of chronic liver problems; liver enzyme tests and bilirubin results are pending. In order to assess for jaundice, where is the best place for the nurse to look for a yellowish discoloration?
    a. Hard palate
    b. Sclera
    c. Palms
    d. Conjunctivae

Matching. Match the terms to the description of the skin lesion configurations.

Terms
a. Annular
b. Universal
c. Serpiginous
d. Coalesced
e. Clustered
f. Diffuse
g. Linear
h. Circumscribed
i. Circinate

Description

_____ 67. Ringlike with raised borders around flat, clear centers of normal skin

_____ 68. Circular

_____ 69. Well-defined with sharp borders

_____ 70. Several lesions grouped together

_____ 71. Lesions that merge with one another and appear confluent

_____ 72. Widespread, involving most of the body with intervening areas of normal skin

_____ 73. Occurring in a straight line

_____ 74. With wavy borders, resembling a snake

_____ 75. All areas of the body involved, with no areas of normal-appearing skin

76. The nurse is collecting a superficial specimen for a suspected fungal infection from the patient's groin area. What is the correct technique to obtain this specimen?
    a. Obtain a small sample of tissue by using a biopsy needle.
    b. Express exudate from a lesion and use a sterile swab to collect the fluid.
    c. Gently scrape scales with a tongue blade into a clean container.
    d. Aspirate fluid from the lesion using sterile technique.

77. The nurse has collected several specimens from patients who have skin conditions. Which specimen must be immediately placed on ice?
    a. Punch biopsy performed with sterile technique for collection of a tissue piece.
    b. Exudate taken by sterile technique and swabbed on a bacterial culture medium.
    c. Aspirate taken by sterile technique, placed in a bacterial culture tube.
    d. Vesicle fluid taken by sterile technique and placed in a viral culture tube.

78. The patient is scheduled to have a punch biopsy for a lesion on the mid-back. The nurse is preparing patient teaching information about this procedure. What does the nurse tell the patient about the procedure?
    a. There will be a small scar similar to any surgical procedure.
    b. The surgeon uses a scalpel to punch through the lesion.
    c. A local anesthetic is used and it causes a temporary burning sensation.
    d. The physician uses a lens that punches the skin to reveal the shape of the lesion.

79. The nurse is caring for the patient who had an excisional biopsy for a skin lesion. What does the post-procedural care for this patient include? *(Select all that apply.)*
    a. Monitor the biopsy site for bleeding.
    b. Instruct the patient to keep the site clean and dry for at least 24 hours.
    c. Teach the patient to clean the site daily after the dressing is removed.
    d. Remove dried blood or crusts with diluted hydrogen peroxide.
    e. Instruct the patient to report any redness or excessive drainage.
    f. Advise the patient that the sutures will be removed in 7 to 10 days.

80. The physician instructs the nurse to prepare the light-skinned patient for examination, which includes evaluation of skin pigment changes. Which piece of equipment does the nurse obtain to assist the physician with this examination?
    a. Wood's light
    b. Glass slide
    c. Biopsy tray
    d. Non-fluorescent light

True or False? *Questions 81 through 89 pertain to skin physiology and assessment. Write T for true or F for false in the blanks provided. If the statement is false, correct the statement to make it true.*

_____ 81. Specialized cells called Langerhans' cells, present in the skin, act as sensory receptors.

_____ 82. When skin is intact, it helps to regulate body temperature and maintains fluid and electrolyte balance.

_____ 83. Emotional stress, systemic disease, and skin injury or disease can alter the function, appearance, and texture of the skin.

_____ 84. The epidermis has a rich blood supply and a capillary network for exchange of oxygen.

_____ 85. Permanent baldness is the result of stress and environmental factors.

_____ 86. The nurse should check the cognitive function of any patient whose hygiene of the skin, hair, and nails appears inadequate.

_____ 87. The nurse should teach the patient to evaluate all skin areas on a daily basis for new lesions and changes to existing lesions.

_____ 88. All patients with skin lesions should be placed into contact isolation.

_____ 89. Pallor, erythema, cyanosis, and other color changes reflective of the physical state are less visible in patients with naturally dark skin tones.

CASE STUDY: THE OLDER ADULT WITH SKIN CHANGES

Use a separate sheet of paper to answer the questions in this Case Study. Answer guidelines for this Case Study are available on your Evolve website at http://evolve. elsevier.com/Iggy/ in the "Prepare for Class" folder.

The older adult patient comes to the clinic for an annual health checkup. The patient reports good general health, but reports that her skin feels very dry and would like recommendations for "a nice skin cream." The patient also expresses some concern about "these ugly age spots" and "a lot of moles and warts as I get older." The patient's friend was recently diagnosed with skin cancer, and asks "Would you look at these moles for me?"

1. What questions may the nurse ask to obtain a good history from the patient?

2. Explain what the ABCD features are that are associated with skin cancer.

3. What type of information and reassurance should be given to this patient about normal changes associated with aging?

4. What additional information would be appropriate to include in the teaching plan for this patient?

27 CHAPTER

Care of Patients with Skin Problems

STUDY/REVIEW QUESTIONS

Matching. *Match the terms with their correct descriptions.*

Terms

a. Xerosis
b. Pruritus
c. Lichenification
d. Erythema
e. Urticaria
f. Debris
g. Débrided
h. Re-epithelialization
i. Granulation
j. Contraction
k. Cellulitis
l. Eschar
m. Maceration

Descriptions

_____ 1. Mushiness

_____ 2. Inflammation of the skin cells

_____ 3. Scar tissue

_____ 4. Redness

_____ 5. Itching

_____ 6. Dead cells and tissues

_____ 7. Black, gray, or brown nonviable, denatured collagen

_____ 8. Pull the wound edges inward along the path of least resistance

_____ 9. Thickening

_____ 10. Dry skin

_____ 11. Hives

_____ 12. Production of new skin cells by undamaged epidermal cells

_____ 13. Remove exudate and dead tissue

14. The nurse is directing the home health aide in the care of an older adult patient. The patient reports dry skin and wants help in applying an emollient cream. What does the nurse direct the aide to do?
   a. Assist the patient to soak for 20 minutes in a warm bath and then apply the cream to slightly damp skin within 2 to 3 minutes after bathing.
   b. Generously apply the cream and leave it on for 15 to 20 minutes, then bathe the patient, especially the genital and axillary areas.
   c. Use an antimicrobial skin soap and wash the patient carefully, then apply the emollient cream, especially to the leg area.
   d. Use extra warm water with added bath oil, then gently pat the patient dry and apply more oil and cream to the skin.

15. Which patients are at risk for pressure ulcers? *(Select all that apply.)*
   a. A confused patient who likes to wander through the halls.
   b. A middle-aged quadriplegic patient who is alert and conversant.
   c. A bedridden patient who is in the late stage of Alzheimer's.
   d. A very heavy patient who must be assisted to move in the bed.
   e. An ambulatory patient who has occasional urinary incontinence.
   f. A thin patient who sits for long periods and refuses meals.

16. The nurse is caring for an obese patient who has been on bedrest for several days. The nurse observes that the patient is beginning to develop redness on the sacral area. What intervention is used to decrease the shearing force?
   a. Place the patient in a high Fowler's position.
   b. Instruct the patient to use arms and legs to push when moving self in bed.
   c. Obtain an order for the patient to be up 3 to 4 times per day in a recliner chair.
   d. Place the patient in a side-lying position.

17. The nurse is reviewing the results of a pressure mapping on the patient at high risk for pressure ulcers. The map shows a red area over the hips. How does the nurse interpret this evidence?
   a. Normal finding because there is always pressure on the hip area
   b. Greater heat production associated with greater pressure
   c. Cooler skin associated with lower pressure
   d. Validation of observable skin redness and breakdown

18. The nurse is assessing the nutritional status of the patient at risk for skin breakdown who has been refusing to eat the hospital food. Which indicator is the most sensitive in identifying inadequate nutrition for this patient?
   a. Serum albumin level of 3.0 mg/dL
   b. Prealbumin level of 17.5 mg/dL
   c. Lymphocyte count of 1700/mm^3
   d. Weight loss of 10% of total body weight

19. Seeing a reddened area on the patient's skin, the nurse presses firmly with fingers at the center of the area and sees that the area blanches with pressure. The nurse interprets this finding as changes related to which factor?
   a. Inflammation
   b. Infection
   c. Blood vessel dilation
   d. Tissue damage

20. The nurse is assessing a wound on the patient's abdomen. What is the correct technique?
   a. Stand on the right side of the bed and lay a sterile cotton swab across the width and the length of the wound.
   b. Read the previous nursing documentation and follow the same pattern that other nurses are using for standardization.
   c. Assess the wound as a clock face with 12 o'clock in the direction of the patient's head and 6 o'clock in the direction of the patient's feet.
   d. Observe the wound after the dressing is removed and estimate the shape and record the appearance.

21. The nurse is assessing the patient's wound every day for signs of healing or infection. Which finding is a positive indication that healing is progressing as expected?
    a. Eschar starts to lift and separate from the tissue beneath which appears dry and pale.
    b. Area appears pale pink, progressing to a spongy texture with a beefy red color.
    c. Tissue is softer and more yellow and wound exudate increases substantially.
    d. Ulcer surface is excessively moist with a deep reddish-purple color.

22. The student nurse is irrigating a large pressure ulcer on the patient's hip, and notes a small opening in the skin with purulent drainage. Which technique does the student use to check for tunneling?
    a. Ask the primary nurse if the physician will order an ultrasound.
    b. Palpate the surface of the wound to identify spongy areas.
    c. Continue to flush the wound and watch the flow of the fluid.
    d. Use a cotton-tipped applicator to probe gently for a tunnel.

True or False? *Write T for true or F for false in the blanks provided. If the statement is false, correct the statement to make it true.*

_____ 23. Pruritus is worse at night.

_____ 24. Xerosis is worse in humid climates.

_____ 25. For second intention wound healing, the wound is closed surgically after it was open for several days.

_____ 26. A full-thickness wound requires necrotic tissue to be removed for healing to occur.

_____ 27. Progressive flattening of cells at the dermal-epidermal junction predisposes older adults to skin tears from mechanical shearing forces.

_____ 28. A successful skin graft must be irrigated frequently.

_____ 29. Herpes zoster (shingles) is usually painless.

_____ 30. Pediculosis capitis is self-limiting.

_____ 31. Psoriasis is a scaling disorder with underlying dermal inflammation.

32. The mother reports that her child has dry skin with itching that seems to worsen at night. What nonpharmacologic interventions does the nurse teach to the mother? *(Select all that apply.)*
    a. Keep the child's fingernails trimmed short and filed, to reduce skin damage.
    b. Place mittens or splints on the child's hands at night if the scratching is causing skin tears during sleep.
    c. Ensure a warm and moderately humid sleeping environment.
    d. Read the child a relaxing and familiar story to reduce stress.
    e. Colloidal oatmeal bath may give temporary relief.

33. After eating a food that triggered an allergic reaction, the patient developed hives. In addition to over-the-counter diphenhydramine (Benadryl), what does the nurse suggest to the patient for self-care?
    a. Avoid alcohol consumption which can potentiate the sedative effect of Benadryl.
    b. Warm environments and warm showers will accelerate metabolism and recovery.
    c. Use an emollient cream or lotion after bathing to reduce the itching.
    d. Apply a topical antibiotic cream after bathing in the evening.

34. The nurse is examining the patient's skin and sees large, sore-looking, raised bumps with pustular heads. Which method does the nurse use to obtain a specimen to test for a bacterial infection?
    a. Take a culture swab of the purulent material.
    b. Take cells from the base of a lesion for a Tzanck's smear.
    c. Scrape scales from the lesions and prepare a slide with KOH.
    c. Assist the physician with a skin biopsy.

35. The nurse is teaching the patient about self-care for a minor bacterial skin infection. What is the most important aspect the nurse emphasizes?
    a. Apply warm compresses twice a day.
    b. Do not squeeze any pustules or crusts.
    c. Apply astringent compresses.
    d. Bathe daily with an antibacterial soap.

36. The patient is diagnosed with psoriasis. Which description of the characteristic lesions of psoriasis would the nurse expect to see in the patient's documentation?
    a. Plaques surmounted by silvery-white scales
    b. Circular areas of redness
    c. Multiple blisters with a yellowish crust
    d. Patches of tender, raised areas limited to extremities

37. What does the treatment for psoriasis include? *(Select all that apply.)*
    a. UV light therapy
    b. Calcipotriene (Dovonex) topical cream
    c. Topical methotrexate
    d. Oral ciprofloxacin
    e. Corticosteroids

38. What is the most common symptom of pruritus?
    a. Blisters
    b. Itching
    c. Flaking
    d. Tenderness

39. The nurse is teaching the older adult about how to deal with and prevent dry skin. What information does the nurse include? *(Select all that apply.)*
    a. Use a room humidifier during the winter months or whenever the furnace is in use.
    b. Take a complete bath or shower every day.
    c. Maintain a daily fluid intake of 1000 mL unless contraindicated.
    d. Use a superfatted, nonalkaline soap instead of deodorant soap.
    e. Rinse the soap thoroughly from the skin.
    f. Vigorously rub the skin until it is free of moisture.
    g. Avoid clothing that continuously rubs the skin, such as tight belts or pantyhose.

Matching. Match each tinea infection with its corresponding location.

Infection

a. Tinea capitis
b. Tinea manus
c. Tinea cruris
d. Tinea pedis
e. Tinea corporis

Location

_____ 40. Feet

_____ 41. Hands

_____ 42. Groin (jock itch)

_____ 43. Scalp

_____ 44. Smooth skin surfaces

45. The nurse is teaching the patient about treatment of pediculosis corporis. What information does the nurse include?
    a. Proper use of topical sprays or creams, such as permethrin or lindane
    b. Abstinence of sexual intercourse with the infected person
    c. Treatment of the patient's social contacts
    d. Side effects of ciprofloxacin (Cipro) or doxycycline (Doryx, Vibramycin)

46. The school nurse is examining a child and observes linear ridges in the skin. The child reports intense itching, especially at night. The nurse scrapes the lesion and examines it under a microscope. For which condition should the child be treated?
    a. Head lice
    b. Scabies
    c. Body lice
    d. Dermatitis

47. The school nurse discovers a child has tinea capitis. What does the nurse instruct the parents to do?
    a. Treat the family pet and temporarily isolate the pet.
    b. Refrain from sharing items like combs or hats.
    c. Scrub the shower area and keep the feet dry.
    d. Ensure all family members carefully wash their hands.

48. The nurse is assessing the pedicle flap that has been used to cover the patient's wound, and observes a pale flap with delayed capillary filling when blanched. How does the nurse interpret this finding?
    a. Inadequate venous drainage
    b. Inadequate lymphatic drainage
    c. Inadequate arterial perfusion
    d. Expected flap condition

49. The patient returns from surgery with a large graft site on the sacral area. Which task is delegated to unlicensed assistive personnel?
    a. Turn the patient every 2 hours.
    b. Explain to the patient that he will be in a side-lying or prone position for 7 to 10 days.
    c. Give the patient a backrub.
    d. Trim the gauze close to the skin surface to prevent accidental removal of the dressing.

50. The nurse is giving discharge instructions to the patient and family who must continue dressing changes and wound care at home. Which point does the nurse emphasize to help the family prevent infection and minimize cost?
    a. Scrupulous handwashing before and after wound care
    b. Use of sterile water for flushing and sterile dressing materials
    c. Use of clean gloves for performing dressing changes
    d. Careful disposal of contaminated dressings in a biohazard bag

51. The nurse is caring for a 25-year-old patient who recently had a rhinoplasty as part of reconstruction after cancer treatment. The patient is swallowing repeatedly and belching. What does the nurse suspect?
    a. Postnasal bleeding
    b. Respiratory distress
    c. Edema and swelling
    d. Anxiety

52. The patient has been prescribed isotretinoin (Accutane) for a skin condition. What information does the nurse tell the patient about this drug? *(Select all that apply.)*
    a. It may cause dry, chapped lips.
    b. It is the first choice for acne treatment.
    c. Strict birth control measures are necessary.
    d. Liver function studies should be monitored while on this therapy.
    e. It is used for superficial lesions.

53. The nurse is caring for the patient with toxic epidermal necrolysis (TEN). Which nursing action is included in the nursing care plan?
    a. Assessing input and output
    b. Administering antibiotics as prescribed
    c. Monitoring for hyperthermia
    d. Managing inflammation with steroid creams

54. The patient is prescribed a topical steroid for treatment of contact dermatitis. Which instruction does the nurse provide to the patient about this drug?
    a. Moisten dressings with warm tap water; place over topical steroids for short periods.
    b. Apply topical steroids then cover with an occlusive dressing.
    c. Apply a topical corticosteroid sparingly on the face.
    d. Discontinue the use of topical steroids when symptoms subside.

55. Which statement is true about the application and use of topical preparations?
    a. A stiff paste should be applied to large areas such as the trunk or legs.
    b. Using a water-soluble cream in the groin area could cause maceration.
    c. Using an oil-based ointment in the axillary area could cause folliculitis.
    d. An oil-based gel should be massaged into hairy areas.

Matching. Match the disorders with their descriptions. Disorders may be used more than once.

Disorders

a. Toxic epidermal necrolysis
b. Stevens-Johnson syndrome
c. Contact dermatitis
d. Lichen planus
e. Hansen's disease
f. Acne
g. Pemphigus vulgaris
h. Cutaneous anthrax
i. Seborrheic keratoses
j. Pilonidal cyst
k. Keloid
l. Nevus

Descriptions

_____ 56. A rash caused by toxic injury to the skin as a result of contact with an irritant substance

_____ 57. A chronic, contagious, systemic mycobacterial infection of the peripheral nervous system with skin involvement

_____ 58. A drug-induced skin reaction that may include a mix of vesicles, erosions, and crusts

_____ 59. Painless lesions and eschar that form regardless of treatment used

_____ 60. A rare, chronic blistering disease with high morbidity and mortality

_____ 61. A rare, acute drug reaction of the skin that gradually heals in 2 to 3 weeks with widespread peeling of the epidermis

_____ 62. Purple, flat-topped, itchy papules over the wrists and inner surfaces of the forearms

_____ 63. Also known as leprosy

_____ 64. Comedone lesions

_____ 65. Removed for cosmetic reasons or if a lesion becomes irritated from friction

_____ 66. A lesion of the sacral area that often has a sinus tract extending into deeper tissue structures

_____ 67. Overgrowth of a scar with excessive accumulation of collagen and ground substance

_____ 68. Mole, a benign growth of the pigment-forming cells

69. The patient has a partial-thickness wound. How long does the nurse anticipate the healing by epithelialization will take?
   a. 24 hours
   b. 2 to 3 days
   c. 5 to 7 days
   d. 12 to 14 days

70. The toddler is miserable with itching from chickenpox. Which type of bath is the best to help relieve the toddler's discomfort?
   a. Milk
   b. Emollient
   c. Tar with Polytar formula
   d. Aveeno colloidal oatmeal

71. The nurse is performing daily wound care and dressing changes on a patient with a full-thickness wound. The patient protests when the nurse attempts to débride the wound. What is the nurse's best response?
    a. "Re-epithelialization, granulation, and contraction are natural body processes that will occur if this tissue is removed."
    b. "I know this is uncomfortable, but don't you want your wound to heal as fast as possible? This treatment allows the body to heal itself."
    c. "Harmful bacteria can grow in the dead tissue and it also interferes with the body's attempt to fill in the wound with new cells and collagen."
    d. "I would never force a patient to do anything, but this really is the best treatment for the wound that you have."

72. The patient has a stage III pressure ulcer over the left trochanter area that has a thick exudate. The wound bed is visible and beefy red, and the edges are surrounded with swollen, pink tissue. The exudate has an odor. Which dressing is best for this wound?
    a. Transparent
    b. Alginate
    c. Continuous dry gauze
    d. Pigskin or cadaver skin

73. The nurse is caring for a patient with arterial insufficiency in the lower right leg. In order to prevent leg ulcers, what does the nurse do?
    a. Elevates the leg frequently.
    b. Places the leg in a dependent position.
    c. Places a heel protector on the right foot.
    d. Encourages the patient to walk briskly.

74. The nurse is caring for a patient who had surgical débridement with a skin graft on the leg. The patient returns from the operating room with the graft site immobilized and a bulky cotton pressure dressing in place. What does the nurse do next?
    a. Encourages elevation and complete rest of the grafted area.
    b. Removes the dressing and cleans the wound every shift.
    c. Encourages the patient to get up and ambulate as soon as he is awake and alert.
    d. Monitors the dressing for a small amount of bleeding which is expected.

75. Place the physiologic steps of healing of partial-thickness wounds in the correct order using the numbers 1 through 8.
    _____ a. Skin injury is followed immediately by local inflammation.
    _____ b. The protective barrier is re-established.
    _____ c. The cell layer thickens and stratifies to resemble normal skin.
    _____ d. New skin cells move into open spaces on the wound surface.
    _____ e. Regrowth across the opening area is only one cell layer thick at first.
    _____ f. Fibrin clot acts as a frame or scaffold to guide cell movement.
    _____ g. Growth factors are released to stimulate epidermal cell division.
    _____ h. There is formation of a fibrin clot.

76. The nurse is caring for several patients who are incontinent of stool and urine. Which task is delegated to unlicensed assistive personnel?
    a. Inspect the skin daily for any areas of redness.
    b. Massage the reddened areas after cleaning.
    c. Wash the skin with a pH-balanced soap to maintain normal acidity.
    d. Change the absorbent pads or garments every 4 hours.

77. The nurse is caring for a patient in a prolonged coma after a serious head injury. The nurse uses which interventions to prevent the development of pressure ulcers for this patient? *(Select all that apply.)*
    a. Use pillows or padding devices to keep heels pressure-free.
    b. Assess heel positioning every 8 hours.
    c. Delegate turning and positioning every 2 hours.
    d. Obtain an order for a pressure-relief device.
    e. Give special attention to fleshy or muscular areas.

78. The nurse is assessing the patient's skin and observes a superficial infection with a raised, red rash with small pustules. How does the nurse interpret this finding?
    a. Minor skin trauma
    b. Folliculitis
    c. Furuncles
    d. Cellulitis

79. The patient has a painful and unsightly herpes simplex blister on her lip, and would like to have her school photo delayed until after the lesion has resolved. How long does the nurse tell the patient the outbreak may last?
    a. 2 to 3 days
    b. 3 to 5 days
    c. 3 to 10 days
    d. Up to 2 weeks

80. The nurse is caring for the patient who needs frequent oral hygiene and endotracheal suctioning. In this particular circumstance, the nurse wears gloves to prevent contracting and spreading which organism?
    a. Herpetic whitlow
    b. Herpes zoster
    c. Methicillin-resistant *Staphylococcus aureus*
    d. Streptococcus

81. The nurse hears in report that a patient admitted for an elective surgery also has herpes zoster. Which factor causes contact isolation to be initiated for this patient?
    a. Fever and malaise are present as accompanying symptoms.
    b. Other patients or staff members have never had chickenpox.
    c. Lesions are present as fluid-filled blisters.
    d. Lesions are present and crusted over.

82. The patient is diagnosed with a primary herpetic infection. The nurse questions an order for which drug?
    a. Acyclovir (Zovirax)
    b. Valacyclovir (Valtrex)
    c. Ketoconazole (Nizoral)
    d. Famciclovir (Famvir)

83. The public health nurse is reviewing case files of people who were exposed and treated for cutaneous anthrax. Which patient who develops the disease warrants further investigation as a possible bioterrorism exposure?
    a. Farmer
    b. Veterinarian
    c. Tannery worker
    d. Construction worker

84. The patient reported painless raised vesicles that itched. Within a few days, there was bleeding in the center and then it sank inwards. Now it looks black and leathery. Which question does the nurse ask in order to elicit more information about this patient's condition?
    a. "Do you remember being bitten by an insect?"
    b. "Do you work with or around animals?"
    c. "Have you noticed any mite or lice infestations?"
    d. "Have you had exposure to new soaps, lotions, or foods?"

85. The patient underwent cryosurgery for removal of a small lesion. The nurse teaches the patient to clean the area to prevent infection. What does the patient use for cleaning?
    a. Soap and water
    b. Hydrogen peroxide
    c. Alcohol
    d. Betadine

86. The patient is diagnosed with chronic psoriasis and is prescribed a topical therapy of anthralin (Lasan). What does the nurse teach the patient about proper use of this drug?
    a. Apply the paste every night before going to bed.
    b. Check for local tissue reaction.
    c. Apply the drug generously to the lesion and surrounding skin.
    d. Use two forms of contraception.

87. What does the nurse teach the patient about ultraviolet (UV) therapy for psoriasis?
    a. Use a commercial tanning bed service but limit exposure to 2 to 3 times per week.
    b. Use the sun as an inexpensive source of UV; inspect skin daily for overexposure.
    c. Wear dark glasses during and after treatment if psoralen is prescribed.
    d. Expect generalized redness with edema and tenderness after the treatment.

88. Which are examples of benign skin tumors? *(Select all that apply.)*
    a. Pilonidal cyst
    b. Nevus
    c. Hemangioma
    d. Actinic keratoses
    e. Keloid
    f. Seborrheic keratoses
    g. Melanoma

Matching. Match the skin disorder with its description.

Skin Disorder
a. Melanoma
b. Basal cell carcinoma
c. Actinic keratosis
d. Squamous cell carcinoma

Description

_____ 89. Most common cause: ultraviolet exposure; metastasis is rare.

_____ 90. Invades locally and is potentially metastatic; arises from epidermis.

_____ 91. Pigmented skin cancer that is highly metastatic.

_____ 92. Premalignant lesions of the cells of the epidermis.

93. The nurse is examining the nevi on the patient's back and neck. Because about 50% of malignant melanomas arise from moles, which finding is a concern to warrant further investigation?
    a. Regular, well-defined borders
    b. Uniform dark brown color
    c. Rough surface
    d. Sudden report of itching

94. *Koebner's phenomenon* is known as a greater risk for which disorder/condition?
    a. Skin cancer
    b. Psoriasis
    c. Nevus
    d. Keloids

95. Which statement is true about Mohs' surgery used to treat squamous cell carcinoma?
    a. Cure rates are high and there is less removal of healthy tissue compared with other surgical methods.
    b. The surgeon places an electric probe on the wound, and remnants of the tumor are destroyed by thermal energy.
    c. Local anesthesia is seldom needed because most patients have only minor discomfort during the procedure.
    d. Wounds created by this treatment heal by second intention, and scarring is usually minimal.

96. The nurse is talking to the patient who is planning to have cosmetic plastic surgery. Which patient statement prompts the nurse to report concerns to the surgeon?
    a. "Having this surgery is going to help increase my self-confidence."
    b. "I know this surgery is going to solve my marital problems."
    c. "I have been thinking about having this surgery for a long time."
    d. "I am nervous about having the surgery, but I can't wait to see the outcome."

97. The nurse is doing preoperative teaching for the patient who is scheduled to have cosmetic plastic surgery. The nurse decides the surgeon must be notified when the patient adamantly refuses to comply with which instruction?
    a. Take NSAIDs for pain associated with the procedure.
    b. Stop drinking an evening alcoholic cocktail prior to the procedure.
    c. Maintain a moderate calorie, low-fat diet after the procedure.
    d. Stop smoking cigarettes either before or after the procedure.

98. The nurse is caring for the patient who had facial reconstruction surgery. In order to decrease pressure in the head region, what does the nurse instruct the patient to do?
    a. Rest in bed in a supine position and log roll to change position.
    b. Chew, talk, and smile to normally use and exercise the facial muscles.
    c. Avoid bending over, blowing the nose, sneezing with the mouth closed.
    d. Take small and frequent sips of fluid through a straw.

99. The older patient who is receiving chemotherapy is diagnosed with toxic epidermal necrolysis. In addition to identifying the causative agent, what does the nurse monitor for?
    a. Fluid and electrolyte imbalance, caloric intake, and hypothermia
    b. Shortness of breath, hypertension, and cardiac dysrhythmias
    c. Nausea, vomiting, diarrhea, and severe abdominal pain
    d. Severe itching with tenderness and edema of the skin

100. The nurse is caring for the patient with localized leprosy who recently immigrated to the U.S. The patient is fearful because she has seen others with leprosy deformity. What is the nurse's best response?
    a. "The progression of the disease is limited to the current area of skin involvement."
    b. "Widespread, faintly red macules suggest that your body is limiting the disease."
    c. "One or two isolated red plaques suggest that your body has high immunity."
    d. "There are drugs that can reverse the physical deformities and cure the disease."

CASE STUDY: THE PATIENT WITH MALIGNANT MELANOMA

Use a separate sheet of paper to answer the questions in this Case Study. Answer guidelines for this Case Study are available on your Evolve website at http://evolve. elsevier.com/Iggy/ in the "Prepare for Class" folder.

A 44-year-old Caucasian woman is admitted for local wide excision of a large mole that has been diagnosed as malignant melanoma on her upper thigh. Her past history is negative for serious illness. She was hospitalized for the birth of her three children. She admits to being an "avid sun worshipper" and is noted to have very dark brown skin and some premature aging of the facial skin.

1. Considering the possible etiology of melanoma, what effect does the exposure to sunlight have on this form of cancer?

2. During her preoperative instructions, the patient asks why she is going to have a 4-inch circle of skin and tissue removed to get rid of a "mole." What information should the nurse consider before responding to her question?

3. The patient has a wide excision of the melanoma, and the surgical site is closed with a split-thickness skin graft from the opposite thigh. Following surgery, the wound is dressed with a bulky dressing, and the donor site is covered with a pressure dressing. When the nurse is assessing the dressings, the patient asks to "peek" at the surgical site so that she can see where the mole had been. How should the nurse respond?

4. On the following morning, the patient reports that the donor site "hurts worse than the cancer site." What should the nurse say and what interventions are appropriate?

5. On the third day after surgery, the bulky dressing is removed. The wound appears wet with cloudy fluid oozing from it, and the skin graft is unattached to the wound. The surrounding tissues are red and swollen. What is the likely cause of these features in the graft site?

28 CHAPTER

Care of Patients with Burns

STUDY/REVIEW QUESTIONS

Matching. *Match each term with its corresponding definition.*

Terms

a. Dermal appendages
b. Anesthetic
c. Avascular
d. Eschar
e. Desquamation
f. Fasciotomy
g. Viable
h. Hyperkalemia
i. Hyponatremia
j. Hemoconcentration
k. Catabolism

Definitions

_____ 1. Decreased sodium levels

_____ 2. Peeling of dead skin

_____ 3. Living

_____ 4. Sweat and oil glands and hair follicles

_____ 5. Burn crust

_____ 6. Elevated potassium levels

_____ 7. Without a blood supply

_____ 8. Incision through the eschar and fascia

_____ 9. Does not transmit sensation

_____ 10. Fat and protein breakdown

_____ 11. Elevated blood osmolarity, hemoglobin, and hematocrit

12. The patient was burned on the forearm after tripping and falling against a wood-burning stove. There are currently several small blisters over the burn area. What does the nurse advise the patient to do about the blisters?
    a. Leave the blisters intact because they protect the wound from infection
    b. Use a sterile needle to open a tiny hole in each blister to drain the fluid
    c. Allow blisters to increase in size; then open them to prevent immunosuppression
    d. Leave the blisters intact unless the pain and pressure increase

13. The nurse is caring for the patient who has 30% total body surface area (TBSA) burn. During the first 12 to 36 hours, the nurse carefully monitors the patient for which status changes related to capillary leak syndrome?
    a. Bradycardia and pitting edema
    b. Hypertension and decreased urine output
    c. Tachycardia and hypotension
    d. Respiratory depression and lung crackles

14. The home health nurse is visiting the older couple for the initial visit. In observing the household, the nurse identifies several behaviors and environmental factors to address. Which identified factors increase the risk for burns and/or household fires? *(Select all that apply.)*
    a. Several potholders hanging within easy reach from the stove
    b. Ashtray with old cigarette butts on the bedside table
    c. Space heater very close to the bed
    d. Single smoke detector in the kitchen
    e. Back exit hall of the house used as a storage space

15. The nurse is caring for several patients on the burn unit who have sustained extensive tissue damage. The nurse should monitor for which electrolyte imbalance that is typically associated with the initial third spacing fluid shift?
    a. Hypercalcemia
    b. Hypernatremia
    c. Hypokalemia
    d. Hyperkalemia

16. The nurse is reviewing the hemoglobin and hematocrit results for the patient recently admitted for a severe burn. Which result is most likely related to vascular dehydration?
    a. Hematocrit of 58%
    b. Hemoglobin of 14 g/dL
    c. Hematocrit of 42%
    d. Hemoglobin of 10 g/dL

17. The nurse is performing a morning assessment on the patient admitted for serious burns to the extremities. For what reason does the nurse assess the patient's abdomen?
    a. To perform a daily full head-to-toe assessment
    b. To assess for nausea and vomiting related to pain medication
    c. To assess for a paralytic ileus secondary to reduced blood flow
    d. To monitor increased motility that may result in cramps and diarrhea

18. The nurse is interviewing and assessing an electrician who was brought to the emergency department (ED) after being "electrocuted." Bystanders report that he was holding onto the electrical source "for a long time." The patient is currently alert with no respiratory distress. During the interview, what does the nurse assess for?
    a. Knowledge of electrical safety
    b. Burn marks on the dominant hand
    c. Injuries based on reports of pain
    d. Entrance and exit wounds

19. The patient was involved in a house fire and suffered extensive full-thickness burns. In the long term, what issue may this patient have trouble with?
    a. Intolerance for vitamin C
    b. Metabolism of vitamin K
    c. Activation of vitamin D
    d. Absorption of vitamin A

20. During shift report, the nurse learns that a new patient was admitted for an inhalation injury. The auscultation of the lungs has revealed wheezing over the mainstream bronchi since admission. During the nurse's assessment of the patient, the wheezing sounds are absent. What does the nurse do next?
    a. Document these findings because it indicates that the patient is improving.
    b. Assess for respiratory distress because of potential airway obstruction.
    c. Obtain an order to discontinue oxygen therapy because it is no longer needed.
    d. Encourage use of incentive spirometry to prevent atelectasis.

21. What is the maximum temperature that the skin can tolerate without injury?
    a. 102° F
    b. 104° F
    c. 110° F
    d. 120° F

22. The nurse is caring for several patients who have sustained burns. The patient with which initial injury is the *least* likely to experience severe pain when a sharp stimulus is applied?
    a. Severe sunburn after lying in the sun for several hours
    b. Deep full-thickness burn from an electrical accident
    c. Partial-thickness burn from picking up a hot pan
    d. Deep partial-thickness burn after a motorcycle accident

23. The nurse is reviewing arterial blood gas (ABG) results for the patient with 35% TBSA burn in the emergent phase: pH is 7.26; P_{CO_2} is 36 mm Hg; and HCO_3^- is 19 mEq/L. What condition does the nurse suspect the patient has?
    a. Metabolic alkalosis
    b. Metabolic acidosis
    c. Respiratory acidosis
    d. Respiratory alkalosis

24. The patient comes to the clinic to be treated for burns from a barbeque fire. Although the patient does not appear to be in any respiratory distress, the nurse suspects an inhalation injury after observing which findings? *(Select all that apply.)*
    a. Burns to the face
    b. Bright cherry red color to lips
    c. Singed nose hairs
    d. Edema of the nasal septum
    e. Black carbon particles around the mouth
    f. Sweet, sugary smell to the breath

25. The nurse is caring for the burn patient who received rigorous fluid resuscitation in the ED for hypotension and hypovolemic shock. In assessing renal function for the first 24 hours, what finding does the nurse anticipate?
    a. Output will be approximately equal to fluid intake.
    b. Output will be decreased compared to fluid intake.
    c. Urine will have a very low specific gravity and a pale yellow color.
    d. Output will be managed with diuretics.

26. The patient sustained a superficial-thickness burn over a large area of the body. The patient is crying with discomfort and is very concerned about the long-term effects. What does the nurse tell the patient to expect to see?
    a. Desquamation of the involved area
    b. Blanching of the involved area
    c. Eschar over the involved area
    d. Blistering over the involved area

27. The nurse is caring for the patient brought to the ED after bending over the engine of his car when it exploded in his face. What is the priority for this patient?
    a. Initiate fluid resuscitation
    b. Secure the airway
    c. Manage pain and discomfort
    d. Prevent infection

28. The nurse is caring for the patient who sustained carbon monoxide poisoning while working on his car engine in an enclosed space. What assessment finding does the nurse anticipate?
    a. Patient will be cyanotic because of hypoxia.
    b. Blood gas value of Pa_{O_2} will be very low.
    c. Patient will report a headache.
    d. Patient will report a dry and irritated throat.

29. For which patient would the Rule of Nines method of calculating burn size be most appropriate?
    a. Child who weighs at least 50 pounds
    b. Adult whose weight is proportionate to height
    c. Adult who weighs under 300 pounds
    d. Child whose weight is proportionate to height

True or False? Read the statements about burn pathophysiology and write T for true or F for false in the blanks provided.

_____ 30. The depth of dermal appendages is equal across body areas.

_____ 31. Full-thickness burn is identified by the total destruction of the dermis.

_____ 32. Full-thickness burn results in loss of excretory ability.

_____ 33. All burn injuries are painful.

_____ 34. Cell destruction is so rapid at 158° F that even brief exposure damages the skin and tissues below.

_____ 35. The magnitude of the injury is based on the depth and extent of the total body surface burn.

_____ 36. Blood transfusions are critical in the first 24 hours for all burns.

_____ 37. The degree of tissue damage is related to the agent that caused the burn and the temperature of the heat source as well as how long the skin was exposed to it.

_____ 38. When a burn injury occurs, the skin can regenerate as long the epidermis layer is present.

_____ 39. Hypovolemic shock occurs in burned patients as a result of a marked increase in capillary permeability.

40. The patient has severe burns to the anterior surface of the body from a short exposure to high temperatures at a worksite furnace. Which area of the body is most vulnerable to a deep burn injury?
    a. Anterior chest
    b. Upper arms
    c. Palmar surface of hands
    d. Eyelids

41. The patient has sustained a burn which appears red and moist. The nurse gently applies pressure to the area to assess for what sign/symptom?
    a. Intensity of pain
    b. Blanching
    c. Pitting edema
    d. Fluid-filled blisters

42. What is the primary reason to avoid infection with burn injuries?
    a. Prevent extensive scar formation
    b. Prevent sepsis
    c. Avert worsening of pain
    d. Avoid fever and inflammation

43. The nurse is caring for several patients on the burn unit. Which patients have the greatest risk for developing respiratory problems? *(Select all that apply.)*
    a. Patient who was in a storage room where chemicals caught fire
    b. Patient who was working in an area where steam escaped from a pipe
    c. Patient who sustained a circumferential burn to the chest area
    d. Patient who was burned when a firecracker exploded prematurely
    e. Patient who was found unconscious in a slow-burning house fire

44. The nurse is caring for a firefighter who was trapped for a prolonged period of time by burning debris. During the shift, the nurse notes a progressive hoarseness, a brassy cough, and the patient reports increased difficulty with swallowing. How does the nurse interpret these changes?
    a. Temporary discomfort that can be treated with sips of cool fluids
    b. Signs and symptoms of probable carbon monoxide poisoning
    c. Signs indicating a pulmonary injury and possible airway obstruction
    d. Expected findings considering the mechanism of injury

45. The nurse has just received report on the patient admitted for steam inhalation burns. The patient is alert and conversant, but reports that his throat feels raw. His wife says that he sounds hoarse compared to usual. Considering these findings, which order does the nurse question?
    a. Continuous pulse oximetry
    b. Vital signs and airway assessment every shift
    c. Intubation equipment at the bedside
    d. Oxygen 2 L via nasal cannula to maintain saturation of greater than 90%

46. The nurse is caring for the burn patient who was stabilized by and transferred from a small rural hospital. The patient develops a new complaint of shortness of breath. On auscultation, the nurse hears crackles throughout the lung fields. What does the nurse suspect is causing this patient's symptoms?
    a. Pulmonary fluid overload due to fluid resuscitation
    b. Exposure to carbon monoxide that was undiagnosed
    c. Fat emboli secondary to extensive injury
    d. Excessive oxygen therapy at the first facility

47. The nurse is caring for several patients on the burn unit. Which of these patients has the most acute need for cardiac monitoring?
    a. Older adult woman who spilled hot water over her legs while boiling noodles
    b. Teenager with facial burns that occurred when he threw gasoline on a campfire
    c. Young woman who was struck by lightning while jogging on the beach
    d. Middle-aged man who fell asleep while smoking and sustained burns to the chest

48. The patient is transported to the ED for severe and extensive burns that occurred while he was trapped in a burning building. The patient is severely injured with respiratory distress and the resuscitation team must immediately begin multiple interventions. Which task is delegated to unlicensed assistive personnel (UAP)?
    a. Position the patient's head to open the airway and assist with intubation.
    b. Assist the respiratory therapist to maintain a seal during bag-valve-mask ventilation.
    c. Prepare the intubation equipment and set up the oxygen flowmeter.
    d. Elevate the head of the bed to achieve a high Fowler's position.

49. The nursing student notes on the care plan that the burn patient she is caring for is at risk for Ineffective Tissue Perfusion, Renal. Based on her knowledge of the pathophysiology of burns, which etiology does the nursing student select?
    a. Related to hypovolemia and myoglobin release
    b. Related to fluid overload and peripheral edema
    c. Related to prolonged resuscitation and hypoxia
    d. Related to direct blunt trauma to the kidneys

50. The student nurse is caring for the patient who has been in the burn unit for several weeks. The patient needs assistance with the bedpan to have a bowel movement, and the student nurse notes that the stool is black with a tarry appearance. What does the student nurse do next?
    a. Report this finding to the primary nurse or the instructor.
    b. Obtain a stool specimen to be sent to the laboratory for analysis.
    c. Test for the presence of occult blood with a hemocult card and reagent.
    d. Perform a dietary assessment to determine if the stool color is related to food.

51. The patient who lives in a rural community sustained severe burns during a house fire at 10 AM. The rural EMS started a peripheral IV at 11:00 AM at a keep vein open (KVO) rate. The patient was admitted to the hospital at 1:00 PM. In calculating the fluid replacement, at what time is the fluid for the first 8-hour period completed?
    a. 6:00 PM
    b. 7:00 PM
    c. 8:00 PM
    d. 9:00 PM

52. The patient in the burn intensive care unit weighed 80 kg (preburn weight). The physician orders titration of IV fluid to achieve 0.5 mL/kg/hr urine output. What is the minimal hourly urine output for this patient? _____ mL/hr

53. The burn patient with which condition is most likely to have mannitol (Osmitrol) ordered as part of the drug therapy?
    a. Peripheral edema associated with burns on the lower extremities
    b. Inhalation burns around the mouth causing mucosal swelling
    c. Electrical burn and myoglobin in the urine
    d. Smoke inhalation and superficial burns to the forearms

54. The patient was admitted to the burn unit approximately 6 hours ago after being rescued from a burning building. In the ED, he reported a dry, irritated throat "from breathing in the fumes," but otherwise had no airway complaints. During the shift, the nurse notes that the patient has suddenly developed marked stridor. The nurse anticipates preparing the patient for which emergency procedure?
    a. Bronchoscopy
    b. Intubation
    c. Needle thoracotomy
    d. Escharotomy

55. The patient was admitted for burns to the upper extremities after being trapped in a burning structure. The patient is also at risk for Impaired Gas Exchange related to inhalation of smoke and superheated fumes. Which diagnostic test best monitors this patient's gas exchange?
    a. Complete blood count
    b. Myoglobin level
    c. Carboxyhemoglobin level
    d. Chest x-ray

56. The patient in the burn intensive care unit is receiving vecuronium (Norcuron). What is the priority nursing intervention for this patient?
    a. Have emergency intubation equipment at the bedside.
    b. Ensure that all the equipment alarms are on and functional.
    c. Closely monitor the patient's urinary output every hour.
    d. Ensure that daily drug levels and electrolyte values are obtained.

True or False? *Read the statements about the acute phase of burn injury and write T for true or F for false in the blanks provided.*

_____ 57. It begins 24 hours after the injury and lasts until the wound closure is complete.

_____ 58. During the acute phase, the patient is at a high risk for infection.

_____ 59. Caloric requirements are decreased during this phase.

_____ 60. Pneumonia is a potential complication during this phase.

_____ 61. Active and passive range of motion for all joints should be assessed.

_____ 62. All patients are at risk for Disturbed Body Image.

63. The burn patient refuses to eat. The nursing diagnosis of Imbalanced Nutrition: Less than Body Requirements related to increased metabolic rate; reduced calorie intake is identified for this patient. What method does the nurse use to correctly weigh this patient?
    a. Weigh once a week after morning hygiene and compare to previous weight.
    b. Weigh daily at the same time of day and compare to preburn weight.
    c. Use a bed scale and subtract the estimated weight of linens.
    d. Weigh daily without dressings or splints and compare to preburn weight.

64. The student nurse is preparing to assist with hydrotherapy for a burn patient. The supervising nurse instructs the student to obtain the necessary equipment before beginning the procedure. What equipment does the student nurse obtain? *(Select all that apply.)*
    a. Scissors and forceps
    b. Hydrogen peroxide
    c. Mild soap or detergent
    d. Pressure dressings
    e. Washcloths and gauze sponges
    f. Chlorhexidine sponges

65. The nurse is applying a dressing to cover a burn on the patient's left leg. What technique does the nurse use?
    a. Consider the depth of the injury and amount of drainage, and work distal to proximal.
    b. Change the dressing every 4 hours or when the drainage leaks through the dressing.
    c. Consider the patient's mobility and the area of injury, and work proximal to distal.
    d. Use multiple gauze layers and roller gauze to pad and protect the joint areas.

66. The nurse has just received a phone report on the burn patient being transferred from the burn intensive care unit to the step-down burn unit. Which task is appropriate to delegate to unlicensed assistive personnel (UAP) in order to prepare the room?
    a. Place sterile sheets and a sterile pillowcase on the bed.
    b. Place a new disposable stethoscope in the room.
    c. Clear a space in the corner for the patient's flowers.
    d. Hang a sign on the door to prohibit entry of visitors.

67. The nurse is monitoring the nutritional status of the burn patient. Which indicators does the nurse use? *(Select all that apply.)*
    a. Amount of food the patient eats
    b. Weight to height ratio
    c. Serum albumin
    d. Amount of water the patient drinks
    e. Blood glucose
    f. Serum potassium

68. The nurse is educating the patient who has sustained burns to the dominant hand. What kind of active range of motion exercises does the nurse instruct the patient to perform?
    a. Exercise the hand, thumb, and fingers every hour while awake.
    b. Exercise the fingers and thumb at least three times a day.
    c. Use the hands to perform activities of daily living.
    d. Squeeze a soft rubber ball several times a day.

69. The burn patient must have pressure dressings applied to prevent contractures and reduce scarring. For maximum effectiveness, what procedure pertaining to the pressure garments is implemented?
    a. Changed every 24 to 48 hours to prevent infection
    b. Worn at least 23 hours a day until the scar tissue matures
    c. Removed for hygiene and during sleeping
    d. Applied with aseptic technique

70. The family reports that the burn patient is unable to perform self-care measures, so someone has been "doing everything for her." The nurse finds that the patient has the knowledge and the physical capacity to independently perform self-care. What is the nurse's best response?
    a. "What can your family do to help you feel better and stronger?"
    b. "You should be doing these things for yourself to increase your self-esteem."
    c. "What has been happening since you were discharged from the hospital?"
    d. "Let's review the principles of self-care that you learned in the hospital."

71. The patient who sustained severe burns to the face with significant scarring and disfigurement will soon be discharged from the hospital. Which intervention is best to help the patient make the transition into the community?
    a. Discuss cosmetic surgery that could occur over the next several years.
    b. Focus on the positive aspects of going home and being with family.
    c. Encourage the patient to look at the disfigurement and participate in self-care.
    d. Role play the scenario where a child asks about the scarring and disfigurement.

72. Complete the chart below about the characteristics of burns according to burn depth.

Characteristic	Superficial	Partial-Thickness Superficial	Deep Partial-Thickness	Full-Thickness	Deep Full-Thickness
Color					
Edema					
Pain					
Blisters					
Eschar					
Healing time					
Grafts required					
Example					

73. What does the process of full-thickness wound healing include? *(Select all that apply.)*
    a. Healing occurs by wound contraction.
    b. Eschar must be removed.
    c. Large blisters are protective and left undisturbed.
    d. Skin grafting may be necessary.
    e. Fasciotomy may be needed to relieve pressure and allow normal blood flow.

74. Which statement about the third spacing or capillary leak syndrome in the patient with severe burns is true?
    a. It usually happens in the first 36 to 48 hours.
    b. It is a leak of plasma fluids into the interstitial space.
    c. It is present only in the burned tissues.
    d. It can usually be prevented with diuretics.

75. As a result of third spacing, during the acute phase, which electrolyte imbalances may occur? *(Select all that apply.)*
    a. Hyperkalemia
    b. Hypokalemia
    c. Hypernatremia
    d. Hyponatremia
    e. Hypokalemia
    f. Hypercalcemia

76. Because of the fluid shifts in burn patients, what effects on cardiac output does the nurse expect to see?
    a. An initial increase, then normalized in 24 to 48 hours
    b. Depressed up to 36 hours after the burn
    c. Improved with fluid restriction
    d. Responsive to diuretics as evidenced by urinary output

77. The patient with burn injuries is being discharged from the hospital. What important points does the nurse include in the discharge teaching? *(Select all that apply.)*
    a. Signs and symptoms of infection
    b. Drug regimens and potential medication side effects
    c. Definition of full-thickness burns
    d. Correct application and care of pressure garments
    e. Comfort measures to reduce scarring
    f. Dates for follow-up appointments

78. The patient has sustained significant burns which have created a hypermetabolic state. In planning care for this patient, what does the nurse consider?
    a. Increased retention of sodium
    b. Decreased secretion of catecholamines
    c. Increased caloric needs
    d. The decrease in core temperature

79. The nurse is reviewing the laboratory results for several burn patients who are approximately 24 to 36 hours postinjury. What laboratory results related to the fluid remobilization these patients are currently experiencing does the nurse expect to see?
    a. Anemia
    b. Metabolic alkalosis
    c. Hypernatremia
    d. Hyperkalemia

80. Local tissue resistance to electricity varies in different parts of the body. Which tissue has the *most* resistance?
    a. Skin epidermis
    b. Tendons and muscle
    c. Fatty tissue
    d. Nerve tissue and blood vessels

81. The patient was rescued from a burning house and treated with oxygen. Initially, the patient had audible wheezing and wheezing on auscultation, but after approximately 30 minutes the wheezing stopped. The patient now demonstrates substernal retractions and anxiety. What action does the nurse take at this time?
    a. Recognize an impending airway obstruction and prepare for immediate intubation.
    b. Continue to monitor the patient's respiratory status and initiate pulse oximetry.
    c. Document this finding as evidence of improvement and continue to observe.
    d. Stay with and encourage the patient to remain calm and breathe deeply.

82. The nurse is caring for the young woman who sustained burns on the upper extremities and anterior chest while attempting to put out a kitchen grease fire. Which laboratory results does the nurse expect to see during the emergent period? *(Select all that apply.)*
    a. Potassium level of 3.2 mEq/L
    b. Glucose level of 180 mg/dL
    c. Hematocrit of 49%
    d. pH of 7.20
    e. Sodium level of 139 mEq/L

True or False? *Read the statements about the correct procedure for débridement and write T for true or F for false in the blanks provided.*

_____ 83. Eschar and other cellular debris are removed from the wound.

_____ 84. Nonviable tissue is removed during hydrotherapy.

_____ 85. Sterile saline is used during débridement.

_____ 86. Small blisters are usually opened.

_____ 87. Includes both mechanical and enzymatic actions.

88. The patient has sustained a burn to the right ankle. The physician has applied the initial dressing to the ankle, and the nurse assists the patient into bed and positions the ankle to prevent contracture. What is the correct position the nurse uses?
    a. Dorsiflexion
    b. Adduction
    c. External rotation
    d. Hyperextension

89. The patient has sustained a severe burn greater than 30% TBSA. What is the best way to assess renal function in this patient?
    a. Measure urine output and compare this value with fluid intake.
    b. Weigh the patient every day and compare that to the dry weight.
    c. Note the amount of edema and measure abdominal girth.
    d. Assist the patient with a urinal or bedpan every 2 hours.

90. The nurse is caring for the African-American patient with a burn injury. The patient appears to be having severe pain and discomfort that are unrelated to the burned areas. The nurse advocates that the physician order which additional test?
    a. Sickle cell for trait
    b. Drug screen for opiate abuse
    c. X-rays to identify bone injuries
    d. ECG to identify cardiac dysrhythmias

91. The physician has ordered an escharotomy for the patient because of constriction around the patient's chest. The nurse is teaching the patient and family about the procedure. Which statement by the family indicates a need for additional teaching?
    a. "He doesn't do well under general anesthesia."
    b. "He'll be awake for the procedure."
    c. "He will receive medication for sedation and pain."
    d. "We could stay with him at the bedside during the procedure."

92. The nurse is caring for the firefighter who was brought in for burns around the face and upper chest. Airway maintenance for this patient with respiratory involvement includes what action?
    a. Monitoring for signs and symptoms of upper airway edema during fluid resuscitation
    b. Inserting a nasopharyngeal or oropharyngeal airway when the patient's airway is completely obstructed
    c. Obtaining an order for PRN oxygen per nasal cannula
    d. Frequently suctioning the mouth with a Yankauer suction

93. At what point does fluid mobilization occur in patients with burns?
    a. After the scar tissue is formed and fluids are no longer being lost.
    b. Within the first 4 hours after the burns were sustained.
    c. After 36 hours when the fluid is reabsorbed from the interstitial tissue.
    d. Immediately after the burns occur.

94. The nurse is caring for the patient with chronic pain associated with an old burn injury. Which nonpharmacologic intervention does the nurse use to help relieve the patient's pain?
    a. Nitrous oxide
    b. Cool room temperature to reduce discomfort
    c. Massaging nonburned areas
    d. Intravenous narcotics due to delayed tissue absorption

Matching. Match the different types of dressing materials with their descriptions.

Dressing Materials
a. Artificial skin
b. Xenograft
c. Allograft
d. Biobrane
e. Cultured skin
f. Amniotic membrane
g. Synthetic dressing

Descriptions

_____ 95. Biologic dressing from a cadaver provided by a skin bank

_____ 96. Membrane obtained from an animal donor

_____ 97. Does not develop a blood supply; it disintegrates in about 48 hours

_____ 98. Cells are grown in a laboratory to produce cell sheets

_____ 99. Silastic epidermis and a porous dermis made from beef collagen and shark cartilage

_____ 100. Made up of a nylon fabric that is partially embedded into a silicone film

_____ 101. Made of solid silicone and plastic membranes

102. The patient with a burn injury had an autograft. The nurse learns in report that the donor site is on the upper thigh. What type of wound does the nurse expect to find at donor site?
    a. Stage 1
    b. Partial thickness
    c. Full thickness
    d. Stage 4

103. To prevent the complication of Curling's ulcer, what does the nurse anticipate the physician will order?
    a. Nasogastric tube insertion
    b. H_2 histamine blockers
    c. Abdominal assessment every 4 hours
    d. Systemic antibiotic

104. Several patients are transported from an industrial fire to a local ED. Which factors increase the risk of death for these patients? *(Select all that apply.)*
    a. Male gender
    b. Age greater than 60 years
    c. Burn greater than 40% TBSA
    d. Presence of an inhalation injury
    e. Presence of contact burns

105. What is the most essential patient data needed for calculating the fluid rates, energy requirements, and drug doses for the burn patient?
    a. Age
    b. Previous health history
    c. Preburn weight
    d. Current weight

106. Which drug therapy reduces the risk of wound infection for burn patients?
    a. Large doses of oral antifungal medications every 4 hours
    b. Silver nitrate solution covered by dry dressings applied every 4 hours
    c. Silver sulfadiazine (Silvadene) on full-thickness injuries every 4 hours
    d. Broad-spectrum antibiotics given intravenously

107. The patient has sustained a relatively large burn. The nurse anticipates that the patient's nutritional requirements may exceed how many kcal/day?
    a. 1500
    b. 2000
    c. 3000
    d. 5000

108. Which feelings are most typically expressed by the burn patient? *(Select all that apply.)*
    a. Suspicion
    b. Regression
    c. Apathy
    d. Denial
    e. Suicidal ideations
    f. Anger

109. The patient has been depressed and withdrawn since her injury and has expressed that "life will never be the same." Which nursing intervention best promotes a positive image for this burn patient?
    a. Discussing the possibility of reconstructive surgery with the patient
    b. Allowing the patient to choose a colorful scarf to cover the burned area
    c. Playing cards or board games with the patient
    d. Encouraging the patient to consider how fortunate she is to be alive

110. The 28-year-old male patient sustained second- and third-degree burns on his legs (30%) when his clothing caught fire while he was burning leaves. He was hosed down by his neighbor and has arrived at the ED in severe discomfort. What is the priority nursing diagnosis for this patient at this time?
    a. Acute Pain related to damaged or exposed nerve endings
    b. Deficient Fluid Volume related to electrolyte imbalance
    c. Risk for Pulmonary Edema
    d. Disturbed Body Image related to the appearance of legs

111. Which patient has the highest risk for a fatal burn injury?
    a. 4-year-old child
    b. 32-year-old man
    c. 45-year-old woman
    d. 77-year-old man

112. **Crossword Puzzle.** Complete the crossword puzzle by answering the questions below.

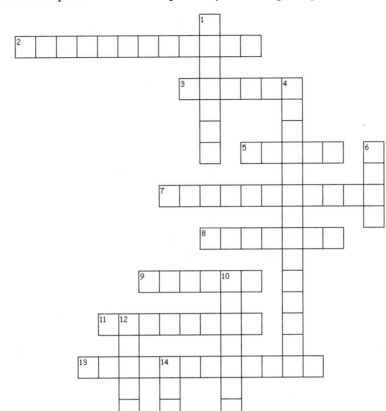

Across

2. A patient has noticed that the skin is peeling off 3 days after a severe sunburn. What is this called?

3. Also known as "burn crust."

5. The nurse monitors for this severe complication of a full-thickness burn by watching for tachycardia, decreased blood pressure, decreased peripheral pulses, and other signs of decreased cardiac output.

7. After spending the day at the beach, a teenage girl has a severe sunburn. This is an example of a _____-thickness burn.

8. _____-thickness burn involves the entire epidermis and varying parts of the dermis.

9. To assess whether a superficial partial-thickness wound is present, the nurse notes that the wound is red, moist, and _____ when pressure is applied.

11. A patient is admitted to a burn trauma unit after suffering a severe electrical shock. He is in the _____ phase of burn injury.

13. The patient in Question 11 has severe edema. This is due to a fluid shift, known as _____ _____ (two words).

Down

1. A patient who was admitted with a severe burn after spilling hot liquid on his legs will be receiving a heterograft. The most common heterograft, which is compatible with human skin, is made from _____.

4. After 48 hours, the patient in Question 11 begins to produce large amounts of urine. This is known as fluid _____.

6. A patient is admitted after a house fire with severe burns across her body. The burns have destroyed the entire epidermis and dermis layers. This is known as a _____-thickness wound.

10. A camper spills bacon grease on his foot while cooking breakfast. This type of burn is a ____ burn.

12. An older adult man tips over a tea kettle with boiling water and burns the skin of his abdomen and thighs. This type of heat injury is a _____ burn, or a scald.

14. A patient suffers burns on her arms after the sleeves of her robe catch fire while she is cooking breakfast. This type of burn injury is known as a _____ heat injury.

CASE STUDY: THE OLDER ADULT WITH SEVERE BURNS

Use a separate sheet of paper to answer the questions in this Case Study. Answer guidelines for this Case Study are available on your Evolve website at http://evolve. elsevier.com/Iggy/ in the "Prepare for Class" folder.

An older adult woman arrives in the ED at 11:00 AM. According to her family, she was cooking and accidentally spilled a pot of boiling liquids while trying to move the pan from the stove to the table. She sustained severe burns on her arms, anterior trunk, and legs. The injury occurred at 9:00 AM, but she was home alone and tried to administer first aid before notifying her family. She weighs 70 kg and the burns are estimated at 50% TBSA.

1. Identify the age-related changes that increase morbidity and mortality in the older adult.
2. Identify information that should be included in a history.
3. Why is it important to evaluate the size and extent of the burn?
4. Using the Parkland (Baxter) formula, calculate the fluids needed for the first 8 hours after injury.
5. What time does the first 8-hour period end?
6. How much fluid is required for the 24 hours?
7. Hourly urine output is adjusted to _____ mL/kg.
8. Tissue destruction caused by a burn injury causes local and systemic problems. Identify six of these potential problems.
9. Early detection of wound infection is important. The wound should be examined for which six signs of infection?
10. Identify priority nursing diagnoses for patients with burn injuries in the emergent phase who have sustained a burn injury greater than 25% TBSA.

Assessment of the Respiratory System

CHAPTER

29

STUDY/REVIEW QUESTIONS

Matching. *Match each function/description of the airway with its corresponding location.*

Locations

a. Upper airway
b. Lower airway

Functions/Descriptions

_____ 1. Traps particles not filtered by nares

_____ 2. Traps organisms entering nose and mouth

_____ 3. Trachea

_____ 4. Contains cilia to move mucus to trachea

_____ 5. Composed of alveoli for gas exchange

_____ 6. Pharynx, or throat

_____ 7. Place where the trachea divides into the right and left bronchi

_____ 8. Larynx

_____ 9. Dividing point where solid foods and fluids are separated from air

_____ 10. Epiglottis

_____ 11. Pleura

_____ 12. Alveoli

Matching. *Match each process of respiration with its description.*

Processes

a. Diffusion
b. Perfusion
c. Ventilation

Descriptions

_____ 13. Movement of air in and out of the lungs

_____ 14. Exchange of oxygen and carbon dioxide in the capillary-alveolar network

_____ 15. Pumping of oxygenated blood through the body

16. The patient comes to the physician's office for an annual physical. The patient reports having a persistent nagging cough. Which question does the nurse ask first about this symptom?
    a. "When did the cough start?"
    b. "Do you have a family history of lung cancer?"
    c. "Have you been running a fever"
    d. "Do you have sneezing and congestion?"

17. The patient reports smoking a pack of cigarettes a day for 9 years. He then quit for 2 years, then smoked 2 packs a day for the last 30 years. What are the pack-years for this patient?
    a. 39 years
    b. 69 years
    c. 19.5 years
    d. 41 years

18. Pulmonary function tests are scheduled for a patient with a history of smoking who reports dyspnea and chronic cough. What will patient teaching information about this procedure include?
    a. Do not smoke for at least 2 weeks before the test.
    b. Bronchodilator drugs may be withheld 2 days before the test.
    c. The patient will breathe through the mouth and wear a nose clip during the test.
    d. The patient will be expected to walk on a treadmill during the test.

19. The patient is scheduled to have a pulmonary function test (PFT). Which type of information does the nurse include in the nursing history so that PFT results can be appropriately determined?
    a. Age, gender, race, height, weight, and smoking status
    b. Occupational status, activity tolerance for activities of daily living
    c. Medication history and history of allergies to contrast media
    d. History of chronic medical conditions and surgical procedures

Matching. *Match each PFT with its description.*

PFTs
a. Forced expiratory volume (FEV)
b. Functional residual capacity (FRC)
c. Forced vital capacity (FVC)
d. Residual volume (RV)
e. Total lung capacity (TLC)
f. Vital capacity (VC)
g. Diffusion

Descriptions

_____ 20. Maximal amount of forced air that can be exhaled after maximal inspiration

_____ 21. Amount of air in lungs at the end of maximal inhalation

_____ 22. Amount of air remaining in lungs after normal exhalation

_____ 23. Maximal amount of air that can be exhaled over a specific time

_____ 24. Amount of air remaining in lungs at the end of full, forced exhalation

_____ 25. Measure of carbon monoxide uptake across alveolar-capillary membrane

_____ 26. Maximum amount of gas that can be exhaled after maximal inspiration

27. The nurse is caring for the older adult who is temporarily confined to bed. Which intervention is important in promoting pulmonary hygiene related to age and decreased mobility?
    a. Obtain an order for PRN oxygen via nasal cannula.
    b. Encourage the patient to turn, cough, and deep breathe.
    c. Reassure the patient that immobility is temporary.
    d. Monitor the respiratory rate and check pulse oximetry readings.

28. The nurse is assessing an older adult patient who reports a decreased tolerance for exercise and that she must work harder to breathe. Which question assists the nurse in determining if these are normal changes related to aging?
    a. "How old are you?"
    b. "When did you first notice these symptoms?"
    c. "Do you or have you ever smoked cigarettes?"
    d. "How often do you exercise?"

29. The patient has had a bronchoscopy and was NPO for several hours before the test. Now a few hours after the test, the patient is hungry and would like to eat a meal. What will the nurse do?
    a. Order a meal because the patient is now alert and oriented.
    b. Check pulse oximetry to be sure oxygen saturation has returned to normal.
    c. Check for a gag reflex before allowing the patient to eat.
    d. Assess for nausea from the medications given for the test.

30. After a bronchoscopy procedure, the patient coughs up sputum which contains blood. What is the best nursing intervention for this patient?
    a. Assess vital signs and respiratory status and notify the physician of the findings.
    b. Monitor the patient for 24 hours to see if blood continues in the sputum.
    c. Send the sputum to the lab for cytology for possible lung cancer.
    d. Reassure the patient this is a normal response after a bronchoscopy.

31. Before a bronchoscopy procedure, the patient received benzocaine spray as a topical anesthetic to numb the oropharynx. The nurse is assessing the patient after the procedure. Which finding suggests that the patient is developing methemoglobinemia?
    a. The patient has a decreased hematocrit level.
    b. The patient does not respond to supplemental oxygen.
    c. The blood sample is a bright cherry red color.
    d. The patient experiences sedation and amnesia.

32. The nurse is caring for several patients who had diagnostic testing for respiratory disorders. Which diagnostic test has the highest risk for the postprocedure complication of pneumothorax?
    a. Bronchoscopy
    b. Laryngoscopy
    c. Computed tomography of lungs
    d. Percutaneous lung biopsy

33. The patient's pulse oximetry reading is 89%. What is the nurse's priority action?
    a. Recheck the reading with a different oximeter.
    b. Apply supplemental oxygen and recheck the oximeter reading in 15 minutes.
    c. Assess the patient for respiratory distress and recheck the oximeter reading.
    d. Place the patient in the recovery position and monitor frequently.

34. The patient demonstrates labored shallow respirations and a respiratory rate of 32/min with a pulse oximetry reading of 85%. What is the priority nursing intervention?
    a. Notify respiratory therapy to give the patient a breathing treatment.
    b. Start oxygen via nasal cannula at 2 L/min.
    c. Obtain an order for a stat arterial blood gas (ABG).
    d. Encourage coughing and deep-breathing exercises.

35. The older patient is confined to bed and is therefore prone to decreased alveolar surface and elastic recoil. Which intervention is best to address these physiologic changes?
    a. Adequate nutritional intake
    b. Coughing and deep breathing
    c. Fluids to thin secretions
    d. Periods of rest and sleep

36. The nurse is reviewing ABG results from an 86-year-old patient. Which results would be considered normal findings for a patient of this age?
    a. Normal pH, normal Pao_2, normal $Paco_2$
    b. Normal pH, decreased Pao_2, normal $Paco_2$
    c. Decreased pH, decreased Pao_2, normal $Paco_2$
    d. Decreased pH, decreased Pao_2, decreased $Paco_2$

37. The nurse is caring for an older patient and identifies a nursing diagnosis of Ineffective Airway Clearance. Which etiology for this diagnosis is related to the normal aging process?
    a. Decreased muscle strength and cough
    b. Increased carbon dioxide exchange
    c. Decreased residual volume
    d. Increased elastic recoil of the lungs

38. The nurse is performing a physical assessment of the respiratory system. Although the patient is currently confined to bed, he has the strength and mobility to move and reposition himself. The nurse instructs him to assume which position for the assessment?
    a. Side-lying
    b. Semi-Fowler's
    c. Supine
    d. Sitting upright

39. Upon performing a lung sound assessment of the anterior chest, the nurse hears moderately loud sounds on inspiration that are equal in length with expiration. In what area is this lung sound considered normal?
    a. Trachea
    b. Primary bronchi
    c. Lung fields
    d. Larynx

40. Which sounds in the smaller bronchioles and the alveoli indicate normal lung sounds?
    a. Harsh, hollow, and tubular blowing
    b. Nothing; normally no sounds are heard
    c. Soft, low rustling; like wind in the trees
    d. Flat and dull tones with a moderate pitch

41. What is the characteristic of normal lung sounds that should be heard throughout the lung fields?
    a. Short inspiration, long expiration, loud, harsh
    b. Soft sound, long inspiration, short quiet expiration
    c. Mixed sounds of harsh and soft, long inspiration and long expiration
    d. Loud, long inspiration and short, loud expiration

42. Upon assessing the lungs, the nurse hears short, discrete popping sounds "like hair being rolled between fingers near the ear" in the bilateral lower lobes. How is this assessment documented?
    a. Rhonchi
    b. Wheezes
    c. Fine crackles
    d. Coarse crackles

43. The nurse is taking a history on a patient who reports sleeping in a recliner chair at night because lying on the bed causes shortness of breath. How is this documented?
    a. Orthopnea
    b. Paroxysmal nocturnal dyspnea
    c. Orthostatic nocturnal dyspnea
    d. Tachypnea

44. On the diagram below, indicate the correct sequence for percussion and auscultation for the anteroposterior assessment of the lungs.

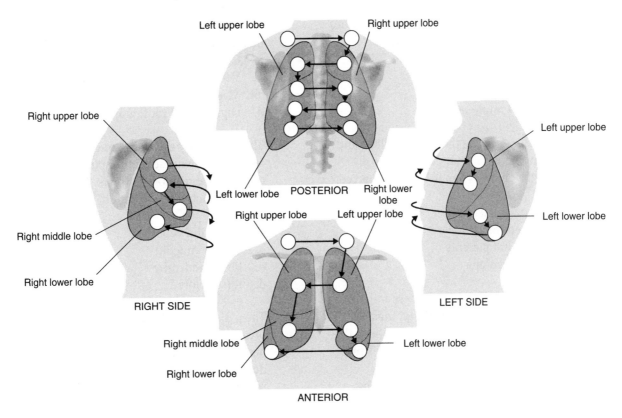

45. Which patient has an increased risk for problems of the respiratory system?
    a. 45-year-old man who breeds and raises racing pigeons
    b. 25-year-old woman who enjoys body surfing in the ocean
    c. 68-year-old woman who does needlework for relaxation
    d. 56-year-old man who ties flies for trout fishing

46. What observations does the nurse make when performing a general assessment of the patient's lungs and thorax? *(Select all that apply.)*
    a. Symmetry of chest movement
    b. Rate, rhythm, and depth of respirations
    c. Use of accessory muscles for breathing
    d. Comparison of the anteroposterior diameter with the lateral diameter
    e. Measurement of the length of the chest cavity
    f. Assessment of chest expansion and respiratory excursion

47. Which assessment finding is an objective sign of chronic oxygen deprivation?
    a. Continuous cough productive of clear sputum
    b. Audible inspiratory and expiratory wheeze
    c. Chest pain that increases with deep inspiration
    d. Clubbing of fingernails and a barrel-shaped chest

48. The nurse is palpating the patient's chest and identifies an increased tactile fremitus or vibration of the chest wall produced when the patient speaks. What does the nurse do next?
    a. Observe for other findings associated with subcutaneous emphysema.
    b. Document the observation as an expected normal finding.
    c. Observe the patient for other findings associated with a pneumothorax.
    d. Document the observation as a pleural friction rub.

49. The nurse reviews the complete blood count results for the patient who has chronic obstructive pulmonary disease (COPD) and lives in a high mountain area. What lab results does the nurse expect to see for this patient?
    a. Increased red blood cells
    b. Decreased neutrophils
    c. Decreased eosinophils
    d. Increased lymphocytes

50. The nurse is inspecting the patient's chest and observes an increase in anteroposterior diameter of the chest. When is this an expected finding?
    a. With a pulmonary mass
    b. Upon deep inhalation
    c. In older adult patients
    d. With chest trauma

51. While percussing the patient's chest and lung fields, the nurse notes a high, loud, musical, drumlike sound similar to tapping a cheek that is puffed out with air. What is the nurse's priority action?
    a. Document this expected finding using words like, "high," "loud," and "hollow."
    b. Immediately notify the physician because the patient has an airway obstruction.
    c. Assess the patient for air hunger or pain at the end of inhalation and exhalation.
    d. Palpate for crackling sensation underneath the skin or for localized tenderness.

52. What is the best position for the patient to assume for a thoracentesis?
    a. Side-lying, affected side exposed, head slightly raised
    b. Lying flat with arm on affected side across the chest
    c. Sitting up, leaning forward on the overbed table
    d. Prone position with arms above the head

53. Which procedure has a risk for the complication of pneumothorax?
    a. Thoracentesis
    b. Bronchoscopy
    c. PFT
    d. Ventilation-perfusion scan

54. The patient is admitted for a deep vein thrombosis (DVT) and later becomes short of breath. A pulmonary embolus is suspected. The nurse should prepare the patient for which type of diagnostic testing?
    a. Computed tomography
    b. Ventilation-perfusion scanning
    c. Magnetic resonance imaging
    d. Digital chest radiography

55. The respiratory therapist consults with and reports to the nurse on the sputum production of several respiratory patients. The patient producing which kind of sputum needs priority attention?
    a. Thick and yellow
    b. Watery mucoid
    c. Pink and frothy
    d. Rust-colored

56. The patient with chronic respiratory disease presents with a decreased level of consciousness, dusky skin, pale mucous membranes, decreased capillary refill, and an increased respiratory rate. What is the priority nursing diagnosis?
    a. Ineffective Airway Clearance
    b. Ineffective Tissue Perfusion
    c. Decreased Cardiac Output
    d. Acute Confusion

57. While caring for a patient who had a routine surgical procedure, the nurse suspects that the patient may be having decreased tissue perfusion. Which assessment finding is considered the earliest sign of decreased oxygenation?
    a. Cyanosis
    b. Unexplained restlessness
    c. Cool, clammy skin
    d. Paleness, shortness of breath

58. The nurse has just received a patient from the recovery room who is somewhat drowsy, but is capable of following instructions. Pulse oximetry has dropped from 95% to 90%. What is the priority nursing intervention?
    a. Administer oxygen at 2 L/min by nasal cannula, then reassess.
    b. Have the patient perform coughing and deep-breathing exercises, then reassess.
    c. Administer Narcan to reverse narcotic sedation effect.
    d. Withhold narcotic pain medication to reduce sedation effect.

Matching. *Match the pulmonary function capacities and functions with the correct corresponding assessment findings. One answer will not be used.*

Capacities and Functions
a. Forced vital capacity (FVC)
b. Forced expiratory volume in 1 sec (FEV$_1$)
c. Forced expiratory flow (FEF)
d. Functional residual capacity (FRC)
e. Total lung capacity (TLC)
f. Residual volume (RV)
g. Diffusion capacity of carbon monoxide (DLCO)

Assessment Findings

_____ 59. Reduced in patients with obstructive disease and increased with exercise or congestive heart failure

_____ 60. Air left in lung after a forced exhalation

_____ 61. Largest amount of air the lungs can hold

_____ 62. After a maximum deep breath, amount of air quickly exhaled

_____ 63. Not used to measure larger airway obstructions

_____ 64. After a maximum deep breath, the maximum amount of air exhaled in the first 1 second

65. The patient is scheduled for a ventilation-perfusion scan. What does the nurse explain to the patient about the procedure?
    a. Being NPO before the examination is necessary to prevent aspiration of the dye.
    b. After the test, isolation is necessary for 8 hours because of the radioactive dye.
    c. The procedure is painless and the radioactive substance leaves the body in about 8 hours.
    d. The test screens for pulmonary embolus; a CT scan will follow if needed.

66. What is a pulse oximeter used to measure?
    a. Oxygen perfusion in the extremities
    b. Pulse and perfusion in the extremities
    c. Generalized tissue perfusion
    d. Oxygen saturation in the red blood cells

67. Which aspect of PFTs would be considered a normal result in the older adult?
    a. Increased forced vital capacity
    b. Decline in forced expiratory volume in 1 second
    c. Decrease in diffusion capacity of carbon monoxide
    d. Increased functional residual capacity

68. In the older adult, there is a loss of elastic recoiling of the lung and decreased chest wall compliance. What is the result of this occurrence?
    a. The thoracic area becomes shorter.
    b. The patient has an increased activity tolerance.
    c. There is an increase in anteroposterior ratio.
    d. The patient has severe shortness of breath.

69. In the older adult, there is a decreased number of functional alveoli. To assist the patient to compensate for this change related to aging, what does the nurse do?
    a. Encourage the patient to ambulate and change positions.
    b. Allow the patient to rest and sleep frequently.
    c. Have face-to-face conversations when possible.
    d. Obtain an order for supplemental oxygen.

70. The nurse teaches the patient about the impact of cigarette smoking on the lower respiratory tract. Which statement by the patient indicates an understanding of the information?
    a. "Smoking increases my susceptibility to respiratory infections."
    b. "If I stop smoking the damage to my lungs will be reversed."
    c. "Cigarette smoke affects my ability to cough out secretions from the lungs."
    d. "Smoking makes the large and small airways get bigger."

71. The patient reports fatigue and shortness of breath when getting up to walk to the bathroom; however, the pulse oximetry reading is 99%. The nurse identifies a diagnosis of Activity Intolerance. Which laboratory value is consistent with the patient's subjective symptoms?
    a. BUN of 15 mg/dL
    b. WBC count of 8000/mm^3
    c. Hemoglobin of 9g/dL
    d. Glucose 160 mg/dL

72. The nurse is performing a respiratory assessment including pulse oximetry on several patients. Which patients or situations may cause an artificially low reading? *(Mark Y for yes or N for no, and provide a rationale for your answers.)*

    _____ a. Patient with peripheral arterial disease

    _____ b. Patient with anemia

    _____ c. Patient with sickle cell disease

    _____ d. Patient with a fever

    _____ e. Patient receiving oxygen via nasal cannula

    _____ f. Patient in severe shock

    _____ g. Patient receiving narcotic pain medication

    _____ h. African-American patient

    _____ i. Female patients versus male patients

    _____ j. Patient with history of respiratory diseases such as cystic fibrosis or tuberculosis

    _____ k. Patient with allergies

73. The patient who had neck surgery for removal of a tumor reports, "not being able to breathe very well." The nurse observes that the patient has decreased chest movement and an elevated pulse. A bronchoscopy is ordered. For what reason did the physician order a bronchoscopy for this patient?
    a. Reverse and relieve any obstruction caused during the neck surgery
    b. Assess the function of vocal cords or remove foreign bodies from the larynx
    c. Aspirate pleural fluid or air from the pleural space
    d. Visualize airway structures and obtaining tissue samples

74. The patient returns to the unit after bronchoscopy. In addition to respiratory status assessment, which assessment does the nurse make in order to prevent aspiration?
    a. Presence of pain or soreness in throat
    b. Time and amount of last oral fluid intake
    c. Type and location of chest pain
    d. Presence or absence of gag reflex

75. The nurse hears fine crackles during a lung assessment of the patient who is in the initial postoperative period. Which nursing intervention helps relieve this respiratory problem?
    a. Monitor the patient with a pulse oximeter.
    b. Encourage coughing and deep breathing.
    c. Obtain an order for a chest x-ray.
    d. Obtain an order for high-flow oxygen.

76. In performing a respiratory assessment, which finding is considered the principal or main sign of respiratory disease?
    a. Sputum production
    b. Continuous cough
    c. Fever with congestion
    d. Increased respiratory rate

77. The patient is admitted for a pneumothorax. Which clinical assessment findings are most likely to be documented in the patient's admission record?
    a. Progressive fatigue and shortness of breath that has been increasing over a period of years
    b. Cough, high fever, rusty-colored sputum production with decreased breath sounds, particularly in lower lobes
    c. Frequent cough and copious sputum production, and wheezing and coarse crackles heard throughout the lung fields
    d. Sudden onset of sharp pain after sneezing with lung sounds diminished over the left upper lobe

78. For a healthy adult, what is the expected normal range for the respiratory rate per minute?
    a. 10 to 12
    b. 12 to 15
    c. 12 to 20
    d. 20 or more

79. The nurse is reviewing partial pressure of arterial oxygen (Pao_2) levels for several adult patients. Which patient has a Pao_2 that is lower than expected for his age?
    a. 40-year-old man with a Pao_2 of 96
    b. 85-year-old man with a Pao_2 of 83.5
    c. 65-year-old man with a Pao_2 of 92
    d. 50-year-old man with a Pao_2 of 84

80. The nurse is performing a respiratory assessment on the older adult patient. Which question is not appropriate to ask when using the Gordon's Functional Health Pattern Assessment approach?
    a. "How has your general health been?"
    b. "Have you had any colds this past year?"
    c. "Do you have sufficient energy to do what you like to do?"
    d. "When was the last time you were hospitalized?"

81. The patient has previously reported several chronic health conditions including hypertension and heart problems, and has stated a new drug was recently added to his drug regimen. Today the patient reports a new onset of cough. Which drug does the nurse suspect the patient has recently been prescribed?
    a. ACE inhibitor
    b. Vasodilator
    c. Diuretic
    d. Calcium channel blocker

82. The nurse makes observations about several respiratory patients' abilities to perform activities of daily living in order to quantify the level of dyspnea. Which patient is considered to have Class V dyspnea?
    a. Experiences subjective shortness of breath when walking up a flight of stairs
    b. Limited to bed or chair and experiences shortness of breath at rest
    c. Can independently shower and dress, but cannot keep pace with similarly aged people
    d. Experiences shortness of breath during aerobic exercise such as jogging

83. The nurse is reviewing the arterial blood gas results for a 25-year-old trauma patient who has new onset of shortness of breath and demonstrates shallow and irregular respirations. The pH is 7.26. What imbalance does the nurse suspect this patient has?
    a. Respiratory acidosis
    b. Respiratory alkalosis
    c. Metabolic acidosis
    d. Metabolic alkalosis

84. The patient is HIV-positive and reports feeling tired with shortness of breath, weight loss, and occasionally coughing up blood-tinged sputum. After considering these symptoms in conjunction with the patient's HIV status, what disorder does the nurse suspect this patient has?
    a. Tuberculosis
    b. Bronchitis
    c. Pneumococcal pneumonia
    d. Lung abscess

CASE STUDY: RESPIRATORY TRACT ASSESSMENT

Use a separate sheet of paper to answer the questions in this Case Study. Answer guidelines for this Case Study are available on your Evolve website at http://evolve. elsevier.com/Iggy/ in the "Prepare for Class" folder.

The adult patient reports to the pulmonary clinic with complaints of a productive cough that "won't go away." She is a 62-year-old married housewife whose children are grown. She smoked two packs of cigarettes per day for 20 years, but she has not smoked for the past 10 years. She contracted a "virus" 4 weeks ago, which "settled in her chest." Her usual remedies have not resulted in improvement in her status.

1. What additional subjective data should the nurse elicit from this patient?
2. What physical assessments should the nurse perform on this patient?
3. What effect does this patient's 10 years of not smoking have on the condition of her lungs?
4. The physician orders a chest x-ray and a sputum specimen. What should the nurse tell this patient about these tests?

After 1 week, this patient reports no improvement, and the chest x-ray results also indicate that there is no change. A bronchoscopy is scheduled to be done in the outpatient surgical unit the following day. (The physician would prefer to do an MRI scan, but the patient has an inner-ear implant.)

5. Prepare a teaching-learning plan for this patient regarding the bronchoscopy. Consider restrictions related to breathing during the procedure.
6. When the patient reports to the outpatient surgical unit the next morning, what assessments should the nurse make?
7. Both the patient and her husband are very anxious. Describe interventions that the nurse should implement to assist the patient and her spouse.

Thirty minutes before the procedure, the patient is given atropine sulfate 0.6 mg IM. An intravenous infusion is begun with $D_5$1/2 NS, and diazepam (Valium) 10 mg IV is given.

8. Why have these medications been ordered?
9. A topical anesthetic agent is applied to the pharynx immediately before the bronchoscopy is to begin. What is the purpose of this agent?
10. What special actions must the nurse take after the procedure is completed and the patient is taken to the PACU?
11. What equipment should be available when she arrives?
12. What are the reasons for having this equipment available?

30 CHAPTER

Care of Patients Requiring Oxygen Therapy or Tracheostomy

STUDY/REVIEW QUESTIONS

True or False? *Read the statements about oxygen therapy and write T for true or F for false in the blanks provided. If the statement is false, correct the statement to make it true.*

_____ 1. Oxygen therapy is needed when the normal 21% oxygen in the air is inadequate and causes hypoxemia and hypoxia.

_____ 2. Examples of conditions that can increase the body's need for more oxygen are infection in the blood, increase in body temperature such as 101° F, Hgb of 9.0, or sickle cell disease.

_____ 3. Hypoxemia and hypoxia can be measured by low Pao_2 and low pulse oximetry.

_____ 4. In order to improve breathing, supplemental oxygen is based on analysis of the patient's symptoms.

_____ 5. A low Pao_2 level is the patient's primary drive for breathing.

_____ 6. Oxygen is a fire hazard because it can spontaneously ignite when in use.

7. The patient requires home oxygen therapy. When the home health nurse enters the patient's home for the initial visit, he observes several issues that are safety hazards related to the patient's oxygen therapy. What hazards do these include? *(Select all that apply.)*
   a. Bottle of wine in the kitchen area
   b. Package of cigarettes on the coffee table
   c. Several decorative candles on the mantlepiece
   d. Grounded outlet with a green dot on the plate
   e. Electric fan with a frayed cord in the bathroom
   f. Computer with a three-pronged plug

8. Before completing the morning assessment, the nurse concludes that the patient is experiencing inadequate oxygenation and tissue perfusion as a result of respiratory problems. Which assessment findings support the nurse's conclusion? *(Select all that apply.)*
   a. Inspiratory and expiratory effort is shallow, even, and quiet.
   b. Patient must take a breath after every third or fourth word.
   c. Skin is pale, pink, and dry.
   d. Patient appears strained and fatigued.
   e. Pulse of 95 beats/min, respiratory rate of 30/min.
   f. Patient does not want to eat.

9. The home health nurse has been caring for a patient with a chronic respiratory disorder. Today the patient seems confused when she is normally alert and oriented x 3. What is the priority nursing action?
    a. Notify the physician about the mental status change.
    b. Take vital signs and check the pulse oximeter readings.
    c. Ask the patient's family when this behavior started.
    d. Perform a mental status examination.

10. The nurse is caring for several patients on a general medical-surgical unit. The nurse would question the necessity of oxygen therapy for the patient with which condition?
    a. Pulmonary edema with decreased arterial Po_2 levels
    b. Valve replacement with increased cardiac output
    c. Anemia with a decreased hemoglobin and hematocrit
    d. Sustained fever with an increased metabolic demand

11. When a patient is requiring oxygen therapy, what is important for the nurse to know?
    a. Patients require 1 to 10 L/min by nasal cannula in order for oxygen to be effective.
    b. Oxygen-induced hypoventilation is the priority when the $Paco_2$ levels are unknown.
    c. Why the patient is receiving oxygen, expected outcomes, and complications.
    d. The goal is the highest Fio_2 possible for the particular device being used.

12. The patient with chronic obstructive pulmonary disease (COPD) is admitted to the hospital with oxygen-induced hypoventilation. What is the respiratory stimulus to breathe for this patient?
    a. High carbon dioxide (60 to 65 mm Hg) level in the blood that rose over time
    b. Low level of carbon dioxide concentration in the blood, as sensed by the chemoreceptors in the brain
    c. Low level of oxygen concentration in the blood, as sensed by the peripheral chemoreceptors
    d. Oxygen narcosis which stimulates central chemoreceptors in the brain

13. The nurse is administering oxygen to the patient who is hypoxic and has chronic high levels of carbon dioxide. Which oxygen therapy prevents a respiratory complication for this patient?
    a. Fio_2 higher than the usual 2 to 4 L/min per nasal cannula
    b. Venturi mask of 40% for the delivery of oxygen
    c. Lower concentration of oxygen (1 to 2 L/min) per nasal cannula
    d. Variable Fio_2 via partial rebreather mask

14. The patient is at high risk or unknown risk for oxygen-induced hypoventilation. What must the nurse monitor for?
    a. Signs of nonproductive cough, chest pain, crackles, and hypoxemia
    b. Change of skin tone from pink to gray color after several minutes of oxygen therapy
    c. Signs and symptoms of hypoventilation rather than hypoxemia
    d. Changes in level of consciousness, apnea, and respiratory pattern

15. The patient is receiving a high concentration of oxygen as a temporary emergency measure. Which nursing action is the most appropriate to prevent complications associated with high-flow oxygen?
    a. Auscultate the lungs every 4 hours for oxygen toxicity.
    b. Increase the oxygen if the PaO_2 level is less than 93 mm Hg.
    c. Monitor the prescribed oxygen level and length of therapy.
    d. Decrease the oxygen if the patient's condition does not respond.

16. Increased risk for oxygen toxicity is related to which factors? *(Select all that apply.)*
    a. Continuous delivery of oxygen at greater than 50% concentration
    b. Delivery of a high concentration of oxygen over 24 to 48 hours
    c. The severity and extent of lung disease
    d. Neglecting to monitor the patient's status and reducing oxygen concentration as soon as possible
    e. Excluding measures such as continuous positive airway pressure (CPAP) or positive end-expiratory pressure (PEEP)

17. The patient is receiving humidified oxygen which places the patient at high risk for which nursing diagnosis?
    a. Risk for Injury related to the moisture in the tube
    b. Risk for Infection related to the condensation in the tubing
    c. Impaired Physical Mobility related to reliance on equipment
    d. Risk for Impaired Skin Integrity related to the mask

18. The patient is receiving warmed and humidified oxygen. The respiratory therapist informs the nurse that several other patients on other units have developed hospital-acquired infections and *Pseudomonas aeruginosa* has been identified as the organism. What does the nurse do?
    a. Place the patient in respiratory isolation.
    b. Obtain an order for a sputum culture.
    c. Change the humidifier every 24 hours.
    d. Obtain an order to discontinue the humidifier.

19. Nursing interventions to prevent infection in patients with humidified oxygen include which actions?
    a. Use sterile normal saline to provide moisture.
    b. Drain condensation into the humidifier.
    c. Drain condensation from the water trap.
    d. Maintain a sterile closed system at all times.

20. Which factors are considered hazards associated with oxygen therapy? *(Select all that apply.)*
    a. Increased combustion
    b. Oxygen narcosis
    c. Oxygen toxicity
    d. Absorption atelectasis
    d. Hypoxic drive
    e. Oxygen-induced hypoventilation

21. The patient is receiving warmed and humidified oxygen. In discarding the moisture formed by condensation, why does the nurse minimize the time that the tubing is disconnected?
    a. To prevent the patient from desaturating
    b. To reduce the patient's risk of infection
    c. To minimize the disturbance to the patient
    d. To facilitate overall time management

22. What is the best description of the nurse's role in the delivery of oxygen therapy?
    a. Receiving the therapy report from the respiratory therapist
    b. Evaluating the response to oxygen therapy
    c. Contacting respiratory therapy for the devices
    d. Being familiar with the devices and techniques used in order to provide proper care

23. The patient with an oxygen delivery device would like to ambulate to the bathroom but the tubing is too short. Extension tubing is added. What is the maximum length of the tubing that can be added in order to deliver the amount of oxygen needed for that device?
    a. 25 feet
    b. 35 feet
    c. 45 feet
    d. 50 feet

24. The patient is being discharged and requires home oxygen therapy with a reservoir-type nasal cannula. He asks the nurse, "Why can't I just take this nasal cannula that I have been using in the hospital?" What is the nurse's best response?
    a. "The doctor ordered the cannula, so your insurance company should cover the cost."
    b. "With the used cannula there is a risk of a hospital-acquired infection."
    c. "This special nasal cannula allows you to decrease the oxygen flow by 50%."
    d. "This nasal cannula is much better. It is more flexible and comfortable to wear."

25. Complete the chart below on oxygen delivery systems.

Oxygen Delivery System	Nursing Interventions	Rationales
Nasal cannula		
Simple face mask		
Partial rebreather mask		
Non-rebreather mask		
Venturi mask		
Tent and aerosol mask		

26. The patient is receiving oxygen therapy through a non-rebreather mask. What is the correct nursing intervention?
    a. Maintain liter flow so that the reservoir bag is up to one-half full.
    b. Maintain 60% to 75% FiO_2 at 6 to 11 L/min.
    c. Ensure that valves and rubber flaps are patent, functional, and not stuck.
    d. Assess for effectiveness and switch to partial rebreather for more precise FiO_2.

27. The patient with a face mask at 5 L/min is able to eat. Which nursing intervention is performed at mealtimes?
    a. Change the mask to a nasal cannula of 6 L/min or more.
    b. Have the patient work around the face mask as best as possible.
    c. Obtain a physician order for a nasal cannula at 5 L/min.
    d. Obtain a physician order to remove the mask at meals.

28. The physician orders transtracheal oxygen therapy for the patient with respiratory difficulty. What does the nurse tell the patient's family is the purpose of this type of oxygen delivery system?
    a. Delivers oxygen directly into the lungs.
    b. Keeps the small air sacs open to improve gas exchange.
    c. Prevents the need for an endotracheal tube.
    d. Provides high humidity with oxygen delivery.

29. The nursing diagnosis for the patient receiving oxygen therapy is Risk for Impaired Skin Integrity. Which nursing interventions are related to prevention of skin breakdown? *(Select all that apply.)*
    a. Assess the patient's ears, back of neck, and face at least every 4 to 8 hours for irritation.
    b. Apply padding on tubing to prevent pressure on skin.
    c. Use petroleum jelly on nostrils, face, and lips to relieve dryness.
    d. Assess nasal and mucous membranes for dryness and cracks.
    e. Obtain an order for humidification when oxygen is being delivered at 6 L/min or more.
    f. Provide mouth care every 8 hours and as needed.
    g. Position tubing so it will not pull on patient's ears.

30. The patient is receiving oxygen therapy for respiratory problems. According to NIC interventions for administration and monitoring of its effectiveness, what does the nurse do?
    a. Monitor the effectiveness of oxygen therapy at least once every 8 hours.
    b. Monitor for signs of oxygen toxicity and absorption atelectasis.
    c. Instruct the patient to replace the oxygen mask when the device is removed.
    d. Ask the respiratory therapist to monitor the oxygen flow and patient response.

31. The patient requires long-term airway maintenance following surgery for cancer of the neck. The nurse is using a piece of equipment to explain the procedure and mechanism that are associated with this long-term therapy. Which piece of equipment does the nurse most likely use for this patient teaching session?
    a. Tracheostomy tube
    b. Nasal trumpet
    c. Endotracheal tube
    d. Nasal cannula

32. The patient is receiving preoperative teaching for a partial laryngectomy and will have a tracheostomy postoperatively. How does the nurse define a tracheostomy to the patient?
    a. Opening in the trachea that enables breathing
    b. Temporary procedure that will be reversed at a later date
    c. Technique using positive pressure to improve gas exchange
    d. Procedure that holds open the upper airways

33. The patient returns from the operating room and the nurse assesses for subcutaneous emphysema which is a potential complication associated with tracheostomy. How does the nurse assess for this complication?
    a. Checking the volume of the pilot balloon
    b. Listening for airflow through the tube
    c. Inspecting and palpating for air under the skin
    d. Assessing the tube for patency

34. The patient with a tracheostomy develops increased coughing, inability to expectorate secretions, and difficulty breathing. What are these assessment findings related to?
    a. Overinflation of the pilot balloon
    b. Tracheoesophageal fistula
    c. Cuff leak and rupture
    d. Tracheal stenosis

35. The patient returns from the operating room after having a tracheostomy. While assessing the patient, which observations made by the nurse warrant immediate notification of the physician?
    a. Patient is alert but unable to speak and has difficulty communicating his needs.
    b. Small amount of bleeding present at the incision.
    c. Skin is puffy at the neck area with a crackling sensation.
    d. Respirations are audible and noisy with an increased respiratory rate.

36. The patient was intubated for acute respiratory failure, and there is an endotracheal tube in place. Which nursing intervention is *not* appropriate for this patient?
    a. Ensure that the oxygen is warmed and humidified.
    b. Suction the airway, then the mouth, and give oral care.
    c. Suction the airway with the oral suction equipment.
    d. Position the tubing so it does not pull on the airway.

37. To prevent accidental decannulation of a tracheostomy tube, what does the nurse do?
    a. Obtain an order for continuous upper extremity restraints.
    b. Secure the tube in place using ties or fabric fasteners.
    c. Allow some flexibility in motion of the tube while coughing.
    d. Instruct the patient to hold the tube with a tissue while coughing.

38. The patient has a recent tracheostomy. What necessary equipment does the nurse ensure is kept at the bedside?
    a. Pair of wire cutters
    b. Pocket mask and code cart
    c. Ambu bag and oxygen tubing
    d. Tracheostomy tube with obturator

39. Which statement by the nursing student indicates an understanding of the deflation of the tracheostomy cuff?
    a. "The cuff is deflated to allow the patient to speak."
    b. "The cuff is deflated to permit suctioning more easily."
    c. "The cuff should never be deflated because the patient will choke."
    d. "The cuff should be deflated to facilitate access for tracheostomy care."

40. The patient has a temporary tracheostomy following surgery to the neck area to remove a benign tumor. Which nursing intervention is performed to prevent obstruction of the tracheostomy tube?
    a. Provide tracheal suctioning when there are noisy respirations.
    b. Provide oxygenation to maintain pulse oximeter readings.
    c. Inflate the cuff to maximum pressure and check it once per shift.
    d. Suction regularly and PRN with a Yankauer suction.

41. The patient sustained a serious crush injury to the neck and had a tracheostomy tube placed yesterday. As the nurse is performing tracheostomy care, the patient suddenly sneezes very forcefully and the tracheostomy tube falls out onto the bed linens. What does the nurse do?
    a. Ventilate the patient with 100% oxygen and notify the physician.
    b. Quickly and gently replace the tube with a clean cannula kept at the bedside.
    c. Quickly rinse the tube with sterile solution and gently replace it.
    d. Give the patient oxygen; call for assistance and a new tracheostomy kit.

42. The patient required emergency intubation and currently has an artificial airway in place. Oxygen is being administered directly from the wall source. Why would warmed and humidified oxygen be a more appropriate choice for this patient?
    a. Helps prevent tracheal damage
    b. Promotes thick secretions
    c. Is more comfortable for the patient
    d. Is less likely to cause oxygen toxicity

43. The patient has an endotracheal tube and requires frequent suctioning for copious secretions. What is a complication of tracheal suctioning?
    a. Atelectasis
    b. Hypoxia
    c. Hypercarbia
    d. Bronchodilation

44. The nurse has explained the endotracheal suctioning procedure to the patient, gathered equipment, washed hands, and set low wall suction. Indicate the correct steps of completing the suctioning procedure in order using 1 through 9.
    _____ a. Open the suction kit.
    _____ b. Pour sterile saline into sterile container.
    _____ c. Preoxygenate the patient.
    _____ d. Discard supplies, wash hands, and document.
    _____ e. Put on sterile gloves.
    _____ f. Keep catheter sterile; attach to suction.
    _____ g. Withdraw catheter, applying suction and twirling catheter.
    _____ h. Insert catheter into trachea without suctioning.
    _____ i. Lubricate catheter tip in sterile saline solution.

45. The nurse has explained the tracheostomy care procedure to the patient, gathered equipment, and washed hands. Indicate the correct steps of completing the tracheostomy care procedure in order using 1 through 10.
    _____ a. Remove old dressing and excess secretions.
    _____ b. Wash hands, dispose of equipment, and document.
    _____ c. Suction tracheostomy tube if necessary.
    _____ d. Put on sterile gloves.
    _____ e. Reinsert inner cannula into outer cannula.
    _____ f. Open tracheostomy kit and pour peroxide into one side of container and saline into another.

    _____ g. Clean stoma site and plate.
    _____ h. Rinse inner cannula in sterile saline.
    _____ i. Remove inner cannula; place it in peroxide solution use brush to clean.
    _____ j. Change tracheostomy ties if needed and place new tracheostomy dressing.

46. While the nursing student changes the patient's tracheostomy dressing, the nurse observes the student using a pair of scissors to cut a 4 x 4 gauze pad to make a split dressing that will fit around the tracheostomy tube. What is the nurse's best action?
    a. Give the student positive reinforcement for use of materials and technique.
    b. Report the student to the instructor for remediation of the skill.
    c. Change the dressing immediately after the student has left the room.
    d. Direct the student in the correct use of materials and explain the rationale.

47. The nurse is caring for a patient with a tracheostomy who has recently been transferred from the ICU, but he has had no unusual occurrences related to the tracheostomy or his oxygenation status. What does the routine care for this patient include?
    a. Thorough respiratory assessment at least every 2 hours
    b. Maintaining the cuff pressure between 50 and 100 mm Hg
    c. Suctioning as needed; maximum suction time of 20 seconds
    d. Changing the tracheostomy dressing once a day

48. The patient with a tracheostomy is being discharged to home. In patient teaching, what does the nurse instruct the patient to do?
    a. Use sterile technique when suctioning.
    b. Instill tap water into the artificial airway.
    c. Clean the tracheostomy tube with soap and water.
    d. Increase the humidity in the home.

49. The patient with a permanent tracheostomy is interested in developing an exercise regimen. Which activity does the nurse advise the patient to avoid?
    a. Aerobics
    b. Tennis
    c. Golf
    d. Swimming

50. The patient with an endotracheal tube in place has dry mucous membranes and lips related to the tube and the partial open mouth position. What techniques does the nurse use to provide this patient with frequent oral care?
    a. Cleanses the mouth with glycerin swabs.
    b. Provides alcohol-based mouth rinse and oral suction.
    c. Cleanses with a mixture of hydrogen peroxide and water.
    d. Uses toothettes or a soft-bristled brush moistened in water.

51. The patient with a tracheostomy tube is able to speak and is no longer on mechanical ventilation. Which type of tracheostomy tube does this patient have?
    a. Cuffless tube
    b. Standard cuffed tube
    c. Cuffed fenestrated tube
    d. Tube without an obturator

Matching. *Match each type of tracheostomy tube with its description.*

Tracheostomy Tubes
a. Double-lumen tube
b. Single-lumen tube
c. Cuffed tube
d. Cuffless tube
e. Fenestrated tube
f. Cuffed fenestrated tube
g. Metal tracheostomy tube
h. Talking tracheostomy tube

Descriptions

_____ 52. Used with patients who can speak while on a ventilator for a long-term basis

_____ 53. Has a cuff that seals airway when inflated

_____ 54. Used for long-term management of patients not on mechanical ventilation or at high risk for aspiration

_____ 55. Has three parts—outer cannula, inner cannula, and obturator

_____ 56. Used for permanent tracheostomy

_____ 57. Used often with patients with spinal cord paralysis or muscular disease who do not require a ventilator all the time

_____ 58. Has no inner cannula and is used for patients with long or extra-thick necks

_____ 59. Used when weaning a patient from a ventilator; allows the patient to speak

60. The patient has a cuffed tracheostomy tube without a pressure relief valve. To prevent tissue damage of the tracheal mucosa, what does the nurse do?
    a. Deflate the cuff every 2 to 4 hours and maintain as needed.
    b. Change the tracheostomy tube every 3 days or per hospital policy.
    c. Assess and record cuff pressures each shift using the occlusive technique.
    d. Assess and record cuff pressures each shift using minimal leak technique.

61. An older adult patient is at risk for aspirating food or fluids. What is the most appropriate nursing action to assess for and prevent this problem?
    a. Monitor for increased amount of secretions when patient is coughing.
    b. Add food coloring to fluids or enteral feedings and monitor the color of the secretions.
    c. Obtain an order for a clear liquid diet and offer small but frequent amounts.
    d. Obtain an order for a chest x-ray to determine the presence of aspiration pneumonia.

62. An older adult patient sustained a stroke several weeks ago and is having difficulty swallowing. To prevent aspiration during mealtimes, what does the nurse do?
    a. Hyperextend the head to allow food to enter the stomach and not the lungs.
    b. Give thin liquids after each bite of food to help "wash the food down."
    c. Encourage "dry swallowing" after each bite to clear residue from the throat.
    d. Maintain a low Fowler's position during eating and for 2 hours afterwards.

63. The patient with a tracheostomy tube is currently alert and cooperative but seems to be coughing more frequently and producing more secretions than usual. The nurse determines that there is a need for suctioning. Which nursing intervention does the nurse use to prevent hypoxia for this patient?
    a. Allow the patient to breathe room air prior to suctioning.
    b. Avoid prolonged suctioning time.
    c. Suction frequently when the patient is coughing.
    d. Use the largest available catheter.

64. The nurse is suctioning the secretions from a patient's endotracheal tube. The patient demonstrates a vagal response by a drop in heart rate to 54 and a drop in blood pressure to 90/50. After stopping suctioning, what is the nurse's priority action?
    a. Allow the patient to rest for at least 10 minutes.
    b. Monitor the patient and call the Rapid Response Team.
    c. Oxygenate with 100% oxygen and monitor the patient.
    d. Administer atropine according to standing orders.

65. The patient with a tracheostomy is unable to speak. He is not in acute distress, but is gesturing and trying to communicate with the nurse. Which nursing intervention is the best approach in this situation?
    a. Rely on the family to interpret for the patient.
    b. Ask questions that can be answered with a "yes" or "no" response.
    c. Obtain an immediate consult with the speech therapist.
    d. Encourage the patient to rest rather than struggle with communication.

66. Which clinical finding in the patient with a recent tracheostomy is the most serious and requires immediate intervention?
    a. Increased cough and difficulty expectorating secretions
    b. Food particles in the tracheal secretions
    c. Pulsating tracheostomy tube in synchrony with the heartbeat
    d. Set tidal volume on the ventilator not being received by the patient

67. The nurse is providing discharge instructions for the patient who must perform self-care of a tracheostomy. The patient has been cheerful and cooperative during the hospital stay and has demonstrated interest and capability in performing self-care. But now the patient begins crying and refuses to leave the hospital. What is the nurse's best response?
    a. "You have done so well with your self-care. I am sure that you will be okay."
    b. "Let me call your family. They can help you to get home and get settled."
    c. "You have been brave and cheerful, but there is something that is worrying you."
    d. "We'll delay this teaching until later. Let's choose a scarf for you to wear home."

CASE STUDY: THE PATIENT WITH A TRACHEOSTOMY

Use a separate sheet of paper to answer the questions in this Case Study. Answer guidelines for this Case Study are available on your Evolve website at http://evolve.elsevier.com/Iggy/ in the "Prepare for Class" folder.

The nurse is caring for a 75-year-old man who was admitted for laryngeal cancer and surgery. The patient was transferred from the ICU several days ago. He has a tracheostomy and the tracheostomy collar is in place. He is receiving high-flow oxygen at 8 L/min. In shift report, the nurse learns that the patient is alert and oriented to person, place, and time. He is able to feed himself and independently perform most basic ADLs. He appears to be anxious and is having difficulty coping with the tracheostomy. He has some yellow mucus secretions and a specimen has been sent for culture and sensitivity. He is increasingly resistant to tracheostomy care and suctioning, although the need to deal with the excessive secretions has been explained to him. He is frustrated by his inability to communicate verbally. His pulse is 85 beats/min; blood pressure is 135/60; respirations 20/min; temperature 100° F; pulse oximetry reading 95%.

1. Identify at least six nursing diagnoses for this patient.
2. List six complications associated with tracheostomy.
3. What assessment findings would accompany an airway obstruction related to the patient's excessive secretions?
4. List interventions to prevent obstruction.
5. Explain the prevention of tissue damage that could occur because the patient has a tracheostomy.
6. What assessment findings indicate that the patient should be suctioned?
7. Write a dialogue to enlist the patient's cooperation for the suctioning procedure. Include an explanation of the purpose, the procedure, and the patient's role. (Role play this with a classmate.)
8. Discuss special considerations for this older patient who has a tracheostomy.
9. Describe nursing interventions and several alternative communication methods to try with this patient.

31 CHAPTER

Care of Patients with Noninfectious Upper Respiratory Problems

STUDY/REVIEW QUESTIONS

1. The nurse is caring for several patients who are at risk because of problems related to the upper airway. What is the priority assessment for these patients?
   a. Thickness of oral secretions; encourage ingestion of oral fluids
   b. Anxiety and pain; provide reassurance and NSAIDs
   c. Adequacy of oxygenation; ensure an unobstructed air passageway
   d. Evidence of spinal cord injuries; obtain order for x-rays

2. The patient's wife is concerned that her overweight husband has sleep apnea because of his heavy snoring. Which questions are appropriate to ask to elicit information related to sleep apnea? *(Select all that apply.)*
   a. "Is your husband a heavy smoker?"
   b. "Does he have a breathing interruption that lasts at least 10 seconds?"
   c. "Does he complain of waking up feeling tired?"
   d. "Does your husband eat late night snacks and sleep on his back?"
   e. "Is there a history of frequent throat or sinus infections?"
   f. "Have you noticed a change in his personality?"

3. The nurse is instructing the patient about a scheduled polysomnograph. Which patient statement indicates understanding of the procedure?
   a. "The test can be done in the doctor's office and will take 2 to 3 hours."
   b. "I shouldn't eat anything after midnight the night before, and someone must accompany me."
   c. "The test determines the depth and type of sleep and muscle movement."
   d. "The test determines the amount of sleep I need for adequate rest."

4. The patient has been diagnosed with sleep apnea. Which assessment findings indicate that the patient is having complications associated with sleep apnea?
   a. Side effects of hypoxemia, hypercapnia, and sleep deprivation
   b. Decrease in arterial carbon dioxide levels and sleep deprivation
   c. Respiratory alkalosis with retention of carbon dioxide
   d. Irritability, obesity, and enlarged tonsils or adenoids

5. The patient has been diagnosed with airway obstruction during sleep. The nurse most likely includes patient education about which device for home use?
   a. CPAP to deliver a positive airway pressure
   b. Oxygen via face mask to prevent hypoxia
   c. Neck brace to support the head and facilitate breathing
   d. Nebulizer treatments with bronchodilators

6. The patient is at risk for aspiration related to vocal cord paralysis. What does the nurse teach the patient to do?
   a. Raise the chin while swallowing
   b. Breathe slowly through an open mouth immediately after swallowing
   c. Hold the breath during swallowing
   d. Tilt the head backward during and immediately after swallowing

7. The patient has been diagnosed with vocal nodules. The physician recommends conservative treatment that includes lifestyle modifications. What does the nurse teach the patient to do?
   a. Whisper instead of speaking loudly
   b. Avoid humid climate conditions
   c. Use stool softeners to decrease straining
   d. Limit intake of caffeinated beverages

8. The nurse is assessing the patient who reports being struck in the face and head several times. During the assessment, a pink-tinged drainage from the nares is observed. Which nursing action provides relevant assessment data?
   a. Have the patient gently blow the nose and observe for bloody mucus.
   b. Test the drainage with a reagent to check the pH.
   c. Ask the patient to describe the appearance of the face before the incident.
   d. Place a drop of the drainage on a filter paper and look for a yellow ring.

9. While playing football at school, the patient injured his nose resulting in a possible simple fracture. The patient's parents call the nurse seeking advice. What does the nurse tell the parents to do?
   a. Ask the school nurse to insert a nasal airway to ensure patency.
   b. Apply an ice pack and allow the patient to rest in a supine position.
   c. Seek medical attention within 24 hours to minimize further complications.
   d. Monitor the symptoms for 24 hours and contact the physician if there is bleeding.

10. The patient had a rhinoplasty and is preparing for discharge home. A family member is instructed by the nurse to monitor the patient for postnasal drip by using a flashlight to look in the back of the throat. If bleeding is noted, what does the nurse tell the family member to do?
    a. Place ice packs on the back of the neck and apply pressure to the nose.
    b. Hyperextend the neck and apply pressure and ice packs as needed.
    c. Seek immediate medical attention for the bleeding.
    d. Monitor for 24 hours if the bleeding appears to be a small amount.

11. The nurse is teaching the patient about post-rhinoplasty care. Which patient statement indicates an understanding of the instruction?
    a. "I will have a very large dressing on my nose."
    b. "I will have bruising around my eyes, nose, and face."
    c. "There will be swelling that will cause a loss of sense of smell."
    d. "My nose will be three times its normal size for 3 weeks."

12. The patient with an active nosebleed is admitted to the emergency department. How does the nurse attempt to stop the nosebleed?
    a. Administer sedation/relaxation medication, apply ice packs and pressure to the nose, monitor respiratory status.
    b. Immediately pack the nose, apply ice packs, have the patient sit with head forward, monitor the amount of bleeding.
    c. Have the patient sit with head forward, monitor the color and amount of blood, monitor vital signs, apply an ice pack and pressure to the nose.
    d. Apply pressure and ice, have the patient blow the nose hard to remove obstructing clots, administer humidified oxygen.

13. The nurse is caring for the older adult patient with a history of noncompliance with pre-scribed metoprolol (Toprol XL) and recurrent nosebleeds. Which assessment finding is the most significant in relation to this patient's risk for repeated nosebleeds?
    a. Irregular apical pulse of 58 beats/min
    b. Open-mouth breathing with respiratory rate of 28/min
    c. Asymptomatic blood pressure of 180/110 mm Hg
    d. Subjective chills and oral temperature of 97.2° F

14. After being treated in the emergency depart-ment for posterior nosebleed, the patient is admitted to the hospital. The nasal packing is in place and vital signs are stable. The patient has an IV of normal saline at 125 mL/hr. What is the priority nursing diagnosis?
    a. Risk for Impaired Gas Exchange
    b. Risk for Fluid Volume Deficit
    c. Risk for Decreased Cardiac Output
    d. Risk for Infection

15. The patient is admitted for a posterior nose-bleed. Posterior packing is in place and, in addition, the patient is on oxygen therapy, antibiotics, and opioid analgesics. What is the priority assessment?
    a. Tolerance of packing or tubes
    b. Gag and cough reflexes
    c. Mouth breathing
    d. Skin breakdown around the nares

16. The patient reports noticing a change in the character of nasal discharge and speech quality, and a subjective feeling of blockage in the nasal passages. To gather additional relevant infor-mation, which question is the most appropriate to ask this patient?
    a. "Are you experiencing any soreness or tightness in your throat?"
    b. "Do you have a history of nasal polyps?"
    c. "Do you take over-the-counter medica-tions on a regular basis?"
    d. "Do you have a history of frequent nose-bleeds?"

17. The nurse is caring for the patient who has just returned from rhinoplasty surgery. Which assessment finding warrants additional assess-ment and concern?
    a. Bilateral packing of both nares in place
    b. Moustache pad in place
    c. Demonstrated repeated swallowing
    d. Traces of bruising around the eyes

18. The patient returns from surgery following a rhinoplasty. The nursing assistant places the patient in a supine position to encourage rest and sleep. Which action should the nurse take first?
    a. Teach the patient how to use the bed con-trols to position herself.
    b. Explain the purpose of the semi-Fowler's position to the nursing assistant.
    c. Place the patient in a semi-Fowler's posi-tion and assess for aspiration.
    d. Post a notice at the head of the bed to re-mind personnel about positioning.

19. The nurse is caring for the patient who had a nasoseptoplasty. Which action is the best to delegate to the licensed practical nurse?
    a. Administer a stool softener to ease bowel movements.
    b. Assess the patient's airway and breathing after general anesthesia.
    c. Evaluate the patient's emotional reaction to the facial edema and bruising.
    d. Take vital signs every 4 hours as ordered by the physician.

20. After the patient has a rhinoplasty, postopera-tive instructions are given to the patient and family. Which instruction set does the nurse provide?
    a. Place ice packs over the eyes and face, and swelling and discoloration should be re-lieved quickly.
    b. Resume food and fluids as tolerated, but minimize fluids to decrease nasal secre-tions.
    c. Use mild analgesics only, such as Tylenol, Excedrin with aspirin, and Motrin, to re-lieve discomfort.
    d. Avoid constipation for the first few days after surgery to prevent straining, which puts pressure on the incision.

21. The nurse is providing postoperative nursing care for the patient with surgical correction of a deviated septum. Which intervention is part of the standard care for this patient?
    a. Apply ice to the nasal area and eyes to decrease swelling and pain.
    b. Encourage deep coughing to prevent atelectasis and clear secretions.
    c. Administer NSAIDs or Tylenol every 4 to 6 hours for pain relief.
    d. Apply moist heat and humidity to the nasal area for comfort and circulation.

22. The nurse is monitoring the child who has been admitted for a fever of unknown origin. The child also reports a sore throat and demonstrates reluctance to eat and drink. Which assessment finding indicates an upper airway obstruction which requires immediate intervention?
    a. Stridor
    b. Crepitus
    c. Weak cough
    d. Subcutaneous emphysema

23. The patient arrives in the emergency department with a severe crush injury to the face with blood gurgling from the mouth and nose and obvious respiratory distress. The nurse prepares to assist the physician with which procedure to manage the airway?
    a. Performing a needle thoracotomy
    b. Inserting an endotracheal tube
    c. Performing a tracheostomy
    d. Inserting a nasal airway and giving oxygen

24. The patient with facial trauma has undergone surgical intervention to wire the jaw shut. In performing discharge teaching with this patient, which topics does the nurse cover?
    a. Bleeding, oral care and nutrition, pain control, activity
    b. Oral care, nutrition, pain, communication, aspiration prevention
    c. Prevention of airway obstructions, bleeding and oral infection, pain control
    d. Activity, diet, communication, bleeding, shock

25. The nurse is assessing the patient with significant and obvious facial trauma after being struck repeatedly in the face. Which finding is the priority and requires immediate intervention?
    a. Asymmetry of the mandible
    b. Restlessness and gurgling respirations
    c. Nonparallel extraocular movements
    d. Pain upon palpation over the nasal bridge

26. The nurse enters the room and the patient is crying. When the nurse asks the patient what happened, the patient says, "The doctor told me I have a LeFort I fracture of my face." What is the nurse's best response?
    a. "Don't worry; a LeFort I fracture is much less serious than a LeFort III."
    b. "You have an excellent doctor who will take good care of you."
    c. "Let me get you a mirror and you will see that it's not so bad."
    d. "What is your main concern about the LeFort I fracture?"

27. The patient has an inner maxillary fixation. The nurse encourages the patient to eat which kind of food?
    a. Milkshakes
    b. Cottage cheese
    c. Tea and toast
    d. Tuna and noodle casserole

28. The patient enters the emergency department after being punched in the throat. What does the nurse monitor for?
    a. Aphonia
    b. Dry cough
    c. Crepitus
    d. Loss of gag reflex

29. The patient has sustained a mandible fracture and the surgeon has explained that the repair will be made using a resorbable plate. The patient discloses to the nurse that he has not told the surgeon about his substance abuse and illicit drug dependence. What is the nurse's best response?
    a. "Why didn't you talk to your surgeon about this issue?"
    b. "You should tell the surgeon, but it is your choice."
    c. "It is important for your surgeon to know about this information."
    d. "You shouldn't be ashamed; your surgeon will still repair your fracture."

30. The patient has had an inner maxillary fixation for a mandibular fracture. Which piece of equipment should be kept at the bedside at all times?
    a. Water Pik
    b. Wire cutters
    c. Pair of hemostats
    d. Emesis basin

31. The patient who was in a motor vehicle accident and sustained laryngeal trauma is being treated in the emergency department with humidified oxygen and is being monitored every 15 to 30 minutes for respiratory distress. Which assessment finding may indicate the need for further intervention?
    a. Respiratory rate 24, Pao$_2$ 80 to 100, no difficulty with communication
    b. Pulse oximetry 96%, anxious, fatigued, blood in sputum, abdominal breathing
    c. Confused and disoriented, difficulty producing sounds, pulse oximetry 80%
    d. Anxious, respiratory rate 30, talking rapidly about the accident, warm to touch

32. The patient in the emergency department with laryngeal trauma has developed shortness of breath with stridor and decreased oxygen saturation. What is the priority action?
    a. Insert an oral or nasal airway.
    b. Assess for tachypnea, anxiety, and nasal flaring.
    c. Obtain the equipment for a tracheostomy.
    d. Apply oxygen and stay with the patient.

33. The older adult patient who is talking and laughing while eating begins to choke on a piece of meat. What is the initial emergency management for this patient?
    a. Several sharp blows between the scapulae
    b. Call the Rapid Response Team
    c. Nasotracheal suctioning
    d. Abdominal thrusts (Heimlich maneuver)

True or False? Read the statements about head and neck cancers and write T for true or F for false in the blanks provided. If the statement is false, correct the statement to make it true.

_____ 34. Head and neck cancers can be cured when treated early.

_____ 35. Diagnosis is usually not made until the disease is advanced.

_____ 36. Signs and symptoms of the disease are related to the location of the cancer.

_____ 37. Red velvety patches are called leukoplakia.

_____ 38. Many diagnostic tests are performed. CT scan aids in finding the exact location of a tumor, whereas MRI defines soft tissue invasion.

_____ 39. Radiation treatments are the preferred treatment for all locations and sizes of head and neck cancers.

_____ 40. Physical therapy is for postoperative radical neck surgery patients only.

_____ 41. Discharge teaching for all partial or total laryngectomy patients includes tracheostomy care.

_____ 42. Patients may have tubes removed before they are discharged from the hospital.

_____ 43. Discharge teaching for a total laryngectomy patient includes stoma care, which combines wound and airway care.

44. The nursing student is preparing patient teaching materials about head and neck cancer. Which statement is accurate and included in the patient teaching information?
   a. It metastasizes often to the brain.
   b. It usually develops over a short time.
   c. It is often seen as red edematous areas.
   d. It is often seen as white patchy mucosal lesions.

45. The nurse is interviewing the patient to assess for risk factors related to head and neck cancer. Which questions are appropriate to include? _(Select all that apply.)_
   a. "How many servings per day of alcohol would you typically drink?"
   b. "Have you had frequent episodes of acute or chronic visual problems?"
   c. "Have you had a problem with sores in your mouth?"
   d. "When was the last time you saw your dentist?"
   e. "Do you have recurrent laryngitis or frequent episodes of sore throat?"
   f. "How many packs per day do you smoke and for how many years?"

46. Which patient has the highest risk for developing cancer of the larynx and should be alerted about relevant lifestyle modifications to decrease this risk?
   a. 57-year-old male with alcoholism
   b. 18-year-old marijuana smoker
   c. 28-year-old female with diabetes
   d. 34-year-old male who snorts cocaine

47. The nurse is caring for the patient with a laryngeal tumor. In order to facilitate comfort and breathing for the patient, which type of position does the nurse use?
   a. Sims'
   b. Supine
   c. Fowler's
   d. Prone

48. The patient suffers from chronic xerostomia related to past radiation therapy treatments. Which intervention does the nurse use to assist the patient with this symptom?
   a. Offer small frequent meals.
   b. Suggest chewing sugarless gum.
   c. Explain fluid restrictions.
   d. Teach to wash with mild soap and water.

49. The nurse is assessing the patient's skin at the site of radiation therapy to the neck. Which skin condition is expected in relation to the radiation treatments?
   a. Red, tender, and peeling
   b. Shiny, pale, and tight
   c. Puffy and edematous
   d. Pale, dry, and cool

50. Which surgical procedure of the neck area poses no risk postoperatively for aspiration?
   a. Total laryngectomy
   b. Transoral cordectomy
   c. Hemilaryngectomy
   d. Partial laryngectomy

51. The nurse is caring for the postoperative patient who had a radical neck dissection. Which assessment finding is expected?
   a. Bulky gauze dressing is present that is dry and intact over the site.
   b. The patient can speak normally, but reports a sore throat.
   c. Permanent gastrostomy tube is present with continuous tube feedings.
   d. The patient has shoulder muscle weakness and limited range of motion.

52. The nursing student is caring for the older adult patient who sustained a stroke and is confused and having trouble swallowing. Which statement by the nursing student indicates an understanding of aspiration precautions for this patient?
    a. "I will administer pills as whole tablets; they are easier to swallow."
    b. "If the patient coughs, I will discontinue feeding and contact the physician."
    c. "I will keep the head of bed elevated during and after feeding."
    d. "I will encourage small amounts of fluids such as water, tea, or juices."

53. The nurse observes that the patient is having difficulty swallowing and has initiated aspiration precautions. Which procedure does the nurse expect the physician to order for this patient?
    a. Chest x-ray of the neck and chest
    b. CT scan of the head and neck
    c. Barium swallow under fluoroscopy
    d. Direct and indirect laryngoscopy

54. The patient has had a radical neck dissection surgery with a reconstructive flap over the carotid artery. Which intervention is appropriate for the flap care?
    a. Evaluate the flap every hour for the first 72 hours.
    b. Monitor the flap by gently placing a Doppler on the flap.
    c. Position the patient so that the flap is in the dependent position.
    d. Apply a wet-to-dry dressing to the flap.

55. The nurse is caring for several patients who require treatment for laryngeal cancer. Which treatment/procedure requires patient education about aspiration precautions?
    a. Total laryngectomy
    b. Laser surgery
    c. Radiation therapy
    d. Supraglottic laryngectomy

56. Which statement by the patient indicates understanding about radiation therapy for neck cancer?
    a. "My voice will initially be hoarse but should improve over time."
    b. "There are no side effects other than a hoarse voice."
    c. "Dry mouth after radiation therapy is temporary and short-term."
    d. "My throat is not directly affected by radiation."

57. What does the nurse include in the teaching session for the patient who is scheduled to have a partial laryngectomy?
    a. Supraglottic method of swallowing
    b. Presence of a tracheostomy tube and nasogastric tube for feeding due to postoperative swelling
    c. Not being able to eat solid foods
    d. Permanence of the tracheostomy, referred to as a laryngectomy stoma

58. The patient has been transferred from the intensive care unit to the medical surgical unit after a laryngectomy. What does the nurse suggest to encourage the patient to participate in self-care?
    a. Changing the tracheostomy collar
    b. Suctioning the mouth with a Yankauer suction
    c. Checking the stoma with a flashlight
    d. Observing the color of the reconstructive flap

59. The nurse is caring for the patient who had reconstructive neck surgery and observes bright red blood spurting from the tissue flap that is covering the carotid artery. What is the priority action?
    a. Call the surgeon and alert the operating room.
    b. Call the Rapid Response Team.
    c. Apply immediate, direct pressure to the site.
    d. Apply a bulky sterile dressing and secure the airway.

60. The patient is experiencing acute anxiety related to hospitalization stress and an inability to accept changes related to laryngeal cancer. The patient wants to leave the hospital, but agrees to try a medication to "help me calm down." For which medication does the nurse obtain a PRN order?
    a. Amitriptyline (Elavil)
    b. Modafinil (Provigil)
    c. Morphine sulfate (Statex)
    d. Lorazepam (Ativan)

61. The patient with a recent diagnosis of sinus cancer states that he wants another course of antibiotics because he believes he simply has another sinus infection. What is the nurse's best response?
    a. "I'll call the physician for the antibiotic prescription."
    b. "Why are you doubting your doctor's diagnosis?"
    c. "Let me bring you some information about sinus cancer."
    d. "What did the doctor say to you about your condition?"

62. The nurse identifies a nursing diagnosis of Disturbed Body Image related to perceived disfigurement created by tracheostomy for the young female patient. What is the priority action?
    a. Encourage the family to bring several attractive scarves.
    b. Assist the patient to identify realistic goals.
    c. Redirect conversation topics away from body image.
    d. Obtain an order for a psychiatric social services consult.

63. The patient is unable to speak following a cordectomy. Which action is delegated to the nursing assistant to assist the patient in dealing with communication issues?
    a. Politely tell the patient not to communicate.
    b. Teach the patient how to use hand signals.
    c. Allow extra time to accomplish ADLs because of communication limitations.
    d. Give step-by-step instructions during the ADLs and discourage two-way communication.

64. The nurse is assessing the patient who has had a neck dissection with removal of muscle tissue, lymph nodes, and the eleventh cranial nerve. Which assessment finding is anticipated because of the surgical procedure?
    a. Shoulder drop with a decreased limitation of movement
    b. Asymmetrical eye movements and a change of visual acuity
    c. Blood and serous fluid under the reconstructive flap
    d. Facial swelling with discoloration and bruising around the eyes

65. The patient is having radiation therapy to the neck and reports a sore throat and difficulty swallowing. Which statement by the nursing student indicates a correct understanding of symptom relief for this patient?
    a. "The patient should not swallow anything too cold or too hot."
    b. "I will give the patient a mouthwash with an alcohol base."
    c. "I will help the patient with a saline gargle."
    d. "The patient should be reassured that the sore throat is temporary."

66. The physician orders the discontinuation of the nasogastric tube for the patient with a total laryngectomy. Before discontinuing the tube, which action is performed?
    a. The physician and the nurse will assess the patient's ability to swallow.
    b. Reassure the patient that eating and swallowing will be painless and natural.
    c. The nutritionist will evaluate the patient's nutritional status.
    d. The patient will be offered a PRN analgesic or an anxiolytic medication.

67. The patient is learning esophageal speech and reports that he feels bloated after a practice session. To assist the patient with this issue, what does the nurse do?
    a. Refer the patient to the American Cancer Society Visitor Program.
    b. Obtain an order for PRN antacids.
    c. Reassure the patient that the discomfort is worth the long-term benefit.
    d. Notify the speech therapist about the symptom.

68. The patient has had surgery for cancer of the neck. Which behavior indicates that the patient understands how to perform self-care to prevent aspiration?
    a. Chooses thin liquids that cause coughing, but knows to take small sips.
    b. Eats small frequent meals that include a variety of textures and nutrients.
    c. Asks for small frequent sips of nutrition supplement as a bedtime snack.
    d. Positions self upright before eating or drinking anything.

69. The patient is receiving enteral feedings and a nasogastric tube is in place. In order to prevent aspiration, which precautions are used? *(Select all that apply.)*
    a. No bolus feedings are given at night.
    b. Hold the feeding if the residual volume exceeds 20 mL.
    c. Vary the time of feedings according to the patient's preference.
    d. Check the pH of the secretions.
    e. Elevate the head of bed during and after feedings.
    f. Evaluate the patient's tolerance of the feedings.

70. The patient has demonstrated anxiety since a diagnosis of neck cancer. The surgery and radiation therapy are completed. Which behavior indicates that the patient's anxiety is decreasing?
    a. Repeatedly asks the same questions and seeks to revalidate all information.
    b. States that he is less anxious, but is irritable and tense whenever questioned.
    c. Makes a plan to contact the American Cancer Society Visitor Program.
    d. Makes a plan to share personal belongings with friends and family.

71. Complete the table below regarding each of the surgical procedures for laryngeal cancer.

Procedure	Description	Resulting Voice Quality
Laser surgery		
Transoral cordectomy		
Laryngofissure		
Supraglottic partial laryngectomy		
Hemilaryngectomy or vertical laryngectomy		
Total laryngectomy		

CASE STUDY: THE PATIENT WITH AN UPPER RESPIRATORY CONDITION

Use a separate sheet of paper to answer the questions in this Case Study. Answer guidelines for this Case Study are available on your Evolve website at http://evolve. elsevier.com/Iggy/ in the "Prepare for Class" folder.

The patient is a 45-year-old man whose chief complaint is hoarseness and a sensation of a lump in his throat when swallowing. He reports that he can swallow, but it feels like some foods are getting stuck in the back of his throat. There is no bleeding and he denies any trauma or recent illness, although he does note that he wakes in the morning with a vague sore throat which has been going on for several months. The patient expresses guilt and fear related to lifestyle choices. He is fearful that he has cancer.

1. What additional questions should the nurse ask?

The physician determines that the patient may be at risk for cancer. The nurse must explain that the patient will have several kinds of diagnostic testing.

2. What laboratory tests are most likely to be ordered for this patient?

In addition to the laboratory tests, the patient is scheduled to have a bronchoscopy.

3. Explain the purpose and the procedure in terms that the patient will understand.

The patient is diagnosed with vocal cord polyps. The doctor informs him that the condition is not cancerous and that it will be managed conservatively.

4. Prepare a teaching plan for this patient.

32 CHAPTER

Care of Patients with Noninfectious Lower Respiratory Problems

STUDY/REVIEW QUESTIONS

Matching: Match each characteristic of disease that is associated with chronic airflow limitation (CAL). Answers will be used more than once.

Types of Diseases

a.   Asthma
b.   Chronic bronchitis
c.   Pulmonary emphysema

Characteristics of CAL Diseases

_____ 1.   Affects smaller airways

_____ 2.   Chronic thickening of bronchial walls

_____ 3.   Decreased surface area of alveoli

_____ 4.   Destruction of alveolar walls

_____ 5.   Hypercapnia

_____ 6.   Impaired mucociliary clearance

_____ 7.   Increased airway resistance

_____ 8.   Increased eosinophils

_____ 9.   Increased secretions

_____ 10.   Affects work of breathing

_____ 11.   Intermittent bronchospasm

_____ 12.   Intermittent mucosal edema

_____ 13.   Intermittent excess mucus production

_____ 14.   Loss of elastic recoil

_____ 15.   Mast cell destabilization

_____ 16.   Elastin broken down by proteases

_____ 17.   Stimulation of disease process by allergies

_____ 18.   Possibly results in respiratory acidosis

_____ 19.   Narrowed airway lumen due to inflammation

_____ 20.   Narrowing of airway from smooth muscle constriction

_____ 21.   Disease triggered by anti-inflammatory drugs used to treat disease

22. The nurse is caring for the older adult patient with a chronic respiratory disorder. Which interventions are best to use in caring for this patient? *(Select all that apply.)*
    a. Provide rest periods between activities, such as bathing, meals, and ambulation.
    b. Place the patient in a supine position after meals to allow for rest.
    c. Schedule drug administration around routine activities to increase adherence to drug therapy.
    d. Arrange chairs in strategic locations to allow the patient to walk and rest.
    e. Teach the patient to avoid getting the pneumococcal vaccine.
    f. Encourage the patient to have an annual flu vaccination.

23. The nurse is caring for an older adult patient with a history of chronic asthma. Which problem related to aging can influence the care and treatment of this patient?
    a. Asthma usually resolves with age, so the condition is less severe in older adult patients.
    b. It is more difficult to teach older adult patients about asthma than to teach younger patients.
    c. With aging, the beta-adrenergic drugs do not work as quickly or strongly.
    d. Older adult patients have difficulty manipulating handheld inhalers.

24. The nurse is presenting a community education lecture about respiratory disorders. Which statement by a participant indicates a correct understanding of the information?
    a. "Bronchitis is a genetic disease that affects many organs."
    b. "In bronchial asthma, an airway obstruction can be caused by inflammation."
    c. "In chronic bronchitis, the tissue damage is only temporary and is reversible."
    d. "Smoking cessation reverses the tissue damage caused by emphysema."

25. Which statement is true about asthma and chronic obstructive pulmonary disease (COPD) as chronic diseases of the lower respiratory system?
    a. COPD causes respiratory distress episodes with no permanent alveoli damage.
    b. In asthma, the lungs lose elasticity and become hyperinflated.
    c. Asthma manifests as acute episodes of reversible airway distress.
    d. In COPD, a "twitchy airway" can cause an airway obstruction.

26. The nurse is helping the patient learn about managing her asthma. What does the nurse instruct the patient to do?
    a. Keep a symptom diary to identify what triggers the asthma attacks.
    b. Make an appointment with an allergist for allergy therapy.
    c. Take a low dose of aspirin every day for the anti-inflammatory action.
    d. Drink large amounts of clear fluid to keep mucus thin and watery.

27. The nurse is taking a medical history on the new patient who has come to the office for a checkup. The patient states that he was supposed to take a medication called Singulair (montelukast), but that he never got the prescription filled. What is the best response by the nurse?
    a. "When did you first get diagnosed with a respiratory disorder?"
    b. "Why didn't you get the prescription filled?"
    c. "Tell me how you feel about your decision to not fill the prescription."
    d. "Are you having any problems with your asthma?"

28. The nurse teaches the patient with asthma to monitor for which problem while exercising?
    a. Increased peak expiratory flow rates
    b. Wheezing from bronchospasm
    c. Swelling in the feet and ankles
    d. Respiratory muscle fatigue

29. The high school student desires to participate in sports. His mother is very reluctant to give permission because her son has had asthma since early childhood. What does the nurse recommend?
    a. Participating in a sport like basketball would be a good choice.
    b. Premedicating with an inhaler such as salmeterol (Serevent) would help.
    c. Avoid exercising in cold, dry air because this may trigger an attack.
    d. Avoid exercising because exercise itself can trigger attacks.

30. The child attending day camp has asthma, and her parent packed and sent with her all of her medicine in a small carry bag. The child has an asthma attack that is severe enough to warrant a rescue drug. Which medication from the child's bag is best to use for the acute symptoms?
    a. Omalizumab (Xolair)
    b. Fluticasone (Flovent)
    c. Salmeterol (Serevent)
    d. Albuterol (Proventil)

31. Which assessment findings are expected for the patient with chronic airflow limitation? *(Select all that apply.)*
    a. Cyanosis
    b. Cough
    c. Dyspnea
    d. Tachypnea
    e. Wheezing

32. For the patient who is a nonsmoker, which classic assessment finding of chronic airflow limitation is particularly important in diagnosing asthma?
    a. Cough
    b. Dyspnea
    c. Audible wheezing
    d. Tachypnea

33. The patient who is allergic to dogs experiences a sudden "asthma attack." Which assessment findings does the nurse expect for this patient?
    a. Slow, deep, pursed-lip respirations
    b. Breathlessness and difficulty completing sentences
    c. Clubbing of the fingers and cyanosis of the nail beds
    d. Bradycardia and irregular pulse

34. The patient is experiencing an asthma attack and shows an increased respiratory effort. Which arterial blood gas value is more associated with the early phase of the attack?
    a. $Paco_2$ of 60 mm Hg
    b. $Paco_2$ of 30 mm Hg
    c. pH of 7.40
    d. Pao_2 of 98 mm Hg

35. The patient tells the nurse, "The doctor told me I had a 'barrel chest.' Is that a bad thing? I don't know what that means." What is the best response by the nurse?
    a. "Your chest has become barrel shaped because you breathe hard and your muscles have increased the front-to-back ratio of your chest."
    b. "When a person has chronic asthma, air gets trapped in the lungs and this gradually causes a change in the front-to-back shape of your chest."
    c. "It's really nothing to worry about. It just means the shape of your chest has changed to look like a barrel. It's because you have asthma."
    d. "I'll ask the doctor to come back in and explain it to you. It's really frightening when these strange terms are used and you are not sure what they mean."

36. The nurse is teaching the patient how to interpret peak expiratory flow readings and to use this information to manage drug therapy at home. Which statement by the patient indicates a need for additional teaching?
    a. "If the reading is in the green zone, there is no need to increase the drug therapy."
    b. "Red is 50% below my 'personal best'; I should try a rescue drug and seek help."
    c. "If the reading is in the yellow zone, I should increase my use of my inhalers."
    d. "If frequent yellow readings occur, I should see my doctor for a change in medications."

37. The patient with chronic bronchitis often shows signs of hypoxia. Which clinical manifestation is the priority to look out for in this patient?
    a. Chronic, nonproductive, dry cough
    b. Clubbing of fingers
    c. Large amounts of thick mucus
    d. Barrel chest

38. The nurse is taking a history for the patient with chronic pulmonary disease. The patient reports often sleeping in a chair that allows his head to be elevated rather than going to bed. The patient's behavior is a strategy to deal with which condition?
    a. Paroxysmal nocturnal dyspnea
    b. Orthopnea
    c. Tachypnea
    d. Cheyne-Stokes

39. The patient has chronic bronchitis. The nurse plans interventions for impaired gas exchange based on which set of clinical manifestations?
    a. Chronic cough, thin secretions, and chronic infection
    b. Respiratory alkalosis, decreased $Paco_2$, and increased Pao_2
    c. Areas of chest tenderness and sputum production (often with hemoptysis)
    d. Large amounts of thick secretions and repeated infections

40. The patient has COPD with chronic difficult breathing. In planning this patient's care, what condition must the nurse acknowledge is present in this patient?
    a. Decreased need for calories and protein requirements since dyspnea causes activity intolerance
    b. COPD has no effect on calorie and protein needs, meal tolerance, satiety, appetite, and weight
    c. Increased metabolism and the need for additional calories and protein supplements
    d. Anabolic state, which creates conditions for building body strength and muscle mass

41. In obtaining a history for the patient with chronic airflow limitation, which risk factor is not related to potentially causing or triggering the disease process?
    a. Cigarette smoking
    b. Occupational and air pollution
    c. Genetic tendencies
    d. Smokeless tobacco

42. Which statement is true about the relationship of smoking cessation to the pathophysiology of COPD?
    a. Smoking cessation completely reverses the damage to the lungs.
    b. Smoking cessation slows the rate of disease progression.
    c. Smoking cessation is an important therapy for asthma but not for COPD.
    d. Smoking cessation reverses the effects on the airways but not the lungs.

43. The patient has a history of COPD but is admitted for a surgical procedure that is unrelated to the respiratory system. Nevertheless, to prevent any complications related to the patient's COPD, what does the nurse do?
    a. Assess the patient's respiratory system every 8 hours.
    b. Monitor for signs and symptoms of pneumonia.
    c. Give high-flow oxygen to maintain pulse oximetry readings.
    d. Instruct the patient to use a tissue if coughing or sneezing.

44. The nurse is instructing the patient regarding complications of COPD. Which statement by the patient indicates the need for additional teaching?
    a. "I have to be careful because I am susceptible to respiratory infections."
    b. "I could develop heart failure, which could be fatal if untreated."
    c. "My COPD is serious, but it can be reversed if I follow my doctor's orders."
    d. "The lack of oxygen could cause my heart to beat in an irregular pattern."

45. The nurse is reviewing a summary of pulmonary function testing (PFT). The physician has asked the nurse to call the results of the most significant reading related to obstructive pulmonary disease. Which portion of the PFT is of primary interest?
    a. FEV_1/FVC ratio
    b. Functional residual capacity
    c. Total lung capacity
    d. Residual volume

46. The patient with chronic airflow limitation (CAL) is informed by the physician that, over time, there has been a decrease in the FEV_1/FVC ratio. After the physician leaves, the patient appears to be unsure about the meaning of the results and their relationship to her health condition. What does the nurse tell this patient?
    a. Her disease process is stable.
    b. The CAL is progressing.
    c. The CAL is improving.
    d. Further diagnostic testing is needed.

47. What is the purpose of pulmonary function testing?
    a. Determines the oxygen liter flow rates required by the patient
    b. Measures blood gas levels before bronchodilators are administered
    c. Evaluates the movement of oxygenated blood from the lung to the heart
    d. Distinguishes airway disease from restrictive lung disease

48. The patient with respiratory difficulty has completed a pulmonary function test before starting any treatment. The peak expiratory flow (PEF) is 15% to 20% below what is expected for this adult patient's age, gender, and size. The nurse anticipates this patient will need additional information about which topic?
    a. Further diagnostic tests to confirm pulmonary hypertension
    b. How to manage asthma medications and identify triggers
    c. Smoking cessation and its relationship to COPD
    d. How to manage the acute episode of respiratory infection

49. Patients with asthma are taught self-care activities and treatment modalities according to the "step method." Which symptoms and medication routines relate to step III?
    a. Symptoms occur daily; daily use of inhaled corticosteroid, add a long-acting beta agonist
    b. Symptoms occur more than once per week; daily use of anti-inflammatory inhaler
    c. Symptoms occur less than once per week; use of rescue inhalers once per week
    d. Frequent exacerbations with limited physical activity; increased use of rescue inhalers

50. Why is a high-liter flow of oxygen contraindicated in the patient with COPD?
    a. The patient depends on a hypercapnic drive to breathe.
    b. The patient depends on a hypoxic drive to breathe.
    c. Receiving too much oxygen over a short time results in headache.
    d. Tolerance develops; therefore high doses needed later will be ineffective.

51. In assisting the patient with chronic airflow limitation to relieve dyspnea, which sitting position offers the patient no benefit?
    a. On edge of chair, leaning forward with arms folded and resting on a small table
    b. In a low semi-reclining position with the shoulders back and knees apart
    c. Forward in a chair with feet spread apart and elbows placed on the knees
    d. Head slightly flexed, with feet spread apart and shoulders relaxed

52. The nurse is developing a teaching plan for the patient with chronic airflow limitation using the nursing diagnosis of Deficient Knowledge related to energy conservation. What does the nurse advise the patient to avoid?
    a. Performing activities at a relaxed pace throughout the day with rest periods
    b. Working on activities that require using arms at chest level or lower
    c. Eating three large meals per day
    d. Talking and performing activities separately

53. The patient with COPD has meal-related dyspnea. To address this issue, which drug does the nurse offer the patient 30 minutes before the meal?
    a. Albuterol (Ventolin)
    b. Guaifenesin (Organidin)
    c. Fluticasone (Flovent)
    d. Pantoprazole sodium (Protonix)

54. The laboratory result for the patient's theophylline level is 18 mcg/mL. What action does the nurse take?
    a. Place the results in the patient's chart because the value is within therapeutic range.
    b. Immediately alert the physician because the value indicates that the dose is too high.
    c. Contact the physician during AM rounds to get a prescription to increase the dose.
    d. Immediately assess the patient for adverse reactions related to a toxic level.

55. The patient is receiving ipratropium (Atrovent) and reports nausea, blurred vision, headache, and inability to sleep. What action does the nurse take?
    a. Administer a PRN medication for nausea and a mild PRN sedative.
    b. Report these symptoms to the physician as signs of overdose.
    c. Obtain a physician's request for an ipratropium level.
    d. Tell the patient that these side effects are normal and not to worry.

56. The patient with asthma has been prescribed a Flovent inhaler. What is the purpose of this drug for the patient?
    a. Relaxes the smooth muscles of the airway
    b. Acts as a bronchodilator in severe episodes
    c. Reduces obstruction of airways by decreasing inflammation
    d. Reduces the histamine effect of the triggering agent

57. What is the advantage of using the aerosol route for administering short-acting beta$_2$ agonists?
    a. Achieves a rapid and effective anti-inflammatory action
    b. Reduces the risk for fungus infections
    c. Increases patient compliance because it is easy to use
    d. Provides rapid therapy with fewer systemic side effects

58. The nurse is teaching the patient with chronic airflow limitation about his medications. What is the correct sequence for administering aerosol treatments?
    a. Bronchodilator should be taken 5 to 10 minutes after the steroid.
    b. Bronchodilator should be taken at least 5 minutes before other inhaled drugs.
    c. Bronchodilator should be taken immediately after the steroid.
    d. Bronchodilator and steroid are two different classes of drugs, so sequence is irrelevant.

59. The patient has been prescribed cromolyn sodium (Intal) for the treatment of asthma. Which statement by the patient indicates a correct understanding of this drug?
    a. "It opens my airways and provides short-term relief."
    b. "It is the medication that should be used 30 minutes before exercise."
    c. "It is not intended for use during acute episodes of asthma attacks."
    d. "It is a steroid medication, so there are severe side effects."

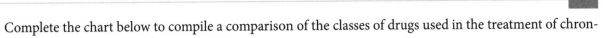

60. Complete the chart below to compile a comparison of the classes of drugs used in the treatment of chronic airflow limitation (CAL).

Drug Classification/ Drug Name	Usual Route/ Dose	Nursing Interventions	Rationale
Short-Acting Beta Agonist (SABA) Albuterol (Proventil, Ventolin)			
Long-Acting Beta Agonist (LABA) Salmeterol (Serevent)			
Cholinergic Antagonist Ipratropium (Atrovent, Apo-Ipravent			
Methylxanthines Theophylline (Elixophyllin, Theo-Dur, Uniphyl, Theolair, many others)			
Corticosteroid Fluticasone (Flovent)			

61. After the nurse has instructed the patient with COPD in the proper coughing technique, which action the next day by the patient indicates the need for additional teaching or intervention?
    a. Coughing upon rising in the morning
    b. Coughing before meals
    c. Coughing after meals
    d. Coughing at bedtime

62. A family member of the patient with COPD asks the nurse, "What is the purpose of making him cough on a routine basis?" What is the nurse's best response?
    a. "We have to check the color and consistency of his sputum."
    b. "We don't want him to feel embarrassed when coughing in public, so we actively encourage it."
    c. "It improves air exchange by increasing airflow in the larger airways."
    d. "If he cannot cough, the physician may elect to do a tracheostomy."

63. The nurse is teaching and assisting the patient with controlled coughing. Place the steps for the "controlled coughing" in the correct order using the numbers 1 through 7.

    _____ a. Turns shoulders inward, bends head downward, and hugs pillow to stomach

    _____ b. Repeats the procedure at least twice

    _____ c. Returns to a sitting position and then takes a comfortable deep breath

    _____ d. Takes three to five deep breaths

    _____ e. Bends forward slowly while coughing two or three times from the same breath

    _____ f. Rests and performs mouth care

    _____ g. Sits in a chair or on the side of a bed with feet placed firmly on the floor

64. The patient has COPD and develops cor pulmonale. Which assessment finding does the nurse expect to observe with this condition?
    a. Left ventricular hypertrophy
    b. Weak pulse
    c. Fatigue
    d. Dehydration

65. The patient is admitted with asthma. Which assessment findings are most likely to indicate that the patient's asthma condition is deteriorating and progressing toward respiratory failure?
    a. Rales, rhonchi, and productive cough with yellow sputum
    b. Tachypnea; thick, tenacious sputum; and hemoptysis
    c. Inaudible breath sounds, wheezing, and use of accessory muscles
    d. Respiratory alkalosis; slow, shallow respiratory rate

66. The patient has returned several times to the clinic for treatment of respiratory problems. Which action does the nurse perform first?
    a. Obtain a history of the patient's previous respiratory problems and response to therapy.
    b. Ask the patient to describe his compliance to the prescribed therapies.
    c. Obtain a request for diagnostic testing, including a tuberculosis and human immune deficiency virus (HIV) evaluation.
    d. Listen to the patient's lungs, obtain a pulse oximetry reading, and count the respiratory rate.

67. The patient is undergoing diagnostic testing for possible cystic fibrosis (CF). Which non-pulmonary assessment findings does the nurse expect to observe in a patient with CF?
    a. Abdominal distention, gastroesophageal reflux, and steatorrhea
    b. Diarrhea, nausea, vomiting, anorexia, and a thin, slender body frame
    c. Cough, congestion, sputum production, and use of accessory muscles
    d. Peripheral edema, weight gain, and water retention

68. The nurse is caring for the patient who has cystic fibrosis. Which assessment findings indicate the need for exacerbation therapy? *(Select all that apply.)*
   a. New-onset crackles
   b. Increased activity tolerance
   c. Increased frequency of coughing
   d. Increased chest congestion
   e. Increased Sao$_2$
   f. At least a 10% decrease in FEV$_1$

69. The patient with cystic fibrosis (CF) is admitted to the medical-surgical unit for an elective surgery. Which infection control measure is best for this patient?
   a. It is best to put two patients with CF in the same room.
   b. Standard Precautions including handwashing are sufficient.
   c. The patient is to be placed on Contact Isolation.
   d. Measures that limit close contact between people with CF are needed.

70. The nurse is working for a manufacturing company and is responsible for routine employee health issues. Which primary prevention is most important for those employees at high risk for occupational pulmonary disease?
   a. Screen all employees by use of chest x-ray films twice a year.
   b. Advise employees not to smoke and to use masks and ventilation equipment.
   c. Perform pulmonary function tests once a year on all employees.
   d. Refer at-risk employees to a social worker for information about pensions.

71. The patient had prolonged occupational exposure to petroleum distillates and subsequently developed a chronic lung disease. This patient is advised to seek frequent health examinations because there is a high risk for developing which respiratory disease condition?
   a. Tuberculosis
   b. Cystic fibrosis
   c. Lung cancer
   d. Pulmonary hypertension

72. The nurse has completed a community presentation about lung cancer. Which statement from a participant demonstrates an understanding of the information presented?
   a. "The primary prevention for reducing the risk of lung cancer is to stop smoking and avoid secondhand smoke."
   b. "The overall 5-year survival rate for all patients with lung cancer is 85%."
   c. "The death rate for lung cancer is less than prostate, breast, and colon cancer combined."
   d. "Cures are most likely for patients who undergo treatment for stage III disease."

True or False? Read the statements about lung cancer and write T for true or F for false in the blanks provided. If the statement is false, correct the statement to make it true.

_____ 73. There are two primary classifications of lung cancer—small cell and non–small cell.

_____ 74. Non–small cell lung cancer is further divided into three types—squamous, adenocarcinoma, and large cell.

_____ 75. Metastasis occurs via three routes—obstruction/direct invasion, blood, and lymph nodes.

_____ 76. Common metastasis sites include bone, liver, brain, and adrenal glands.

_____ 77. Hypoglycemia could be one manifestation of paraneoplastic syndrome.

_____ 78. The risk of lung cancer after 5 years of not smoking approaches that of someone who has never smoked.

_____ 79. The number of cigarettes and years of smoking do not contribute to the risk; it is the tar and nicotine that contribute to the risk.

_____ 80. African Americans are at less risk for lung cancer than are whites.

_____ 81. For smoking cessation, the decrease for women has been less than it has for men.

_____ 82. Wearing a specialized mask can decrease the risk of developing occupation-related lung cancer.

_____ 83. Female smokers are at a lower risk of developing lung cancer than are men because they have a protective gene.

_____ 84. Onset of symptoms is a positive sign of early disease.

_____ 85. A chest x-ray film is a good screening tool for lung cancer.

_____ 86. Lung cancer is always diagnosed by sputum specimens.

_____ 87. Surgical intervention for non–small cell cancer is the goal for curing the patient.

_____ 88. A wedge resection is a form of surgical intervention that removes a small localized section of the diseased lung.

89. The patient presents with the common signs and symptoms that are often associated with lung cancer. Which clinical manifestations does the nurse expect to observe in this patient?
   a. Hemoptysis, hoarseness, cough, and shortness of breath
   b. Abdominal distention, steatorrhea, and dyspnea
   c. Wheezing, clubbing of the nail beds, cyanosis, and dyspnea
   d. Fever, fatigue, dyspnea, and peripheral edema

90. Which statement is true about radiation therapy for lung cancer patients?
   a. It is given daily in "cycles" over the course of several months.
   b. It causes hair loss, nausea, and vomiting for the duration of treatment.
   c. It causes dry skin at the radiation site, fatigue, and changes in appetite with nausea.
   d. It is the best method of treatment for systemic metastatic disease.

91. The nurse is taking a report on the patient who had a pneumonectomy 4 days ago. Which question is the best to ask during the shift report?
   a. "Does the physician want us to continue encouraging use of the spirometer?"
   b. "How much drainage did you see in the Pleur-Evac during your shift?"
   c. "Do we have a request to 'milk' the patient's chest tube?"
   d. "Does the surgeon want the patient placed on the nonoperative side?"

92. The nurse is caring for the patient with a chest tube. What is the correct nursing intervention for this patient?
   a. The patient is encouraged to cough and do deep-breathing exercises frequently.
   b. "Stripping" of the chest tubes is done routinely to prevent obstruction by blood clots.
   c. Water level in the suction chamber need not be monitored—just the collection chamber.
   d. Drainage containers are positioned upright or on the bed next to the patient.

93. Upon observation of a chest tube setup, the nurse reports to the physician that there is a leak in the chest tube and system. How has the nurse identified this problem?
   a. Drainage in the collection chamber has decreased.
   b. The bubbling in the suction chamber has suddenly increased.
   c. Fluctuation in the water seal chamber has stopped.
   d. There was onset of vigorous bubbling in the water seal chamber.

94. The physician's prescriptions indicate an increase in the suction to 20 mL for the patient with a chest tube. To implement this, the nurse performs which intervention?
    a. Increases the wall suction to the medium setting, and observes gentle bubbling in the suction chamber
    b. Adds water to the suction and drainage chambers to the level of 20 mL
    c. Stops the suction, adds sterile water to level of 20 mL to the water seal chamber, and resumes the wall suction
    d. Has the patient cough and deep breathe, and monitors level of fluctuation to achieve 20 mL

95. The patient is fearful that she might develop lung cancer because her father and grandfather died of cancer. She seeks advice about how to modify lifestyle factors that contribute to cancer. How does the nurse advise this patient?
    a. Not to worry about air pollution unless there is hydrocarbon exposure
    b. Quit her job if she has continuous exposure to lead or other heavy metals
    c. Avoid situations where she would be exposed to "secondhand" smoke
    d. Not to be concerned because there are no genetic factors associated with lung cancer

96. The nurse has determined that the patient with COPD has a nursing diagnosis of Impaired Gas Exchange related to reduced airway size, ventilatory muscle fatigue, and excessive mucus production. Which action is best to delegate to the nursing assistant?
    a. Observe the patient for fatigue, shortness of breath, or change of breathing pattern during ADLs.
    b. Report a respiratory rate of greater than 24/min at rest or 30/min after ambulating to the nurses' station.
    c. Encourage the patient to cough up sputum, and examine the color, consistency, and amount.
    d. Record and monitor the patient's intake and output, and give fluids to keep the secretions thin.

97. The patient is receiving a chemotherapy agent for lung cancer. The nurse anticipates that the patient is likely to have which common side effect?
    a. Diarrhea
    b. Nausea
    c. Flatulence
    d. Constipation

98. The patient is having pain resulting from bone metastases caused by lung cancer. What is the most effective intervention for relieving the patient's pain?
    a. Support the patient through chemotherapy.
    b. Handle and move the patient very gently.
    c. Administer analgesics around the clock.
    d. Reposition the patient, and use distraction.

99. The patient has a chest tube in place. What does the water in the water seal chamber do when the system is functioning correctly?
    a. Bubbles vigorously and continuously
    b. Bubbles gently and continuously
    c. Fluctuates with the patient's respirations
    d. Stops fluctuation, and bubbling is not observed

100. Which intervention promotes comfort in dyspnea management for the patient with lung cancer?
    a. Administer morphine only when the patient requests it.
    b. Place the patient in a supine position with a pillow under the knees and legs.
    c. Encourage coughing and deep breathing and independent ambulation.
    d. Provide supplemental oxygen via cannula or mask.

101. The patient with repeated pleural effusions as a result of lung cancer is injected with a sclerosing agent. What is the nurse's role?
    a. Position the patient so that the affected lung is dependent while the drug is being injected.
    b. Ensure that the chest tube is securely clamped after the instillation of the drug.
    c. Instruct the patient to remain very still for at least 2 hours after the drug has been injected.
    d. Notify the respiratory therapist to administer respiratory therapy treatments.

102. The patient is diagnosed with cor pulmonale secondary to pulmonary hypertension and is receiving an infusion of epoprostenol (Flolan) through a small portable IV pump. What is the critical priority for this patient?
    a. Strict aseptic technique must be used to prevent sepsis.
    b. Infusion must not be interrupted, even for a few minutes.
    c. The patient must have a daily dose of warfarin (Coumadin).
    d. The patient must be assessed for angina-like chest pain and fatigue.

103. The patient has developed pulmonary hypertension. What is the goal of drug therapy for this patient?
    a. Dilate pulmonary vessels and prevent clot formation.
    b. Decrease pain and make the patient comfortable.
    c. Improve or maintain gas exchange.
    d. Maintain and manage pulmonary exacerbation.

True or False? *Read the statements about pulmonary hypertension and write T for true or F for false in the blanks provided. Correct the false statements so that they are true.*

_____ 104. Conditions such as COPD, pulmonary fibrosis, and pulmonary emboli can result in pulmonary hypertension.

_____ 105. When treating cor pulmonale, collaborative management is designed around the underlying cause of pulmonary hypertension.

_____ 106. When medical management fails, heart-lung or lung transplantation might be necessary.

107. The patient is newly diagnosed with sarcoidosis. Which statement by the patient indicates an understanding of the disease?
    a. "Corticosteroids are the main type of therapy for sarcoidosis."
    b. "Sarcoidosis is a type of lung cancer that is treatable if diagnosed early."
    c. "My condition can be treated with antibiotics."
    d. "Sarcoidosis is a type of pneumonia that is highly contagious."

108. The nurse is caring for the patient who is in the later stage of pulmonary fibrosis in a home care setting. What is the priority goal for this patient?
    a. Prevent respiratory infection.
    b. Encourage independence.
    c. Reduce the sensation of dyspnea.
    d. Help the family contact hospice.

109. The patient with a history of asthma enters the emergency department with severe dyspnea, accessory muscle involvement, neck vein distention, and severe inspiratory/expiratory wheezing. The nurse is prepared to assist the physician with which procedure if the patient does not respond to initial interventions?
    a. Emergency intubation
    b. Emergency needle thoracentesis
    c. Emergency chest tube insertion
    d. Emergency pleurodesis

110. The patient presents to the walk-in clinic with extremely labored breathing and a history of asthma that is unresponsive to prescribed inhalers or medications. What is the priority nursing action?
    a. Establish IV access to give emergency medications.
    b. Obtain the equipment and prepare the patient for intubation.
    c. Place the patient in a high Fowler's position, and start oxygen.
    d. Call 911 and report that the patient has probable status asthmaticus.

111. The nurse is instructing the patient to use a flutter-valve mucus clearance device. What should the patient be taught to do?
    a. Inhale deeply and exhale forcefully through the device.
    b. Use an inhalation technique that is similar to the handheld inhaler.
    c. Use pursed-lip breathing before and after usage.
    d. Exhale slowly through the nose, and then inhale by sniffing.

CASE STUDY: THE PATIENT WITH COPD

Use a separate sheet of paper to answer the questions in this Case Study. Answer guidelines for this Case Study are available on your Evolve website at http://evolve.elsevier.com/Iggy/ in the "Prepare for Class" folder.

The 72-year-old patient is being evaluated in his home by the home health nurse. He was admitted to the hospital for an exacerbation of his COPD and discharged 2 days ago. He states, "I feel a little more out of breath today than I usually do, but I am breathing better than I was when I went to the hospital." He is thin with a barrel-shaped chest. He is slow moving and slightly stooped. He demonstrates rapid, shallow respirations at 30/min. He currently denies chest pain, but he reports feeling exhausted.

1. List at least eight questions the nurse could ask to evaluate this patient's current condition.

2. Describe how the nurse uses the following assessment tools to determine the severity of the dyspnea:
    a. Visual Analog Dyspnea Scale
    b. Peak expiratory flowmeter
    c. Pulse oximetry (assume availability of portable unit)

3. Identify four or five common nursing diagnoses for patients with COPD.

4. Identify at least eight teaching points to help this patient conserve energy.

5. The patient tells the nurse that he has heard about pulmonary rehabilitation. He is not sure why his doctor did not suggest this for him, but he wonders if it is a possibility.
    a. What is pulmonary rehabilitation?
    b. Describe a typical simple rehabilitation plan.

6. Prepare and practice a dialogue for calling the physician to make an inquiry if pulmonary rehabilitation is appropriate for this patient.

33 CHAPTER

Care of Patients with Infectious Respiratory Problems

STUDY/REVIEW QUESTIONS

1. The adult patient diagnosed with rhinitis medicamentosa reports chronic nasal congestion. What does the nurse instruct the patient to do?
   a. Avoid exposure to older adults or immunosuppressed persons when symptoms flare.
   b. Damp dust the house and clean the carpets to remove animal dander or mold.
   c. Discontinue the use of the current nose drops or sprays.
   d. Identify what triggers the hypersensitivity reaction by keeping a symptom diary.

2. The nurse notes that the patient has a disorder that contraindicates drug therapy that the physician has just prescribed for symptomatic relief of allergic rhinitis. Which disorder does the nurse report to the physician as a contraindication?
   a. Sleep apnea
   b. Valvular heart disease
   c. Ménière's disease
   d. Urinary retention

3. The patient has been prescribed several drugs for sinusitis. During the last clinic visit, the nurse performed patient teaching regarding these drugs. Which patient statement indicates the need for further instruction?
   a. "I have been taking the antihistamine at bedtime, because it makes me sleepy."
   b. "I have been taking an antipyretic every other day to prevent fever."
   c. "The mucolytics do help, but I have been trying to drink a lot of water too."
   d. "I use the decongestants if my nose or sinuses feel really stuffed up."

4. The patient comes to the walk-in clinic reporting seasonal nasal congestion, sneezing, rhinorrhea, and itchy watery eyes. The nurse identifies that the patient most likely has rhinitis and should also be assessed for sinusitis. How does the nurse assess for sinusitis?
   a. Observe the color and consistency of nasal secretions, and do a nasal swab.
   b. Ask the patient to speak, and listen for nasal sounds in the voice quality.
   c. Visually inspect the throat for redness or white patches, and take a throat culture.
   d. Use reflection of light through the tissues, and observe for a red glow on the cheek.

5. The patient is an 80-year-old man with a diagnosis of chronic rhinitis. Which statement is relevant to the care of this patient?
   a. Viral rhinitis is self-limiting and rarely leads to complications in the older adult.
   b. Antihistamines and decongestants should be used with caution.
   c. Antipyretics are rarely used because older adults are unlikely to have fever.
   d. Complementary and alternative therapies are not recommended for older adults.

6. The patient reports difficulty breathing, facial pain (especially when head is dependent), sneezing or coughing, green or bloody nasal drainage, productive cough, and low-grade fever. Which disorder does the nurse suspect?
   a. Rhinitis
   b. Tonsillitis
   c. Sinusitis
   d. Pneumonia

7. The older adult patient residing in a long-term care facility demonstrates new onset of coughing and sneezing and rhinorrhea after his grandchildren came to visit him. He denies pain or fever. Which infection control procedures does the nurse instruct the LPN to initiate in order to protect the other residents?
   a. Initiate the use of standard precautions when caring for the patient.
   b. Place the patient on droplet precautions for the first 2 to 3 days.
   c. Use gown and gloves when entering the room and perform hand hygiene.
   d. Instruct the patient to wash his hands after coughing or sneezing.

8. The nurse is assessing the older adult who has been diagnosed with bacterial pharyngitis. Which assessment finding is typically associated with this medical diagnosis, but may not be present in the older adult patient?
   a. Cough and rash
   b. High fever and elevated white blood cell (WBC) count
   c. Pain with speaking or swallowing
   d. Erythema of tonsils with yellow exudate

9. The nurse is performing a physical assessment on the patient who is suspected to have pharyngitis. Which assessment finding is most indicative of a bacterial infection versus a viral infection?
   a. Fever
   b. Erythema of throat
   c. Headache
   d. Positive throat culture

10. The patient reporting a "sore throat" also has a temperature of 101.4° F, scarlatiniform rash, and a positive rapid test throat culture. This patient will most likely be treated for which type of bacterial infection?
   a. Staphylococcus
   b. Pneumococcus
   c. Streptococcus
   d. Epstein-Barr virus

11. The patient reporting a soreness in the throat is diagnosed with "strep throat." To prevent complications such as rheumatic heart disease, this patient should receive antibiotic treatment within what time frame?
   a. 24 hours
   b. 48 hours
   c. 1 week
   d. 1 month

12. The child is diagnosed with a group B Streptococcus throat infection. In teaching the parents about treatment of the infection, what does the nurse instruct the parents?
   a. Need to complete penicillin or penicillin-like antibiotics
   b. Gradual return to activities until there are no physical complaints
   c. Purpose of a clear liquid diet until infection subsides
   d. Signs and symptoms of meningitis which is a common complication

13. A few weeks after having a group A beta-hemolytic streptococcal pharyngitis, the patient reports joint pain, weakness, and a rash on the inner aspects of the upper arm and thigh. These assessment findings are indicative of which complication of group A streptococcal infection?
   a. Acute glomerulonephritis
   b. Arthritis
   c. Rheumatic fever
   d. Scarlet fever

14. The 35-year-old male patient with no health problems states that he had a flu shot last year and asks if it is necessary to have it again this year. What is the best response by the nurse?
   a. "No, because once you get a flu shot, it lasts for several years and is effective against many different viruses."
   b. "Yes, because the immunity against the virus wears off, increasing your chances of getting the flu."
   c. "Yes, because the vaccine guards against a specific virus and reduces your chances of acquiring flu."
   d. "No, flu shots are only for high-risk patients and you are not considered to be at high risk."

15. The active 45-year-old schoolteacher with chronic obstructive pulmonary disease (COPD) taking prednisone asks if it is necessary to get a flu shot. What is the best response by the nurse?
    a. "Yes, flu shots are highly recommended for patients with chronic illness and/or patients who are receiving immunotherapy."
    b. "No, flu shots are only recommended for patients 50 years old and older."
    c. "Yes, it will help minimize the risk of triggering an exacerbation of COPD."
    d. "No, patients who are active, not living in a nursing home, and not health care providers do not need a flu shot."

16. The patient who had sinus surgery has a surgical incision under the upper lip. The nurse intervenes when a well-intentioned family member performs which action in attempting to make the patient feel better?
    a. Uses the bed controls to move the patient to a semi-Fowler's position
    b. Hands the patient a tissue to blow the nose
    c. Brings the patient a special custard dessert from a nearby restaurant
    d. Gently helps the patient with oral hygiene during morning care

17. The nurse is giving discharge instructions to the patient diagnosed with a viral pharyngitis. Which statement by the patient indicates the need for further teaching?
    a. "I should try to rest, increase my fluid intake, and get a humidifier for the house."
    b. "I will wait for my test results, then I can get a prescription for antibiotics."
    c. "Over-the-counter analgesics, like Tylenol or ibuprofen, can be used for pain."
    d. "I should gargle several times a day with warm salt water and use throat lozenges."

18. The physician orders a throat culture for the patient suspected of having bacterial pharyngitis. Which technique does the nurse use to obtain the specimen?
    a. Rub a sterile cotton swab over the right tonsillar area, across the right arch, the uvula, and then across the left arch to the left tonsillar area.
    b. Rub a sterile swab back and forth over the areas with marked inflammation and try to obtain a smear of white patchy exudate.
    c. Extend a sterile swab back towards the uvula without touching it directly and reach as far posterior as possible.
    d. Move the sterile swab towards the back of the throat and use any position that avoids touching the tongue and making the patient gag.

19. The nurse is taking a history on the patient who presents with symptoms of pharyngitis: sore throat with dry sensation, pain on swallowing, and low-grade fever. The patient mentions plans to take an overseas trip. Which immunization does the nurse suggest the patient should have, if not already received, before leaving?
    a. Tetanus toxoid
    b. Hepatitis B
    c. Diphtheria
    d. Yellow fever

20. The patient with a history of frequent and recurrent episodes of tonsillitis now reports a severe sore throat with pain that radiates behind the ear and difficulty swallowing. The nurse suspects the patient may have a peritonsillar abscess. On physical assessment, which deviated structure supports the nurse's supposition?
    a. Uvula
    b. Trachea
    c. Tongue
    d. Mucous membranes

21. The parent calls the emergency department (ED) about her child who complains of severe sore throat and refuses to drink fluids or to take liquid pain medication. What is the most important question for the nurse to ask in order to determine the need to seek immediate medical attention?
    a. "Does the child seem to be refusing fluids and medications because of the sore throat?"
    b. "Is the child drooling or do you hear stridor, a raspy rough sound when the child breathes?"
    c. "When did the symptoms start and how long have you been encouraging fluids?"
    d. "Is the throat red or do you see any white patches in the back of the throat?"

22. In a long-term care facility for older adults and immunocompromised patients, one employee and several patients have been diagnosed with influenza (flu). What does the supervising nurse do to decrease risk of infection to other patients?
    a. Ask employees who have flu to stay at home for at least 24 hours.
    b. Place any patient with a sore throat, cough, or rhinorrhea into isolation for 1 to 2 weeks.
    c. Ask employees with flu symptoms to stay at home for up to 5 days after onset of symptoms.
    d. Recommend that all patients and employees be immediately vaccinated for flu.

23. The nurse is giving discharge instructions to the adult patient diagnosed with the flu. The patient says, "I am generally pretty healthy, but I am concerned because my wife has several serious chronic health problems. What can I do to protect her from getting my flu?" What does the nurse instruct the patient to do? (Select all that apply.)
    a. Wash hands thoroughly after sneezing, coughing, or blowing nose.
    b. Avoid kissing, hugging, close face-to-face proximity, or hand-holding.
    c. If there is no tissue immediately available, cough or sneeze into your upper sleeve.
    d. Have the wife wear a respiratory filter mask until you stop coughing.
    e. Use disposable tissues rather than cloth handkerchiefs, and immediately dispose of tissues.

24. Number the events in sequential order as they pertain to the pathophysiologic process of pneumonia using the numbers 1 through 12.
    _____ a. Atelectasis
    _____ b. Possible septicemia
    _____ c. Decreased surfactant production and compliance
    _____ d. Arterial hypoxemia
    _____ e. Edema formation and inflammation
    _____ f. Tachypnea and tachycardia
    _____ g. Migration of WBCs to alveoli
    _____ h. Spread of organisms to other alveoli
    _____ i. Shunting of unoxygenated blood
    _____ j. Thickening of alveolar wall and stiffening of lungs
    _____ k. Diminished capillary blood flow in alveoli
    _____ l. Invasion of pulmonary tissue by pathogens

25. Which patient is at highest risk of developing pneumonia?
    a. Any hospitalized patient between the ages of 18 and 65 years
    b. 32-year-old trauma patient on a mechanical ventilator
    c. Disabled 54-year-old with osteoporosis; discharged to home
    d. Any patient who has not received the vaccine for pneumonia

26. Which statement best describes pneumonia?
    a. An infection of just the "windpipe" because the lungs are "clear" of any problems
    b. A serious inflammation of the bronchioles from various causes
    c. Only an infection of the lungs with mild to severe effects on breathing
    d. An inflammation resulting from lung damage caused by long-term smoking

27. The patient is seen in the physician's office for a complaint of chest pleuritic discomfort, chills, fever, cough, dyspnea, and sputum production. The nurse prepares patient information about diagnostic testing of the respiratory system. Which diagnostic test is most likely to be performed first?
    a. Lung scan
    b. Pulmonary function test
    c. Fluorescein bronchoscopy
    d. Sputum gram stain

28. The nurse is reviewing laboratory results for the patient who has pneumonia. Which laboratory value does the nurse expect to see for this patient?
    a. Decreased hemoglobin
    b. Increased red blood cells (RBCs)
    c. Decreased neutrophils
    d. Increased WBCs

29. The patient is diagnosed with pneumonia. During auscultation of the lower lung fields, the nurse hears coarse crackles. The nursing diagnosis of Impaired Gas Exchange is identified. What is the underlying physiologic condition associated with the patient's condition?
    a. Hypoxemia
    b. Hyperemia
    c. Hypocapnia
    d. Hypercapnia

30. Which patient is the least likely to be at risk for developing pneumonia?
    a. Patient with a 5-year history of smoking
    b. Renal transplant patient
    c. Postoperative patient with a bedside commode
    d. Postoperative patient with a hip replacement

31. The older adult patient who is several days postoperative develops chest pain, dyspnea, generalized fatigue, and confusion. Which common diagnostic test for pneumonia does the nurse expect to be ordered for this patient?
    a. Continuous pulse oximetry
    b. Sputum specimen
    c. Complete blood cell count
    d. Chest x-ray

32. The patient is admitted to the hospital with pneumonia. What does the nurse expect the chest x-ray results to reveal?
    a. Patchy areas of consolidation
    b. Tension pneumothorax
    c. Thick secretions causing airway obstruction
    d. Large hyperinflated airways

33. What nursing intervention prevents the complication of pneumonia for the surgical patient?
    a. Monitoring chest x-rays and white cell counts for early signs of infection
    b. Monitoring lung sounds every shift and encouraging fluids
    c. Teaching coughing, deep-breathing exercises, and use of incentive spirometry
    d. Encouraging hand hygiene among all caregivers, patients, and visitors

34. The nurse is conducting an in-service for the hospital staff about practices that help prevent pneumonia among at-risk patients. Which nursing intervention is encouraged as standard practice?
    a. Administering vaccines to patients at risk
    b. Implementing isolation for debilitated patients
    c. Restricting foods from home in immunosuppressed patients
    d. Decontaminating respiratory therapy equipment weekly

35. The patient hospitalized for pneumonia has a nursing diagnosis of Ineffective Airway Clearance related to fatigue, chest pain, excessive secretions, and muscle weakness. What nursing intervention helps to correct these problems?
    a. Administer oxygen to prevent hypoxemia and atelectasis.
    b. Push fluids to greater than 3000 mL/day to ensure adequate hydration.
    c. Administer respiratory therapy in a timely manner to decrease bronchospasms.
    d. Maintain semi-Fowler's position to facilitate breathing and prevent further fatigue.

36. The patient is admitted to the hospital for treatment of pneumonia. Which nursing assessment finding best indicates that the patient is responding to antibiotics?
    a. Wheezing, oxygen at 2 L/min, respiratory rate 26, no shortness of breath or chills
    b. Temperature 99° F, lung sounds clear, pulse oximetry on 2 L/min at 98%, cough with yellow sputum
    c. Cough, clear sputum, temperature 99° F, pulse oximetry at 96% on room air
    d. Feeling tired, respiratory rate 28 on 2 L/min of oxygen, audible breath sounds

37. The nurse is reviewing the laboratory results for the older adult patient with pneumonia. Which laboratory value frequently seen in patients with pneumonia may not be seen in this patient?
    a. RBC 4.0 to 5.0
    b. Hgb 12 to 16
    c. Hct 36 to 48
    d. WBC 12 to 18

38. The patient is admitted to the hospital to rule out pneumonia. Which infection control technique does the nurse maintain?
    a. Strict respiratory isolation and use of a specially designed face mask
    b. Respiratory isolation and contact isolation for sputum
    c. Respiratory isolation with a stock surgical mask
    d. Standard precautions and no respiratory isolation

39. A critical concern for the patient returning to the unit after a surgical procedure is related to Impaired Gas Exchange caused by inadequate ventilation. Which arterial blood gas value and assessment finding indicates to the nurse that oxygen and incentive spirometry must be administered?
    a. Pao_2 is 90 mm Hg with crackles.
    b. Pao_2 is 90 mm Hg with wheezing.
    c. Pco_2 is 38 mm Hg with clear lung sounds.
    d. Pco_2 is 45 mm Hg with atelectasis.

40. The nurse has identified a nursing diagnosis of Ineffective Airway Clearance with bronchospasms for the patient with pneumonia. The patient has no previous history of chronic respiratory disorders. The nurse obtains an order for which nursing intervention?
    a. Increased liters of humidified oxygen per face mask
    b. Scheduled and PRN aerosol nebulizer bronchodilator treatments
    c. Handheld bronchodilator inhaler as needed
    d. Prednisone via inhaler or IV to reduce the inflammation

41. The patient is admitted to the hospital with pneumonia. Which approach to the administration of antibiotics does the nurse expect the physician to order?
    a. Start any antibiotic that is immediately available and follow up on culture results.
    b. Start broad spectrum IV antibiotic therapy without delay.
    c. Wait for sputum culture results with specificity before starting antibiotic therapy.
    d. Obtain three sputum specimens before starting IV antibiotics to reduce risk of toxicity.

42. The older adult patient asks the nurse how often one should receive the pneumococcal vaccine for pneumonia prevention. What is the nurse's best response?
    a. "Every year, when the patient is receiving the 'flu shot.'"
    b. "The standard is vaccination every 3 years."
    c. "The recommendation is every 5 years; older adults may need it more frequently."
    d. "There is no set schedule; it depends on the patient's history and risk factors."

43. The nurse is providing discharge instructions about pneumonia to the patient and family. Which discharge information is the nurse sure to include?
    a. Complete antibiotics as prescribed, rest, drink fluids, and minimize contact with crowds.
    b. Take all antibiotics as ordered, resume diet and all activities as before hospitalization.
    c. No restrictions regarding activities, diet, and rest because the patient is fully recovered when discharged.
    d. Continue antibiotics only until no further signs of pneumonia are present; avoid exposing immunosuppressed individuals.

44. The patient is admitted for pneumonia. Which kind of drug therapy does the nurse anticipate will be ordered by the physician?
    a. Cough suppressants
    b. Antibiotics
    c. Mucolytic agents
    d. Corticosteroids

45. The patient has been treated for pneumonia and the nurse is preparing discharge instructions. The patient is capable of performing self-care and is anxious to return to his job at the construction site. Which instructions does the nurse give to this patient?
    a. "You are not contagious to others, so you can return to work as soon as you like."
    b. "You will continue to feel tired and will fatigue easily for the next several weeks."
    c. "Try to drink 4 quarts of water per day, especially if you are very physically active."
    d. "You should be able to return to work full-time in 2 weeks when your energy returns."

46. Which complication of pneumonia creates pain that increases on inspiration because of inflammation of the parietal pleura?
    a. Pleuritic chest pain
    b. Pulmonary emboli
    c. Pleural effusion
    d. Meningitis

47. Which conditions may cause patients to be at risk for aspiration pneumonia? *(Select all that apply.)*
    a. Continuous tube feedings
    b. Bronchoscopy procedure
    c. MRI procedure
    d. Decreased level of consciousness
    e. Stroke
    f. Chest tube

48. The older adult patient often coughs and chokes while eating or trying to take medication. The patient insists that he is okay, but the nurse identifies a nursing diagnosis of Risk for Aspiration. Which nursing interventions are used to prevent aspiration pneumonia? *(Select all the apply.)*
    a. Head of bed should always be elevated during feeding.
    b. Monitor the patient's ability to swallow small bites.
    c. Give thin liquids to drink in small frequent amounts.
    d. Consult a nutritionist and obtain swallowing studies.
    e. Monitor the patient's ability to swallow saliva.
    f. Place the patient on NPO status until swallowing is normal.

49. Which condition causes a patient to have the greatest risk for community-acquired pneumonia?
    a. Tube feedings
    b. History of tobacco use
    c. Poor nutritional status
    d. Altered mental status

50. In the event of a new SARS outbreak, what is the nurse's primary role?
    a. Immediately report new cases of SARS to the Centers for Disease Control and Prevention.
    b. Administer oxygen, standard antibiotics, and supportive therapies to patients.
    c. Prevent the spread of infection to other employees and patients.
    d. Initiate and strictly enforce contact isolation procedures.

51. The nurse is preparing a community information packet about "bird flu." What information does the nurse include for public dissemination? *(Select all that apply.)*
    a. In the event of an outbreak, do not eat any cooked or uncooked poultry products.
    b. Prepare a minimum of 2 weeks supply of food, water, and routine prescription drugs.
    c. Listen to public health announcements and early warning signs for disease outbreaks.
    d. Avoid traveling to areas where there has been a suspected outbreak of disease.
    e. Obtain a supply of antiviral drugs such as oseltamivir (Tamiflu).
    f. In the event of an outbreak, avoid going to public areas such as churches or schools.

52. The patient reports experiencing mild fatigue and a dry, harsh cough. There is a possibility of exposure to inhalation anthrax, but the patient currently reports feeling much better. What does the nurse advise the patient to do?
    a. Have a complete blood count to rule out the disease.
    b. Monitor for and immediately seek attention for respiratory symptoms.
    c. Consult a physician for diagnostic testing and antibiotic therapy.
    d. Stay at home, rest, increase fluid intake, and avoid public places.

53. The patient with HIV is admitted to the hospital with a temperature of 99.6° F, and reports of bloody sputum, night sweats, feeling of tiredness, and shortness of breath. What are these assessment findings consistent with?
    a. Pneumocystic pneumonia (PCP)
    b. Tuberculosis
    c. Superinfection as a result of a low CD4 count
    d. Bacterial pneumonia

54. Which statement about the transmission of tuberculosis (TB) is true?
    a. Exposure to a person with TB results in active disease within 2 to 10 weeks.
    b. The causative agent of TB is transmitted via aerosolization (airborne).
    c. If a person has had the disease, there is no risk for reoccurrence.
    d. Any "exposed" person is considered as having active TB.

55. Which patient is at the greatest risk for developing TB?
    a. 22-year-old college student living in a double room in a dormitory
    b. 82-year-old retired schoolteacher living in a house with her widowed sister
    c. 42-year-old alcoholic homeless man who occasionally stays in a shelter
    d. 53-year-old homemaker who does volunteer work in a homeless shelter

56. The most substantial impact in incidence of TB is from which high-risk population?
    a. Older adults, the homeless, minorities
    b. Lower socioeconomic groups
    c. Those in constant frequent contact with untreated individuals
    d. Those with immune dysfunction, particularly HIV

57. After several weeks of "not feeling well," the patient is seen in the physician's office for possible TB. If TB is present, which assessment findings does the nurse expect to observe?
    a. Fatigue, night sweats, low-grade fever
    b. Weight gain, bloody streaked sputum, night sweats
    c. Hemoptysis, loss of appetite, high fever
    d. Nonproductive cough, fatigue, anorexia

58. Which test result indicates the patient has clinically active TB?
    a. Induration of 12 mm and positive sputum
    b. Positive chest x-ray for TB
    c. Positive chest x-ray and clinical symptoms
    d. Sputum tests positive for blood

59. After receiving the subcutaneous Mantoux skin test, the patient with no risk factors returns to the clinic in the required 48 to 72 hours for the test results. Which assessment finding indicates a positive result?
    a. Test area is red, warm, and tender to touch
    b. Induration or a hard nodule of any size at the site
    c. Induration/hardened area measures 5 mm or greater
    d. Induration/hardened area measures 10 mm or greater

60. The patient has a positive skin test result for TB. What explanation does the nurse give to the patient?
    a. "There is active disease, but you are not yet infectious to others."
    b. "There is active disease and you need immediate treatment."
    c. "You have been infected but this does not mean active disease is present."
    d. "A repeat skin test is necessary because the test could give a false-positive result."

61. What is the minimum time period for treatment of TB?
    a. 7 to 10 days
    b. 3 weeks
    c. 3 months
    d. 6 months

62. The patient has been compliant with drug therapy for TB and has returned as instructed for follow-up. Which result indicates that the patient is no longer infectious/communicable?
    a. Negative chest x-ray
    b. No clinical symptoms
    c. Negative skin test
    d. Three negative sputum cultures

63. The patient diagnosed with TB agrees to take the medication as instructed and to complete the therapy. When does the nurse tell the patient is the best time to take the medication?
    a. Before breakfast
    b. After breakfast
    c. Midday
    d. Bedtime

64. The patient has an HIV infection, but the TB skin test shows an induration of less than 10 mm and no clinical symptoms of TB are present. Which medication does the patient receive for a period of 12 months to prevent TB?
    a. Bacille Calmette-Guérin (BCG) vaccine
    b. Isoniazid (INH)
    c. Ethambutol
    d. Streptomycin

65. The nurse is teaching the patient about the combination drug therapy that is used in the treatment of TB. Which patient statement indicates the nurse's instruction was effective?
    a. "I will take three drugs: isoniazid, rifampin, and pyrazinamide, then ethambutol may be added later."
    b. "Combining the drugs in one pill is a convenient way for me to take all the medications."
    c. "The isoniazid combines with the TB bacteria. I can take the rifampin and pyrazinamide if I continue to have symptoms."
    d. "Combining the medications means to take the isoniazid, rifampin, and pyrazinamide all at the same time."

66. The patient diagnosed with TB has been receiving treatment for 3 weeks and has clinically shown improvement. The family asks the nurse if the patient is still infectious. What is the nurse's reply?
    a. "The patient is still infectious until the entire treatment is completed."
    b. "The patient is not infectious but needs to continue treatment for at least 6 months."
    c. "The patient is infectious until there is a negative chest x-ray."
    d. "The patient may or may not be infectious; a PPD must be done."

Matching. *Match the nursing interventions with the medications to treat TB. Answers may be used more than once.*

TB Medications
a. Isoniazid (INH)
b. Rifampin
c. Pyrazinamide
d. Ethambutol

Nursing Interventions

_____ 67. Teach women that this drug reduces the effectiveness of oral contraceptives and that another form of birth control should be used while on this therapy.

_____ 68. Teach the patient that urine will be orange in color.

_____ 69. Consult the physician for dose reduction when the patient complains of blurry vision after starting treatment.

_____ 70. Teach the patient not to take medications such as Maalox with this medication.

_____ 71. Avoid drinking alcoholic beverages.

_____ 72. Take a multivitamin with B-complex.

_____ 73. Teach the patient to take in the morning, preferably before eating unless it causes an "upset stomach."

_____ 74. Teach to take with food to decrease GI upset.

_____ 75. If going out into the sun, wear protective clothing and sunscreen.

_____ 76. Teach patients to identify changes in the ability to differentiate colors.

77. The patient with suspected TB is admitted to the hospital. Along with a private room, which nursing intervention is appropriate related to isolation procedures?
   a. Respiratory isolation and contact isolation for sputum only
   b. Strict respiratory isolation and use of specially designed face masks
   c. Respiratory isolation with surgical masks until diagnosis is confirmed
   d. No respiratory isolation necessary until diagnosis is confirmed

78. The patient is admitted to the hospital to rule out TB. What type of mask does the nurse wear when caring for this patient?
   a. Surgical face mask
   b. Surgical face mask with eye shield
   c. HEPA respirator mask
   d. Any type of mask that covers the nose and mouth

79. After being discharged from the hospital, the patient is diagnosed with TB at the outpatient clinic. What is the correct procedure regarding public health policy in this case?
    a. Contact the infection control nurse at the hospital because the hospital is responsible for follow-up of this case.
    b. There are no regulations because the patient was diagnosed at the clinic and not during hospitalization.
    c. Contact the public health nurse so that all individuals who have come in contact with the patient can be screened.
    d. Have the patient sign a waiver regarding the hospital and clinic's liability for treatment.

80. Which diagnostic test is *not* used to diagnose TB?
    a. Chest radiography
    b. Complete blood count
    c. Mantoux skin test
    d. Sputum culture

81. The patient is at high risk for TB. Which question does the nurse ask to elicit information about a physical symptom that is associated with TB?
    a. "Are you experiencing unusual fatigue?"
    b. "Have you recently gained any weight?"
    c. "Have you had a high-grade fever?"
    d. "Are you experiencing a nonproductive cough?"

82. After a motor vehicle accident, the patient is dependent on mechanical ventilation. The nurse initiates "ventilator bundle" precautions to prevent ventilator-associated pneumonia. Which actions does the nurse perform to initiate these precautions? *(Select all that apply.)*
    a. Elevate head of the bed to between 30 and 45 degrees whenever possible.
    b. Continuously remove subglottic secretions.
    c. Change the ventilator circuit every 24 hours.
    d. Perform handwashing before and after contact with each patient.
    e. No rings are worn when caring for ventilator patients.
    f. Perform meticulous oral care no less frequently than every 12 hours.

83. The nurse is making home visits to the older adult recovering from a hip fracture and identifies a nursing diagnosis of Risk for Infection, Respiratory. Which condition represents a factor of normal aging that would contribute to this increased risk?
    a. Inability to force a cough
    b. Decreased strength of respiratory muscles
    c. Increased elastic recoil of alveoli
    d. Increased macrophages in alveoli

CASE STUDY: THE OLDER ADULT PATIENT WITH TUBERCULOSIS

Use a separate sheet of paper to answer the questions in this Case Study. Answer guidelines for this Case Study are available on your Evolve website at http://evolve.elsevier.com/Iggy/ in the "Prepare for Class" folder.

The patient is a 65-year-old woman who shares a three-room inner-city apartment with two of her daughters and their seven children. She comes into the neighborhood walk-in clinic reporting extreme fatigue, a 30-pound weight loss, and a cough of 4 months' duration. A Mantoux test, sputum culture, and chest x-ray confirm a diagnosis of tuberculosis (TB). She is to begin a 12-month course of medication therapy with isoniazid (INH) 300 mg orally once a day, and rifampin (Rifadin) 600 mg orally once a day.

1. Discuss why one or more pharmacologic agents are used to treat TB.
2. When is the best time for this patient to take the chemotherapeutic agents to minimize the side effects?
3. Why should rifampin (Rifadin) be taken on an empty stomach?
4. What type of follow-up care should be planned for this patient?
5. How long will this patient be considered contagious?
6. What measures should be taken with the other family members? Explain your answer.
7. Develop a teaching-learning plan for this patient.

Three weeks after diagnosis, the patient returns to the clinic stating that she has stopped taking her medications because they made her sick to her stomach. She is unable to eat and has continued to lose weight.

8. Identify the relevant nursing diagnoses for this patient based on the above information.
9. Discuss what the nurse should do to assist this patient in taking her medications and eating a balanced diet.

CASE STUDY: THE YOUNG PATIENT WITH TUBERCULOSIS

Use a separate sheet of paper to answer the questions in this Case Study. Answer guidelines for this Case Study are available on your Evolve website at http://evolve. elsevier.com/Iggy/ in the "Prepare for Class" folder.

The patient is a 25-year-old inner-city woman with AIDS. She is hospitalized now for active TB. She has four young children who are currently being cared for by her mother, a 42-year-old unemployed woman with diabetes mellitus.

1. What kind of isolation must this patient be placed in and why?
2. Sputum cultures for acid-fast bacilli (AFB) are ordered. When is the best time to collect sputum?
3. Can sputum that contains saliva be sent to the laboratory?
4. Before the patient is discharged, what interventions must be done at her home in preparation for her return?

CASE STUDY: THE PATIENT WITH PNEUMONIA

Use a separate sheet of paper to answer the questions in this Case Study. Answer guidelines for this Case Study are available on your Evolve website at http://evolve. elsevier.com/Iggy/ in the "Prepare for Class" folder.

A 75-year-old married woman comes to the outpatient clinic with her husband reporting a severe cough, left-sided chest pain, and she holds her left side while coughing. She appears anxious and her face is flushed. Vital signs are temperature 102.6° F, pulse 118, apical; respirations 32, shallow; and blood pressure 120/80. A diagnosis of pneumonia is suspected. A sputum specimen, chest x-ray, arterial blood gases, and complete blood count are ordered.

1. What should this patient and her husband be taught about the sputum collection and x-ray?
2. What will likely be heard when the patient's lungs are auscultated? Explain your answer.

A diagnosis of pneumonia is confirmed by the chest x-ray and sputum cultures. Because the patient's blood gases are within normal limits, she will be managed on an outpatient basis.

3. Identify the relevant nursing diagnoses for this patient based on above information.

The physician orders cefaclor (Ceclor) 500 mg orally every 8 hours and wants the patient to return to the clinic in 1 week. If her condition does not improve within 48 hours or she becomes short of breath, she should call or return to the clinic.

4. Develop teaching-learning and discharge care plans for the patient and her husband.

34 CHAPTER

Care of Critically Ill Patients with Respiratory Problems

STUDY/REVIEW QUESTIONS

True or False? *Read the statements about pulmonary embolus (PE) and deep vein thrombosis (DVT) and write T for true or F for false in the blanks provided. If the statement is false, correct the statement to make it true.*

_____ 1. Any substance can cause an embolism, but septic clots are the most common cause.

_____ 2. In PE, platelets collect on the embolus, triggering the release of substances that cause blood vessel constriction.

_____ 3. Additional risk factors for PE and DVT include smoking, pregnancy, estrogen therapy, heart failure, stroke, cancer (particularly lung or prostate), Trousseau's syndrome, and trauma.

_____ 4. With PE, some patients could have more vague symptoms resembling the flu, such as nausea, vomiting, and general malaise.

_____ 5. Some patients with PE will not have hypoxemia.

_____ 6. Amniotic fluid embolus has a high mortality rate and occurs as a rare complication of childbirth, abortion, or amniocentesis.

_____ 7. The most common site of origin for a PE is clots in the right side of the heart.

8. The nurse's young neighbor who smokes is going on an overseas flight. The neighbor knows he is at risk for DVT and PE, and asks the nurse for advice. What does the nurse suggest?
   a. Exercise regularly and walk around before boarding the flight.
   b. Get a prescription for heparin therapy and take it before the flight.
   c. Drink water; get up every hour for at least 5 minutes during the flight.
   d. Elevate the legs as much as possible during and after the flight.

9. The nurse is caring for several postoperative patients at risk for developing PE. Which interventions does the nurse use to help prevent the development of PE in these patients? *(Select all that apply.)*
   a. Start passive and active range-of-motion exercises for the extremities.
   b. Ambulate postoperative patients soon after surgery.
   c. Use antiembolism devices postoperatively.
   d. Elevate legs in an extended position.
   e. Change patient position every 4 to 6 hours.
   f. Massage leg muscles.
   g. Administer drugs to prevent episodes of Valsalva maneuver.

10. The nurse suspects the patient has a PE and notifies the physician who orders an arterial blood gas. The physician is en route to the facility. The nurse anticipates and prepares the patient for which additional diagnostic test?
    a. Spiral CT scan
    b. Pulmonary angiography
    c. 12-lead ECG
    d. Ventilation and perfusion scan

11. The physician orders heparin therapy for the patient with a relatively small PE. The patient states, "I didn't tell the doctor my complete medical history." Which condition may affect the physician's decision to immediately start heparin therapy?
    a. Type 2 diabetes mellitus
    b. Recent cerebral hemorrhage
    c. Newly diagnosed osteoarthritis
    d. Asthma since childhood

12. The patient with a PE asks for an explanation of heparin therapy. What is the nurse's best response?
    a. "It keeps the clot from getting larger by preventing platelets from sticking together to improve blood flow."
    b. "It will improve your breathing and decrease chest pain by dissolving the clot in your lung."
    c. "It promotes the absorption of the clot in your leg that originally caused the PE."
    d. "It increases the time it takes for blood to clot, therefore preventing further clotting and improving blood flow."

13. The patient is being treated with heparin therapy for a PE. The patient has a nursing diagnosis of Risk for Injury (bleeding). What does the nurse monitor in relation to the heparin therapy?
    a. Lab values for any elevation of PT or PTT value
    b. PTT values for greater than 2.5 times the control and/or the patient for bleeding
    c. Occurrence of a pulmonary infarction by blood in sputum
    d. PT values for international normalized ratio (INR) for a therapeutic range of 2 to 3 and/or the patient for bleeding

14. The nurse is reviewing the lab values for the patient on heparin therapy for a PE. The nurse discovers that the relevant lab values are above the therapeutic range for this therapy. Which physician's order does the nurse obtain for this patient?
    a. Temporarily stop heparin infusion or slow the rate of administration.
    b. Change the concentration of heparin in the IV bag.
    c. Administer the antidote protamine sulfate stat.
    d. Administer a dose of vitamin K by IM injection.

15. Upon diagnosis of a PE, the nurse expects to perform which therapeutic intervention for the patient?
    a. Oral anticoagulant therapy
    b. Bedrest in the supine position
    c. Oxygen therapy via mechanical ventilator
    d. Parenteral anticoagulant therapy

16. The nurse is caring for the patient with a postoperative complication of PE. The patient has been receiving treatment for several days. Which factors are indicators of adequate perfusion in the patient? *(Select all that apply.)*
    a. Pulse oximetry of 95%
    b. Arterial blood gas, pH of 7.28
    c. Patient's subjective desire to go home
    d. Absence of pallor or cyanosis
    e. Mental status at patient's baseline

Indicate which patients the nurse monitors for PE and provides preventive measures. Mark Y for yes or N for no, and provide a brief rationale for your answer.

_____ 17. Patient with total hip or knee replacement, postoperative

_____ 18. Patient with multiple trauma

_____ 19. Patient who had surgery at an outpatient clinic

_____ 20. Patient with previous history of deep vein thrombosis

_____ 21. Older adult patient hospitalized with dehydration

_____ 22. Patient with sickle cell anemia

_____ 23. Patient with pneumonia able to get out of bed into a chair

_____ 24. Patient who weighs 250 pounds with a height of 5' 5"

_____ 25. Patient who is being evaluated for endometriosis

_____ 26. Patient in labor about to deliver a baby

_____ 27. Patient with a dislocated shoulder

_____ 28. Patient with abdominal surgery, postoperative

_____ 29. Patient with atrial fibrillation

_____ 30. Patient with spinal cord injury and paralysis

_____ 31. Any patient with the nursing diagnosis of Impaired Mobility

32. The nurse is caring for several postoperative patients with high risk for a PE. All of these patients have pre-existing chronic respiratory problems. What is a unique assessment finding for a clot in the lung?
a. Dyspnea
b. Sudden dry cough
c. Pursed-lip breathing
d. Audible wheezing

33. The nurse is caring for several patients at risk for DVT and PE. Which condition causes the patient to be the most likely candidate for placement of a vena cava filter?
a. Massive PE causing the patient to experience shock symptoms
b. Multiple emboli with deteriorating cardiopulmonary status
c. Recurrent bleeding while receiving anticoagulants
d. No response to oxygen therapy and conservative management

34. The patient with a massive PE has hypotension and shock, and is receiving IV crystalloids. However, the patient's cardiac output is not improving. The nurse anticipates an order for which drug?
a. Hydromorphone (Dilaudid)
b. Alteplase (Activase, tPA)
c. Diltiazem (Cardizem)
d. Dobutamine (Dobutrex)

35. The older adult patient on anticoagulation therapy for a PE is somewhat confused and requires assistance with ADLs. Which instruction specific to this therapy does the nurse give to the unlicensed assistive personnel?
a. Count and report episodes of urinary incontinence.
b. Use a lift sheet when moving or turning the patient in bed.
c. Assist with ambulation because the patient is likely to have dizziness.
d. Give the patient an extra blanket, because the patient is likely to feel cold.

36. The patient with a PE is receiving anticoagulant therapy. Which assessment related to the therapy does the nurse perform?
    a. Measure abdominal girth because the medication causes fluid retention.
    b. Check skin turgor because dehydration contributes to anticoagulation.
    c. Monitor for nausea, vomiting, and diarrhea.
    d. Examine skin every 2 hours for evidence of bleeding.

37. What does the nurse monitor for in the patient with a PE? *(Select all that apply.)*
    a. Nausea and vomiting
    b. Cyanosis
    c. Rapid heart rate
    d. Dyspnea
    e. Paradoxical chest movement
    f. Crackles in the lung fields

38. After receiving IV heparin anticoagulant therapy, patients are generally not discharged from the hospital without a prescription and instructions for which drug?
    a. Protamine sulfate
    b. Prednisone (Deltasone)
    c. Warfarin (Coumadin)
    d. Oral heparin

39. The patient is following up on a postoperative complication of PE. The patient must have blood drawn to determine the therapeutic range for Coumadin. Which lab test determines this therapeutic range?
    a. PTT level
    b. Platelets
    c. PT and INR
    d. Coumadin peak and trough

40. The nurse is reviewing lab results for the patient with a new-onset PE. What is the INR therapeutic range?
    a. 1.0 to 1.5 times the normal value
    b. 2.0 to 3.0 times the normal value
    c. 3.0 to 4.5 times the normal value
    d. 5 times the normal value

41. The patient demonstrates chest pain, dyspnea, dry cough, and change in level of consciousness. The nurse suspects PE and notifies the physician who orders an arterial blood gas (ABG). In the early stage of a PE, what would ABG results probably indicate?
    a. Respiratory alkalosis
    b. Respiratory acidosis
    c. Metabolic acidosis
    d. Metabolic alkalosis

42. The patient recently received anticoagulant therapy for complications of PE after knee surgery. The patient is now in a rehabilitation facility and is receiving Coumadin. What is the nursing responsibility related to Coumadin?
    a. Having protamine sulfate available as an antidote
    b. Administering NSAIDs or aspirin for pain related to the knee
    c. Teaching the patient about foods high in vitamin K
    d. Monitoring platelets for thrombocytopenia

True or False? Read the statements regarding ventilatory and oxygen failure and acute respiratory distress syndrome (ARDS) and write T for true or F for false in the blanks provided. If the statement is false, correct the statement to make it true.

_____ 43. In ventilatory failure, ventilation-perfusion (V/Q) mismatch is found in conditions where perfusion is inadequate and ventilation is also inadequate.

_____ 44. Ventilatory failure is often the result of a physical problem of the lungs or chest wall, a defect in the respiratory control center in the brain, or poor function of the diaphragm.

_____ 45. In oxygenation failure, there is V/Q mismatch in which air movement and oxygen intake are normal and lung perfusion is normal.

_____ 46. Oxygenation failure occurs when blood shunts from right to left in pulmonary vessels.

_____ 47. The patient who is having an asthma attack is at risk for combined ventilatory and oxygenation failure.

_____ 48. In ARDS, the main trigger is a systemic inflammatory response.

_____ 49. The lung tissue is normally moist, but in patients with ARDS, the lung dries out and becomes stiff.

_____ 50. In ARDS, lung volume is increased and there is increased compliance.

_____ 51. Transfusion-related acute lung injury (TRALI) is a noncardiogenic pulmonary edema associated with the activation of the inflammatory response due to a recent transfusion of plasma-containing products.

_____ 52. In ARDS, especially after trauma, clot production is increased and fibrinolysis is reduced.

53. The nurse is reviewing the ABG results for the patient. The latest ABGs show pH 7.48, HCO_3^- 23 mEq/L, $Paco_2$ 25 mm Hg, Pao_2 98 mm Hg. What is the correct interpretation of these lab findings?
   a. Normal ABGs indicating adequate ventilation
   b. Acute respiratory alkalosis and hyperventilation
   c. Acute respiratory acidosis and hypoventilation
   d. Chronic respiratory acidosis and hypoventilation

54. The nurse is caring for the patient with acute hypoxemia. Which nursing interventions are best for the care of this patient? *(Select all that apply.)*
   a. Minimal self-care
   b. PRN sedatives
   c. Upright position
   d. Oxygen therapy
   e. Keep NPO while dyspneic
   f. Prescribed metered dose inhalers

55. The patient reports pain with inspiration after falling off a skateboard. The physician makes the diagnosis of rib fracture. The nurse prepares to do patient teaching for which treatment?
   a. Mechanical ventilation
   b. Tight bandage around chest
   c. Coughing and deep breathing
   d. Potent analgesics for pain

56. The nurse is assessing the patient who sustained significant chest trauma during a motor vehicle accident. What significant assessment finding suggests tension pneumothorax?
   a. Tracheal deviation to the unaffected side
   b. Inspiratory stridor and respiratory distress
   c. Diminished breath sounds over the affected hemothorax
   d. Hyperresonant percussion note over the affected side

57. The nurse is assessing the patient with a hemothorax. When the nurse performs percussion of the chest on the affected side, what type of sound is expected?
   a. Hypertympanic
   b. Dull
   c. Hyperresonant
   d. Crackles

58. On arrival to the ED, the patient develops extreme respiratory distress and the physician identifies a tension pneumothorax. The nurses prepares to assist with which urgent procedure?
    a. Endotracheal intubation with mechanical ventilation
    b. Placement of a chest tube to reduce pneumothorax on the affected side
    c. Insertion of a 8-inch (20.3-cm), 16- or 18-gauge pericardial needle
    d. Insertion of a large-bore needle into the intercostal space on the affected side

59. The nurse is performing patient teaching for the patient who will be taking anticoagulants at home. What does the nurse include in the instructions? *(Select all that apply.)*
    a. Use a soft-bristled toothbrush and floss frequently.
    b. Do not take aspirin or any aspirin-containing products.
    c. Do not participate in activities that will cause bumps, scratches, or scrapes.
    d. If you are bumped, apply ice to the site for at least 24 hours.
    e. Eat warm, cool, or cold foods to avoid burning your mouth.
    f. Check your skin and mouth monthly for bruising or bleeding.
    g. If you must blow your nose, do so gently without blocking either nasal passage.

60. Which patient has the greatest risk for developing ARDS?
    a. 74-year-old who aspirates a tube feeding
    b. 34-year-old with chronic renal failure
    c. 56-year-old with uncontrolled diabetes mellitus
    d. 18-year-old with a fractured femur

61. Which assessment finding is considered an early sign of ARDS?
    a. Adventitious lung sounds
    b. Hyperthermia and hot, dry skin
    c. Intercostal and suprasternal retractions
    d. Heightened mental acuity and surveillance

62. The patient with which condition is a potential candidate for autotransfusion, should the need arise?
    a. Tension pneumothorax
    b. Hemothorax
    c. Abdominal bleeding
    d. Esophageal bleeding

63. Identify the acid-base problems and the necessary interventions for each set of ABG data given below.
    a. pH = 7.40, Po_2 = 74 mm Hg, Pco_2 = 40 mm Hg, HCO_3 25 mEq/L

    _____

    b. pH = 7.30, Po_2 = 90 mm Hg, Pco_2 = 40 mm Hg, HCO_3 19 mEq/L

    _____

    c. pH = 7.30, Po_2 = 87 mm Hg, Pco_2 = 50 mm Hg, HCO_3 27 mEq/L

    _____

    d. pH = 7.60, Po_2 = 94 mm Hg, Pco_2 = 21 mm Hg, HCO_3 22 mEq/L

    _____

    e. pH = 7.43, Po_2 = 92 mm Hg, Pco_2 = 40 mm Hg, HCO_3 24 mEq/L

    _____

    f. pH = 7.28, Po_2 = 59 mm Hg, Pco_2 = 40 mm Hg, HCO_3 26 mEq/L

    _____

64. The patient sustained a chest injury resulting from a motor vehicle accident. The patient is asymptomatic at first, but slowly develops decreased breath sounds, crackles, wheezing, and blood in the sputum. The mechanism of injury and physical findings are consistent with which condition?
    a. Flail chest
    b. Rib fractures
    c. Pneumothorax
    d. Pulmonary contusion

65. The patient is admitted after a near-drowning and develops ARDS which is confirmed by the physician. The nurse prepares equipment for which treatment?
    a. Oxygen therapy via CPAP
    b. Mechanical ventilation and endotracheal tube
    c. High-flow oxygen via face mask
    d. Tracheostomy tube

66. A 19-year-old was seen in the ED after a motorcycle accident for multiple rib fractures that resulted in free-floating ribs, paradoxical breathing, and impaired gas exchange. What is this condition called?
    a. Tension pneumothorax
    b. Flail chest
    c. Pulmonary contusion
    d. Subcutaneous emphysema

67. Before suctioning the patient with an endotracheal or tracheostomy tube, the nurse preoxygenates the patient with what percent oxygen concentration?
    a. 21%
    b. 40%
    c. 70%
    d. 100%

68. The patient has been intubated and has copious secretions. The nurse identifies a need for endotracheal suctioning. What is the maximum length of time that suction should be applied?
    a. 5 to 10 seconds
    b. 10 to 15 seconds
    c. 20 to 30 seconds
    d. 40 to 60 seconds

69. The nurse is caring for several patients with acute or chronic respiratory problems. The patient with which condition needs immediate intervention because of impending acute respiratory failure?
    a. Orthopnea
    b. Tachypnea
    c. Dyspnea on exertion
    d. Status asthmaticus

70. The patient with ARDS is currently in the phase 1 management stage. What is the focus of the nursing assessment?
    a. Monitor closely for progressive hypoxemia.
    b. Note early changes in dyspnea and tachypnea.
    c. Review the x-ray reports for evidence of patchy infiltrates.
    d. Monitor for multiple organ dysfunction syndrome.

71. The nurse is caring for the patient at risk for pulmonary contusion. Why is this is a potentially lethal chest injury?
    a. The patient could have broken ribs.
    b. The patient could develop laryngospasm.
    c. Respiratory failure develops over time.
    d. There is a risk of infection from chest tubes.

Matching. Match each disorder or event that can cause patients to be at risk for acute respiratory failure with its corresponding type of respiratory failure. Answers may be used more than once.

Types of Respiratory Failure

a. Ventilatory failure
b. Oxygenation failure
c. Combination of ventilatory and oxygenation failure

Disorders and Events

_____ 72. Lung tumors

_____ 73. Cerebral edema

_____ 74. Bronchial asthma

_____ 75. Near-drowning

_____ 76. Sleep apnea

_____ 77. Multiple sclerosis

_____ 78. Pneumonia

_____ 79. Chronic bronchitis

_____ 80. Atelectasis

_____ 81. Gross obesity

_____ 82. Poliomyelitis

_____ 83. Smoke inhalation

_____ 84. Myasthenia gravis

_____ 85. Meningitis

_____ 86. Pulmonary emphysema

_____ 87. Carbon monoxide poisoning

_____ 88. Opioid overdose

_____ 89. Guillain-Barré syndrome

_____ 90. Liquid aspiration

91. The patient has been successfully intubated by the physician, and the nurse and respiratory therapist are securing the tube in place. What does the nurse include in the documentation regarding the intubation procedure? *(Select all that apply.)*
    a. Presence of bilateral and equal breath sounds
    b. Level of the tube
    c. Changes in vital signs during the procedure
    d. Rate of the IV fluids
    e. Presence (or absence) of dysrhythmias
    f. Patient's speech quality during and after procedure
    g. Placement verification by end-tidal carbon dioxide levels

92. The nurse is assisting with an emergency intubation for the patient in severe respiratory distress. Although the physician is experienced, the procedure is difficult because the patient has severe kyphosis. At what point does the nurse intervene?
    a. First intubation attempt lasts longer than 15 seconds.
    b. First intubation attempt lasts longer than 30 seconds.
    c. Second intubation attempt is unsuccessful.
    d. Second intubation attempt causes the patient to struggle.

93. The patient in the ED required emergency intubation for status asthmaticus. Immediately after the insertion of an ET tube, how does the nurse and/or physician verify correct placement?
    a. Observe for chest excursion.
    b. Listen for expired air from the ET tube.
    c. Auscultate for bilateral breath sounds.
    d. Wait for the results of the chest x-ray.

94. The nurse is caring for several patients on the medical-surgical unit who are experiencing acute respiratory problems. Which conditions may eventually require a patient to be intubated? *(Select all that apply.)*
    a. Trouble maintaining a patent airway because of mucosal swelling
    b. History of congestive heart failure and demonstrating orthopnea
    c. Copious secretions and lacking muscular strength to cough
    d. Pulse oximetry of 93% with a high-flow oxygen face mask
    e. Increasing fatigue because of the work of breathing

95. The nurse hears in report that the patient with ARDS has been intubated for 6 days and has progressive hypoxemia that responds poorly to high levels of oxygen. This patient is in which phase of ARDS case management?
    a. Phase 1
    b. Phase 2
    c. Phase 3
    d. Phase 4

96. The postoperative patient reports sudden onset of shortness of breath and pleuritic chest pain. Assessment findings include diaphoresis, hypotension, crackles in the left lower lobe, and pulse oximetry of 85%. What does the nurse suspect this patient has?
    a. Atelectasis
    b. Pneumothorax
    c. Pulmonary embolism
    d. Flail chest

97. The nurse hears in shift report that the patient has been agitated and pulling at the ET. Restraints have recently been ordered and placed, but the patient continues to move his head and chew at the tube. What does the nurse do to ensure proper placement of the ET tube?
    a. Suction the patient frequently through the oral airway.
    b. Talk to the patient and tell him to calm down.
    c. Mark the tube where it touches the patient's teeth.
    d. Auscultate for breath sounds every 4 hours.

98. The nurse is caring for the patient on a mechanical ventilator. What does the nurse monitor to assess for the most likely cardiac problem associated with this therapy?
    a. Check blood pressure.
    b. Check for ventricular arrythmias.
    c. Take an apical pulse before giving medications.
    d. Ask the patient about chest pain.

Matching. Match the parts of an endotracheal tube (ET) with their descriptions.

Parts of ET
a. Shaft
b. Cuff
c. Pilot balloon
d. Adapter

Descriptions

_____ 99. Device to provide a seal between the trachea and tube

_____ 100. Device to allow attachment of ET tube to ventilation source

_____ 101. Hollow tube extending from naso-oral cavity to just above the carina

_____ 102. Access site for inserting air into the cuff

103. The patient in the critical care unit requires an emergency ET intubation. The nurse immediately obtains and prepares which supplies to perform this procedure? *(Select all that apply.)*
    a. Tracheostomy tube or kit
    b. Resuscitation Ambu bag
    c. Source for 100% oxygen
    d. Suction equipment
    e. Insertion equipment (i.e., larnygoscope)
    f. Oral airway
    g. Bronchodilator inhaler

104. The patient on a ventilator is biting and chewing at the ET tube. Which nursing intervention is used for ET management?
    a. Reassure the patient that everything is okay.
    b. Administer a paralyzing agent.
    c. Insert an oral airway.
    d. Frequently suction the mouth.

105. The nurse is performing a check of the ventilator equipment. What is included during the equipment check?
    a. Drain the condensed moisture back into the humidifier.
    b. Empty the humidifier and the drainage tubing.
    c. Note the prescribed and actual settings.
    d. Turn off the alarms during the system check.

106. The nursing student is assisting in the care of the critically ill patient on a ventilator. Which action by the student nurse requires intervention by the supervising nurse?
    a. Deflates the cuff on the ET tube to check placement.
    b. Applies soft wrist restraints as ordered.
    c. Suctions the patient for 10 seconds at a time.
    d. Maintains the correct placement of the ET tube.

107. The patient has a history of chronic obstructive pulmonary disease (COPD) and had to be intubated for respiratory failure. The patient is currently on a mechanical ventilator. The nurse obtains an order for which type of dietary therapy for this patient?
    a. High-fat nutritional supplement
    b. High-protein nutritional supplement
    c. High-carbohydrate nutritional supplement
    d. High-calorie nutritional supplement

108. The nursing student is assisting in the care of the patient on a mechanical ventilator. Which action by the student contributes to the prevention of ventilator-assisted pneumonia?
    a. Suctions the patient frequently
    b. Performs oral care every 2 hours
    c. Encourages visitors to wear a mask
    d. Obtains a sputum specimen for culture

109. The nurse is caring for the patient on a mechanical ventilator. During the shift, the nurse hears the patient talking to himself. What does the nurse do next?
    a. See if the patient has a change of mental status.
    b. Check the inflation of the pilot balloon.
    c. Assess the pulse oximetry for saturation level.
    d. Evaluate the patient's readiness to be weaned.

110. The nurse notices that the patient has a gradual increase in peak inspiratory pressure over the last several days. What is the best nursing intervention for this patient?
    a. Assess for a reason such as ARDS or pneumonia.
    b. Continue to increase peak airway pressure as needed.
    c. Change to another mode such as IMV.
    d. Make arrangements for permanent ventilatory support.

111. The patient is intubated and has mechanical ventilation with positive end-expiratory pressure (PEEP). Because this patient is at risk for a tension pneumothorax, what is the nurse's priority action?
    a. Assess lung sounds every 30 to 60 minutes.
    b. Obtain an order for an arterial blood gas.
    c. Have chest tube equipment on standby.
    d. Direct the unlicensed assistive personnel to turn the patient every 2 hours.

112. The nurse is caring for the patient on a mechanical ventilator. Which assessments does the nurse perform for this patient? *(Select all that apply.)*
    a. Observe the patient's mouth around the tube for pressure ulcers.
    b. Auscultate the lungs for crackles, wheezes, equal breath sounds, and decreased or absent breath sounds.
    c. Assess the placement of the endotracheal tube.
    d. Check at least every 24 hours to be sure the ventilator settings are as prescribed.
    e. Check to be sure alarms are set.
    f. Ensure the endotracheal cuff is deflated.
    g. Observe the patient's need for tracheal, oral, or nasal suctioning every 2 hours.

Matching. *Match the characteristics of ventilators with their types. Some characteristics may apply to more than one type of ventilator. Indicate all types to which a characteristic applies.*

Ventilator Types
a. Pressure-cycled
b. Time-cycled
c. Volume-cycled

Ventilator Characteristics

_____ 113. Positive-pressure ventilator

_____ 114. Administers consistent volume and gas (oxygen concentration) regardless of the patient's lung status until preset tidal volume is reached

_____ 115. Preset inspiration and expiration rate with possible variation of tidal volume and pressure

_____ 116. Pushes air into the lungs until preset airway pressure is reached

_____ 117. Needs an artificial airway such as a tracheostomy or endotracheal tube

_____ 118. Tidal volumes and inspiratory time are variable

Matching. *Match the ventilator terms and settings with their descriptions.*

Terms and Settings

a. Assist-control mode (AC)
b. Rate or breaths/minute (BPM)
c. Continuous positive airway pressure (CPAP)
d. Bi-level positive airway pressure (BiPAP)
e. Fraction of inspired oxygen (Fio_2)
f. Peak airway inspiratory pressure (PIP)
g. Positive end-expiratory pressure (PEEP)
h. Tidal volume (V_T)
i. Synchronized intermittent mandatory ventilation (SIMV)
j. Microprocessor ventilator

Descriptions

_____ 119. Pressure needed to deliver a set tidal volume

_____ 120. Positive pressure throughout the entire respiratory cycle to prevent alveolar collapse

_____ 121. Number of ventilations delivered per minute

_____ 122. Volume of air the patient receives with each breath

_____ 123. Set tidal volume and set rate delivered to the patient

_____ 124. Positive pressure exerted during expiration to keep lungs partially inflated

_____ 125. Oxygen concentration delivered to the patient

_____ 126. Noninvasive pressure support ventilation by nasal mask or face mask

_____ 127. Ventilator delivers mandatory breaths at a preset rate and allows the patient to breathe spontaneously between set rate

_____ 128. A computer monitors ventilatory functions, alarms, and patient condition

129. The physician instructs the nurse to watch for and report signs and symptoms of improvement so the patient can be weaned from the ventilator. Which assessment finding indicates the patient is ready to be weaned?
    a. Indications that respiratory infection is resolving
    b. Showing signs of becoming ventilator-dependent
    c. Maintaining blood gases within normal limits
    d. Patient insisting that the ventilator is not necessary anymore

130. The older adult patient arrives in the ED after falling off a roof. The nurse observes "sucking inward" of the loose chest area during inspiration and a "puffing out" of the same area during expiration. ABG results show severe hypoxemia and hypercarbia. Which procedure does the nurse prepare for?
    a. Chest tube insertion
    b. Endotracheal intubation
    c. Needle thoracotomy
    d. Tracheostomy

131. The charge nurse in the intensive care unit is reviewing patient census and caseload to identify staffing needs and potential transfers. Which patient might take the longest time to wean from a ventilator?
    a. 54-year-old man with metastatic colon cancer who has been intubated for 6 days
    b. 32-year-old woman recovering from a general anesthetic following a tubal ligation
    c. 25-year-old man intubated for 28 hours after an anaphylactic reaction
    d. 49-year-old man with a gunshot wound to the chest who was intubated for 8 hours

132. The patient is being extubated and the nurse has emergency equipment at the bedside. Which intervention is implemented during extubation?
    a. Ensure that the cuff is inflated at all times.
    b. Remove the tube during expiration.
    c. Instruct the patient to pant while the tube is removed.
    d. Instruct the patient to cough after tube is removed.

133. The nurse is caring for the patient who was recently extubated. What is an expected assessment finding for this patient?
    a. Stridor
    b. Dyspnea
    c. Restlessness
    d. Hoarseness

134. Place the steps for extubating the patient in the correct order using the numbers 1 through 8.
    _____ a. Hyperoxygenate the patient.
    _____ b. Rapidly deflate the cuff of the ET tube.
    _____ c. Immediately instruct the patient to cough.
    _____ d. Thoroughly suction both the ET tube and the oral cavity.
    _____ e. Give oxygen by facemask or nasal cannula.
    _____ f. Explain the procedure.
    _____ g. Set up oxygen; bring emergency reintubation equipment.
    _____ h. Remove the tube at peak inspiration.

135. Which patients on mechanical ventilators are at high risk for barotraumas? (Select all that apply.)
    a. Patient with ARDS
    b. Patient with underlying chronic airflow limitation
    c. Patient on BiPAP
    d. Patient on PEEP
    e. Patient on SIMV

136. The nurse is caring for the patient who has just been extubated. What interventions does the nurse use in caring for this patient? (Select all that apply.)
    a. Monitor vital signs every 30 minutes at first.
    b. Assess the ventilatory pattern for manifestations of respiratory distress.
    c. Place the patient in a recumbent position.
    d. Instruct the patient to take deep breaths every half hour.
    e. Encourage use an incentive spirometer every 2 hours.
    f. Advise the patient to limit speaking right after extubation.

137. The nurse is assessing the patient who was extubated several hours ago. Which patient finding warrants notification of the Rapid Response Team?
    a. Hoarseness
    b. Report of sore throat
    c. Inability to expectorate secretions
    d. 90% saturation on room air

138. The patient is admitted to the trauma unit following a front-end motor vehicle collision. The patient is currently asymptomatic, but the physician advises the nurse that the patient has a high risk for pulmonary contusion. What does the nurse carefully monitor for?
    a. Tracheal deviation
    b. Paradoxical chest movements
    c. Progressive chest pain
    d. Decreased breath sounds

139. Which finding might delay weaning the patient from mechanical ventilation support?
    a. Hematocrit = 42%
    b. Arterial Po_2 = 70 mm Hg on a 40% Fio_2
    c. Apical heart rate = 72 beats per minute
    d. Oral temperature = 101° F

140. The patient in respiratory failure is diagnosed with a flail chest. After the patient is intubated, which treatment does the nurse expect to be implemented?
    a. PEEP
    b. SIMV
    c. BiPap
    d. PIP

141. The patient in a motor vehicle accident was unrestrained and appears to have hit the front dashboard. The patient has severe respiratory distress, inspiratory stridor, and extensive subcutaneous emphysema. The ED physician identifies tracheobronchial trauma. Which procedure does the nurse immediately prepare for?
    a. Cricothyroidotomy
    b. Chest tube insertion
    c. Cardiopulmonary resuscitation
    d. Pericardiocentesis

CASE STUDY: CHEST TRAUMA AND ADULT RESPIRATORY DISTRESS SYNDROME (ARDS)

Use a separate sheet of paper to answer the questions in this Case Study. Answer guidelines for this Case Study are available on your Evolve website at http://evolve. elsevier.com/Iggy/ in the "Prepare for Class" folder.

A 36-year-old woman is brought to the hospital following a head-on car accident. She was unrestrained and sustained a blunt injury to the chest from hitting the steering wheel. Initially, she is asymptomatic. Initial orders include a stat chest x-ray, arterial blood gases, and oxygen at 4 L/minute via Venturi mask.

1. What other assessments should be made when she arrives in the ED?

2. Gradually over the next 24 hours, she develops difficulty breathing, hypoxemia, and secretions increase. The nurse notifies the physician who orders an arterial blood gas and a chest x-ray. The chest x-ray obtained in the ED showed no abnormalities; however, the repeat x-ray now shows a hazy opacity in the lobes and the physician makes a diagnosis of pulmonary contusion. What physical assessments will accompany this diagnosis?

3. Arterial blood gas results show: Pao_2 68 mm Hg, $Paco_2$ 32 mm Hg, and pH 7.53. What do these values suggest?

4. What interventions should be implemented based on the laboratory results?

5. The patient temporarily responds to the high-flow oxygen therapy, but later the nurse notes that the patient demonstrates hyperpnea, grunting respiration, cyanosis, pallor, and intercostal and substernal retractions, with a change in mental status. The nurse suspects ARDS and calls the physician to obtain an order for which primary laboratory study used to establish this diagnosis?

6. Discuss the pathophysiology of ARDS.

7. The patient is intubated for respiratory failure. Describe how the nurse would secure the ET in place.

8. The patient is placed on a respirator with PEEP. Why is PEEP necessary?

9. Explain the rationale for the use of corticosteroids, antibiotics, and colloids in the management of the patient with ARDS.

35 CHAPTER

Assessment of the Cardiovascular System

STUDY/REVIEW QUESTIONS

Matching. *Match each structure of the heart with its description.*

Structures of the Heart

a. Aortic valve
b. Atria
c. Chordae tendineae
d. Coronary arteries
e. Mitral valve
f. Pulmonic valve
g. Septum
h. Tricuspid valve
i. Ventricle

Descriptions

_____ 1. Muscular wall dividing the heart into halves

_____ 2. Upper heart chamber

_____ 3. Lower heart chamber

_____ 4. Valve between right atrium and ventricle

_____ 5. Valve between right ventricle and pulmonary artery

_____ 6. Valve between left atrium and ventricle, bicuspid value

_____ 7. Filaments that secure the AV valve leaflets

_____ 8. Vessels that supply the heart with oxygenated blood

_____ 9. Valve from the left ventricle to the aorta

10. What are the three pacemaker sites in the heart? Name the pacer rate for each site.

     a. _____

     b. _____

     c. _____

Matching. Match each variable that affects cardiac output with its description.

Cardiac Output Variables
a. Afterload
b. Contractility
c. Heart rate
d. Impedance
e. Preload

Descriptions

_____ 11. Number of times ventricles contract per minute

_____ 12. Degree of myocardial fiber stretch at end of diastole and just before heart contracts

_____ 13. Amount of pressure or resistance that the ventricles must overcome to eject blood through the semilunar valves and into the peripheral blood vessels

_____ 14. Pressure that ventricle must overcome to open aortic valve

_____ 15. Force of contraction independent of preload

16. Which are risk factors for cardiovascular disease (CVD) in women? *(Select all that apply.)*
    a. Waist and abdominal obesity
    b. Excess fat in the buttocks, hips, and thighs
    c. Postmenopausal
    d. Diabetes mellitus
    e. Asian ethnicity

17. The nurse is assessing the patient's nicotine dependency. Which questions does the nurse ask for an accurate assessment? *(Select all that apply.)*
    a. "How soon after you wake up in the morning do you smoke?"
    b. "What kind of cigarettes do you smoke?"
    c. "Do you inhale deeply when you smoke?"
    d. "Do you find it difficult not to smoke in places where smoking is prohibited?"
    e. "Do you smoke when you are ill?"
    f. "What happened the last time you tried to quit smoking?"

18. The nurse is talking to the patient who has been trying to quit smoking. Which statement by the patient indicates an understanding of cigarette usage as it relates to reducing cardiovascular risks?
    a. "I need to be completely cigarette-free for at least 3 years."
    b. "I don't smoke as much as I used to; I'm down to one pack a day."
    c. "I started smoking a while ago, but I'll quit in a couple of years."
    d. "I only smoke to relax, when I drink, or when I go out with friends."

19. Which repetitive patient behavior causes the nurse to plan interventions to reduce psychological factors that increase risk for CVD?
    a. Withdrawal and quietness
    b. Inattentiveness and easy distraction
    c. Defensiveness and hostility
    d. Excessive cheerfulness and energy

20. The nurse is providing health teaching for the patient at risk for heart disease. Which factor is the most modifiable, controllable risk factor?
    a. Obesity
    b. Diabetes mellitus
    c. Ethnic background
    d. Family history of cardiovascular disease

21. The nurse is giving a community presentation about heart disease in women. What information does the nurse include in the presentation? *(Select all that apply.)*
    a. Dyspnea on exertion may be the first and only symptom of heart failure.
    b. Symptoms are subtle or atypical.
    c. Pain is often relieved by rest.
    d. Having waist and abdominal obesity is a higher risk factor than having fat in buttocks and thighs.
    e. Pain always responds to nitroglycerin.
    f. Common symptoms include back pain, indigestion, nausea, vomiting, and anorexia.

22. Which blood pressure readings require further prehypertensive assessment? *(Select all that apply.)*
    a. 125 mm Hg systolic
    b. 139 mm Hg systolic
    c. 115 mm Hg systolic
    d. 60 mm Hg diastolic
    e. 100 mm Hg diastolic

23. The nurse working in the public health department is reviewing data for populations at risk for CVD. Which group has the greatest need for intervention to reduce CVD risk?
    a. Government employees who make approximately $40,000 a year
    b. Part-time fast food workers who make approximately $9,000 a year
    c. Hospital-employed nurses who make approximately $52,000 a year
    d. Chain retail employees who make approximately $18,000 a year

True or False? *Read the statements about the various components of blood pressure and write T for true or F for false in the blanks provided. For statements that are false, rewrite the statement to make it true.*

_____ 24. Systolic blood pressure is the lowest pressure during the relaxation phase of the cardiac cycle.

_____ 25. Diastolic blood pressure is the highest pressure during contraction of the ventricles.

_____ 26. Diastolic blood pressure is primarily determined by the amount of peripheral vasoconstriction.

_____ 27. Pulse pressure is the difference between the systolic and diastolic pressures.

_____ 28. Fluid moves from the vascular system into the interstitial spaces when the capillary endothelium is impaired.

_____ 29. S_1 results from tricuspid and mitral valve closure.

_____ 30. The right ventricle of the heart generates the greatest amount of blood pressure.

_____ 31. To maintain adequate blood flow through the coronary arteries, diastolic blood pressure must be at least 60 mm Hg.

32. Place the steps for checking the patient for postural hypotension in the correct order, using the numbers 1 through 5.

    _____ a. Patient changes position to sitting or standing.

    _____ b. Measure the blood pressure when the patient is supine.

    _____ c. Have the patient remain supine for at least 3 minutes.

    _____ d. Observe and record any signs or symptoms of dizziness.

    _____ e. Wait for at least 1 minute before auscultating blood pressure and counting the radial pulse.

33. While taking the patient's blood pressure, the nurse observes a weak pulse that alternates with a strong pulse despite a regular heart rhythm. What does the nurse do to exclude a false reading?
    a. Repeat the blood pressure on the other arm with a different cuff.
    b. Palpate the radial or brachial artery.
    c. Repeat the blood pressure and ask the patient to hold his or her breath.
    d. Place the patient on a cardiac monitor.

34. In the hypovolemic patient, stretch receptors in the blood vessels sense a reduced volume or pressure and send fewer impulses to the central nervous system. As a result, which sign/symptoms does the nurse expect to observe in the patient?
    a. Reddish mottling to skin and a blood pressure elevation
    b. Cool, pale skin and tachycardia
    c. Warm, flushed skin with low blood pressure
    d. Pale, pink skin with bradycardia

35. What term describes the difference between systolic and diastolic values, which is an indirect measure of cardiac output?
    a. Paradoxical blood pressure
    b. Pulse pressure
    c. Ankle-brachial index
    d. Normal blood pressure

36. The nurse is performing a dietary assessment on the 45-year-old business executive at risk for CVD. Which assessment method used by the nurse is the most reliable and accurate?
    a. Ask the patient to identify foods he or she eats that contain sodium, sugar, cholesterol, fiber, and fat.
    b. Ask the patient's spouse, who does the cooking and shopping, to identify the types of foods that are consumed.
    c. Ask the patient how cultural beliefs and economic status influences the choice of food items.
    d. Ask the patient to recall the intake of food, fluids, and alcohol during a typical 24-hour period.

37. Based on the physiologic force that propels blood forward in the veins, which patient has the greatest risk for venous stasis?
    a. Older adult patient with hypertension who rides a bicycle daily
    b. Middle-aged construction worker taking Coumadin
    c. Bedridden patient in the end stage of Alzheimer's disease
    d. Teenage patient with a broken leg who sits and plays videogames

38. Which statement about the peripheral vascular system is true?
    a. Veins are equipped with valves that permit one-way flow of blood toward the heart.
    b. The velocity of blood flow depends on the diameter of the vessel lumen.
    c. Blood flow decreases and blood tends to clot as the viscosity decreases.
    d. The parasympathetic nervous system has the largest effect on blood flow to organs.

39. The patient comes to the clinic stating "my right foot turns a darkish red color when I sit too long, and when I put my foot up, it turns pale." Which conditions does the nurse suspect?
    a. Central cyanosis
    b. Peripheral cyanosis
    c. Arterial insufficiency
    d. Venous insufficiency

40. Which exercise regimen for the older adult meets the recommended guidelines for physical fitness to promote heart health?
    a. 6-hour bike ride every Saturday
    b. Golfing for 4 hours two times a week
    c. Running for 15 minutes three times a week
    d. Brisk walk 30 minutes every day

41. Calculate the number of pack-years for the patient who has smoked half a pack of cigarettes per day for 2 years. _____

42. In assessing the patient who has come to the clinic for a physical exam, the nurse sees that the patient has pallor. What is this finding most indicative of?
    a. Anemia
    b. Thrombophlebitis
    c. Heart disease
    d. Stroke

43. Emergency personnel discovered the patient lying outside in the cool evening air for an unknown length of time. The patient is in a hypothermic state and the metabolic needs of the tissues are decreased. What other assessment finding does the nurse expect to see?
    a. Blood pressure and heart rate lower than normal
    b. Heart rate and respiratory rate higher than normal
    c. Normal vital signs due to compensatory mechanisms
    d. Gradually improved vital signs with enteral nutrition

44. The advanced practice nurse is assessing the vascular status of the patient's lower extremities using the ankle-brachial index. What is the correct technique for this assessment method?
    a. A blood pressure cuff is applied to the lower extremities and the systolic pressure is measured by Doppler ultrasound at both the dorsalis pedis and posterior tibial pulses.
    b. The dorsalis pedis and posterior tibial pulses are manually palpated and compared bilaterally for strength and equality and compared to the standard index.
    c. A blood pressure cuff is applied to the lower extremities to observe for an exaggerated decrease in systolic pressure by more than 10 mm Hg during inspiration.
    d. Measure blood pressure on the legs when the patient is supine; then have the patient stand for several minutes and repeat blood pressure measurement in the arms.

45. What is the correct technique for assessing the patient with arterial insufficiency in the right lower leg?
    a. Use the Doppler to find the dorsalis pedis and posterior tibial pulses on the right leg.
    b. Palpate the peripheral arteries in a head-to-toe approach with a side-to-side comparison.
    c. Check all the pulse points in the right leg in dependent and supine positions.
    d. Palpate the major arteries, such as the radial and femoral, and observe for pallor.

46. The nurse is performing a cardiac assessment on the older adult. What is a common assessment finding for this patient?
    a. S_4 heart sound
    b. Leg edema
    c. Pericardial friction rubs
    d. Change in point of maximum impulse location

47. The patient's chart notes that the examiner has heard S_1 and S_2 on auscultation of the heart. What does this documentation refer to?
    a. First and second heart sounds
    b. Pericardial friction rub
    c. Murmur
    d. Gallop

48. The nurse is taking report on the patient who will be transferred from the cardiac intensive care unit to the general medical-surgical unit. The reporting nurse states that S_4 is heard on auscultation of the heart. This indicates that the patient has which condition?
    a. Heart murmur
    b. Pericardial friction rub
    c. Ventricular hypertrophy
    d. Normal heart sounds

49. Which patient has an abnormal heart sound?
    a. S_1 in a 45-year-old patient
    b. S_2 in a 30-year-old patient
    c. S_3 in a 15-year-old patient
    d. S_3 in a 54-year-old patient

50. The nurse is caring for the patient at risk for heart problems. What are normal findings for the cardiovascular assessment of this patient? *(Select all that apply.)*
   a. Presence of a thrill
   b. Splitting of S$_2$; decreases with expiration
   c. Jugular venous distention to level of the mandible
   d. Point of maximal impulse (PMI) in fifth intercostal space at midclavicular line
   e. Paradoxical chest movement with inspiration and expiration

51. The nurse practitioner reads in the patient's chart that a carotid bruit was heard during the last two annual checkups. Today on auscultation, the bruit is not present. How does the nurse practitioner evaluate this data?
   a. The problem has resolved spontaneously.
   b. There may have been an anomaly in previous findings.
   c. The occlusion of the vessel may have progressed past 90%.
   d. The antiplatelet therapy is working.

52. In assessing the patient, the nurse finds that the PMI appears in more than one intercostal space, and has shifted lateral to the midclavicular line. How does the nurse interpret this data?
   a. Left ventricular hypertrophy
   b. Superior vena cava obstruction
   c. Pulmonary hypertension
   d. Constrictive pericarditis

53. In the illustration below, locate and describe the sites for auscultation of the heart sounds and pulse points listed.
   a. Aortic area
   b. Pulmonic area
   c. Erb's point
   d. Right ventricular area
   e. Epigastric area
   f. Mitral area
   g. Tricuspid area

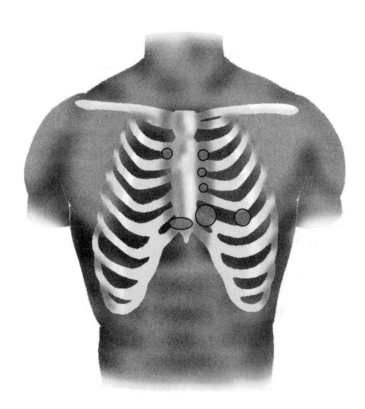

True or False? *Read the following statements about performing a pericardium assessment and write T for true or F for false in the blanks provided. If the statement is false, correct the statement to make it true.*

_____ 54.   The assessment begins with auscultation.

_____ 55.   The patient is in a supine position with the head of bed elevated for comfort and ease of breathing.

_____ 56.   Inspect for PMI or pulsations at the apex of the heart.

_____ 57.   Murmurs and rubs are detected by palpation.

_____ 58.   Inspect the chest from the side, at a right angle, and downward over areas of the precordium where vibrations are visible.

_____ 59.   The first heart sound is heard best at the base of the heart.

_____ 60.   When auscultating, use the diaphragm of the stethoscope to listen for low-frequency sounds.

_____ 61.   The skill of accurately auscultating sounds requires a good stethoscope and lots of practice.

Matching. *Match each source of chest pain with its assessment findings. Each source of chest pain may be used more than once.*

Sources of Chest Pain
a.   Angina
b.   Myocardial infarction
c.   Pericarditis
d.   Esophageal-gastric
e.   Anxiety
f.   Pleuropulmonary

Assessment Findings

_____ 62.   Sudden onset

_____ 63.   Moderate ache, worse on inspiration

_____ 64.   Substernal, may spread to shoulders or abdomen

_____ 65.   Intermittent, relieved with sitting upright

_____ 66.   Substernal, may spread across chest, back, arms

_____ 67.   Usually lasts less than 15 minutes

_____ 68.   Continuous until underlying condition is treated

_____ 69.   Intense, stabbing, vice-like pain

_____ 70.   Dull ache to sharp stabbing, may have numbness of fingers

_____ 71.   Sudden onset, often in early morning

_____ 72.   May be in response to stress

_____ 73.   Sharp stabbing, moderate to severe

_____ 74.   Squeezing, heartburn, variable in severity

75. The nurse working in a women's health clinic is reviewing the risk factors for several patients for stroke and myocardial infarction (MI). Which patient has the highest risk for MI?
    a. 49-year-old on estrogen replacement therapy
    b. 40-year-old taking oral contraceptives who smokes
    c. 23-year-old with diabetes that is currently not well-controlled
    d. 60-year-old with well-controlled hypertension

76. The patient comes to the emergency department (ED) reporting chest pain. In evaluating the patient's pain, which questions does the nurse ask the patient? *(Select all that apply.)*
    a. "How long does the pain last and how often does it occur?"
    b. "How do you feel about the pain?"
    c. "Is the pain different from any other episodes of pain you've had?"
    d. "What activities were you doing when the pain first occurred?"
    e. "Where is the chest pain? What does it feel like?"
    f. "Have you had other signs and symptoms that occur at the same time?"
    g. "How can we help you to alleviate the pain?"

77. The nurse is taking a history on the patient with congestive heart failure. Which patient behavior indicates the most severe case of orthopnea?
    a. Becoming short of breath after minor exertion
    b. Routinely sleeping at night in a recliner chair
    c. Feeling of fatigue and weariness after activity
    d. Waking at night with a feeling of breathlessness

78. The 65-year-old patient comes to the clinic reporting fatigue and tiredness. The patient would like to start an exercise program, but thinks "anemia might be causing the fatigue." What is the nurse's first action?
    a. Advise the patient to start out slowly and gradually build strength and endurance.
    b. Obtain an order for a complete blood count and nutritional profile.
    c. Assess the onset, duration, and circumstances associated with the fatigue and tiredness.
    d. Perform a physical assessment to include testing of muscle strength and tone.

79. The young patient reports having frequent episodes of palpitations but denies having chest pain. Which follow-up question does the nurse ask to assess the patient's symptom of palpitations?
    a. "Have you noticed a worsening of shortness of breath when you are lying flat?"
    b. "Do your shoes feel unusually tight, or are your rings tighter than usual?"
    c. "Do you feel dizzy or have you lost consciousness with the palpitations?"
    d. "Does anyone in your family have a history of palpitations?"

True or False? *Read each statement and write T for true or F for false in the blanks provided.*

_____ 80. Dyspnea can occur with both cardiac disease and pulmonary disease.

_____ 81. Dyspnea that is associated with activity, such as climbing stairs, is referred to as *dyspnea on exertion.*

_____ 82. Paroxysmal nocturnal dyspnea occurs when the patient has been sitting for a prolonged period of time.

_____ 83. Severity of orthopnea is measured by the length of time it takes to recover after exertion.

_____ 84. Dyspnea on exertion may be the only sign of early heart failure in women.

85. The nurse performing a physical assessment on the patient with a history of CVD observes that the patient has ascites, jaundice, and anasarca. How does the nurse interpret these findings?
    a. Late signs of severe right-sided heart failure
    b. Early signs of mild right-sided heart failure
    c. Late signs of mild left-sided heart failure
    d. Early signs of left and right-sided heart failure

86. The nurse is performing an assessment on the patient brought in by emergency personnel. The nurse immediately observes that the patient has spontaneous respirations and the skin is cool, pale, and moist. What is the priority nursing diagnosis?
    a. Risk for Imbalanced Body Temperature
    b. Ineffective Tissue Perfusion
    c. Impaired Skin Integrity
    d. Risk for Peripheral Neurovascular Dysfunction

87. The nurse is caring for the patient at risk for MI. For what primary reason does the nurse plan interventions to prevent anxiety or overexertion?
    a. An increase in heart rate increases myocardial oxygen demand.
    b. A release of epinephrine and norepinephrine causes MI.
    c. An increase in activity or emotion effects preload and afterload.
    d. Cardiac output is decreased by anxiety or physical stress.

88. The nurse is caring for the patient with a nursing diagnosis of Decreased Cardiac Output. Which situation may result in decreased myocardial contractility that will further lower cardiac output?
    a. Administration of a positive inotropic medication
    b. Hyperventilation to correct respiratory acidosis
    c. Frequent endotracheal suctioning that results in hypoxemia
    d. Administration of IV fluids to correct underlying hypovolemia

89. The patient reports severe cramping in the legs while attempting to walk for exercise. The physician diagnoses the patient with intermittent claudication. What does the nurse advise the patient to do?
    a. Elevate the legs on a pillow.
    b. Buy and wear supportive shoes.
    c. Massage the legs before walking.
    d. Rest the legs in a dependent position.

90. The patient entering the cardiac rehabilitation unit seems optimistic and at times unexpectedly cheerful and upbeat. Which statement by the patient causes the nurse to suspect a maladaptive use of denial in the patient?
    a. "I am sick and tired of talking about these dietary restrictions. Could we talk about it tomorrow?"
    b. "Oh, I don't really need that medication information. I'm sure that I'll soon be able to get by without it."
    c. "This whole episode of heart problems has been an eye-opener for me, but I really can't wait to get out of here."
    d. "That doctor is really driving me crazy with all his instructions. Could you put all that information away in my suitcase?"

91. The nurse taking a medical history of the patient makes a special notation to follow up on valvular abnormalities of the heart. Which recurrent condition in the patient's history causes the nurse to make this notation?
    a. Streptococcal infections of the throat
    b. Staphylococcal infections of the skin
    c. Vaginal yeast infections
    d. Fungal infections of the feet or inner thighs

Matching. *Match each serum lipid value with the serum lipid laboratory test used to determine the value in an adult.*

Name of Lipid Test

a. Total cholesterol
b. Triglycerides
c. Plasma high-density lipoproteins (HDLs)
d. Plasma low-density lipoproteins (LDLs)
e. HDL:LDL ratio

Normal Laboratory Value

_____ 92. Less than 70 mg/dL in high-risk cardiovascular patients, less than 100 mg/dL in patients with moderate risk factors, and less than 130 mg/dL in patients with no risk factors

_____ 93. Less than 150 mg/dL

_____ 94. 122 to 200 mg/dL; older adults is 144 to 280 mg/dL

_____ 95. 3:1

_____ 96. greater than 45 mg/dL

97. What is the most significant laboratory cardiac marker in the patient who has had an MI?
    a. Presence of troponin T and I
    b. Elevation of myoglobin levels
    c. Creatine kinase levels
    d. Elevation of the white count

98. The patient in the ED with chest pain has a possible MI. Which laboratory test is done to determine this diagnosis?
    a. Troponin T and I
    b. Serum potassium
    c. Homocysteine
    d. Highly sensitive C-reactive protein

99. Which laboratory tests are used to predict the patient's risk for coronary artery disease (CAD)? *(Select all that apply.)*
    a. Cholesterol level
    b. Triglyceride level
    c. Prothrombin time
    d. Low-density lipoprotein level
    e. Albumin level

100. The patient is undergoing diagnostic testing for reports of chest pain. Which test is done to determine the location and extent of CAD?
    a. Electrocardiogram (ECG)
    b. Echocardiogram
    c. Cardiac catheterization
    d. Chest x-ray

101. Microalbuminuria has been shown to be a clear marker of widespread endothelial dysfunction in cardiovascular disease. Which conditions should prompt patients to be tested annually for microalbuminuria? *(Select all that apply.)*
    a. Hypertension
    b. Metabolic syndrome
    c. Smoker
    d. Diabetes mellitus
    e. Use of anticoagulant therapy

102. The patient is being discharged with a prescription for warfarin (Coumadin). Which test does the nurse instruct the patient to routinely have done for follow-up monitoring?
    a. Prothrombin time (PT) and International Normalized Ratio (INR)
    b. Partial thromboplastin time (PTT)
    c. Complete blood count and platelet count
    d. Sodium and potassium levels

103. What is the significance of a sodium level of 130 mEq/L for the patient with heart failure?
    a. Increased risk for ventricular dysrhythmias
    b. Dilutional hyponatremia and fluid retention
    c. Potential for electrical instability of the heart
    d. Slowed conduction of impulse through the heart

104. Which test is performed to determine valve disease of the mitral valve, left atrium, or aortic arch?
    a. Transesophageal echocardiogram
    b. ECG
    c. Myocardial nuclear perfusion imaging (MNPI)
    d. Phonocardiography

105. The patient is scheduled to have an exercise electrocardiography test. What instruction does the nurse provide to the patient before the procedure takes place?
    a. Have nothing to eat or drink after midnight.
    b. Avoid smoking or drinking alcohol for at least 2 weeks before the test.
    c. Wear comfortable, loose clothing and rubber-soled, supportive shoes.
    d. Someone must drive you home because of possible sedative effects of the medications.

106. The nurse is monitoring the patient's blood pressure and ECG during a stress test. Which parameter indicates the patient should stop exercising?
    a. Increase in heart rate
    b. Increase in blood pressure
    c. ECG showing the PQRS complex
    d. ECG showing ST-segment depression

True or False? *Read each statement and write T for true or F for false in the blanks provided. If the statement is false, correct it to make it true.*

_____ 107. There is no follow-up care for patients who undergo echocardiograms.

_____ 108. Echocardiograms require an informed consent.

_____ 109. MNPI is a radioactive technique used to view cardiovascular abnormalities.

_____ 110. Technetium scanning is effective for diagnosing old infarctions.

_____ 111. After an MNPI, the patient is placed in isolation because of radioactive isotopes.

_____ 112. Thallium imaging can be done with the patient at rest or during exercise.

_____ 113. For patients who cannot perform a treadmill stress test, vasodilating drugs can simulate the effects of exercise.

_____ 114. Patients should be aware that thallium can cause flushing, headache, dyspnea, and chest tightness a few moments after the injection.

_____ 115. An echocardiogram is a risk-free, pain-free test that uses sound waves to assess cardiac structure and mobility, particularly that of the valves.

_____ 116. A PET scan takes 2 to 3 hours and a patient may be asked to use a treadmill.

_____ 117. During multigated blood pool scanning, several blood samples are taken for measurement of oxygen saturation.

_____ 118. Electronic beam computed tomography (EBCT) can look for calcifications within the arteries.

_____ 119. During a electrophysiologic study (EPS), programmed electrical stimulation of the heart is used to induce and evaluate lethal dysrhythmias and conduction abnormalities.

_____ 120. MRI is not useful in evaluating disorders of the cardiac system.

121. The patient will be receiving a pulmonary artery catheter. What position does the nurse place the patient in?
    a. Semi-Fowler's
    b. Side-lying
    c. Trendelenburg
    d. Sitting slightly hunched forward

122. The patient is being hemodynamically monitored via a pulmonary artery catheter. There is a right atrial pressure (RAP) reading of less than 3 cm H_2O. How does the nurse interpret this finding?
    a. Right-sided heart failure
    b. Left-sided heart failure
    c. Cardiac tamponade
    d. Hypovolemia

123. The patient's Svo_2 (mixed venous oxygen saturation) is 70%. What is the nurse's interpretation of this finding?
    a. Oxygen demand is balanced by the oxygen supply.
    b. Oxygen demand exceeds the available oxygen supply.
    c. Available oxygen supply exceeds the current oxygen demand.
    d. Venous oxygen saturation is equal to the arterial oxygen saturation.

124. What is the purpose of an angiogram?
    a. Determine the size, silhouette, and position of the heart
    b. Identify abnormal structures and calcifications of the heart by fluoroscopy
    c. Assess cardiovascular response to an increased workload
    d. Determine arterial obstruction, narrowing, or aneurysm in specific locations

125. What is included in postprocedural care of the patient after a cardiac catheterization? *(Select all that apply.)*
    a. Patient remains on bedrest for 12 to 24 hours.
    b. Patient is placed in a high Fowler's position.
    c. Dressing is assessed for bloody drainage or hematoma.
    d. Peripheral pulses in the affected extremity, as well as skin temperature and color, are monitored with every vital sign check.
    e. Patient is assessed for pain at the insertion site.
    f. Adequate oral and IV fluids are provided for hydration.
    g. Intake and output are monitored because the dye is an osmotic diuretic.
    h. Vital signs are monitored every hour for 24 hours.

126. Which assessment finding in the patient who has had a cardiac catheterization does the nurse report immediately to the physician?
    a. Pain at the catheter insertion site
    b. Catheterized extremity dusky with decreased peripheral pulses
    c. Small hematoma at the catheter insertion site
    d. Pulse pressure of 40 mm Hg with a slow, bounding pulse

127. The critical care nurse has just taken a reading of the patient's pulmonary artery wedge pressure (PAWP). The balloon remains in the wedge position after the reading. What does the nurse do next?
    a. Elevate the head of the bed to 45 degrees.
    b. Ask the patient to cough or change body position.
    c. Notify the physician immediately.
    d. Place the transducer at the level of the phlebostatic axis.

CASE STUDY: ASSESSMENT OF THE CARDIOVASCULAR SYSTEM

Use a separate sheet of paper to answer the questions in this Case Study. Answer guidelines for this Case Study are available on your Evolve website at http://evolve. elsevier.com/Iggy/ in the "Prepare for Class" folder.

The patient is a 72-year-old man who had an extensive left ventricular myocardial infarction (MI) at 36 years of age. At the time of his MI, he was overweight by 50 pounds and smoked two packs of unfiltered cigarettes per day. He had smoked for 20 years. Alcohol consumption was part of his ethnic background; it was customary for him to drink one or two beers per day and several mixed drinks per week. His father had also suffered an MI at the age of 48, and was a chain smoker. The patient slowly recovered from his MI, gave up smoking, and lost weight. His weight stabilized within 15 pounds of the upper limit of his ideal weight. His wife became an active participant in his recovery by changing her style of cooking and virtually eliminating saturated fats from their diets. He no longer drank beer, but he continued to consume an average of two mixed drinks per day. He began a moderate exercise program that included walking several miles at least three times a week. He has had stable angina for many years and has annual physical checkups and ECGs at the cardiologist's office. He took up the hobby of downhill skiing at the age of 66, with his cardiologist's approval. He is a retired accountant with a type A personality. Over the past 6 months, he has experienced infrequent periods of lightheadedness. He has "blacked out" on at least one occasion and was unable to remember any details of what happened. A second episode of loss of consciousness occurred on a clear, cold winter day while he was skiing. He revived spontaneously. The next day, he scheduled an appointment with his physician.

1. Which lifestyle changes decreased the patient's risk status after his MI? Which habits increased his risk status?

2. Compare and contrast the risk factors of CV disease for a 36-year-old man and a 72-year-old man.

3. The cardiologist performs an ECG and orders blood work drawn for serum lipids, troponins, AST, CK and CK-MB, LDH and isoenzymes, serum potassium, and C-reactive protein. What is the purpose for these tests?

4. The ECG and blood work are inconclusive, but the physician is concerned about the patient's symptoms. Discuss why there is reason for concern.

5. The patient is scheduled for an inpatient cardiac catheterization. The physician tells him that, based on the findings at the time of the catheterization, he may go ahead and perform an angioplasty. Develop a teaching-learning plan for this patient.

6. What are postprocedural nursing responsibilities?

7. What are home instructions and risk factor modifications the nurse should relay to the patient before discharge?

Continued

CASE STUDY: ASSESSMENT OF THE CARDIOVASCULAR SYSTEM *(Cont'd)*

8. The cardiac catheterization is completed, and a 95% blockage of the left anterior descending (LAD) artery is seen along with an 80% blockage of the circumflex artery. A balloon angioplasty is performed in the catheterization laboratory. After the procedure, the LAD has a 40% blockage, and the circumflex has a 25% blockage. The physician counsels the patient to resume activity gradually. A stress test will be scheduled in several weeks for further evaluation of his exercise tolerance and cardiac status. Develop a teaching-learning plan for this patient to prepare him for the upcoming tests.

36

CHAPTER

Care of Patients with Dysrhythmias

STUDY/REVIEW QUESTIONS

Fill in the blank.

1. The primary pacemaker of the heart is the _____.

2. The electrical impulse of the heart moves through the ventricles from the _____ to right and left bundle branches to the _____.

3. The function of the atrioventricular (AV) node is to _____ impulses between the atria and ventricles.

4. The ability of all cardiac cells to initiate an impulse spontaneously and repetitively is called _____.

5. _____ is the ability of atrial and ventricular muscle cells to shorten their fiber length in response to electrical stimulation.

6. The transmitting of electrical impulses from cardiac cell to cardiac cell is called _____.

7. The ability of a cell to respond to a stimulus by initiating an impulse is called _____.

8. _____ contributes additional blood volume for a greater cardiac output.

9. What does stimulation of the sympathetic nervous system produce?
   a. Delayed electrical impulse that causes hypotension and bradypnea
   b. Contractility and dilation of coronary vessels and increased heart rate
   c. Virtually no effect on the ventricles of the heart or the vitals signs
   d. A slowed AV conduction time that results in a slow heart rate

10. The primary pacemaker of the heart, the sinoatrial (SA) node, is functional if the patient's pulse is at what regular rate?
    a. Less than 60 beats/min
    b. 60 to 100 beats/min
    c. 80 to 100 beats/min
    d. Greater than 100 beats/min

11. The nurse is taking vital signs and reviewing the electrocardiogram (ECG) of the patient who is training for a marathon. The heart rate is 45 beats/min and the ECG shows sinus bradycardia. How does the nurse interpret this data?
    a. A rapid filling rate that lengthens diastolic filling time and leads to decreased cardiac output
    b. The body's attempt to compensate for a decreased stroke volume by decreasing the heart rate
    c. An adequate stroke volume that is associated with cardiac conditioning
    d. A common finding in the healthy adult that would be considered normal

12. The nurse is performing the shift assessment on a cardiac patient. In order to determine if the patient has a pulse deficit, what does the nurse do?

   a. Take the patient's blood pressure and subtract the diastolic from the systolic pressure.

   b. Take the patient's pulse in a supine position and then in a standing position.

   c. Assess the apical and radial pulses for a full minute and observe for differences.

   d. Take the radial pulse, have the patient rest for 15 minutes, and then retake the pulse.

Matching. *Match the placements with the correct limb leads for ECG monitoring.*

Limb Lead

a. Lead I
b. Lead II
c. Lead III
d. aVr
e. aVL
f. aVF

Placement

_____ 13. Right arm (+)

_____ 14. Right arm (−), left arm (+)

_____ 15. Left arm (−), left leg (+)

_____ 16. Left leg (+)

_____ 17. Left arm (+)

_____ 18. Right arm (−), left leg (+)

19. Identify the components of a normal ECG.

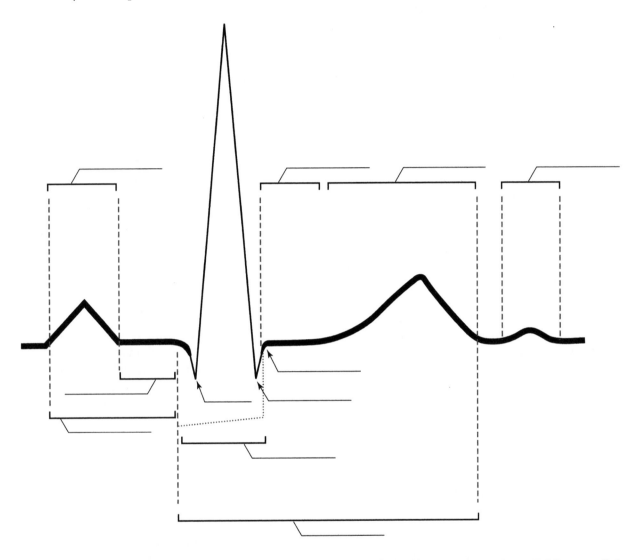

20. What does the P wave in an ECG represent?
    a. Atrial depolarization
    b. Atrial repolarization
    c. Ventricular depolarization
    d. Ventricular repolarization

21. What is the normal measurement of the PR interval in an ECG?
    a. Less than 0.11 second
    b. 0.06 to 0.10 second
    c. 0.12 to 0.20 second
    d. 0.16 to 0.26 second

22. What is the QRS complex in an ECG normally?
    a. Less than 0.12 second
    b. 0.10 to 0.16 second
    c. 0.12 to 0.20 second
    d. 0.16 to 0.24 second

23. What is the ST segment in an ECG normally?
    a. Isoelectric
    b. Elevated
    c. Depressed
    d. Biphasic

24. What is the total time required for ventricular depolarization and repolarization as represented on the ECG?
    a. PR interval
    b. QRS complex
    c. ST segment
    d. QT interval

25. The nurse is performing a 12-lead ECG on the patient with chest pain. Because the positioning of the electrodes is crucial, how does the nurse place the ECG components?
    a. Four leads are placed on the limbs and six are placed on the chest.
    b. The negative electrode is placed on the left arm and the positive electrode is placed on the right leg.
    c. Four leads are placed on the limbs and four are placed on the chest.
    d. The negative electrode is placed on the right arm and the positive electrode is placed on the left leg.

26. Where does the nurse place the electrodes on the patient who requires continuous ECG monitoring?
    a. On the right arm, left arm, and left foot
    b. On the left arm, left leg, and right arm
    c. Below the clavicles and on the lowest ribs
    d. With regular spacing across the anterior chest

27. The patient is admitted for chest pain and requires continuous ECG monitoring. How does the nurse prepare the patient's skin before placing the electrodes?
    a. Apply fresh lotion to soften the skin.
    b. Clean the skin with alcohol and Betadine.
    c. Moisten the skin with a damp sponge.
    d. The skin is left dry.

28. The nurse is caring for several patients in the telemetry unit who are being remotely watched by a monitor technician. What is the nurse's primary responsibility in the monitoring process of these patients?
    a. Watching the bank of monitors on the unit
    b. Printing ECG rhythm strips routinely and as needed
    c. Interpreting rhythms
    d. Assessment and management

29. The patient in the telemetry unit is having continuous ECG monitoring. The patient is scheduled for a test in the radiology department. Who is responsible for determining when monitoring can be suspended?
    a. Telemetry technician
    b. Charge nurse
    c. Physician
    d. Primary nurse

30. The nurse is reviewing preliminary ECG results of the patient admitted for mental status changes. The nurse alerts the provider about ST elevation or depression in the patient because it is an indication of which condition?
    a. Myocardial injury or ischemia
    b. Ventricular irritability
    c. Subarachnoid hemorrhage
    d. Prinzmetal's angina

31. The nurse is reviewing ECG results of the patient admitted for fluid and electrolyte imbalances. The T waves are tall and peaked. The nurse reports this finding to the provider and obtains an order for which serum level test?
    a. Sodium
    b. Glucose
    c. Potassium
    d. Phosphorus

32. The nurse is notified by the telemetry monitor technician about the patient's heart rate. Which method does the nurse use to confirm the technician's report?
    a. Count QRS complexes in a 6-second strip and multiply by 10.
    b. Analyze an ECG rhythm strip by using an ECG caliper.
    c. Run an ECG rhythm strip and use the memory method.
    d. Assess the patient's heart rate directly by taking an apical pulse.

33. Place the six steps of analyzing an ECG rhythm strip in the correct order using the numbers 1 through 6.

    _____ a. Interpret the rhythm

    _____ b. Analyze the P waves

    _____ c. Determine the heart rate

    _____ d. Measure the QRS duration

    _____ e. Measure the PR interval

    _____ f. Determine the heart rhythm

34. The patient's ECG rhythm strip is irregular. Which method does the nurse use for an accurate assessment?
    a. 6-second strip method
    b. Memory method
    c. Big block method
    d. Commercial ECG rate ruler

35. The nurse is assessing the patient's ECG rhythm strip and checking the regularity of the atrial rhythm. What is the correct technique?
    a. Place one caliper point on a QRS complex; place the other point on the precise spot on the next QRS complex.
    b. Place one caliper point on a P wave; place the other point on the precise spot on the next P wave.
    c. Place one caliper point at the beginning of the P wave; place the other point at the end of the P-R segment.
    d. Place one caliper point at the beginning of the QRS complex; place and the other point where the S-T segment begins.

36. The nurse is assessing the patient's ECG rhythm strip and analyzing the P waves. Which questions does the nurse use to evaluate the P waves? *(Select all that apply.)*
    a. Are P waves present?
    b. Are the P waves occurring regularly?
    c. Does one P wave follow each QRS complex?
    d. Are the P waves greater than 0.20 second?
    e. Do all the P waves look similar?
    f. Are the P waves smooth, rounded, and upright in appearance?

37. The nurse is assessing the patient's ECG rhythm strip and notes that occasionally the QRS complex is missing. How does the nurse interpret this finding?
    a. A junctional impulse
    b. A supraventricular impulse
    c. Ventricular tachycardia
    d. A dysrhythmia

38. The student nurse is looking at the patient's ECG rhythm strip and suspects a normal sinus rhythm (NSR). Which ECG criteria are included for NSR? *(Select all that apply.)*
    a. Rate: Atrial and ventricular rates of 40 to 120 beats/min
    b. Rhythm: Atrial and ventricular rhythms regular
    c. P waves: Present, consistent configuration, one P wave before each QRS complex
    d. P-R interval is nondetermined
    e. QRS duration: 0.04 to 0.10 second and constant

True or False? Read the following statements about characteristics of an ECG complex and write T for true or F for false in the blanks provided. If the statement is false, correct the statement to make it true.

_____ 39. The P wave represents atrial depolarization followed by atrial contraction.

_____ 40. The P-R interval is the period of time from the firing of the SA node to just before ventricular depolarization.

_____ 41. When depolarization occurs in the ventricles, the T wave is formed on the ECG.

_____ 42. The period between ventricular depolarization and the beginning of ventricular repolarization is the S-T segment.

_____ 43. The T wave represents ventricular repolarization.

_____ 44. Q-T interval is the total time it takes the depolarization and repolarization of atria and ventricles to occur.

_____ 45. The amplitude of the wave reflects the muscular strength of the contraction.

46. The remote telemetry technician calls the nurse to report that the patient's ECG signal transmission is not very clear. What does the nurse do to enhance the transmission?
    a. Clean the skin with povidone-iodine solution before applying the electrodes.
    b. Ensure that the area for electrode placement is dry and non-hairy.
    c. Apply tincture of benzoin to the electrode sites and allow it to dry.
    d. Abrade the skin by rubbing briskly with a rough washcloth.

47. With the speed set for 25 mm/second, the segment between the dark lines on a monitor ECG strip represents how many seconds?
    a. 3
    b. 6
    c. 10
    d. 20

48. Which components measure ECG waveforms?
    a. Blood pressure (BP) and cardiac output (CO)
    b. Seconds (sec) and minutes (min)
    c. Heart rate per minute (HR/min)
    d. Amplitude (voltage) and duration (time)

49. Calculate the heart rate from an ECG strip when there are 25 small blocks from one R wave to the next R wave. _____

50. Calculate the heart rate shown on a 6-second ECG strip when the number of R-R intervals is 5. What is this rhythm? _____

51. How does the nurse interpret the measurement of the P-R interval when the interval to be measured is six small boxes on the ECG strip?
    a. Atrium is taking longer to repolarize.
    b. Longer than normal impulse time from the SA node to the ventricles is shown.
    c. There is a problem with the length of time the ventricles are depolarizing.
    d. This is the normal length of time for the P-R interval.

52. The nurse is reviewing the patient's ECG and interprets a wide distorted QRS complex of 0.14 second followed by a P wave. What does this finding indicate?
    a. Wide but normal complex, and no cause for concern
    b. Premature ventricular contraction
    c. Problem with the speed set on the ECG machine
    d. Delayed time of the electrical impulse through the ventricles

53. The monitor technician notifies the nurse that the patient's monitor is showing artifact. What does the nurse do next?
    a. Monitor and document the artifact.
    b. Troubleshoot the equipment.
    c. Check the status of the patient.
    d. Notify the physician for orders.

Matching. Match each type of dysrhythmia with its description. Answers may be used more than once.

Types of Dysrhythmias

a. Sinus tachycardia
b. Atrial flutter
c. Atrial fibrillation
d. First-degree atrioventricular block
e. Ventricular tachycardia
f. Ventricular fibrillation
g. Asystole
h. Third-degree heart block

Descriptions

_____ 54. A straight line or wavy line on the cardiac monitor

_____ 55. Sinus impulses are delayed, but all eventually reach the ventricles

_____ 56. A ventricular rhythm that in most cases results in loss of consciousness

_____ 57. Rapidly fatal if not corrected in 3 to 5 minutes

_____ 58. Complete heart block

_____ 59. Results in asynchrony of atrial contraction and decreased cardiac output

_____ 60. May result from sympathetic nervous system stimulation of the heart or vagal inhibition

_____ 61. Characterized by rapid atrial depolarization occurring at a rate of 250 to 350 times per minute

_____ 62. Causes the ventricles to quiver, resulting in absence of cardiac output

63. The nurse hears in report that the patient has sinus arrhythmia. In order to validate that this is associated with the changes in intrathoracic pressure, what does the nurse do next?
    a. Count the respiratory and pulse rate at rest and then count both rates after moderate exertion.
    b. Observe that the heart rate increases slightly during inspiration and decreases slightly during exhalation.
    c. Ask the patient to hold the breath and take an apical pulse; then have the patient resume normal breathing.
    d. Have the patient take a deep breath and count the patient's apical pulse rate while the patient slowly exhales.

64. The nurse is caring for the patient with coronary artery disease (CAD). The patient reports palpitations and chest discomfort and the nurse notes a tachydysrhythmia on the ECG monitor. What does the nurse do next?
    a. Analyze the ECG strip.
    b. Notify the health care provider.
    c. Give supplemental oxygen.
    d. Administer a narcotic analgesic.

65. The nurse is taking the initial history and vital signs on the patient with fatigue. The nurse notes a regular apical pulse of 130 beats/min. Which contributing factors does the nurse assess for? *(Select all that apply.)*
    a. Anxiety or stress
    b. Fever
    c. Hypovolemia
    d. Anemia or hypoxemia
    e. Hypothyroidism
    f. Constipation

66. The nurse is taking a history and vital signs on the patient who has come to the clinic for a routine checkup. The patient has a pulse rate of 50 beats/min, but denies any distress. What does the nurse do next?
    a. Give supplemental oxygen.
    b. Establish IV access.
    c. Complete the health history.
    d. Check the blood pressure.

67. The nurse is reviewing the monitored rhythms of several patients in the cardiac stepdown unit. The patient with which cardiac anomaly has the greatest need of immediate attention?
    a. Chronic atrial fibrillation
    b. Paroxysmal supraventricular tachycardia that is suddenly terminated
    c. Sustained rapid ventricular response
    d. Sinus tachycardia with premature atrial complexes

68. The patient is diagnosed with recurrent supraventricular tachycardia (SVT). What does the nurse do in order to accomplish the preferred treatment?
    a. Place the patient on the cardiac monitor and perform carotid massage.
    b. Give oxygen and establish IV access for antidysrhythmic drugs.
    c. Assist the physician in attempting atrial overdrive pacing.
    d. Provide information about radiofrequency catheter ablation therapy.

69. Based on the prevalence and risk factors for atrial fibrillation (AF), which patient group is at highest risk for AF?
    a. Older adults
    b. Diabetics
    c. Substance abusers
    d. Pediatric cardiology patients

70. The patient with AF suddenly develops shortness of breath, chest pain, hemoptysis, and a feeling of impending doom. The nurse recognizes these symptoms as which complication?
    a. Pulmonary embolism
    b. Embolic stroke
    c. Absence of atrial kick
    d. Increased cardiac output

71. The patient scheduled to have elective cardioversion for AF will receive drug therapy for about 6 weeks before the procedure. What information about the drug therapy does the nurse teach the patient?
    a. Managing orthostatic hypotension
    b. Watching for bleeding signs
    c. Eating potassium food sources
    d. Reporting muscle weakness or tremors

72. The bedside cardiac monitor of the postoperative patient who becomes confused shows sinus rhythm, but there is no palpable pulse. How does the nurse interpret these findings?
    a. ECG monitor artifact or dysfunction
    b. Pulseless electrical activity with inadequate perfusion
    c. A paced rhythm with hypotension
    d. Idioventricular rhythm as seen in the dying heart

73. The remote telemetry technician alerts the nurse to the presence of premature ventricular contractions (PVCs) in the newly admitted patient. How does the nurse assess whether the premature complexes perfuse to the extremities?
    a. Palpate peripheral arteries while observing the monitor for widened complexes.
    b. Auscultate for the apical heart sounds and listen for irregularities or pauses.
    c. Check the color and temperature of extremities, and capillary refill of fingers and toes.
    d. Assess the ECG strip for regularity and width of QRS complexes.

74. What is the primary significance of ventricular tachycardia (VT) in the cardiac patient?
    a. It increases the ventricular filling time, therefore increasing cardiac output.
    b. It signals that the patient needs potassium supplement for replacement.
    c. It warrants immediate initiation of cardiopulmonary resuscitation.
    d. It is commonly the initial rhythm before deterioration into ventricular fibrillation.

75. The nurse is interviewing the patient who suddenly becomes faint, immediately loses consciousness, and becomes pulseless and apneic. There is no blood pressure, and heart sounds are absent. What does the nurse do next?
    a. Request the defibrillator.
    b. Start cardiopulmonary resuscitation (CPR).
    c. Establish or ensure IV access.
    d. Give supplemental oxygen.

76. The patient is in full cardiac arrest and CPR is in progress. The ECG monitor shows ventricular asystole. What does the nurse do next?
    a. Assist with or administer defibrillation.
    b. Assess another ECG lead to ensure the rhythm is asystole and not fine VF.
    c. Assist the physician with noninvasive pacing or invasive transvenous pacing.
    d. Encourage the family's presence during the resuscitation.

77. The patient is being treated for chronic atrial fibrillation (AF). Which medication is the patient most likely to be prescribed?
    a. Propranolol (Lopressor)
    b. Mexiletine hydrochloride (Mexitil)
    c. Diltiazem hydrochloride (Cardizem)
    d. Amiodarone (Cordarone)

78. The patient is diagnosed with torsade de pointes. The nurse prepares to administer which emergency medication?
    a. Magnesium sulfate
    b. Epinephrine (Adrenalin)
    c. Adenosine (Adenocard)
    d. Calcium chloride

79. In the patient's record, the nurse notes frequent episodes of bradycardia and hypotension related to unintended vagal stimulation. Which instruction for this patient's care does the nurse relay to the unlicensed assistive personnel (UAP)?
    a. Avoid raising the patient's arms above the head during hygiene.
    b. Ambulate the patient slowly and stop frequently for brief rests.
    c. Generously lubricate rectal thermometer probes and insert very cautiously.
    d. Monitor the heart rate and rhythm if the patient is vomiting.

True or False? Read the following statements about heart block and write T for true or F for false in the blanks provided. If the statement is false, correct the statement to make it true.

_____ 80. In *second-degree* heart block, some sinus impulses reach the ventricles, but others do not because they are blocked.

_____ 81. First-degree heart block is the complete blockage of impulses from the SA node.

_____ 82. Third-degree AV block results in ventricular rhythm.

_____ 83. Oxygen, drug therapy, pacing, and/or permanent pacemakers may be used, depending on the degree of the AV block.

_____ 84. A characteristic feature of third-degree block is that none of the sinus impulses reaches the ventricles.

_____ 85. All heart blocks require intervention.

86. The nurse is caring for several patients who have a dysrhythmia. What does the nurse instruct these patients to do?
    a. Stay at least 4 feet away from a microwave oven that is operating.
    b. Avoid electronic metal detectors, such as those at airports.
    c. Learn the procedure for assessing the apical pulse.
    d. Purchase an automatic external defibrillator for home use.

87. The patient reports chest pain and dizziness after exertion, and the family reports a concurrent new onset of mild confusion in the patient as well as difficulty concentrating. What is the best nursing diagnosis for this patient?
   a. Activity Intolerance
   b. Decreased Cardiac Output
   c. Acute Confusion
   d. Impaired Gas Exchange

Matching. Using the Vaughn-Williams classification of antidysrhythmics, match the class of drug with its action.

Class
a. Class I
b. Class II
c. Class III
d. Class IV

Action

_____ 88. Lengthens the absolute refractory period and prolongs repolarization and the action potential duration of ischemic cells

_____ 89. Impedes the flow of calcium into the cell during depolarization, thereby depressing the automaticity of SA and AV nodes and decreasing heart rate

_____ 90. Membrane-stabilizing agents used to decrease automaticity

_____ 91. Controls dysrhythmias associated with excessive beta-adrenergic stimulation by competing for receptor sites, and thereby decreasing heart rate and conduction velocity

92. According to the Vaughn-Williams classification of antidysrhythmics, which class II drug controls dysrhythmias associated with excessive beta-adrenergic stimulation?
   a. Amiodarone hydrochloride (Cordarone)
   b. Propranolol hydrochloride (Inderal)
   c. Diltiazem (Cardizem)
   d. Verapamil hydrochloride (Calan)

93. Which drug for symptomatic bradycardia does the nurse prepare to administer to the patient with a bradydysrhythmia?
   a. Epinephrine
   b. Atropine
   c. Calcium
   d. Lidocaine

94. Which medication does the adult patient with ventricular fibrillation or pulseless ventricular tachycardia receive?
   a. Propranolol (Inderal)
   b. Adenosine (Adenocard)
   c. Diltiazem hydrochloride (Cardizem)
   d. Epinephrine (Adrenalin Chloride)

95. The respiratory therapist (RT) and the medical student are ventilating the patient in cardiac arrest, while the nurse and physician are preparing the patient and equipment for intubation. At which point does the nurse intervene?
   a. The RT inserts an oropharyngeal airway.
   b. The medical student sets the oxygen flow meter at 2 L/min.
   c. The RT ventilates with a manual resuscitation bag and mask.
   d. The medical student uses the chin-lift position on the patient.

96. After advanced cardiac life support (ACLS) is performed, the patient who experienced ventricular fibrillation has a return of spontaneous circulation. To protect the patient's nervous system, which intervention does the nurse anticipate will be performed?
    a. Neurologic checks every 4 hours
    b. Administration of IV mannitol
    c. Application of a cooling blanket
    d. Continuous ECG monitoring

97. The nurse discovers the patient is unconscious and without palpable pulses and immediately initiates CPR. For what reason is CPR started on this patient?
    a. To identify the underlying heart rhythm
    b. For the rapid return of a pulse, blood pressure, and consciousness
    c. To prevent rib fractures or lacerations of the liver and spleen
    d. To mimic cardiac function until the defibrillator arrives

98. Automatic external defibrillator (AED) electrodes are placed on the patient who is unconscious and pulseless. The nurse prepares to immediately defibrillate if the monitor shows which cardiac anomaly?
    a. Third-degree heart block
    b. Pulseless electrical activity
    c. Ventricular fibrillation
    d. Idioventricular rhythm

99. The patient is found pulseless and the cardiac monitor shows a rhythm that has no recognizable deflections, but instead has coarse "waves" of varying amplitudes. What is the priority ACLS intervention for this rhythm?
    a. Immediate defibrillation
    b. Administration of epinephrine IVP
    c. Administration of lidocaine IVP
    d. Noninvasive temporary pacing

100. The patient has no pulse and the cardiac monitor shows ventricular fibrillation. Which drugs does the nurse prepare to administer during the resuscitation? *(Select all that apply.)*
    a. Lidocaine
    b. Epinephrine
    c. Calcium chloride
    d. Amiodarone hydrochloride (Cordarone)
    e. Dopamine hydrochloride (Intropin)
    f. Magnesium sulfate
    g. Dobutamine hydrochloride (Dobutrex)
    h. Vasopressin (Pitressin)

101. The nurse is placing the electrodes on the patient for cardioversion. What is the correct placement for the electrodes?
    a. One electrode is placed on the upper left chest and the other is placed on the lower left chest in a midaxillary line.
    b. One electrode is placed the upper right chest below the clavicle and the other is placed on the back.
    c. One electrode is placed to the left of the precordium, and the other is placed on the right next to the sternum and below the clavicle.
    d. One electrode is placed on the sternum and the other is placed on the lower left chest in a midaxillary line.

102. The patient is in ventricular fibrillation. The nurse sets the biphasic defibrillator to deliver how many joules?
    a. 100
    b. 200
    c. 300
    d. 360

103. The patient is about to undergo elective cardioversion. The nurse sets the defibrillator for synchronized mode so that the electrical shock is not delivered on the T wave. This is done to avoid which complication?
    a. Electrical burns to the skin
    b. Ventricular standstill
    c. Arcing from the electrodes
    d. Ventricular fibrillation

104. The nurse is performing external defibrillation. Which step is most vital this procedure?
    a. Place the gel pads anterior over the apex and posterior for better conduction.
    b. Do not administer a second shock for 1 minute to allow for recharging.
    c. No-one must touch the patient at the time a shock is delivered.
    d. Continuously ventilate the patient via endotracheal tube during the defibrillation.

Matching. Match the terms with their correct definitions.

Terms

a. Capture
b. Atrial overdrive pacing
c. Synchronous (demand) pacing mode
d. Asynchronous (fixed-rate) pacing mode
e. Noninvasive temporary pacing (NTP)
f. Invasive temporary pacemaker

Definitions

_____ 105. The pacemaker continues to fire at a fixed rate as set on the generator.

_____ 106. Electrical pulses are transmitted through two large external electrodes, then transcutaneously to stimulate ventricular depolarization.

_____ 107. Indicating that the pacemaker has successfully depolarized, or captured, the chamber.

_____ 108. Rapidly pacing the atrium to control depolarization, followed by no pacing, to allow the sinus node to regain control of the heart.

_____ 109. External battery-operated pulse generator on one end and wires in contact with the heart on the other end.

_____ 110. The pacemaker's sensitivity is set to sense the patient's own beats.

111. The nurse is assisting the physician perform temporary pacing for the patient who has third-degree heart block. What is the desired outcome for this patient as evidenced by the cardiac monitor?
    a. Capture
    b. Pacemaker spike
    c. Pacemaker artifact
    d. Second-degree heart block

112. The physician has completed the placement of lead wires for the invasive temporary pacemaker in the patient who is asystolic. In turning on the pacing unit, which setting does the nurse use?
    a. Synchronous pacing mode
    b. Demand pacing mode
    c. Asynchronous pacing mode
    d. Temporary pacing mode

113. The nurse in the telemetry unit may have to perform NTP in nonemergent situations. Place the steps of this procedure in sequential order using the numbers 1 through 7.

_____ a. Explain NTP to the patient and family and prepare the equipment.

_____ b. Apply the electrodes on the chest according to package instructions.

_____ c. Set milliamperes (mA) output 2 mA above where consistent capture is observed.

_____ d. Turn the pacer on; set the pacing rate as ordered.

_____ e. Establish the stimulation threshold.

_____ f. Palpate the right radial or carotid pulse and assess the blood pressure.

_____ g. Wash the skin with soap and water.

114. The nurse in the telemetry unit must perform NTP. How does the nurse position the electrodes?
    a. One over breast tissue on the right side and one over breast tissue on left side
    b. One on the upper chest to the left of the sternum and one beneath the left scapula
    c. One on the upper chest to the right of the sternum and one over the heart apex
    d. One over the sternum and one on the left anterior lateral chest

115. The nurse has been taking postprocedure vital signs of the patient with NTP. The patient is now stable and vital sign monitoring can be delegated to UAP. Which instruction does the nurse give the UAP regarding this patient's vital signs?
    a. Assess blood pressure using the patient's right arm and check the right radial pulse.
    b. Assess blood pressure using the patient's left arm and check the left carotid pulse.
    c. Set the automatic blood pressure cuff to cycle every 15 minutes on either arm.
    d. Do not use the pulse oximeter because of the danger of electromagnetic interference.

116. The patient has an invasive temporary pacemaker. In what ways does the nurse ensure the patient's safety related to electrical issues with the pacemaker? (Select all that apply.)
    a. Ensure that external ends of the lead wires are insulated with rubber gloves.
    b. Loop the wire ends and cover with nonconductive tape.
    c. Ensure that no electrical equipment is used in the patient's room.
    d. Report frayed wire to the biomedical engineering department.
    e. Wash hands before touching any of the wires.

True or False? Write T for true or F for false in the blanks provided. If the statement is false, correct it to make it true.

_____ 117. The implantable cardioverter defibrillator (ICD) treats bradydysrhythmias.

_____ 118. Dobutamine is a beta-adrenergic agent used to improve contractility.

_____ 119. Ventricular aneurysms are a complication of myocardial infarction.

_____ 120. Cardioversion shock is synchronized with the T wave.

_____ 121. Class III antidysrhythmics lengthen the absolute refractory period and prolong repolarization.

_____ 122. Confusion, drowsiness, and slurring of speech are signs of lidocaine toxicity.

123. The patient with atrial fibrillation is scheduled to have an elective cardioversion. The nurse ensures that the patient has a prescription for a 4 to 6 week supply of which type of medication?
    a. Anticoagulants
    b. Digitalis
    c. Diuretics
    d. Potassium supplements

124. The nurse is teaching the patient with an implantable cardioverter defibrillator (ICD). What instruction does the nurse emphasize to the patient?
    a. Rest for several hours after an internal defibrillator shock before resuming activities.
    b. Have family members step away during the internal defibrillator shock for safety.
    c. Expect that the shock may feel like a thud or a painful kick in the chest.
    d. Report any pulse rate higher than what is set on the pacemaker.

125. The patient has had synchronized cardioversion for unstable ventricular tachycardia. Which interventions does the nurse include in this patient's care after the procedure? *(Select all that apply.)*
    a. Administer therapeutic hypothermia.
    b. Assess vital signs and the level of consciousness.
    c. Administer antidysrhythmic drug therapy.
    d. Monitor for dysrhythmias.
    e. Monitor for loss of capture.
    f. Assess for chest burns from electrodes.

126. The nurse is teaching a community group how to use an automatic external defibrillator (AED). Place the steps of using an AED in sequential order using the numbers 1 through 5.

    _____ a. Rescuer presses the "analyze" button on the machine.

    _____ b. Place the patient on a firm, dry surface.

    _____ c. Rescuer stops CPR and directs anyone present to move away.

    _____ d. The machine advises if a shock is necessary.

    _____ e. Place two large adhesive-patch electrodes on the patient's chest.

127. The patient has had a permanent pacemaker surgically implanted. What are the nursing responsibilities for the care of this patient related to the surgery? *(Select all that apply.)*
    a. Administer short-acting sedatives.
    b. Assess the implantation site for bleeding, swelling, redness, tenderness, or infection.
    c. Teach about and monitor for the initial activity restrictions.
    d. Observe for overstimulation of the chest wall which could lead to pneumothorax.
    e. Monitor the ECG rhythm to check that the pacemaker is working correctly.

128. The nurse is interviewing the patient with spontaneous ventricular tachycardia who may be a possible candidate for an implantable cardioverter/defibrillator (ICD). The nurse senses that the patient is anxious. What is the nurse's most therapeutic response?
    a. "Your feelings are natural; patients report psychological distress related to ICD."
    b. "ICD is similar to defibrillation which saved your life during the last episode."
    c. "You seem anxious. What are your concerns about having this therapy?"
    d. "Would you like to talk to the doctor about the details of the procedure?"

129. The nurse is teaching the patient with a permanent pacemaker. What information about the pacemaker does the nurse tell the patient? *(Select all that apply.)*
    a. Report any pulse rate lower than what is set on the pacemaker.
    b. If the surgical incision is near the shoulder, avoid overextending the joint.
    c. Keep handheld cellular phones at least 6 inches away from the generator.
    d. Avoid sources of strong electromagnetic fields, such as magnets.
    e. Avoid strenuous activities that may cause the device to discharge inappropriately.
    f. Carry a pacemaker identification card and wear a medical alert bracelet.

Interpret each ECG strip below. Write your answers in the blanks provided.

130. _____

RATE _____ RHYTHM _____ P WAVES _____

PR INTERVAL _____ QRS DURATION _____

INTERPRETATION _____

131. _____

RATE _____ RHYTHM _____ P WAVES _____

PR INTERVAL _____ QRS DURATION _____

INTERPRETATION _____

132. _____

RATE _____ RHYTHM _____ P WAVES _____

PR INTERVAL _____ QRS DURATION _____

INTERPRETATION _____

133. _____

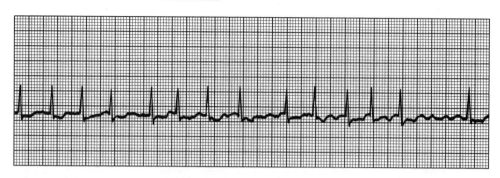

RATE _____   RHYTHM _____   P WAVES _____

PR INTERVAL _____   QRS DURATION _____

INTERPRETATION _____

134. _____

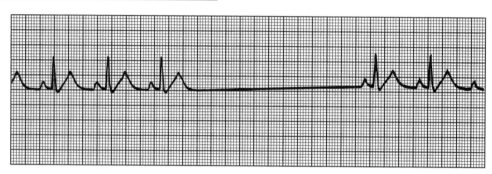

RATE _____   RHYTHM _____   P WAVES _____

PR INTERVAL _____   QRS DURATION _____

INTERPRETATION _____

135. _____

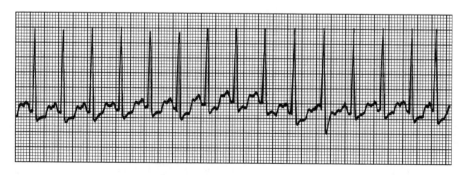

RATE _____   RHYTHM _____   P WAVES _____

PR INTERVAL _____   QRS DURATION _____

INTERPRETATION _____

136. _____

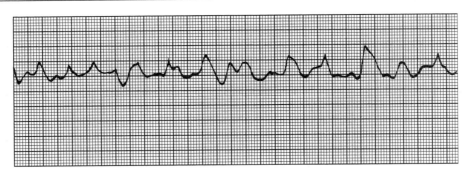

RATE _____   RHYTHM _____   P WAVES _____

PR INTERVAL _____   QRS DURATION _____

INTERPRETATION _____

137. _____

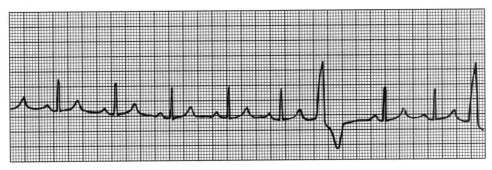

RATE _____   RHYTHM _____   P WAVES _____

PR INTERVAL _____   QRS DURATION _____

INTERPRETATION _____

138. _____

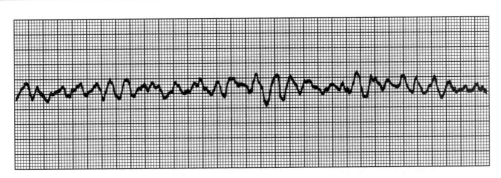

RATE _____   RHYTHM _____   P WAVES _____

PR INTERVAL _____   QRS DURATION _____

INTERPRETATION _____

139. _____

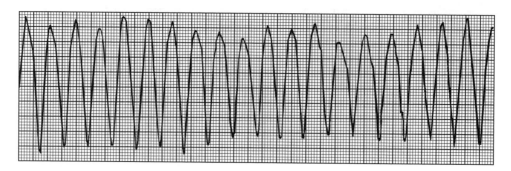

RATE _____   RHYTHM _____   P WAVES _____

PR INTERVAL _____   QRS DURATION _____

INTERPRETATION _____

140. _____

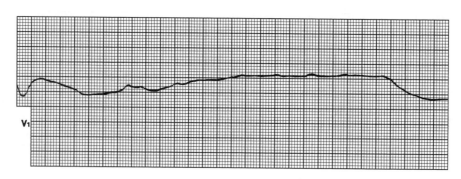

RATE _____   RHYTHM _____   P WAVES _____

PR INTERVAL _____   QRS DURATION _____

INTERPRETATION _____

141. _____

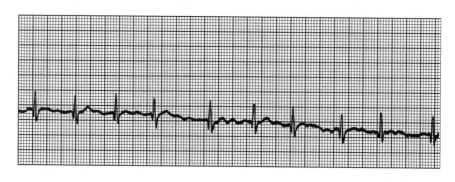

RATE _____   RHYTHM _____   P WAVES _____

PR INTERVAL _____   QRS DURATION _____

INTERPRETATION _____

142. _____

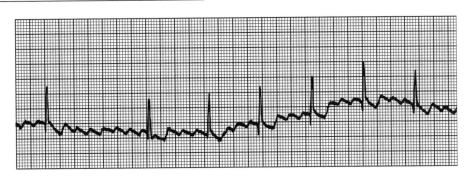

RATE _____   RHYTHM _____   P WAVES _____

PR INTERVAL _____   QRS DURATION _____

INTERPRETATION _____

143. _____

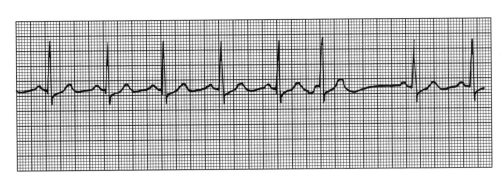

RATE _____   RHYTHM _____   P WAVES _____

PR INTERVAL _____   QRS DURATION _____

INTERPRETATION _____

144. _____

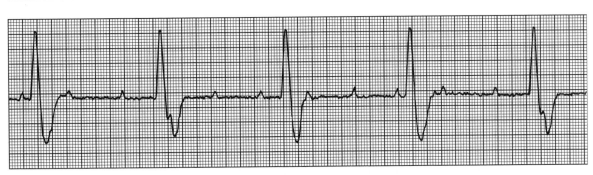

RATE _____   RHYTHM _____   P WAVES _____

PR INTERVAL _____   QRS DURATION _____

INTERPRETATION _____

CASE STUDY: THE PATIENT WITH BRADYCARDIA

Use a separate sheet of paper to answer the questions in this Case Study. Answer guidelines for this Case Study are available on your Evolve website at http://evolve. elsevier.com/Iggy/ in the "Prepare for Class" folder.

A patient in a critical care unit on telemetry develops the following rhythm: normal P waves at a regular rate of 88 beats per minute. There is a separate ventricular regular rate of 55 with a normal QRS complex.

1. What can be determined about the relationship of the P wave and the QRS complexes?

2. Based on this ECG, what assessment findings might be identified with this dysrhythmia?

3. What would make a difference in the physical findings?

4. What type of heart block has been identified?

5. What interventions are necessary for this patient?

6. Differentiate between invasive and noninvasive temporary pacing. Describe the two types of invasive temporary pacing.

7. Identify the three complications that can occur with noninvasive pacemaker therapy.

8. Briefly describe what the synchronous, or demand, mode means regarding pacemaker therapy.

9. Would the patient have a temporary or permanent pacemaker?

10. What would be included in a teaching plan for a patient with a pacemaker?

CASE STUDY: THE PATIENT WITH A DYSRHYTHMIA

Use a separate sheet of paper to answer the questions in this Case Study. Answer guidelines for this Case Study are available on your Evolve website at http://evolve. elsevier.com/Iggy/ in the "Prepare for Class" folder.

A 78-year-old woman is admitted to a telemetry unit directly from her physician's office for evaluation and management of congestive heart failure. She has a history of systemic hypertension and chronic moderate mitral regurgitation. Her medication orders include furosemide (Lasix) 80 mg orally four times a day, digoxin 0.125 mg orally daily, and diltiazem (Cardizem) 60 mg orally three times a day. The initial assessment of the patient reveals a pulse rate that is rapid and very irregular. The patient is restless, her skin is pale and cool, she states she is dizzy when she stands up, and she is slightly short of breath and anxious. Her blood pressure is 106/88. Her ECG monitor pattern shows uncontrolled atrial fibrillation, with a rate ranging from 150 to 170 beats/min. Her oxygen saturation level is 90%.

1. Given the assessment findings, what should the nurse do first?

2. What additional physical assessment techniques would the nurse perform?

3. Because the length of time the patient has been in atrial fibrillation is unknown, what potential complication may occur if cardioversion is attempted?

4. What should be done before elective cardioversion is attempted?

5. Later that evening, the patient calls the nurse because she feels "like something terrible is going to happen." She reports chest pain, has increased shortness of breath, and has coughed up blood-tinged sputum. What should the nurse suspect? What is the first thing the nurse should do, and what further assessments should be performed at this time?

37

CHAPTER

Care of Patients with Cardiac Problems

STUDY/REVIEW QUESTIONS

Matching. *Match the terms with their correct definitions.*

Terms
a. Right-sided heart (ventricular) failure
b. Left-sided heart (ventricular) failure
c. High-output failure
d. Ejection fraction
e. Pulsus alternans
f. Renin-angiotensin system (RAS)

Definitions
_____ 1. Decreased tissue perfusion from poor cardiac output and pulmonary congestion from increased pressure in the pulmonary vessels

_____ 2. Alternate in strength

_____ 3. Can occur when cardiac output remains normal or above normal

_____ 4. Percentage of blood ejected from the heart during systole

_____ 5. Activated by reduced blood flow to the kidneys

_____ 6. Increased volume and pressure develop and result in peripheral edema

Fill in the blanks.

7. Most heart failure begins with failure of the _____ and progresses to failure of both ventricles.

8. As the ejection fraction decreases, tissue perfusion _____ and blood accumulates in the _____ vessels.

9. B-type natriuretic peptide (BNP) is produced and released by the ventricles when the patient has _____ as a result of heart failure.

10. Cardiac output (CO) is the product of heart rate (HR) and stroke volume (SV), and an increase in HR results in an immediate _____ in cardiac output.

11. The initial compensatory mechanism of the heart that maintains cardiac output is increased _____

_____.

12. The nurse is taking a history on the patient recently diagnosed with heart failure. The patient admits to "sometimes having trouble catching my breath," but is unable to provide more specific details. What question does the nurse ask to gather more data about the patient's symptoms?
    a. "Do you have any medical problems, such as high blood pressure?"
    b. "What did your doctor tell you about your diagnosis?"
    c. "What was your most strenuous activity in the past week?"
    d. "How do you feel about being told that you have heart failure?"

13. The night shift nurse is listening to report and hears that the patient has paroxysmal nocturnal dyspnea. What does the nurse plan to do next?
    a. Instruct the patient to sleep in a side-lying position and then check on the patient every 2 hours to help with switching sides.
    b. Make the patient comfortable in a bedside recliner with several pillows to keep the patient more upright throughout the night.
    c. Check on the patient several hours after bedtime and assist the patient to sit upright and dangle the feet when dyspnea occurs.
    d. Check the patient frequently because the patient has insomnia due to a fear of suffocation.

14. The nurse is assessing the patient with right-sided heart failure. Which assessment findings does the nurse expect to see in this patient? *(Select all that apply.)*
    a. Dependent edema
    b. Weight loss
    c. Polyuria at night
    d. Hypotension
    e. Hepatomegaly
    f. Angina

15. The nurse is assessing the patient with left-sided heart failure. Which assessment findings does the nurse expect to see in this patient? *(Select all that apply.)*
    a. Displacement of the apical impulse to the left
    b. S_3 heart sound
    c. Paroxysmal nocturnal dyspnea
    d. Jugular venous distention
    e. Oliguria during the day
    f. Wheezes or crackles

16. Based on the etiology and the main cause of heart failure, which patient has the greatest need for health promotion measures to prevent heart failure?
    a. Alzheimer's patient
    b. Patient with cystitis
    c. Patient with asthma
    d. Patient with hypertension

17. What is an early sign of left ventricular failure that the patient is most likely to report?
    a. Nocturia
    b. Weight gain
    c. Swollen legs
    d. Nocturnal coughing

18. The nurse is reviewing diagnostic test results for the patient who is hypertensive. Which laboratory result is an early warning sign of decreased heart compliance, and prompts the nurse to immediately notify the health care provider?
    a. Normal B-type natriuretic peptide
    b. Decreased hemoglobin and hematocrit
    c. Elevated thyroxine (T_4)
    d. Presence of microalbuminuria

19. The nurse is interviewing the patient with a history of high blood pressure and heart problems. Which statement by the patient causes the nurse to suspect the patient may have heart failure?
    a. "I noticed a very fine red rash on my chest."
    b. "I had to take off my wedding ring last week."
    c. "I've had fever quite frequently."
    d. "I have pain in my shoulder when I cough."

20. What is the best way for the nurse to assess the patient for orthopnea?
    a. Ask how many times the patient voids at night.
    b. Assess for a dry, hacking cough.
    c. Ask if the patient uses two or more pillows to sleep.
    d. Ask if the patient suddenly wakes up with a feeling of breathlessness at night.

21. The patient's bilateral radial pulses are occasionally weak and irregular. Which assessment technique does the nurse use first to investigate this finding?
    a. Check the color and the capillary refill in the upper extremities.
    b. Check the peripheral pulses in the lower extremities.
    c. Take the apical pulse for 1 minute, noting any irregularity in heart rhythm.
    d. Check the cardiac monitor for irregularities in rhythm.

22. The patient is at risk for heart failure, but currently has no official medical diagnosis. While assessing the patient's lungs, the nurse hears fine profuse crackles. What does the nurse do next?
    a. Report the finding to the health care provider.
    b. Document the finding as a baseline for later comparison.
    c. Give the patient low-flow supplemental oxygen.
    d. Ask the patient to cough and reauscultate the lungs.

23. The patient is admitted for heart failure and has edema, neck vein distention, and ascites. What is the most reliable way to monitor fluid gain or loss in this patient?
    a. Check for pitting edema in the dependent body parts.
    b. Auscultate the lungs for crackles or wheezing.
    c. Assess skin turgor and the condition of mucous membranes.
    d. Weigh the patient daily at the same time with the same scale.

24. The home health nurse is evaluating the patient being treated for heart failure. Which statement by the patient is the best indicator of hope and well-being as a desired psychological outcome?
    a. "I'm taking the medication and following the doctor's orders."
    b. "I'm looking forward to dancing with my wife on our wedding anniversary."
    c. "I'm planning to go on a long trip; I'll never go back to the hospital again."
    d. "I want to thank you for all that you have done. I know you did your best."

25. The nurse is reviewing the laboratory results for the patient whose chief complaint is dyspnea. Which diagnostic test best differentiates between heart failure and lung dysfunction?
    a. Arterial blood gas
    b. B-type natriuretic peptide
    c. Hemoglobin and hematocrit
    d. Serum electrolytes

26. The nursing student is assisting in the care of the patient with advanced right-sided heart failure. In addition to bringing a stethoscope, what additional piece of equipment does the student bring in order to assess this patient?
    a. Tape measure
    b. Glasgow Coma Scale
    c. Portable Doppler
    d. Bladder ultrasound scanner

27. Which test is the best tool for diagnosing heart failure?
    a. Echocardiography
    b. Pulmonary artery catheter
    c. Radionuclide studies
    d. Multigated angiographic (MUGA) scan

28. The nurse identifies a nursing diagnosis of In-effective Tissue Perfusion in the patient with heart failure. Which nursing interventions are included in the plan of care for this patient? *(Select all that apply.)*
   a. Monitor respiratory rate, rhythm, and quality every 1 to 4 hours.
   b. Auscultate breath sounds every 4 to 8 hours.
   c. Provide supplemental oxygen to maintain oxygen saturation at 90% or greater.
   d. Place the patient in a supine position with pillows under each leg.
   e. Assist the patient in performing cough-ing and deep-breathing exercises every 2 hours.

29. Which interventions are effective for the pa-tient with fluid volume excess caused by heart failure? *(Select all that apply.)*
   a. Sodium and fluid restriction
   b. Slow infusion of hypotonic saline
   c. Administration of potassium
   d. Administration of loop diuretics
   e. Position in semi-Fowler's to high Fowler's position
   f. Weekly weight monitoring

30. The older adult patient with heart failure is volume depleted and has a low sodium level. The health care provider has ordered valsartan (Diovan), an angiotensin-receptor blocker (ARB). After the initial dose, what does the nurse carefully monitor this patient for?
   a. Hypotension
   b. Cough
   c. Fluid retention
   d. Chest pain

31. The health care provider has ordered an ARB for the patient with heart failure. The param-eters are to maintain a systolic blood pressure ranging from 90 to 110 mm Hg. Today the patient has a blood pressure of 110/80 mm Hg, but shows acute confusion. What is the nurse's priority action?
   a. Give the medication because blood pres-sure is within the parameters.
   b. Call the health care provider about the new onset of confusion.
   c. Hold the medication and document the new findings.
   d. Assess the patient for other symptoms of decreased tissue perfusion.

32. The patient with heart failure has excessive al-dosterone secretion and is therefore experienc-ing thirst and continuously asking for water. What does the nurse instruct the unlicensed assistive personnel (UAP) to do?
   a. Severely restrict fluid to 500 mL plus out-put from the previous 24 hours.
   b. Give the patient as much water as desired to prevent dehydration.
   c. Restrict fluid to a normal 2 L daily, with accurate intake and output.
   d. Frequently offer the patient ice chips and moistened toothettes.

33. The patient is prescribed diuretics for treat-ment of heart failure. Because of this therapy, the nurse pays particular attention to which laboratory test level?
   a. Peak and trough of medication
   b. Serum potassium
   c. Serum sodium
   d. PT and PTT

34. The older adult patient is taking digoxin for treatment of heart failure. What is the priority nursing action for this patient related to the medication therapy?
   a. Give the medication in conjunction with an antacid.
   b. Keep the patient on the cardiac monitor and observe for ventricular dysrhythmias.
   c. Check that the dose is in the lowest pos-sible range for therapeutic effect.
   d. Advise the patient that there is increased mortality related to toxicity.

35. The patient is receiving digoxin therapy for heart failure. What assessment does the nurse perform before administering the medication?
    a. Auscultate the apical pulse rate and heart rhythm.
    b. Assess for nausea and abdominal distention.
    c. Auscultate the lungs for crackles.
    d. Check for increased urine output.

36. The nurse is reviewing the ECG of the patient on digoxin therapy. What early sign of digitalis toxicity does the nurse look for?
    a. Tachycardia
    b. Peaked T wave
    c. Atrial fibrillation
    d. Loss of P wave

37. Which laboratory test monitors for potential cardiac problems and digoxin toxicity?
    a. Complete blood count
    b. BUN and creatinine level
    c. Serum potassium level
    d. Prothrombin time and INR

38. The patient is receiving an infusion of nesiritide (Natrecor) for treatment of heart failure. What is the priority nursing assessment while administering this medication?
    a. Monitor for hypotension.
    b. Assess for cardiac dysrhythmias.
    c. Observe for respiratory depression.
    d. Monitor for peripheral vasoconstriction.

39. The patient has recently been diagnosed with acute heart failure. Which medication order does the nurse question?
    a. Dobutamine (Dobutrex), a beta-adrenergic agonist
    b. Milrinone (Primacor), a phosphodiesterase inhibitor
    c. Levosimendan (Simdax), a positive inotropic
    d. Carvedilol (Coreg), a beta blocker

40. The patient has an ejection fraction of less than 30%. The nurse prepares to provide patient education about which potential treatment?
    a. Automatic implantable cardio-defibrillator
    b. Heart transplant
    c. Mechanical implanted pump
    d. Ventricular reconstructive procedures

41. The nurse identifies a nursing diagnosis of Activity Intolerance for the patient with heart failure. After ambulating 200 feet down the hall, the patient's blood pressure change is more than 20 mm Hg. How does the nurse interpret this data?
    a. The patient is building endurance.
    b. The activity is too stressful.
    c. The patient could walk farther.
    d. The activity is appropriate.

42. The patient with heart failure is anxious to recover quickly. After ambulating with the UAP, the nurse observes that the patient has dyspnea. The nurse asks the patient to rate her exertion on a scale of 1 to 20 and the patient says, "I can keep going. It's only about a 15." What is the nurse's best response?
    a. "Slow down a bit; ideally you should be less than 12."
    b. "As long as you are less than 18, you can keep going."
    c. "Stop right now; you should not tax your heart beyond 5."
    d. "You should go slower; you cannot reach level 0 in one day."

43. Why does the nurse document the precise location of crackles auscultated in the lungs of the patient with heart failure?
    a. Crackles will eventually change to wheezes as the pulmonary edema worsens.
    b. The level of the fluid spreads laterally as the pulmonary edema worsens.
    c. The level of the fluid ascends as the pulmonary edema worsens.
    d. Crackles will eventually diminish as the pulmonary edema worsens.

44. The patient comes to the ED extremely anxious, tachycardiac, and struggling for air with a moist cough productive of frothy, blood-tinged sputum. What is the priority nursing intervention?
    a. Apply a pulse oximeter and cardiac monitor.
    b. Administer high-flow oxygen therapy via face mask.
    c. Prepare for continuous positive airway pressure ventilation.
    d. Prepare for intubation and mechanical ventilation.

45. The patient is treated for acute pulmonary edema. Which medications does the nurse prepare to administer to this patient? *(Select all that apply.)*
    a. Sublingual nitroglycerin
    b. IV Lasix
    c. IV morphine sulfate
    d. IV beta blocker
    e. IV nitroglycerin

46. What is the expected outcome for the collaborative problem Potential for Pulmonary Edema?
    a. No dysrhythmias
    b. Clear lung sounds
    c. Less fatigue
    d. No disorientation

47. The nurse is teaching the patient with heart failure about signs and symptoms that suggest a return or worsening of heart failure. What does the nurse include in the teaching? *(Select all that apply.)*
    a. Rapid weight loss of 3 lbs in a week
    b. Increase in exercise tolerance lasting 2 to 3 days
    c. Cold symptoms (cough) lasting more than 3 to 5 days
    d. Excessive awakening at night to urinate
    e. Development of dyspnea or angina at rest or worsening angina
    f. Increased swelling in the feet, ankles, or hands

48. The patient is prescribed bumetanide (Bumex). What is an important teaching point for the nurse to include about this medication?
    a. Caution to move slowly when changing positions, especially from lying to sitting
    b. Information about potassium-rich foods to include in the diet
    c. Written instructions on how to count the radial pulse rate
    d. Information about low-sodium diets and reading food labels for sodium content

49. The nurse is teaching the patient about the treatment regimen for heart failure. Which statement by the patient indicates a need for further instruction?
    a. "I must weigh myself once a month and watch for fluid retention."
    b. "If my heart feels like it is racing, I should call the doctor."
    c. "I'll need to consider my activities for the day and rest as needed."
    d. "I'll need periods of rest and activity, and I should avoid activity after meals."

True or False? *Read the following statements about valvular disease and write T for true or F for false in the blanks provided. If the statement is false, correct the statement to make it true.*

_____ 50. *Stenosis* refers to the narrowing of the heart valve opening.

_____ 51. *Regurgitation* refers to the heart valves no longer being able to close completely.

_____ 52. Aortic stenosis has been associated with conditions such as Marfan syndrome.

_____ 53. In aortic stenosis, when the surface area of the valve becomes less than or equal to 1 cm, medication therapy is indicated.

_____ 54. In mitral insufficiency, incomplete closure of the valve allows the backflow of blood into the left atrium when the left ventricle contracts.

_____ 55. The most common cause of mitral stenosis is rheumatic carditis.

_____ 56. The tricuspid valve is not frequently affected but can be damaged following endocarditis resulting from intravenous drug use.

_____ 57. Women are diagnosed with mitral regurgitation of rheumatic origin more often than are men.

_____ 58. Nitrates can cause decreased preload and dizziness in patients with aortic stenosis.

Matching. *Match the types of valvular disease with their characteristics. Answers may be used more than once.*

Types of Valvular Disease
a.   Mitral valve stenosis
b.   Mitral valve insufficiency
c.   Mitral valve prolapse
d.   Aortic stenosis
e.   Aortic insufficiency

Characteristics

_____ 59. Usually coexists with some degree of mitral stenosis

_____ 60. Classic signs of dyspnea, angina, and syncope

_____ 61. Hepatomegaly is a late sign

_____ 62. A high-pitched, blowing decrescendo diastolic murmur

_____ 63. Irregular rhythm; atrial fibrillation can cause emboli

_____ 64. Most patients are asymptomatic

_____ 65. Right-side heart failure; later cardiac output fails

_____ 66. The patient may experience palpitations while lying on left side

_____ 67. Symptom-free for decades, later related to left ventricle failure

_____ 68. Rumbling apical diastolic murmur

_____ 69. Right-sided failure results in neck vein distention

_____ 70. Leaflets enlarge and fall back into left atrium during systole

_____ 71. Normal heart rate and blood pressure

_____ 72. Becoming a disorder of aging populations

_____ 73. Murmur, systolic crescendo-decrescendo

_____ 74. S_3 often present due to severe regurgitation

75. The patient is diagnosed with mild mitral valve stenosis. Which finding is the nurse most likely to encounter during the physical assessment of this patient?
    a. Dyspnea on exertion
    b. Orthopnea
    c. Palpitations
    d. Asymptomatic

76. The nurse hears in report that the patient has been diagnosed with mitral insufficiency. Which early symptom is most likely to be first reported by the patient?
    a. Atypical chest pain
    b. Chronic weakness
    c. Anxiety
    d. Dyspnea

77. The patient is diagnosed with mitral valve stenosis. Which finding warrants immediate notification of the health care provider because of potential for decompensation?
    a. Rumbling, apical diastolic murmur on auscultation signifying atrial fibrillation
    b. Slow, bounding peripheral pulses associated with bradycardia
    c. An increase and decrease in pulse rate that follows inspiration and expiration
    d. An increase in pulse rate and blood pressure after exertion

78. The nurse is assessing the pulses of the patient with valvular disease and finds "bounding" arterial pulses. What is this finding most characteristic of?
    a. Aortic regurgitation
    b. Aortic stenosis
    c. Mitral valve prolapse
    d. Mitral insufficiency

79. The patient with a history of valvular heart disease requires a routine colonoscopy. The nurse notifies the health care provider to obtain a patient prescription for which type of medication?
    a. Anticoagulants
    b. Antihypertensives
    c. Antibiotics
    d. Antianginals

80. What is the most common preventable cause of valvular heart disease?
    a. Congenital disease or malformation
    b. Calcium deposits and thrombus formation
    c. Beta-hemolytic streptococcal infection
    d. Hypertension or Marfan syndrome

81. The nurse is assessing the patient at risk for valvular disease and finds pitting edema. This finding is a sign for which type of valvular disease?
    a. Mitral valve stenosis and insufficiency
    b. Aortic valve stenosis and insufficiency
    c. Tricuspid valve prolapse
    d. Mitral valve prolapse

82. The health care provider recommends to the patient that diagnostic testing be performed to assess for valvular heart disease. The nurse teaches the patient about which test that is commonly used for this purpose?
    a. Echocardiography
    b. Electrocardiography
    c. Exercise testing
    d. Thallium scanning

83. Long-term anticoagulant therapy for the patient with valvular heart disease and chronic atrial fibrillation includes which drug?
    a. Heparin sodium
    b. Warfarin sodium (Coumadin)
    c. Diltiazem (Cardizem)
    d. Enoxaparin (Lovenox)

84. The surgical noninvasive intervention of a balloon valvuloplasty is often used for which type of patient?
    a. Young adults with a genetic valve defect
    b. Older adults who are nonsurgical candidates
    c. Adults whose open-heart surgery failed
    d. Older adults who need replacement valves

85. The nurse is caring for the patient who had a valvuloplasty. The nurse monitors for which common complication in the postprocedural period?
    a. Myocardial infarction
    b. Angina
    c. Bleeding and emboli
    d. Infection

86. The patient with a prosthetic valve replacement must understand that postoperative care will include lifelong therapy with which type of medication?
    a. Antibiotics
    b. Anticoagulants
    c. Immunosuppressants
    d. Pain medication

87. The patient is a candidate for a xenograft valve. The nurse emphasizes that this type of valve does not require anticoagulant therapy, but will require which intervention?
    a. Replacement in about 7 to 10 years
    b. An exercise program to develop collateral circulation
    c. Daily temperature checks to watch for signs of rejection
    d. Frequent monitoring for pulmonary edema

88. The patient is scheduled for valve surgery. Which medication does the nurse advise the patient to discontinue for several days before the procedure?
    a. Antihypertensives
    b. Diuretics
    c. Anticoagulants
    d. Antibiotics

89. What is the most common nursing diagnosis for the patient with valvular heart disease?
    a. Decreased Cardiac Output
    b. Ineffective Coping
    c. Ineffective Breathing Pattern
    d. Disturbed Body Image

90. The nurse is giving discharge instructions to the patient who had valve surgery. Which home care instructions does the nurse include in the teaching plan? *(Select all that apply.)*
    a. Increase consumption of foods high in vitamin K.
    b. Use an electric razor to avoid skin cuts.
    c. Report any bleeding or excessive bruising.
    d. Avoid invasive dental procedures unless absolutely necessary.
    e. Watch for and report any fever, drainage, or redness at the site.
    f. Avoid heavy lifting for 3 to 6 months.
    g. Report dyspnea, syncope, dizziness, edema, and palpitations.
    h. Avoid any procedure using magnetic resonance if a prosthetic valve was used.

Matching. Match each description to its corresponding key feature/finding of cardiac disease.

Key Features/Findings
a. Percardial friction rub
b. Splinter hemorrhages
c. Petechiae
d. Systemic emboli
e. Pulsus paradoxus
f. Aschoff's bodies
g. Cardiac tamponade

Descriptions

_____ 91. Vegetation fragments in circulation resulting in a cerebrovascular accident (CVA) or transient ischemic attack (TIA)

_____ 92. Red, flat pinpoint spots/lesions in mucous membrane and conjunctivae

_____ 93. Small red streaks or black longitudinal lines of nail beds

_____ 94. Having a systolic blood pressure higher on expiration than on inspiration

_____ 95. Scratchy, high-pitched sound heard at left lower sternal border

_____ 96. Small nodules on myocardium replaced by scar tissue

_____ 97. Excess fluid in the pericardial cavity

Matching. *Match each assessment finding with its corresponding inflammatory cardiac disease. Answers will be used more than once.*

Inflammatory Cardiac Disease
a. Endocarditis
b. Pericarditis
c. Rheumatic carditis

Assessment Finding

_____ 98. Grating pain that is aggravated by breathing

_____ 99. A new, regurgitant murmur

_____ 100. Janeway's lesions

_____ 101. Streptococcal infection

_____ 102. Osler's nodes

_____ 103. Scratchy, high-pitched sound heard on auscultation over left lower sternal border

_____ 104. Petechiae

_____ 105. Aschoff's bodies

106. Which patients are at greatest risk of developing infective endocarditis? *(Select all that apply.)*
a. IV drug user
b. Patient with pancreatitis
c. Patient with a myocardial infarction
d. Patient with a prosthetic mitral valve replacement, postoperative
e. Patient with mitral stenosis who recently had an abscessed tooth removed
f. Older adult patient with urinary tract infection and valve damage
g. Patient with cardiac dysrhythmias

107. The patient with aortic valve endocarditis reports fatigue and shortness of breath. Crackles are heard on lung auscultation. What do these assessment findings likely indicate?
a. Emboli to the lung
b. Valve incompetence resulting in heart failure
c. Valve stenosis resulting in increased chamber size
d. Coronary artery disease

108. The patient is admitted for possible infective endocarditis. Which test does the nurse anticipate will be performed to confirm a positive diagnosis?
a. CT scan
b. MRI
c. Blood cultures
d. Echocardiogram

109. The patient is diagnosed with new onset infective endocarditis. Which recent procedure is the patient most likely to report?
a. Teeth cleaning
b. Urinary bladder catheterization
c. Chest radiography
d. ECG

110. In what way does arterial embolization to the brain manifest itself in the patient with infective endocarditis?
a. Dysarthria
b. Dysphagia
c. Atelectasis
d. Electrolyte imbalances

111. Which treatment intervention applies to the patient with infective endocarditis?
a. Administration of oral penicillin for 6 weeks or more.
b. Hospitalization for initial IV antibiotics, possibly with a central line.
c. Complete bedrest for the duration of treatment.
d. Long-term anticoagulation therapy with heparin.

True or False? *Read the statements about assessment findings of pericarditis and write T for true or F for false in the blanks provided. If the statement is false, correct the statement to make it true.*

_____ 112. The definitive treatment for chronic constrictive pericarditis is antibiotic therapy.

_____ 113. Dressler's syndrome occurs from 1 to 12 weeks after the infarction and is characterized by pericarditis, fever, and pericardial and pleural effusions.

_____ 114. Acute pericarditis is usually short-term, lasting approximately 2 to 6 days.

_____ 115. In chronic constrictive pericarditis, the pericardium becomes rigid, preventing adequate filling of the ventricles and eventually resulting in cardiac failure.

_____ 116. Tuberculosis can be a cause of chronic constrictive pericarditis.

_____ 117. Pericardiocentesis is a treatment for pericardial effusion.

118. The nurse is assessing the patient with pericarditis. In order to hear a pericardial friction rub, which technique does the nurse use?
    a. Place the diaphragm at the apex of the heart.
    b. Place the diaphragm at the right upper sternal border.
    c. Place the bell just below the left clavicle.
    d. Place the bell at several points while the patient holds his or her breath.

119. The patient is admitted for pericarditis. In order to assist the patient to feel more comfortable, what does the nurse instruct the patient to do?
    a. Sit in a semi-Fowler's position with pillows under the arms.
    b. Lie on the side in a fetal position.
    c. Sit up and lean forward.
    d. Lie down and bend the legs at the knees.

120. The nurse is reviewing the ECG of the patient admitted for acute pericarditis. Which ECG change does the nurse anticipate?
    a. Normal ECG
    b. ST-T spiking
    c. Peaked T waves
    d. Wide QRS complexes

121. The patient is admitted for pericarditis. How will the patient likely describe his pain?
    a. Grating substernal pain that is aggravated by inspiration.
    b. Sharp pain that radiates down the left arm.
    c. Dull ache that feels vaguely like indigestion.
    d. Continuous boring pain that is relieved with rest.

122. Which patient is at greatest risk for developing viral pericarditis?
    a. 35-year-old woman with tuberculosis
    b. 45-year-old man who has had radiation therapy for lung cancer
    c. 30-year-old man with a respiratory infection
    d. 50-year-old woman with chest trauma

123. What is the common treatment for rheumatic carditis?
    a. Pericardiocentesis
    b. Antibiotics for 10 days
    c. Pain medication for substernal pain control
    d. Rest with observation for further necessary treatment

124. Which medication is used to treat rheumatic carditis?
    a. Antibiotic (penicillin)
    b. NSAIDs
    c. Pain medications (opioids)
    d. Steroids

125. Assessment findings for the patient with acute pericarditis indicate neck vein distention, clear lungs, muffled heart sounds, tachycardia, tachypnea, and a greater than 10 mm Hg difference in systolic pressure on inspiration than on expiration. What is the nurse's first response to these assessment findings?
    a. Continue to monitor the patient; these are normal signs of pericarditis.
    b. Administer oxygen and immediately report the findings to the health care provider.
    c. Monitor oxygen saturation and seek order for pain medication to control symptoms.
    d. Check ECG, administer morphine for pain, and administer diuretics.

126. The patient had an emergency pericardiocentesis for cardiac tamponade. Which nursing interventions are included in the postprocedural care for this patient? *(Select all that apply.)*
    a. Closely monitor for the recurrence of tamponade.
    b. Be prepared to provide adequate fluid volumes to increase cardiac output.
    c. Be prepared to assist in emergency sternotomy if tamponade recurs.
    d. Administer diuretics to decrease fluid volumes around the heart.
    e. Send the pericardial effusion specimen to the laboratory for culture.

True or False? Read the statements about cardiomyopathies and write T for true or F for false in the blanks provided.

_____ 127. Dilated cardiomyopathy results in symptoms of left ventricular failure.

_____ 128. Arrhythmogenic right ventricular cardiomyopathy (dysplasia) results from replacement of myocardial tissue with fibrous and fatty tissue.

_____ 129. Sudden death may be the first manifestation of hypertrophic cardiomyopathy.

_____ 130. The earliest sign of restrictive cardiomyopathy is edema.

_____ 131. Dilated cardiomyopathy and restricted cardiomyopathy are initially managed in the same way as heart failure.

_____ 132. Heart transplantation is the treatment of choice for hypertrophic cardiomyopathy.

133. The patient who reports having a sore throat 2 weeks ago now reports chest pain. On physical assessment, the nurse hears a new murmur, pericardial friction rub, and tachycardia. ECG shows a prolonged P-R interval. What condition does the nurse suspect in this patient?
    a. Rheumatic carditis
    b. Heart failure
    c. Cardiomyopathy
    d. Aortic stenosis

134. The patient has received a heart transplant for dilated cardiomyopathy. Because the patient has a high risk for cardiac tamponade, for which sign/symptoms does the nurse immediately notify the provider?
    a. Crackles and wheezes of the lungs
    b. Pulsus paradoxus and muffled heart sounds
    c. Hepatomegaly and ascites
    d. Dependent edema and fluid retention

135. The nurse is assessing the patient who has received a heart transplant. Which clinical manifestations suggest transplant rejection? *(Select all that apply.)*
    a. Shortness of breath
    b. Depression
    c. Fluid loss or dehydration
    d. Severe abdominal pain
    e. New bradycardia
    f. Hypotension
    g. Decreased ejection fraction

CASE STUDY: THE PATIENT WITH HEART FAILURE

Use a separate sheet of paper to answer the questions in this Case Study. Answer guidelines for this Case Study are available on your Evolve website at http://evolve. elsevier.com/Iggy/ in the "Prepare for Class" folder.

A 74-year-old woman is admitted to the hospital with heart failure. She had been growing progressively weaker and had ankle edema, dyspnea on exertion, and three-pillow orthopnea. On admission, she is severely dyspneic and can answer questions only with one-word phrases. She is diaphoretic, with a heart rate of 132 beats/min, and blood pressure 98/70. She is extremely anxious.

1. Because this patient cannot breathe or talk easily, prioritize the immediate nursing assessments upon admission.

2. Considering the process of congestive heart failure, explain the symptoms she is having.

3. Based on assessment, identify priority nursing diagnoses for this patient.

4. The physician orders a treatment plan for this patient: Start an IV, then give dobutamine 3 mg/kg/hr IV; furosemide (Lasix) 40 mg IV stat; digoxin 0.5 mg orally stat, then 0.125 every 6 hours for three doses, with ECG before doses 3 and 4; morphine 2 mg IV stat and then 2 mg IV every 1 to 2 hours PRN; oxygen 4 L/min per nasal cannula; schedule for an echocardiogram; no added salt diet; weigh daily and monitor input and output.

Explain the rationale for these medications and treatments.

5. What should the nurse include in the discharge instructions for self-care for patients with heart failure? What will the nurse teach about the digoxin therapy?

6. The home health nurse is making an initial visit to the patient. What would the nurse include in the home care assessment?

38 CHAPTER

Care of Patients with Vascular Problems

STUDY/REVIEW QUESTIONS

True or False? *Read each statement and write T for true or F for false in the blanks provided. If the statement is false, correct the statement to make it true.*

_____ 1. Atherosclerosis usually affects the larger arteries, such as the coronary artery beds, the aorta, carotid and vertebral arteries, renal, iliac, or femoral arteries.

_____ 2. Atherosclerosis progresses for years before clinical manifestations are evident.

_____ 3. An example of a step one diet is 630 calories a day of fat in a 2100 calorie/day diet.

_____ 4. Any factor producing an increase in peripheral vascular resistance, heart rate, or stroke volume decreases the systemic arterial pressure.

_____ 5. Patients with low-density lipoprotein (LDL) values of 130 to 159 are advised to follow a fat-modified diet.

_____ 6. Intimal arterial damage may result from the effects of hypoglycemia.

_____ 7. Patients with severe diabetes mellitus frequently have premature and severe atherosclerosis from microvascular damage.

_____ 8. Generally, medications for hyperlipidemia should be taken with meals.

_____ 9. The systemic arterial pressure is a product of cardiac output (CO) and total peripheral vascular resistance (PVR).

_____ 10. Hypertension is a nonmodifiable factor that can be a major factor attributing to injury to the intimal layer.

11. The patient's cholesterol screening shows an high-density lipoprotein (HDL) value greater than 40, and a total serum cholesterol level of 188. The patient has no other cardiac or vascular risk factors. What does the nurse advise the patient to do?
    a. Modify the diet to exclude fats and increase fiber, then repeat tests.
    b. Contact the physician for a prescription of antilipemic medication.
    c. Repeat total and HDL cholesterol testing in 6 to 12 weeks.
    d. Repeat total and HDL cholesterol testing during the next routine exam.

12. The nurse is counseling a group of women about triglyceride levels. For women, what is a normal triglyceride level?
    a. Over 150 mg/dL
    b. Under 135 mg/dL
    c. Over 100 mg/dL
    d. Under 70 mg/dL

13. The patient has an elevated homocysteine level. Potentially, this may be lowered by what type of nutritional modification?
    a. Including enriched cereals that contain folic acid, vitamin B_6, and vitamin B_{12}
    b. A total fat intake of less than 30% of total calories
    c. Up to 10% of total calories from polyunsaturated fat
    d. Increasing fiber up to 25 to 35 g in the daily diet

14. The nurse is conducting dietary teaching with the patient. Which statement by the patient indicates an understanding of fat sources and the need to limit saturated fats?
    a. "Coconut oil has a rich flavor and is a good cooking oil."
    b. "Sunflower oil is high in saturated fats, so I should avoid it."
    c. "Meat and eggs mostly contain unsaturated fats."
    d. "Canola oil has monounsaturated fat and is recommended."

15. The nurse educates and advises the patient to follow the National Cholesterol Education Program (NCEP) Therapeutic Lifestyle Changes (TLC) diet. Which instruction does the nurse give to the patient?
    a. Review the literature and see what aspects of the program fit into the patient's current lifestyle.
    b. Return for serum cholesterol levels at 6 and 12 weeks after starting the diet.
    c. Record dietary intake and weight for 12 weeks and then call the physician.
    d. Weigh self once a week for 6 weeks and consult the physician if not losing weight.

16. The patient is prescribed atorvastatin (Lipitor). The nurse instructs the patient to watch for and report which side effect?
    a. Nausea and vomiting
    b. Cough
    c. Headaches
    d. Muscles cramps

17. The patient gets a new prescription for Pravigard for treatment of high cholesterol. Because this is a combination drug, the nurse alerts the physician when the patient discloses an allergy to which drug?
    a. Sulfa
    b. Aspirin
    c. Some calcium channel blockers
    d. Some diuretics

18. The patient is prescribed niacin (Niaspan) to lower low-density lipoprotein cholesterol (LDL-C) and very-low-density lipoprotein (VLDL). Why are lower doses prescribed to the patient?
    a. To prevent an elevation of hepatic enzymes
    b. To prevent muscle myopathies
    c. To prevent elevation of blood pressure
    d. To prevent undesirable hypokalemia

19. Complete the chart below by indicating target levels for cholesterol.

Cholesterol Test	Target Levels
Total serum cholesterol	
LDL-C level (for healthy people)	
LDL-C level (for people with CVD or diabetes)	
HDL-C level	

20. The nurse is conducting an initial cardiac-vascular assessment on a middle-aged patient. What techniques does the nurse include in the assessment? *(Select all that apply.)*
    a. Take blood pressure on the dominant arm.
    b. Palpate pulses at all of the major sites.
    c. Palpate for temperature differences in the lower extremities.
    d. Perform bilateral but separate palpation on the carotid arteries.
    e. Auscultate for bruits in the radial and brachial arteries.

21. The nurse is performing blood pressure screening at a community center. Which patients are referred for evaluation of their blood pressure? *(Select all that apply.)*
    a. Diabetic patient with a blood pressure of 118/78 mm Hg
    b. Patient with heart disease with a blood pressure of 134/90 mm Hg
    c. Patient with no known health problems who has a blood pressure of 125/86 mm Hg
    d. Diabetic patient with a blood pressure of 180/80 mm Hg
    e. Patient with no known health problems who has a blood pressure of 106/70 mm Hg

22. The home health nurse is making the initial visit to the older adult patient with hypertension. The nurse recommends that the patient obtain which item for home use?
    a. Ambulatory blood pressure monitoring device
    b. Exercise bicycle
    c. Blood glucose monitor scale
    d. Food scale

23. The nurse is evaluating the blood pressure of a 75-year-old woman. Based on current research, which finding is the better indicator of heart disease risk for this patient?
    a. Diastolic of 86 mm Hg
    b. Systolic of 160 mm Hg
    c. Blood pressure of 138/68 mm Hg
    d. Blood pressure of 110/90 mm Hg

24. The 32-year-old patient with diabetes reports sudden onset of headaches, blurred vision, and dyspnea. The patient's blood pressure is normally 120/80 mm Hg, but today is 200/130 mm Hg. What condition does the nurse suspect?
    a. Sustained hypertension
    b. Malignant hypertension
    c. Primary hypertension
    d. Secondary hypertension

25. Which are risk factors for hypertension? *(Select all that apply.)*
    a. Age greater than 40 years
    b. Family history of hypertension
    c. Excessive calorie consumption
    d. Physical inactivity
    e. Excessive alcohol intake
    f. Hypolipidemia
    g. High intake of salt or caffeine
    h. Increased intake of potassium, calcium, or magnesium

26. The patient's blood pressure reading is 128/80 mm Hg. Two weeks later, the patient's blood pressure is 130/84 mm Hg. One month later, the reading is unchanged. How is this patient's blood pressure classified?
    a. Normal
    b. Prehypertension
    c. Stage 1 hypertension
    d. Stage 2 hypertension

27. The nurse is taking a blood pressure on the new patient who reports headaches and dizziness. What technique does the nurse use to perform the blood pressure procedure?
    a. Take blood pressure readings in both arms; two or more readings are averaged as the value for the visit.
    b. Take the blood pressure in sitting and standing positions, with 15 minutes between position changes.
    c. Take the blood pressure with an automatic cuff, then retake it with a manual cuff to validate readings.
    d. Delegate the procedure to the unlicensed assistive personnel (UAP) and direct him or her to record the findings on the graphic sheet.

28. The nurse is reviewing the laboratory results of urine tests for the patient with a medical diagnosis of essential hypertension. The presence of catecholamines in the urine is evidence of which disorder?
    a. Renal failure
    b. Primary aldosteronism
    c. Cushing's syndrome
    d. Pheochromocytoma

29. The nurse is reviewing the electrocardiogram (ECG) for the patient with a medical diagnosis of essential hypertension. What is the first ECG sign of heart disease resulting from hypertension?
    a. Left atrial and ventricular hypertrophy
    b. Right atrial and ventricular atrophy
    c. Malfunction of the sinoatrial (SA) node
    d. Malfunction of the atrioventricular (AV) node

30. Which blood pressure findings for the adult patient with no other medical problems are evaluated further for hypertension? *(Select all that apply.)*
    a. 118/78 mm Hg
    b. 124/86 mm Hg
    c. 138/78 mm Hg
    d. 140/96 mm Hg
    e. 110/90 mm Hg

31. The middle-aged patient with no health insurance has tried lifestyle modifications to control uncomplicated hypertension, but continues to struggle. What is considered a first drug of choice for this patient?
    a. Calcium channel blocker
    b. Alpha blocker
    c. Thiazide-type diuretic
    d. Angiotensin-converting enzyme (ACE) inhibitor

32. Complete the chart below by indicating blood pressure readings for each classification.

Classification	Blood Pressure Measurement	Blood Pressure Readings
Normal	Systolic *and* diastolic	
Prehypertension	Systolic *or* diastolic	
Stage 1: Hypertension	Systolic *or* diastolic	
Stage 2: Hypertension	Systolic *or* diastolic	

33. The nurse is reviewing the medication schedule for the older adult patient who needs medication for hypertension. The patient lives alone, but is able to manage self-care. What frequency of drug therapy does the nurse advocate for this patient?
    a. Once a day
    b. Two times a day
    c. Three times a day
    d. Four times a day

34. The nurse is reviewing prescriptions for the patient recently diagnosed with hypertension. The nurse questions a prescription for which type of drug?
    a. Aldosterone receptor antagonist
    b. Alpha blocker
    c. Thiazide-type diuretic
    d. ACE inhibitor

35. For which patient does the nurse question the use of hydrochlorothiazide (HydroDIURIL)?
    a. Asthmatic patient
    b. Patient with chronic airway limitation
    c. Patient with chronic renal disease
    d. Patient with hyponatremia

36. The nurse is teaching the patient about taking hydrochlorothiazide (HydroDIURIL). Which food does the nurse instruct the patient to eat in conjunction with the use of this drug?
    a. Bananas and oranges
    b. Milk and cheese
    c. Cranberries and prunes
    d. Cabbage and cauliflower

37. The patient reports a sudden onset of cough after taking captopril (Capoten). What does the nurse instruct the patient to do?
    a. Monitor self for elevated temperature, sputum production, or flu-like symptoms.
    b. Use over-the-counter throat lozenges and increase oral fluid intake.
    c. Notify the prescribing physician because the medication should be discontinued.
    d. Call the pharmacist to get recommendations for an over-the-counter cough syrup.

38. Which intervention renders angiotensin II receptor blockers (ARBs) and angiotensin-converting enzyme (ACE) inhibitors effective in African Americans?
    a. Take with diuretics, a beta blocker, or calcium channel blocker.
    b. Give at a much higher dosage than for other ethnic groups.
    c. Combine with a rigorous lifestyle modification compliance.
    d. Take around the clock on a very individualized schedule.

39. The nurse is reviewing antihypertensive medication orders for the patient with asthma. The nurse questions the use of which type of medication?
    a. Cardioselective beta blockers because they reduce cardiac output
    b. Non-cardioselective beta blockers because they may inhibit bronchodilation
    c. ACE inhibitors because they cause a nagging cough
    d. Thiazide diuretics because they promote potassium excretion

40. The nurse prepares to teach the patient recovering from a myocardial infarction (MI) about combination drug therapy based on "best practice" for controlling hypertension. Which drugs does the nurse include in the teaching plan? *(Select all that apply.)*
    a. Beta blockers
    b. ACE inhibitors or ARBs
    c. Aldosterone antagonists
    d. Central alpha agonists
    e. NSAIDs
    f. Aspirin

41. The student nurse is giving the patient with benign prostatic hypertrophy a morning dose of terazosin (Hytrin). The student says, "This is your blood pressure medicine," but the patient responds, "I don't have high blood pressure." What does the student nurse do next?
    a. Explain to the patient that her blood pressure is not high because the drug is controlling it.
    b. Stop and recheck the medication administration record and then do additional drug research.
    c. Recheck the blood pressure, then hold the drug if blood pressure is not elevated.
    d. Contact the charge nurse for advice about how to handle the patient's refusal.

42. The patient admits to difficulty with long-term compliance to antihypertensive therapy. Which nursing intervention is most useful for this patient?
    a. Carefully review all the medication instructions with the patient.
    b. Give the patient written materials that reinforce the important points.
    c. Reinforce the fact that damage to organs occurs even if there are no symptoms.
    d. Teach the patient about the continuous ambulatory blood pressure monitoring device.

43. The nurse is reviewing medical records for several patients with kidney problems and actual or potential for hypertension. Which patient does the nurse expect to be screened for renal artery stenosis?
    a. Patient with a history of kidney stones
    b. Patient taking three categories of antihypertensive drugs at high doses
    c. Patient with newly diagnosed hypertension
    d. Patient with a history of frequent urinary tract infections

44. The patient with hypertension also has heart disease and type 2 diabetes mellitus. What is the blood pressure goal for this patient?
    a. 120/80 mm Hg
    b. 125/80 mm Hg
    c. 135/90 mm Hg
    d. 140/90 mm Hg

45. Which assessment findings are indicative of peripheral arterial disease (PAD) and which are indicative of peripheral vascular disease (PVD)? *(Write A for arterial and V for vascular.)*

    _____ a. Decreased peripheral pulses

    _____ b. Reproducible leg pain when walking that is relieved by rest

    _____ c. Neurologic assessment intact in legs

    _____ d. Edema around ankles

    _____ e. Paresthesia

    _____ f. Loss of hair

    _____ g. Skin is cool-to-cold to touch

    _____ h. Skin color is pale, dusky, mottled

    _____ i. Brown pigmentation of the legs

    _____ j. Dependent rubor

    _____ k. Thickened toenails

    _____ l. Pain in distal portion of extremity

    _____ m. Aching pain

    _____ n. Pain relieved in dependent position

    _____ o. Discomfort relieved with elevation

46. Which patients are at risk for PAD? *(Select all that apply.)*
    a. Hypertensive patient
    b. Patient with diabetes mellitus
    c. Patient who is a cigarette smoker
    d. Anemic patient
    e. Patient who is very thin
    f. African-American patient

47. Which symptom is the most common initial manifestation of PAD?
    a. Intermittent claudication
    b. Pain at rest
    c. Redness in the extremity
    d. Muscle atrophy

48. The nurse is caring for the patient with a medical diagnosis of inflow PAD. Which symptom does the nurse expect the patient to report?
    a. Very frequent episodes of rest pain
    b. Discomfort in the lower back, buttocks, or thighs after walking
    c. Burning or cramping in the calves, ankles, feet, or toes after walking
    d. Waking frequently at night to hang the feet off the bed

49. The nurse is assessing the lower extremity of the patient with PAD. What does the nurse palpate?
    a. Posterior tibial pulse of the affected leg
    b. Pedal pulses in both feet
    c. All pulses in both legs
    d. Strength of the pulses in the affected leg

50. While assessing the patient, the nurse sees a small, round ulcer with a "punched out" appearance and well-defined borders on the great toe. The patient reports the ulcer is painful. How does the nurse interpret this finding?
    a. Venous stasis ulcer
    b. Diabetic ulcer
    c. Gangrenous ulcer
    d. Arterial ulcer

51. The patient is undergoing diagnostic testing for pain and burning sensation in the legs. What does an ankle-brachial index (ABI) of less than 0.9 in either leg indicate?
    a. Normal arterial circulation to the lower extremities
    b. Presence of PAD
    c. Severe venous disease of the lower extremities
    d. Need for immediate surgical intervention

52. The nurse is consulting with the physical therapist to design an exercise program for patients with peripheral vascular disease. Which patient is a candidate for an exercise program?
    a. Patient with severe rest pain
    b. Patient with intermittent claudication
    c. Patient with gangrene
    d. Patient with venous ulcers

53. The patient with PAD asks, "Why should I exercise when walking several blocks seems to make my leg cramp up?" What is the nurse's best response?
    a. "Exercise may improve blood flow to your leg because small vessels will compensate for blood vessels that are blocked off."
    b. "This type of therapy is free and you can do it by yourself to improve the muscles in your legs."
    c. "The cramping will eventually stop if you continue the exercise routine. If you have too much pain, just rest for a while."
    d. "Exercise is a noninvasive nonsurgical technique that is used to increase arterial flow to the affected limb."

54. The nurse is teaching the patient with PAD about positioning and position changes. What suggestion does the nurse give to the patient?
    a. Sit upright in a chair if legs are not swollen.
    b. Sleep with legs above the heart level if legs are swollen.
    c. Avoid crossing the legs at all times.
    d. Change positions slowly when getting out of bed.

55. The nurse is instructing the patient with PAD about ways to promote vasodilation. What information does the nurse include? *(Select all that apply.)*
    a. Maintain a warm environment at home.
    b. Wear socks or insulated shoes at all times.
    c. Apply direct heat to the limb by using a heating pad.
    d. Prevent cold exposure of the affected limb.
    e. Limit fluids to prevent increased blood viscosity.
    f. Completely abstain from smoking or chewing tobacco.

56. The patient reports numbness or burning pain that is severe enough to disturb sleep at night. The patient also has dependent rubor. Which stage of PAD does the nurse suspect in this patient?
    a. I
    b. II
    c. III
    d. IV

57. The nurse is assessing the patient at risk for peripheral vascular disease. Which assessment finding indicates arterial ulcers rather than diabetic or venous ulcers?
    a. Ulcer located over the pressure points of the feet
    b. Ulcer of deep, pale color with even edges and little granulation tissue
    c. Severe pain or discomfort occurring at the ulcer site
    d. Associated ankle discoloration and edema

58. Which are complications that can result from severe PAD? *(Select all that apply.)*
    a. Gangrene
    b. Varicose veins
    c. Septicemia
    d. Amputation
    e. Ulcer formation

59. Which drugs are used to promote circulation in the patient with chronic PAD? *(Select all that apply.)*
    a. Pentoxifylline (Trental)
    b. Propranolol hydrochloride (Inderal)
    c. Aspirin
    d. Clopidogrel (Plavix)
    e. Ezetimibe (Zetia)

True or False? *Read the statements about percutaneous transluminal balloon angioplasty and write T for true or F for false in the blanks provided. For statements that are false, rewrite to make the statement true.*

_____ 60. A laser probe is advanced through a cannula into the stenosed/occluded artery to open the vessel lumen by heat from the laser vaporization.

_____ 61. This procedure is for the purpose of curing the patient of any atherosclerosis of the artery.

_____ 62. Preparation for this procedure is similar to that for a diagnostic angiography.

_____ 63. The nurse monitors for the primary complication of bleeding at the puncture site.

_____ 64. After the procedure, the patient is usually on bedrest with the limb straight for 6 to 8 hours.

_____ 65. The occurrence of reocclusion is rare in most patients.

66. The patient with PAD is scheduled to have percutaneous transluminal angioplasty (PTA). What information does the nurse give the patient about this procedure?
    a. It is usually used when amputation is inevitable.
    b. Reocclusion may occur afterwards and the procedure may be repeated.
    c. Most patients are occlusion-free afterwards, particularly if stents are placed.
    d. It is painless and there are very few risks or dangers.

67. The patient has returned to the unit after having PTA. What does the nurse include in the postprocedural care of this patient? *(Select all that apply.)*
    a. Observe for bleeding at the puncture site.
    b. Observe vital signs frequently.
    c. Perform frequent checks of the distal pulses in both limbs.
    d. Encourage bedrest with the limb straight for about 1 to 2 hours.
    e. Administer anticoagulant therapy such as heparin.
    f. Provide supplemental oxygen via nasal cannula.

68. The patient has returned to the unit after surgery for arterial revascularization with graft placement. The nurse monitors for graft occlusion which is most likely to occur within what time frame?
    a. First 2 hours
    b. First 24 hours
    c. Next 2 days
    d. First week

69. The patient is in the postanesthesia care unit (PACU) after surgery for arterial revascularization with graft placement. Which procedure does the nurse use to check the patency of the graft?
    a. Check the extremity every 15 minutes for the first hour, then hourly, for changes in color, temperature, and pulse intensity.
    b. Check the dorsalis pedis pulse every 15 minutes for the first hour, then hourly.
    c. Ask the patient if there is any pain or loss of sensation anywhere in the extremity, and withhold patient-controlled analgesia.
    d. Gently palpate the site every 15 minutes for the first hour and assess for warmth, redness, and edema.

70. The patient has returned to the unit after a PTA. What is the postprocedural nursing priority?
    a. Pain management
    b. Check the distal pulses
    c. Early ambulation to prevent complications
    d. Monitoring for bleeding at the puncture site

71. The student nurse is assisting in the care of the patient returning from the PACU after aortofemoral bypass. The nurse intervenes when the student performs which action?
    a. Offers to obtain a meal tray for the patient
    b. Demonstrates to the patient how to use the incentive spirometer
    c. Encourages the patient to deep breathe every 1 to 2 hours
    d. Explains to the patient the purpose of 24-hour bedrest

72. The patient has had surgery for arterial revascularization with graft placement. The nurse notes swelling, tenseness to the skin tissue, and the patient reports an increasing pain with numbness and tingling as well as a decrease in the ability to wiggle toes and ankles. What does the nurse suspect is occurring with this patient?
    a. Graft infection
    b. Compartment syndrome
    c. Graft occlusion
    d. Reaction to thrombolytic therapy

73. The patient has had aortoiliac bypass surgery with graft placement. The nurse notes induration, erythema, tenderness, warmth, edema, and drainage at the site. Before calling the physician, what additional assessment does the nurse perform?
    a. Palpates the patient's abdomen and checks for the last bowel movement
    b. Auscultates the patient's lung sounds and checks the pulse oximeter reading
    c. Assesses the patient for signs of occult bleeding and looks at the PT results
    d. Checks the patient's temperature and looks at the white blood cell results

74. The patient is admitted with a medical diagnosis of acute arterial occlusion. What documentation does the nurse expect to see in this patient's medical record?
    a. Acute MI and/or atrial fibrillation within the previous weeks
    b. History of chronic venous stasis disease treated with débridement and wound care
    c. History of Marfan syndrome or Ehlers-Danlos syndrome
    d. Episode of blunt trauma that occurred several months ago

75. The patient with an acute arterial occlusion requires abciximab (ReoPro). What nursing responsibilities are associated with the administration of this platelet inhibitor?
    a. Platelet counts must be monitored at 3, 6, and 12 hours after the start of the infusion.
    b. For platelet counts over 100,000/mm³, infusion must be readjusted or discontinued.
    c. Monitor for manifestations of rash, itching, or swelling.
    d. Monitor for edema, pain on passive movement, or poor capillary refill.

76. Which is a postoperative nursing intervention for the patient with arterial revascularization?
    a. Promote graft patency by limiting IV fluid infusion.
    b. Instruct the patient to avoid bending at the hips or knees.
    c. Resume regular diet immediately after surgery.
    d. Avoid cough and deep-breathing exercises.

Matching. Match the types of aneurysms with their descriptions.

Types of Aneurysms
a. Dissecting aneurysm
b. Saccular
c. Fusiform

Descriptions

_____ 77. Involves the entire circumference of the artery

_____ 78. Involves a distinct portion of the artery

_____ 79. Is caused by blood in the wall of the artery

80. What is the most common location for an aneurysm?
    a. Abdominal aorta
    b. Thoracic aorta
    c. Femoral arteries
    d. Popliteal arteries

81. What is the most common cause of an aneurysm?
    a. Emboli
    b. Trauma
    c. Atherosclerosis
    d. Thrombus formation

82. The patient is suspected to have an abdominal aortic aneurysm (AAA). What does the nurse assess for?
    a. Abdominal, flank, or back pain
    b. Chest pain and shortness of breath
    c. Hoarseness and difficulty swallowing
    d. Disruption of bowel and bladder patterns

83. The 75-year-old man with a history of atherosclerosis comes to the emergency department (ED) with abdominal pain. What findings indicate a possible AAA? *(Select all that apply.)*
    a. Left-sided chest pain
    b. Abdominal, flank, or back pain
    c. Visible pulsation on the upper abdominal wall
    d. Hoarseness
    e. Difficulty swallowing

84. The patient with an AAA is admitted to the hospital. Which test does the physician order to confirm an accurate diagnosis as well as to determine the size and location of the AAA? *(Select all that apply.)*
    a. Abdominal x-rays
    b. Ultrasound
    c. Electrocardiogram
    d. Magnetic resonance imaging
    e. Computed tomography

85. The patient is diagnosed with a small 3 cm AAA. What is the best nonsurgical intervention to decrease the risk of rupture of an aneurysm and to slow the rate of enlargement?
    a. Maintenance of normal blood pressure and avoidance of hypertension
    b. Bedrest until there is shrinkage of the aneurysm
    c. Heparin and Coumadin therapy to decrease clotting
    d. Intra-arterial thrombolytic therapy

86. The patient with a ruptured aneurysm may exhibit which symptoms? *(Select all that apply.)*
    a. Bradypnea
    b. Tachycardia
    c. Increased systolic pressure
    d. Decreased blood pressure
    e. Severe pain
    f. Diaphoresis
    g. Loss of pulses distal to rupture
    h. Decreased level of consciousness

87. Which action does the nurse take first if the patient has a suspected aneurysm rupture?
    a. Start an IV infusion with a large-bore needle.
    b. Assess baseline measurements of blood pressure and pulse rate.
    c. Palpate the pulsating abdominal mass to determine its size.
    d. Assess all peripheral pulses to use as a baseline for comparison.

88. The patient has had a repair of an AAA. For what reason is this patient being monitored postoperatively for urinary output and renal function studies (creatinine and BUN)?
    a. The patient was probably in shock preoperatively, and there may be glomerular damage.
    b. The patient is usually in a critical care nursing unit where this is done routinely.
    c. The aorta was clamped during the surgery and the kidneys may have been inadvertently damaged.
    d. Repair of the aneurysm improves renal perfusion and the urinary output should increase.

89. The patient has had an aneurysm repair. Which activity does the nurse suggest as an example of appropriate exercise during the recovery period?
    a. Playing golf
    b. Washing dishes
    c. Raking leaves
    d. Driving a car

90. The patient is admitted for a medical diagnosis of detectable AAA. What does the nurse expect to find documented in the patient's description of symptoms?
    a. Hematuria and painful urination that started very suddenly
    b. Steady and gnawing abdominal pain unaffected by movement and lasting for days
    c. No subjective complaints of pain, but episodes of dizziness
    d. Pain in the lower extremities exacerbated by walking and relieved by rest

91. While assessing the patient with AAA, the nurse notes a pulsation in the upper abdomen slightly to the left of the midline between the xyphoid process and the umbilicus. What does the nurse do next?
    a. Measure the mass with a ruler.
    b. Palpate the mass for tenderness.
    c. Percuss the mass to determine the borders.
    d. Auscultate for a bruit over the mass.

92. The patient was admitted for AAA with a pulsating abdominal mass. The nurse notes a sudden onset of diaphoresis, decreased level of consciousness, a blood pressure of 88/60 mm Hg, and an irregular apical pulse. Oxygen is in place via mask. What is the priority nursing action?
    a. Establish IV access.
    b. Alert the Rapid Response Team.
    c. Auscultate for a bruit and assess the mass.
    d. Place the patient on the cardiac monitor.

93. The nurse is reviewing the radiologist's report of the abdominal x-ray of the patient suspected of having AAA. The report notes an "eggshell" appearance. How does the nurse interpret this data?
    a. Validates the presence of an aneurysm
    b. Suggests an artifact; therefore, the x-ray must be repeated
    c. Indicates a congenital anomaly that will obscure the aneurysm
    d. Indicates the aneurysm is the size of an egg

94. The nurse is designing a teaching plan for the patient with a small (4 cm) AAA. The patient is currently asymptomatic. What is the nurse's goal for nonsurgical management of this patient?
    a. Teach lifestyle modifications that will minimize the growth of the aneurysm.
    b. Monitor the growth of the aneurysm and follow the antihypertensive medication regimen.
    c. Encourage compliance with anticoagulant drugs and laboratory follow-up appointments.
    d. Stabilize the patient's condition and improve overall health so surgery can be safely performed.

95. The nurse is performing preoperative care for the patient who is having an elective surgery for AAA resection. What is included in this patient's care? (Select all that apply.)
    a. Bowel preparation
    b. Instruction on coughing and deep breathing
    c. Blood type and cross-match
    d. Administration of a large volume IV fluid bolus
    e. Assessment of all peripheral pulses
    f. Use of a marker to note where the pulse is palpated or heard by Doppler

96. The patient who has had AAA surgical repair develops chest pain, shortness of breath, diaphoresis, anxiety, and restlessness. These symptoms are consistent with which postoperative complication?
    a. Myocardial infarction
    b. Graft occlusion
    c. Renal failure
    d. Paralytic ileus

97. The nurse notes a change in pulses, a cool extremity below the graft, bluish discoloration to the flanks, and abdominal distention in the patient who has had AAA surgical repair. These symptoms are consistent with which postoperative complication?
    a. Ischemic colitis
    b. Cerebral and spinal cord ischemia
    c. Graft occlusion or rupture
    d. Thoracic outlet syndrome

98. The patient is admitted through the ED for emergency surgery of a ruptured aneurysm. Why does the nurse monitor the patient for renal failure?
    a. A Foley catheter was inserted under potentially nonsterile conditions.
    b. Aggressive fluid management in the ED could overload the kidneys.
    c. Hypovolemia associated with rupture can result in acute tubular necrosis.
    d. Medications used in the emergency procedure are nephrotoxic.

99. The patient who had surgery for an AAA was just extubated. What does the nurse do in caring for this patient for the next 24 hours?
    a. Assess respiratory rate and depth every hour.
    b. Turn and suction the patient every 2 hours.
    c. Discourage coughing and deep breathing.
    d. Assist the patient to a bedside chair.

100. The nurse is performing an assessment on the patient who had AAA repair the day before. The nurse does not hear any bowel sounds when auscultating the abdomen. What does the nurse do next?
    a. Continue to monitor the patient; paralytic ileus is expected for 2 to 3 days.
    b. Obtain an order for a nasogastric tube set to low suction.
    c. Report assessment findings immediately to the surgeon.
    d. Palpate for distention and ask the patient to ambulate.

101. The nurse is assessing the patient with a ruptured AAA. Which assessment finding is most likely to be present?
    a. Retroperitoneal hemorrhage
    b. Mass may be visible above the suprasternal notch
    c. Hoarseness and difficulty swallowing
    d. Disruption of bowel and bladder patterns

102. The patient who had a thoracic aortic aneurysm repair has been progressing well for several days after the surgery, but today tells the nurse, "My toes and lower legs feel a little numb and tingly." What does the nurse do next?
    a. Encourage the patient to do active range-of-motion exercises in bed.
    b. Help the patient get up, dangle the legs, and then ambulate.
    c. Assess extremities for sensation, movement, or pulse changes.
    d. Instruct UAP to assist the patient in elevating the legs.

103. The nurse is caring for the patient who had a repair of a thoracic aneurysm. What does the nurse monitor for in this patient? (*Select all that apply.*)
    a. Cardiac dysrhythmias
    b. Paraplegia
    c. Respiratory distress
    d. Hemorrhage
    e. Pericarditis

104. The patient has had a repair of a thoracic aneurysm. What does the nurse monitor for in this patient and immediately report to the surgeon?
    a. Productive cough when using the incentive spirometer
    b. Increased drainage from chest tubes
    c. Sternal pain with coughing and deep breathing
    d. Increased urinary output from the indwelling catheter

105. The patient is considering endovascular stent grafts. What is one of the advantages of this procedure?
    a. Decreased length of hospital stay
    b. Less risk for hemorrhage
    c. Decreased incidence of postprocedural rupture
    d. Use of local, rather than general, anesthesia

106. The home health nurse is making the first visit to the patient who had a surgical aneurysm repair. In evaluating the home situation, what does the nurse observe that is cause for concern?
    a. The patient has been having groceries delivered for several weeks.
    b. There is a calendar hanging on the refrigerator with medication times.
    c. The patient's bedroom and bathroom access are on the ground floor.
    d. The patient decides to vacuum the house and clean out the garage.

107. The patient comes to the ED with anterior chest pain described as a "tearing" sensation. The patient is diaphoretic, nauseated, faint, apprehensive, and blood pressure is 200/130 mm Hg. Which medication is most likely to be ordered for this patient?
    a. Antianginal such as nitroglycerin (Nitro-bid)
    b. Antihypertensive such as sodium nitro-prusside (Nipride)
    c. Calcium channel antagonist such as amlo-dipine (Norvasc)
    d. Beta blocker such as propranolol (Inderal)

108. Indicate whether the signs and symptoms below are related to Buerger's disease (BD) or Raynaud's disease (RD).

    _____ a. Occurs in smokers and often in young males

    _____ b. Occurs in both sexes, predominately female

    _____ c. Episodic, causing white then blue fingers

    _____ d. Triggered by exposure to cold or tobacco

    _____ e. Occurs in medium and small arteries and veins

    _____ f. Severe episodes may lead to gangrene

Matching. *Match the physical findings with their related arterial disorders.*

Arterial Disorders
a. Popliteal entrapment
b. Subclavian steal
c. Thoracic outlet syndrome

Physical Findings

_____ 109. Blood pressure different in each arm

_____ 110. Intermittent claudication in one or both legs

_____ 111. Intermittent neck and shoulder pain

112. The young male patient is diagnosed with early stage Buerger's disease. What assessment finding does the nurse expect to find in the patient's record?
    a. Claudication of the arch of the foot
    b. Intolerance of warm environments
    c. Dizziness and lightheadedness
    d. Pain in the lower back with ambulation

113. The nurse is teaching the patient with Buerger's disease about self-care. What is the most important point that the nurse emphasizes?
    a. Lower intake of fat and reducing cholesterol to reverse the disease process.
    b. Perform daily exercise for fingers or toes to slow the progress of the disease.
    c. Limit exposure to extreme or prolonged cold temperatures because of vasoconstriction.
    d. Cease cigarette smoking and tobacco use to arrest the disease process.

114. The patient reports tiredness in the arm with exertion, paresthesia, dizziness, and exercise-induced pain in the forearm when the arms are elevated. The nurse suspects subclavian steal. What physical assessment does the nurse perform?
    a. Check blood pressure in both arms.
    b. Auscultate for a carotid bruit.
    c. Check for orthostatic hypotension.
    d. Observe the arm for redness or edema.

115. The patient who is an avid golfer is diagnosed with thoracic outlet syndrome. What does the nurse advise the patient that is specific to this syndrome?
    a. Rest if shortness of breath occurs.
    b. Avoid walking long distances.
    c. Avoid elevating the arms.
    d. Perform deep-breathing exercises.

116. The patient is a 25-year-old woman who reports bilateral blanching of both upper extremities that occurs in cold temperatures. She reports numbness and cold sensation, and afterwards the arms become very red. What are these symptoms consistent with?
    a. Raynaud's disease
    b. Buerger's disease
    c. Subclavian steal
    d. Raynaud's phenomenon

117. Which medication is the patient with Raynaud's disease most likely to be prescribed?
    a. Lovastatin (Mevacor)
    b. Coumadin (Warfarin)
    c. Nifedipine (Procardia)
    d. Captopril (Capoten)

True or False? Read the statements about venous disorders and write T for true or F for false in the blanks provided. If the statement is false, correct the statement to make it true.

_____ 118. Classic signs and symptoms of deep vein thrombosis (DVT) are always present.

_____ 119. Checking for Homans' sign should be done to assess for a DVT.

_____ 120. The focus of treatment for a DVT is to prevent complications and increase in size of the thrombus.

_____ 121. DVTs are often treated medically with rest, anticoagulants, elevation of legs, and compression stockings.

_____ 122. Thrombolytic therapy must be initiated within 24 hours of symptom onset.

_____ 123. To prevent leg edema, elevate legs when in bed or in a chair.

_____ 124. Thrombus formation has been associated with hyperlipidemia, hyperglycemia, and/or hypertension, known as *Virchow's triad*.

_____ 125. The highest incidence of clot formation occurs in patients who have undergone hip surgery, total knee replacement, or open prostate surgery.

_____ 126. Severe infections, systemic lupus erythematosus, polycythemia vera, oral contraceptives, and trauma have also been linked to thrombosis.

_____ 127. Cancer, especially adenocarcinoma of the visceral organs, is the most common malignancy associated with DVT.

_____ 128. Venograms are the best and most common diagnostic test for DVT.

_____ 129. Unfractionated heparin (UFH) is an anticoagulant agent that will break up the clot.

130. The patient is admitted to the hospital with a DVT. Which drug therapy does the nurse expect the health care provider to order?
    a. Heparin 5000 units subcutaneously twice a day
    b. Loading high dose of Coumadin, then smaller doses on following days
    c. Alternate heparin and Coumadin depending on the laboratory values
    d. Heparin via IV infusion, with Coumadin therapy started at the same time

131. What test is the most definitively preferred noninvasive test to diagnose a DVT?
    a. Venogram
    b. Duplex ultrasonography
    c. X-ray films
    d. CT scan

132. Which sign/symptom in the patient with DVT receiving heparin therapy does the nurse report to the health care provider immediately?
    a. Pruritus
    b. Rash
    c. Hematuria
    d. Tinnitus

133. What is the recommended therapeutic range for the International Normalized Ratio (INR) that is done along with prothrombin time in the patient receiving warfarin sodium (Coumadin)?
    a. 0.5 to 1.0
    b. 1.0 to 1.5
    c. 1.5 to 2.0
    d. 2.0 to 2.5

134. The patient prescribed warfarin sodium (Coumadin) is instructed that certain foods decrease the effect of the drug. Which foods, if eaten, must be consumed in consistent and small amounts each day?
    a. Fresh fruits
    b. Chicken and beef
    c. Spinach and asparagus
    d. Milk and cheese

135. The nurse is teaching the patient who is at risk for venous thromboembolism (VTE). The patient is currently asymptomatic and is living in the community. What interventions does the nurse instruct the patient to do to minimize the risk of VTE? *(Select all that apply.)*
    a. Avoid oral contraceptives.
    b. Drink adequate fluids to avoid dehydration.
    c. Exercise the legs during long periods of bedrest or sitting.
    d. Arise early in the morning for ambulation.
    e. Use a venous plexus foot pump.

136. The nurse is reviewing the diagnostic test results for the patient suspected of having a DVT. The results show a negative D-dimer test. How does the nurse interpret this data?
    a. The test excludes DVT.
    b. Venous duplex ultrasonography is needed.
    c. The patient has arterial disease.
    d. Impedance plethysmography is needed.

137. The health care provider has ordered UFH for the patient with DVT. Before administering the drug, the nurse ensures that which laboratory tests were obtained for baseline measurement? *(Select all that apply.)*
    a. Prothrombin time (PT)
    b. Activated partial thromboplastin time (APTT or aPTT)
    c. International Normalized Ratio (INR)
    d. Complete blood count (CBC) with platelet count
    e. Arterial blood gas
    f. Creatinine level
    g. Urinalysis

138. The nurse notes that the platelet count for the patient who is to receive UFH is 100,000/mm³. How does the nurse interpret this result?
    a. It is slightly lowered and worth monitoring for trends.
    b. It is significantly low, so the health care provider should be notified.
    c. It is insignificant unless other values such as PT or APTT are abnormal.
    d. It is higher than expected, but within normal limits for therapy.

139. The medication order for UFH is for 80 units/kg of body weight. How does the nurse interpret this order?
    a. Appropriate dose for the continuous IV infusion
    b. Higher than expected dose for the initial IV bolus
    c. Appropriate dose for the initial IV bolus
    d. Appropriate dose for maintenance therapy

140. The patient is receiving UFH therapy. The nurse instructs the UAP in which task related to the UFH therapy?
    a. Observe the skin for ecchymosis, bruising, and petechiae during AM hygiene.
    b. Replace the antiembolism devices after bathing or ambulating.
    c. Check on the patient every 2 hours and report changes in mental status.
    d. Watch for and report blood in the stool when assisting the patient with toileting.

141. The patient receiving UFH therapy is ordered to discontinue the therapy and begin low–molecular weight heparin (LMWH) and enoxaparin (Lovenox). What is the priority nursing intervention?
    a. Discontinue the UFH at least 30 minutes before the first LMWH injection.
    b. Check the APTT results after giving the first LMWH injection.
    c. Assess the patient's IV site before starting the LMWH.
    d. Check the PT and INR results before giving the first LMWH injection.

142. What are the contraindications for thrombolytic therapy for DVT? *(Select all that apply.)*
    a. Recent surgery
    b. Trauma
    c. Stroke
    d. Diabetes mellitus
    e. Spinal injury

143. The patient is receiving thrombolytic therapy. How does the nurse monitor for the most serious complication from thrombolytic therapy?
    a. Performing neurologic checks and monitoring for level of consciousness
    b. Auscultating for breath sounds and counting respiratory rates
    c. Assessing the IV site and watching for infiltration and swelling
    d. Checking patency of the Foley catheter and monitoring urinary output

144. The nurse is teaching the patient about the side effects and potential problems associated with taking warfarin sodium (Coumadin). Which statement by the patient indicates a correct understanding of the nurse's instruction?
    a. "If I notice bleeding of the gums, I should skip one or two doses of the medication."
    b. "I should eat a lot of cabbage, cauliflower, and broccoli to prevent bleeding."
    c. "For injury and bleeding, I should apply direct pressure and seek medical assistance."
    d. "I should avoid going to the dentist while I am taking this medication."

145. The patient with a history of vascular disease as a result of diabetes has developed a peripheral neuropathy. This patient is at risk for which nursing diagnoses?
    a. Fatigue
    b. Acute Pain
    c. Risk for Injury
    d. Decreased Cardiac Output

True or False? Read the statements about the use of an Unna boot in patients with venous stasis ulcers and write T for true or F for false in the blanks provided. If the statement is false, rewrite the statement to make it true.

_____ 146. The boot is a type of dressing applied by a health care provider and changed daily.

_____ 147. The boot consists of a gauze dressing that is moistened with Betadine or soaked in hydrogen peroxide.

_____ 148. The boot is covered with elastic wrap that hardens like a cast to promote venous circulation.

_____ 149. The boot promotes healing by forming a sterile environment for the ulcer.

_____ 150. The boot is applied around the ankle.

_____ 151. The ulcer is cleaned with normal saline only before application of dressing.

_____ 152. Instruct the patient to assess for signs and symptoms of arterial occlusion if the boot is too tight.

153. The nurse is assessing the obese patient's lower leg and notes a small irregular-shaped ulcer over the medial malleolus with brownish discoloration. The patient reports that the "leg has been that way for a long time." What do these findings suggest to the nurse?
    a. Varicose vein
    b. Venous stasis ulcer
    c. Phlebitis
    d. Raynaud's phenomenon

154. The nurse is consulting with the nutritionist about diet therapy for the patient with chronic venous stasis ulcers. What are the dietary recommendations to help this patient promote wound healing?
    a. High-protein foods
    b. Vitamin D and B supplements
    c. Low-fat foods
    d. High-calcium foods

155. The patient has a venous stasis ulcer that requires a dressing. Which dressing materials are selected for this type of wound? *(Select all that apply.)*
    a. Oxygen-permeable polyethylene film
    b. Oxygen-impermeable hydrocolloid dressing
    c. Dry gauze dressings
    d. Artificial skin products
    e. Unna boot
    f. Vacuum-assisted wound closure

156. The nurse is assessing the patient with distended, protruding veins. In order to assess for varicose veins, what technique does the nurse use?
    a. Place the patient in a supine position with elevated legs; as the patient sits up, observe the veins filling from the proximal end.
    b. Place the patient in the Trendelenburg position and observe the distention and protruding of the veins.
    c. Ask the patient to stand and observe the leg veins; then ask the patient to sit or lie down and observe the veins.
    d. Ask the patient to walk around the room and observe the veins; then have the patient rest for several minutes and reassess the veins.

157. The patient with varicose veins asks the nurse to provide a list of all available treatment options. What does the nurse include on the list? *(Select all that apply.)*
    a. Elastic stockings and elevation of the extremities
    b. Sclerotherapy
    c. Stab avulsion technique
    d. Vein stripping
    e. Application of radio frequency (RF) energy
    f. Endovenous laser treatment
    g. Anticoagulant therapy

158. The nurse is assessing the IV site of the patient who has been receiving a normal saline infusion. There is redness, warmth radiating up the arm with pain, soreness, and swelling. What does the nurse do next?
    a. Discontinue the IV and apply warm moist soaks.
    b. Slow the infusion rate and reassess within 1 hour.
    c. Discontinue the IV and apply a cold pack.
    d. Contact the health care provider for an order for an antidote.

159. Which patient has the greatest risk for a pulmonary embolus related to a venous disorder?
    a. Patient with bilateral varicose veins
    b. Patient with phlebitis of superficial veins
    c. Patient with thrombophlebitis in a deep vein of the lower extremity
    d. Patient with venous insufficiency throughout the leg

160. What information does the nurse include when teaching the patient with chronic venous stasis? *(Select all that apply.)*
    a. Elevate the legs when sitting.
    b. Avoid crossing the legs.
    c. Wear antiembolic stockings at night during sleep.
    d. Avoid standing still for any length of time.
    e. Avoid wearing tight girdles, tight pants, and narrow-banded knee-high socks.

161. Which patient is at greatest risk for developing varicose veins?
    a. 37-year-old mail carrier
    b. 19-year-old retail store clerk
    c. 40-year-old operating room scrub technician
    d. 25-year-old pregnant woman in the first trimester

162. What is the preferred treatment for phlebitis?
    a. Dry heat
    b. Ice packs
    c. Warm, moist packs
    d. Massage and elevation

163. Which type of vascular injury is most likely to result from blunt trauma?
    a. Arteriovenous fistula
    b. Hematoma
    c. Dissection
    d. Incompetent valves

164. Which patient with vascular trauma is a candidate for immediate emergency surgery?
    a. 54-year-old with fractured humerus
    b. 36-year-old with a ruptured renal artery
    c. 18-year-old with a contusion of the pelvis
    d. 67-year-old with a chronic subdural hematoma

165. The patient arrives in the ED with severe trauma from a gunshot wound. Identify in order of priority the management of vascular trauma using the numbers 1 through 6.
    _____ a. Prepare the patient for arteriography.
    _____ b. Restore of blood flow.
    _____ c. Control bleeding.
    _____ d. Ask about mechanism of injury, blood loss, and symptoms after the injury.
    _____ e. Assess for circulatory, sensory, or motor impairment.
    _____ f. Establish patent airway.

166. The nurse observes diminished pulses, cold skin, and a pulsatile mass over the femoral artery in the patient reporting pain in the right leg. What condition does the nurse suspect in this patient?
    a. Venous thromboembolism
    b. Buerger's disease
    c. Femoral aneurysm
    d. Popliteal entrapment

CASE STUDY: THE PATIENT WITH HYPERTENSION

Use a separate sheet of paper to answer the questions in this Case Study. Answer guidelines for this Case Study are available on your Evolve website at http://evolve. elsevier.com/Iggy/ in the "Prepare for Class" folder.

The patient is a 64-year-old African American man who is diagnosed with hypertension. He is 6 feet tall and weighs 300 pounds. He smokes two packs of cigarettes per day. He works as a salesman and has two to three alcoholic drinks a week. He admits that he does not get as much exercise as he used to when he was 40 years old. His mother and brother have high blood pressure, and his father died of a heart attack at age 68.

1. Does he have essential or secondary hypertension? Can this be determined at this point? Give a rationale for the answer.

2. What diseases would have made this patient at risk for developing secondary hypertension?

3. What cultural aspects need to be considered in controlling his hypertension?

4. How does this patient's age impact the diagnosis and treatment of hypertension?

5. During the initial workup for hypertension, what laboratory testing would be ordered? Explain.

6. An interdisciplinary team consult was completed. What assessment findings would indicate successful outcomes have been met?

7. This patient was later seen in the ED with severe headache, extremely high blood pressure, dizziness, blurred vision, and disorientation. His diagnosis is malignant hypertension. Describe the medical interventions for this problem.

CASE STUDY: THE PATIENT WITH DEEP VEIN THROMBOSIS

Use a separate sheet of paper to answer the questions in this Case Study. Answer guidelines for this Case Study are available on your Evolve website at http://evolve. elsevier.com/Iggy/ in the "Prepare for Class" folder.

A 58-year-old woman was discharged from the hospital 4 days ago after lower abdominal surgery. She has been readmitted for pain and edema in her right calf. She has a tentative diagnosis of thrombophlebitis.

1. Discuss the probable etiology of this patient's thrombophlebitis.

2. The physician prescribes heparin sodium 1000 units per hour intravenously for this patient, and also begins therapy with warfarin (Coumadin). Discuss the purpose of these medications, the nursing precautions, and laboratory tests to monitor their effectiveness.

3. The patient asks, "Which medication dissolves the clot? The IV or the pill?" What does the nurse say to her? How does heparin differ from warfarin in the treatment of thrombophlebitis?

4. This patient is placed on strict bedrest with her legs elevated, and a warm, moist pack is to be applied. What are the purposes of these interventions?

5. The following morning, the patient reports leg cramps and asks the nurse to massage her calf because it is "cramping." Should the nurse comply with this request? Why or why not?

6. The patient's activated partial thromboplastin time is 70 seconds (normal range is 22.1 to 34.1 seconds) and the INR is 1. Discuss the significance of these test results.

7. The patient's laboratory values are now within therapeutic ranges, and the patient is being discharged from the hospital on Coumadin. Develop a teaching-learning plan for this patient.

CASE STUDY: THE PATIENT WITH BYPASS SURGERY FOR PAD

Use a separate sheet of paper to answer the questions in this Case Study. Answer guidelines for this Case Study are available on your Evolve website at http://evolve. elsevier.com/Iggy/ in the "Prepare for Class" folder.

A 77-year-old woman has just had femoral-popliteal bypass surgery to treat severe arterial disease.

1. What are the six Ps that are assessed for after femoral-popliteal bypass surgery in relation to arterial flow and lack of oxygenation to the tissues? Indicate techniques, equipment, and principles that are used by the nurse to assess these findings.

2. Which of the six Ps written above is often the first indicator of a graft site occlusion and requires immediate attention from the physician? Give an explanation for the answer.

3. What is the procedure to be followed if a graft occlusion occurs?

4. What is compartment syndrome? What assessments should be performed to detect compartment syndrome?

5. The patient is discharged home and a home health nurse is coming to make the initial visit. What type of assessments should the nurse make?

39 CHAPTER

Care of Patients with Shock

STUDY/REVIEW QUESTIONS

Matching. Match the terms with their correct definitions.

Terms
a. Dilation
b. Sympathetic tone
c. Exogenous
d. Endogenous
e. Anaphylaxis
f. Sepsis
g. Capillary leak syndrome
h. Anoxic
i. Ischemic
j. Vasoconstriction

Definitions

_____ 1. Allergic reactions that result in widespread loss of blood vessel tone and decreased cardiac output

_____ 2. Increase in diameter of vessel walls by relaxing the smooth muscle

_____ 3. Widespread infection that triggers a whole body inflammatory response

_____ 4. State of partial blood vessel constriction

_____ 5. No oxygen

_____ 6. Originate outside the body

_____ 7. Substances normally found in the body

_____ 8. Cell dysfunction or death from lack of oxygen

_____ 9. Mediators change blood vessel integrity and allow fluid to shift from the vascular space to the interstitial tissues

_____ 10. Decrease in diameter by contracting the muscle

Fill in the blanks.

11. Shock is a condition rather than a disease and represents the "whole-body" response that occurs when too little _____ is delivered to the tissues.

12. Shock is a "syndrome" because the cellular, tissue, and organ events that occur in response to its presence happen in a _____ sequence.

13. During shock, compensation by the _____ nervous system, the _____ system, and the cardiovascular system attempt the continued oxygenation of vital organs.

14. Total blood volume and _____ output are directly related to mean arterial pressure (MAP).

15. Some organs, such as the _____ and _____, can tolerate low levels of oxygen for hours without dying or being damaged.

16. Which hormones are released in response to decreased MAP? *(Select all that apply.)*
    a. Insulin
    b. Renin
    c. Antidiuretic hormone (ADH)
    d. Epinephrine
    e. Aldosterone
    f. Serotonin

17. The patient has decreased oxygenation and impaired tissue perfusion. Which clinical manifestation is evidence that the patient's body is attempting to compensate?
    a. Decreased urine output
    b. Low-grade fever
    c. Change of mental status
    d. Decreased pulse rate

18. Which statement about the systemic effects of shock is correct?
    a. The liver is essentially unaffected, but liver enzymes may be lower than normal.
    b. The current heart rate and blood pressure indicate cardiac system is at baseline.
    c. The brain and neurologic system can withstand 10 to 15 minutes of severe hypoperfusion.
    d. The kidneys can tolerate hypoxia and anoxia up to 1 hour without permanent damage.

19. Which patients are at risk for shock related to fluid shifts? *(Select all that apply.)*
    a. Hypoglycemic patient
    b. Severely malnourished patient
    c. Patient with paralytic ileus
    d. Patient with kidney disease
    e. Patient with minor burns
    f. Patient with large wounds

20. The young woman comes to the emergency department (ED) with lightheadedness and "a feeling of impending doom." Pulse is 110 beats/min; respirations 30/min; blood pressure 140/90 mm Hg. Which factors does the nurse ask about that could contribute to shock? *(Select all that apply.)*
    a. Recent accident or trauma
    b. Prolonged diarrhea or vomiting
    c. History of depression or anxiety
    d. Possibility of pregnancy
    e. Use of over-the-counter medications

21. The nurse is caring for the patient with cardiogenic shock. What is the priority for managing this patient?
    a. Prepare for open heart surgery.
    b. Insert an intra-aortic balloon pump.
    c. Administer a thromboembolic agent.
    d. Determine and treat the cause of the shock.

22. Which patient has the highest risk for cardiogenic shock?
    a. Patient with a history of angina
    b. Patient with a recent myocardial infarction
    c. Patient with chronic atrial fibrillation
    d. Patient with a functional pacemaker

23. The patient has cardiac dysrhythmias and pulmonary problems as a result of receiving an IV antibiotic. What type of shock does this represent?
    a. Hypovolemic
    b. Cardiogenic
    c. Anaphylactic
    d. Septic

24. The patient with a head injury was treated for a cerebral hematoma. After surgery, this patient is at risk for what type of shock?
    a. Obstructive
    b. Cardiogenic
    c. Distributive-chemical
    d. Distributive-neural

25. The nurse is performing the AM shift assessment on several patients. The nurse is immediately concerned about decreased tissue perfusion if the capillary refill time was delayed for which patient?
    a. Patient with diabetes mellitus
    b. Anemic patient
    c. Patient with peripheral vascular disease
    d. Asthmatic patient

26. The nursing student takes the morning blood pressure of the postoperative patient and the reading is 90/50 mm Hg. What does the student do next?
    a. Report the reading to the primary nurse as a possible sign of hypovolemia.
    b. Assess the patient for subjective feelings of dizziness or shortness of breath.
    c. Check the patient's chart for trends of morning vital sign readings.
    d. Notify the instructor to verify the significance of the finding.

27. The patient at risk for shock has had some small and subtle changes in behavior within the past hour. How does the nurse evaluate the patient's mental status throughout the night?
    a. Assess the patient while he or she is awake, and then allow him or her to sleep until morning.
    b. Ask the patient and family to describe the patient's normal sleep and behavioral patterns.
    c. Periodically attempt to awaken the patient and document how easily he or she is aroused.
    d. Allow the patient to sleep, but assess respiratory effort and skin temperature.

Matching. Match the overall pathophysiology response that occurs with various types of shock.

Types of Shock
a. Hypovolemic
b. Cardiogenic
c. Distributive
d. Obstructive

General Pathophysiology Responses

_____ 28. Total body fluid volume not affected

_____ 29. Fluid shifted from central vascular space

_____ 30. Total body fluid decreased (in all fluid compartments)

_____ 31. Direct pump failure

Matching. Match either the colloid or crystalloid solution with each of the indications. Answers will be used more than once.

Solutions
a. Colloid
b. Crystalloid

Indications

_____ 32. Hemorrhagic shock

_____ 33. Fluid replacement

_____ 34. Restore osmotic pressure

_____ 35. Carries oxygen to peripheral tissues

_____ 36. Does not cause allergic reactions

_____ 37. Substitute for blood

38. Identify solutions as colloids (Col) or crystalloids (Cry).

    _____ a. Normal saline

    _____ b. Hetastarch

    _____ c. Packed red cells

    _____ d. Ringer's lactate

    _____ e. Fresh frozen plasma (FFP)

39. The nurse is caring for the patient at risk for hypovolemic shock. Which indicator of shock does the nurse monitor for?
    a. Elevated body temperature
    b. Absent peristalsis
    c. Decreasing urine output
    d. Vasodilation

40. Assessment findings of the patient with trauma injuries reveals cool, pale skin; reported thirst, urine output 100 mL/8 hr, blood pressure 122/78 mm Hg, pulse 102 beats/min, respirations 24/min with decreased breath sounds. This patient is in what phase of shock?
    a. Compensatory/nonprogressive
    b. Progressive
    c. Refractory
    d. Multiple organ dysfunction

41. The patient has been NPO for several hours in preparation for a scheduled procedure and now reports subjective thirst. What is the nurse's priority action?
    a. Get the patient a few ice chips or a moistened toothette.
    b. Obtain an order for a stat hematocrit and hemoglobin.
    c. Take the patient's vital signs and compare to baseline.
    d. Obtain an order to increase the IV rate.

42. The patient is brought to the ED with a gunshot wound. The nurse closely monitors the patient for early signs of hypovolemic shock. What early sign does the nurse look for?
    a. Elevated serum potassium level
    b. Marked decrease in blood pressure
    c. Decreased in oxygen saturation
    d. Increase in heart and respiratory rate

43. The unlicensed assistive personnel (UAP) reports repeatedly and unsuccessfully trying to take the patient's blood pressure with the electronic and manual devices. The nurse notes that the patient's apical pulse is elevated and the patient is at risk for hypovolemic shock. The patient begins to deteriorate. What is the quickest way for the nurse to determine the systolic blood pressure?
    a. Apply the electronic device to a lower extremity.
    b. Instruct the UAP to immediately get the Doppler.
    c. Apply the manual cuff and palpate for the systolic.
    d. Tell the UAP to try the electronic device on the other arm.

44. The nurse identifies signs and symptoms of internal hemorrhage in the postoperative patient. What is included in the care of this patient in hypovolemic shock? *(Select all that apply.)*
    a. Elevate the feet with the head flat or elevated 30 degrees.
    b. Monitor vital signs every 5 minutes until they are stable.
    c. Administer clotting factors or plasma in phase 1.
    d. Administer heparin in phase 2.
    e. Provide oxygen therapy.
    f. Ensure IV access.
    g. Notify the Rapid Response Team.

45. The young trauma patient is at risk for hypovolemic shock related to occult hemorrhage. What baseline indicator allows the nurse to recognize the early signs of shock?
    a. Urine output
    b. Pulse rate
    c. Fluid intake
    d. Skin color

46. Which patient is most likely to show elevated hemoglobin and hematocrit during shock?
    a. Patient with severe vomiting and large watery diarrheal stools
    b. Patient with a large wound with copious drainage
    c. Patient who was stable after surgery, but is now decompensating
    d. Patient with a hemothorax and chest tube

47. The patient in hypovolemic shock is receiving sodium nitroprusside (Nitropress) to enhance myocardial perfusion. What is an important nursing implication for administering this drug?
    a. Assess the patient for headache because it is an early symptom of drug excess.
    b. Assess blood pressure at least every 15 minutes because hypertension is a symptom of overdose.
    c. Assess blood pressure at least every 15 minutes because systemic vasodilation can cause hypotension.
    d. Assess the patient every 30 minutes for extravasation because nitroprusside can cause severe vasoconstriction and tissue ischemia.

48. The patient is at risk for hypovolemia secondary to large amounts of watery diarrhea and vomiting. The patient reports feeling a little thirsty and a slightly lightheaded. What does the nurse do next?
    a. Take the blood pressure and pulse and compare results to the patient's baseline.
    b. Obtain an order to start a sodium nitroprusside (Nipride) IV infusion.
    c. Have the patient rest in bed and take small frequent sips of water.
    d. Compare the patient's intake to the urinary output.

49. The patient with hypovolemia is restless and anxious. The skin is cool and pale, pulse is thready at a rate of 135 beats/min; blood pressure is 92/50 mm Hg; respirations are 32/min. What does the nurse do next?
    a. Give an IV normal saline bolus.
    b. Administer supplemental oxygen.
    c. Notify the Rapid Response Team.
    d. Place the patient in a semi-Fowler's position.

50. The patient is showing early clinical manifestations of hypovolemic shock. The physician orders an arterial blood gas (ABG). Which ABG values in does the nurse expect to see in hypovolemic shock?
    a. Increased pH with decreased Pao_2 and increased $Paco_2$
    b. Decreased pH with decreased Pao_2 and increased $Paco_2$
    c. Normal pH with decreased Pao_2 and normal $Paco_2$
    d. Normal pH with decreased Pao_2 and decreased $Paco_2$

51. The nurse finds the patient on the bathroom floor. There is a large amount of blood on the floor and on the patient's hospital gown. What does the nurse do next?
    a. Elevate the patient's legs.
    b. Establish large-bore IV access.
    c. Look for the source of the bleeding.
    d. Ensure a patent airway.

52. The nurse is caring for the postoperative patient who had major abdominal surgery. Which assessment finding is consistent with hypovolemic shock?
    a. Pulse pressure of 40 mm Hg
    b. A rapid, weak, and thready pulse
    c. Warm, flushed skin
    d. Increased urinary output

53. Which IV therapy results in the greatest increase in oxygen-carrying capacity for the patient with hypovolemic shock?
    a. Lactated Ringer's solution
    b. Hetastarch
    c. FFP
    d. Packed red cells

54. The patient comes to the ED with severe injury and significant blood loss. The nurse anticipates that resuscitation will begin with which fluid?
    a. Whole blood
    b. Ringer's lactate
    c. 0.9% sodium chloride
    d. Plasma protein fractions

55. Which change in the skin is an early indication of hypovolemic shock?
    a. Pallor or cyanosis in the mucous membranes
    b. Color changes in the trunk area
    c. Axilla and groin feel moist or clammy
    d. Generalized mottling of skin

56. The patient is in hypovolemic shock related to hemorrhage from a large gunshot wound. Which order does the nurse question?
    a. Establish a large-bore peripheral IV and give crystalloid bolus.
    b. Give furosemide (Lasix) 20 mg slow IVP.
    c. Insert a Foley catheter and monitor intake and output.
    d. Give high-flow oxygen via mask at 10 L/min.

57. After discharge from the hospital, what is a common psychosocial problem faced by the patient who has suffered from hypovolemic shock?
    a. Confusion related to loss of fluids
    b. Anxiety regarding recurrence of shock or fear of dying
    c. Inability to perform activities of daily living
    d. Acceptance of resulting self-care limitations

58. Complete the chart below with parameters that are associated with sepsis and septic shock.

Parameter	Normal	Early Sepsis	Late Sepsis	Septic Shock
Cardiac output	normal 3-5 L/min			
Stroke volume	normal 60-80 mL			
Serum lactate (arterial)	< 2 mmol/L			
Blood glucose	< 110 mg/dL			
Oxygen saturation	95-100%			

59. The patient has a systemic infection with a fever, increased respiratory rate, and change in mental status. Which laboratory values does the nurse seek out that are considered "hallmark" of sepsis?
    a. Increased white blood count and increased glucose level
    b. Increased serum lactate level and rising band neutrophils
    c. Increased oxygen saturation and decreased clotting times
    d. Decreased white blood count with increased hematocrit

60. The nurse is caring for the older adult patient at risk for shock. What is an early sign of shock in this patient?
    a. Cool, clammy skin
    b. Decreased urinary output
    c. Restlessness
    d. Hypotension

61. The nurse is caring for the patient with sepsis. At the beginning of the shift, the patient is in a hypodynamic state. Several hours later, the patient's blood pressure is elevated and pulse is bounding. How does the nurse interpret this change?
    a. A positive response and a signal of recovery
    b. Temporary situation that is likely to normalize
    c. Worsening of the condition rather than improvement
    d. Expected response to standard therapies

62. The nurse is caring for the patient with sepsis. What is a late clinical manifestation of shock?
    a. Drop in blood pressure
    b. MAP is decreased by less than 10 mm Hg
    c. Tachycardia with a bounding pulse
    d. Increased urine output

63. The nurse is caring for the patient at risk for sepsis. Why does the nurse closely monitor the patient for early signs of shock?
    a. The patient is unable to self-identify or report these early signs.
    b. Distributive shock usually begins as a bacterial or fungal infection.
    c. Prevention of septic shock is easier to achieve in the early phase.
    d. There is widespread vasodilation and pooling of blood in some tissues.

64. The patient has a localized infection. What assessment findings are considered evidence of a beneficial inflammatory response?
    a. Decreased urine output which normalizes after fluid bolus
    b. Pulse rate of 120 beats/min related to increased metabolic activity
    c. Decreased oxygen saturation which responds to supplemental O_2
    d. Redness and edema that appear but subside in several days

65. The student nurse is assessing the patient's mental status because of the patient's risk for decreased tissue perfusion. The supervising nurse intervenes when the student nurse asks the patient which question?
    a. "What is today's date?"
    b. "Who is the president of this country?"
    c. "Where are we right now?"
    d. "Is your name Mr. John Smith?"

66. The nurse is caring for the patient at risk for septic shock from a wound infection. In order to prevent systemic inflammatory response syndrome, the nurse's priority is to monitor which factor?
    a. Patient's pulse rate and quality
    b. Patient's electrolyte imbalance
    c. Localized infected area
    d. Patient's intake and output

67. The nurse is evaluating the care and treatment for the patient in shock. Which finding indicates that the patient is having an appropriate response to the treatment?
    a. Blood pH of 7.28
    b. Arterial Po_2 of 65 mm Hg
    c. Distended neck veins
    d. Increased urinary output

68. The nurse is caring for the patient with septic shock. Which therapy specific to the management of shock for this patient does the nurse anticipate will be used?
    a. Inotropics
    b. Antibiotics
    c. Colloids
    d. Antidysrhythmics

69. The patient receives dopamine 20 mcg/kg/min IV for the treatment of shock. What does the nurse assess for while administering this drug?
    a. Decreased urine output and decreased blood pressure
    b. Increased respiratory rate and increased urine output
    c. Chest pain and hypertension
    d. Bradycardia and headache

70. When administering norepinephrine (Levophed), what does the nurse monitor for in the patient?
    a. Extravasation
    b. Profuse sweating
    c. High output renal failure
    d. Chest pain

71. The nurse is caring for the patient in septic shock. The nurse notes that the rate and depth of respirations is markedly increased. The nurse interprets this as a possible manifestation of the respiratory system compensating for which condition?
    a. Metabolic acidosis
    b. Metabolic alkalosis
    c. Respiratory acidosis
    d. Respiratory alkalosis

72. The ICU nurse observes petechiae, ecchymoses, and blood oozing from gums and other mucous membranes of the patient with septic shock. How does the nurse interpret this finding?
    a. Pulmonary emboli (PE)
    b. Acute respiratory distress syndrome (ARDS)
    c. Systemic inflammatory response syndrome (SIRS)
    d. Disseminated intravascular coagulation (DIC)

73. The nurse is reviewing the laboratory results of the patient with a systemic infection. What is the significance of a "left shift" in the differential leukocyte count?
    a. Expected finding because the patient has a serious infection.
    b. Indication that the infection is progressing toward resolution.
    c. Indication that the infection is outpacing the white cell production.
    d. Important to watch for trends, but otherwise not urgently significant.

74. The ICU nurse is caring for the patient with septic shock. Which IV infusion order for this patient does the nurse question?
    a. Antibiotics
    b. Insulin
    c. Heparin
    d. Synthetic activated C protein

75. The nurse has identified in the patient the nursing diagnosis of Deficient Knowledge related to prevention of septic shock. What does the nurse include in the teaching plan for this at-risk patient? *(Select all that apply.)*
    a. Wash hands frequently using antimicrobial soap.
    b. Avoid aspirin and aspirin-containing products.
    c. Avoid large crowds or gatherings where people might be ill.
    d. Do not share utensils; wash toothbrushes in a dishwasher.
    e. Take temperature once a week.
    f. Do not change pet litter boxes.

76. The patient is at risk for sepsis. Which assessment finding is most indicative of the hyperdynamic activity that occurs in septic shock?
    a. Crackles in lung bases
    b. Weak, rapid peripheral pulses
    c. Cool, clammy, and cyanotic skin
    d. Increased pulse rate with warm, pink skin

77. The home health nurse is visiting a frail older adult patient at risk for sepsis because of failure to thrive and immunosuppression. What does the nurse assess this patient for? *(Select all that apply.)*
    a. Signs of skin breakdown and presence of redness or swelling
    b. Cough or any other symptoms of a cold or the flu
    c. Appearance and odor of urine, and pain or burning during urination
    d. Patient's and family's understanding of isolation precautions
    e. Presence of pets, especially cats, rodents, or reptiles
    f. Availability and type of facilities for handwashing

78. The postoperative hospitalized patient has a decrease in MAP of greater than 20 mm Hg from baseline value; elevated, thready pulse; decreased blood pressure; shallow respirations of 26/min; pale skin; moderate acidosis; and moderate hyperkalemia. This patient is in what phase of shock?
    a. Compensatory/nonprogressive
    b. Progressive
    c. Refractory
    d. Multiple organ dysfunction

79. The 70-year-old man is admitted to the hospital with an infected finger of several days' duration. He is lethargic, confused, and has a temperature of 101.3° F. Other assessment findings include blood pressure of 94/50 mm Hg, pulse 105 beats/min, respirations 40, and shallow breathing. Pulmonary arterial wedge pressure (PAWP) is 4 mm Hg. These assessment findings indicate what type of shock?
    a. Hypovolemic
    b. Cardiogenic
    c. Anaphylactic
    d. Septic shock

80. The clinical manifestations in the first phase of sepsis-induced distributive shock results from the body's reaction to which factor?
    a. Leukocytes
    b. Endotoxins
    c. Hemorrhage
    d. Hypovolemia

81. What factor increases the older adult's risk for distributive (septic) shock?
    a. Reduced skin integrity
    b. Diuretic therapy
    c. Cardiomyopathy
    d. Musculoskeletal weakness

True or False? *Read the statements about shock and write T for true or F for false in the blanks provided. If the statement is false, correct the statement to make it true.*

_____ 82. Regardless of the cause, the pathophysiologic cellular response is the same for all types of shock.

_____ 83. When shock occurs, the body fails and death is the inevitable result.

_____ 84. The most reliable indicator that causes the nurse to suspect shock in the patient is changes in the systolic blood pressure.

_____ 85. Anaphylaxis results in widespread loss of blood vessel tone and decreased cardiac output.

_____ 86. Oxygen administration is appropriate therapy for any type of shock.

_____ 87. Examples of external causes of hypovolemic shock are trauma, wounds, and surgery.

_____ 88. Dehydration as a result of decreased fluid intake or increased fluid loss can cause hypovolemic shock.

_____ 89. Distributive shock is a result of a decrease in the MAP caused by a loss of sympathetic tone, blood vessel dilation, pooling of blood in venous and capillary beds, and increased blood vessel permeability (leak).

_____ 90. During the hyperdynamic phase of septic shock, the endotoxins cause a decrease in cardiac output.

_____ 91. The clinical manifestations of the first phase of septic shock are unique, often opposite to other types of shock, and therefore can be misinterpreted by the health care provider as a shock state.

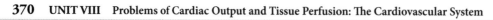

Matching. Match each type of patient who may be at risk with the corresponding type of shock. Answers may be used more than once.

Types of Shock
a. Hypovolemic
b. Cardiogenic
c. Distributive-neurogenic
d. Obstructive
e. Distributive-chemical
f. Distributive-septic

Types of Patients

_____ 92. Patient with cardiac tamponade

_____ 93. Older adult with urinary tract infection

_____ 94. Patient who had an allergic reaction to a medication

_____ 95. Patient who had a myocardial infarction

_____ 96. Patient who had a ruptured aortic aneurysm

_____ 97. Patient with tension pneumothorax

_____ 98. Patient with insect bites

_____ 99. Patient with ruptured spleen resulting from trauma

_____ 100. Patient with pneumonia

_____ 101. Patient with pulmonary hypertension

_____ 102. Patient receiving heparin therapy

_____ 103. Older adult who has a spinal cord re-union

_____ 104. Patient with dehydration

_____ 105. Patient with diabetes insipidus

_____ 106. Older adult with sacral pressure ulcers

_____ 107. Patient who has cancer of the head and neck, with a nasogastric tube

_____ 108. Patient with methicillin-resistant *Staphylococcus aureus* (MRSA) infection

_____ 109. Patient receiving excessive diuretic therapy

CASE STUDY: THE PATIENT WITH HYPOVOLEMIC SHOCK

Use a separate sheet of paper to answer the questions in this Case Study. Answer guidelines for this Case Study are available on your Evolve website at http://evolve. elsevier.com/Iggy/ in the "Prepare for Class" folder.

A 38-year-old female patient returned to the postanesthesia recovery area 2 hours ago after undergoing a tubal ligation by colposcopy (through the back wall of the vagina behind the cervix). Her last documented vital signs taken 30 minutes ago were blood pressure = 102/80 mm Hg, pulse = 88 beats/min, and respirations = 22/min. The nurse now notes that her face is pale and the skin around her lips has a bluish cast. She reports some back pain. Her vital signs are now blood pressure = 90/76 mm Hg, pulse = 98 beats/min, and respirations = 28/min.

1. What additional assessment techniques would the nurse perform?
2. Where would the nurse look for the hemorrhage?
3. What other data would the nurse gather?

The nurse reassesses the patient 15 minutes later. Vital signs are blood pressure = 88/70 mm Hg, pulse = 102 beats/min, and respirations = 30/min. She awakens when the nurse shakes her arm and reports increased back pain and thirst.

4. Given these findings, what are the priority nursing actions?
5. What expected outcomes would be specific to this situation?

CASE STUDY: THE PATIENT WITH SEPTIC SHOCK

Use a separate sheet of paper to answer the questions in this Case Study. Answer guidelines for this Case Study are available on your Evolve website at http://evolve. elsevier.com/Iggy/ in the "Prepare for Class" folder.

A 72-year-old male patient has been living in an assisted living center. He is generally alert, cheerful, and ambulatory with a walker. He has had frequent bouts of urinary tract infections secondary to prostate problems and is being treated for high blood pressure. He was discovered today by one of the UAPs in his room in a lethargic and confused state. He was easily aroused, but irritable and uncooperative with simple commands. He is transported to the ED for an acute change in mental status. On arrival to the ED, vital signs are 110/70 mm Hg, pulse = 120 beats/min, respirations = 30/min, and temperature is 101° F.

1. What factors increase the older adult's risk for septic shock?

2. What conditions predispose to sepsis and septic shock?

3. Does this patient meet the criteria for SIRS? If so, what are the initial indicators of SIRS for this patient? Based on the criteria, what additional assessments and diagnostic tests should be performed?

4. Explain why a patient in severe septic shock could "look" better and have a warm flushed appearance?

5. Explain why the patient can have a massive infection with a low white count.

6. What is the purpose of the sepsis resuscitation and management bundles? Discuss the care and interventions of the patient using the bundle approach.

7. The patient recovers and is discharged back to the assisted living facility. What types of information would the hospital nurse give to the nurse at the assisted living facility regarding the patient?

40 Care of Patients with Acute Coronary Syndromes

CHAPTER

STUDY/REVIEW QUESTIONS

Matching. Match the terms with their correct descriptions.

Terms

a. Ischemia
b. Infarction
c. Angina pectoris
d. New-onset angina
e. Variant (Prinzmetal's) angina
f. Pre-infarction angina
g. Transmural myocardial infarction (MI)
h. Ventricular remodeling
i. Zone of necrosis
j. Zone of injury
k. Zone of ischemia

Descriptions

_____ 1. Chest pain that occurs in the days or weeks before an MI

_____ 2. Necrosis or cell death

_____ 3. All three layers of heart are involved

_____ 4. First angina symptoms, usually after exertion or other increased demands on the heart

_____ 5. "Strangling of the chest"

_____ 6. Scar tissue permanently changes the size and shape of the entire left ventricle

_____ 7. Tissue that is oxygen-deprived

_____ 8. Around the initial area of infarction

_____ 9. Chest pain or discomfort from coronary artery spasm; typically occurs after rest

_____ 10. Tissue that is injured but not necrotic

_____ 11. Occurs when insufficient oxygen is supplied to meet the requirements of the myocardium

Fill in the blanks.

12. In acute coronary syndrome (ACS), it is believed that the atherosclerotic plaque in the coronary artery _____, resulting in platelet _____, thrombus _____, and vasoconstriction.

13. The artery has to have at least _____% plaque accumulation before it starts to occlude the artery wall.

14. Between 10% and 30% of patients with *unstable* angina progress to having a _____ in 1 year, and 29% die of this in _____ years.

15. According to the American Heart Association, the average age of a person having a first MI is _____ years for men and _____ years for women.

16. Infarction is a dynamic process that does not occur instantly; rather, it evolves over a period of several _____.

17. The actual extent of the zone of infarction depends on three factors:

    _____,

    _____, and workload demands on the myocardium.

18. The nurse is interviewing the patient reporting chest discomfort that occurs with moderate to prolonged exertion. The patient describes the pain as being "about the same over the past several months and going away with nitroglycerin or rest." Based on the patient's description of symptoms, what does the nurse suspect in this patient?
    a. Chronic stable angina (CSA)
    b. Unstable angina
    c. Acute coronary syndrome (ACS)
    d. Acute myocardial infarction (MI)

19. The patient with a history of angina is admitted for surgery. The patient reports nausea, pressure in the chest radiating to the left arm, appears anxious, skin is cool and clammy, blood pressure is 150/90 mm Hg, pulse is 100, and respiratory rate is 32. What is the priority nursing diagnosis?
    a. Ineffective Tissue Perfusion
    b. Anxiety
    c. Peripheral Neurovascular Dysfunction
    d. Nausea

20. The patient has been admitted for acute angina. Which diagnostic test identifies if the patient will benefit from further invasive management after acute angina or an MI?
    a. Exercise tolerance test
    b. Cardiac catheterization
    c. Thallium scan
    d. Multigated angiogram (MUGA) scan

21. The nurse is talking to the patient with angina about resuming sexual activity. Which statement by the patient indicates a correct understanding about the effects of angina on sexual activity?
    a. "I won't be able to resume the same level of physical exertion as I did before I had chest pain."
    b. "I will discuss alternative methods with my partner since I will no longer be able to have sexual intercourse."
    c. "If I cannot walk a mile, I am not strong enough to resume intercourse."
    d. "I can resume sexual activity after a rest period."

22. The patient with angina is prescribed nitroglycerin tablets. What information does the nurse include when teaching the patient about this drug? *(Select all that apply.)*
    a. "If one tablet does not relieve the angina after 5 minutes, take two pills."
    b. "You can tell the pills are active when your tongue feels a tingling sensation."
    c. "Keep your nitroglycerin with you at all times."
    d. "The prescription should last about 6 months before a refill is necessary."
    e. "If pain doesn't go away, just wait; the medication will eventually take effect."
    f. "The medication can cause a temporary headache or a flushed face."

23. The patient reports chest pain that is unrelieved with sublingual nitroglycerin. What drug does the nurse administer to this patient next?
    a. Valium intramuscularly
    b. Morphine sulfate IV
    c. Supplemental oxygen
    d. Chewable aspirin

24. The patient is hypertensive and continues to have angina despite therapy with beta blockers. The nurse anticipates which type of drug will be prescribed for this patient?
    a. Calcium channel blocker
    b. Digoxin
    c. Angiotensin-converting enzyme (ACE) inhibitor
    d. Dopamine

25. The nurse has just given the patient two doses of sublingual nitroglycerin for anginal pain. The patient's blood pressure is typically 130/80 mm Hg. Which finding warrants immediate notification of the health care provider?
    a. Patient reports a headache.
    b. Systolic pressure is 140 mm Hg.
    c. Systolic pressure is 100 mm Hg.
    d. Anginal pain continues but is somewhat relieved.

26. The patient is admitted for unstable angina. The patient is currently asymptomatic and all vital signs are stable. Which position does the nurse place the patient in?
    a. Any position of comfort
    b. Supine
    c. Sitting in a chair
    d. Fowler's

27. Place the steps for administering sublingual nitroglycerin to the patient with episodes of angina in the correct order using the numbers 1 through 5.

    _____ a. In 5-minute increments, a total of three doses may be administered in an attempt to relieve angina pain.

    _____ b. For no relief after dosing, immediately inform the health care provider and prepare the patient for transfer to a specialized unit.

    _____ c. Hold the tablet under the tongue so the tablet can dissolve.

    _____ d. After 5 minutes, recheck pain intensity and vital signs.

    _____ e. If the patient is experiencing some, but not complete, relief and vital signs remain stable, another tablet may be used.

28. Indicate whether the characteristics listed below are angina (A) or myocardial infarction (MI).

    _____ a. Pain is precipitated by exertion or stress.

    _____ b. Pain occurs without cause, usually in the morning.

    _____ c. Pain is relieved only by opioids.

    _____ d. Pain is relieved by nitroglycerin or rest.

    _____ e. Nausea, diaphoresis, feelings of fear, and dyspnea may occur.

    _____ f. There are few associated symptoms.

    _____ g. Pain lasts less than 15 minutes.

    _____ h. Pain lasts 30 minutes or more.

    _____ i. Pain radiates to left arm, back, or jaw.

True or False? Read each statement and write T for true or F for false in the blanks provided. If the statement is false, correct the statement to make it true.

_____ 29. Ischemia that occurs with angina is limited in duration and does not cause permanent damage of myocardial tissue.

_____ 30. Some women may experience atypical angina as indigestion or a choking sensation.

_____ 31. Angina in women has often been misdiagnosed.

_____ 32. Cardiac disease is the leading cause of death for men in the most prevalent ethnic groups, but not for women.

_____ 33. Premenopausal women have a lower incidence of MI than men do.

_____ 34. Postmenopausal women in their 70s have a higher incidence of MI than men.

_____ 35. More women than men die within 1 year of initial recognition of an MI.

_____ 36. For women, impaired glucose tolerance (e.g., diabetes) seriously increases the risk of coronary artery disease (CAD).

_____ 37. Catecholamines are released in response to hypoxia and pain which decrease the heart rate, contractility, and afterload.

_____ 38. The scarred tissue does not contract nor does it conduct electrically.

39. The patient is admitted for acute MI, but the nurse notes that the traditional manifestation of ST elevation MI (STEMI) is not occurring. What other evidence for acute MI does the nurse expect to find in the patient? *(Select all that apply.)*
    a. Positive troponin markers
    b. Chronic stable angina
    c. Non-ST elevation MI (non-STEMI)
    d. Cardiac dysrhythmia
    e. Heart failure

40. People should seek treatment for symptoms of MI rather than delay because physical changes will occur approximately how many hours after an infarction?
    a. 3
    b. 6
    c. 12
    d. 24

41. Place in order the steps that occur in cardiac tissues after an infarction using the numbers 1 through 5.
    _____ a. Granulation tissue forms at the edges of the necrotic tissue.
    _____ b. Infarcted region appears blue and swollen.
    _____ c. Scar tissue permanently changes the size and shape of the entire left ventricle.
    _____ d. Neutrophils invade the tissue and begin to remove the necrotic cells.
    _____ e. Necrotic area eventually develops into a shrunken, thin, firm scar.

42. The nurse is auscultating the heart of the patient who had an MI. Which finding most strongly indicates heart failure?
    a. Murmur
    b. S_3 gallop
    c. Split S_1 and S_2
    d. Pericardial friction rub

43. Which diagnostic test is used to assess myocardial damage caused by an MI?
    a. Positive chest x-ray
    b. Creatine kinase (CK) elevation
    c. ECG: ST depression
    d. CK-MB isoenzymes elevation

44. The patient has heart failure related to MI. What intervention does the nurse plan for this patient's care?
    a. Administering digoxin (Lanoxin) 1.0 mg as a loading dose and then daily
    b. Infusing IV fluids to maintain a urinary output of 60 mL/hr
    c. Titrating vasoactive drugs to maintain a sufficient cardiac output
    d. Observing for such complications as hypertension and flushed, hot skin

45. Which patient has the highest risk for death because of ventricular failure and dysrhythmias related to damage to the left ventricle?
    a. Patient with an anterior wall MI (AWMI)
    b. Patient with a posterior wall MI (PWMI)
    c. Patient with a lateral wall MI (LWMI)
    d. Patient with an inferior wall MI (IWMI)

46. The patient had an IWMI. The nurse closely monitors the patient for which dysrhythmia associated with IWMI?
    a. Bradycardia and second-degree heart block
    b. Premature ventricular contractions
    c. Supraventricular tachycardia
    d. Atrial fibrillation

47. The nurse is giving a community presentation about heart disease. Because 95% of sudden cardiac arrest victims die of ventricular fibrillation before reaching the hospital, which teaching point does the nurse emphasize?
    a. Controlling alcohol consumption and quitting cigarette smoking
    b. Modifying risk factors such as diet and weight, and blood pressure medication compliance
    c. Recognizing the difference between chronic stable angina and unstable angina
    d. Learning to operate the automatic external defibrillators (AEDs) in the workplace

48. What are indicators of metabolic syndrome, which increases the risk for coronary heart disease? *(Select all that apply.)*
    a. Triglyceride level of 170 mg/dL
    b. HDL cholesterol level of 45 mg/dL in a male
    c. HDL cholesterol level of 45 mg/dL in a female
    d. Blood pressure of 130/86 mm Hg
    e. Fasting blood sugar level of 120 mg/dL

49. The patient has high risk for CAD. What is the goal for this patient's LDL level?
    a. Less than 70 mg/dL
    b. Less than 100 mg/dL
    c. Below 135 mg/dL
    d. Below 200 mg/dL

50. The patient is trying to make dietary modifications to reduce lipid levels. The patient would like information about omega-3 fatty acid food sources. What best source does the nurse recommend?
    a. Flaxseed
    b. Flaxseed oil
    c. Fish
    d. Walnuts

True or False? *Read the statements about CAD and write T for true or F for false in the blanks provided. If the statement is false, correct the statement to make it true.*

_____ 51. Tobacco use, especially cigarette smoking, accounts for over 90% of deaths from CAD.

_____ 52. A person who stops smoking may decrease the risk of CAD by as much as 80% in 1 year.

_____ 53. Reducing the tar and nicotine content of the cigarettes smoked reduces the risk of CAD.

_____ 54. Less active, less fit people have a 30% to 50% greater risk of developing high blood pressure which predisposes to CAD.

_____ 55. Physical inactivity is more prevalent among women than men, among African Americans and Hispanics than Euro-Americans, among older than younger adults, and among the less affluent than the more affluent.

_____ 56. Intense exercise contributes to a major reduction in CAD risk.

_____ 57. Physical activity increases collateral circulation and reduces the size of existing plaques.

_____ 58. Work stress in particular may be associated with left ventricular hypertrophy.

59. Fill in the chart below for the Killip classification of heart failure.

Class	Description
I	
II	
III	
IV	

60. The patient comes to the walk-in clinic reporting left anterior chest discomfort with mild shortness of breath. The patient is alert, oriented, diaphoretic, and anxious. What does the nurse do next?
    a. Obtain a complete cardiac history to include a full description of the presenting symptoms.
    b. Place the patient in Fowler's position and start supplemental oxygen.
    c. Instruct the patient to go immediately to the closest full-service hospital.
    d. Immediately alert the physician and establish IV access.

61. The patient reports having chest discomfort that started during exercise. The patient is currently pain-free, but "is concerned." What questions does the nurse ask to assess the patient's pain episode? *(Select all that apply.)*
    a. "When did the pain start and how long did it last?"
    b. "What were you doing when the pain started?"
    c. "What did you do to alleviate the pain?"
    d. "How did you feel about the pain?"
    e. "Did the pain radiate to other locations?"
    f. "Was the pain sharp and stabbing?"
    g. "On a scale of 0 to 10 with 10 as the worst pain, what number would you use to categorize the pain?"

62. The patient is currently pain- and symptom-free, but reports having intermittent episodes of chest pain over the past week. The nurse asks about which associated symptoms? *(Select all that apply.)*
    a. Nausea
    b. Diarrhea
    c. Diaphoresis
    d. Dizziness
    e. Joint pain
    f. Palpitations
    g. Shortness of breath

63. The emergency department (ED) nurse is assessing the 86-year-old patient with acute confusion, increased respiratory rate, anxiety, and chest pain. The nurse finds a respiratory rate of 36/min with crackles and wheezes on auscultation. How does the nurse interpret these findings?
    a. Left sided-heart failure
    b. Atypical angina
    c. CAD
    d. Unstable angina

64. The nurse is assessing the middle-aged woman with diabetes who denies any history of known heart problems. However, on auscultation of the heart the nurse hears an S_4 heart sound. The nurse alerts the physician and obtains an order for which diagnostic test?
    a. Blood glucose level
    b. ECG
    c. Chest x-ray
    d. Echocardiogram

65. The nurse receives a phone call from the patient who says, "I'm having a little chest pain, some mild shortness of breath, and I have indigestion. Do you think I should take an antacid or an aspirin?" The nurse interprets these comments as evidence of which nursing diagnosis?
    a. Knowledge Deficit related to over-the-counter medication
    b. Powerlessness related to unfamiliar symptoms and situation
    c. Ineffective Denial which is a common early reaction to chest discomfort
    d. Readiness for Enhanced Self-Care related to cardiac symptoms

66. The middle-aged African-American patient with no known medical problems has acute onset chest pain and dyspnea. In order to rule out acute MI, the nurse obtains orders for which diagnostic tests?
    a. Triglyceride levels and C-reactive protein
    b. Chest x-ray, arterial blood gas, pulmonary function testing
    c. Total serum cholesterol, low-density lipoprotein, high-density lipoprotein
    d. Troponin T and I, creatine kinase-MB, myoglobin

67. The patient had severe chest pain several hours ago but is currently pain-free and has a normal ECG. Which statement by the patient indicates a correct understanding of the significance of the ECG results?
    a. "I'll go home and make an appointment to see my family doctor next week."
    b. "The ECG could be normal since I am currently pain-free."
    c. "A normal ECG means I am okay."
    d. "I have always had a strong heart, low blood pressure, and a normal ECG."

68. Which statement about silent MI is correct?
    a. In a silent MI, the patient does not have any pain, so there is less myocardial damage.
    b. Diabetic patients are prone to silent MI that goes undiagnosed without complications.
    c. Silent MI increases the incidence of new coronary events.
    d. In silent MI, the myocardium is oxygenated by increased collateral circulation.

69. The ED nurse is caring for the patient with acute pain associated with MI. What is the purpose of collaborative management for this patient?
    a. Return the vital signs and cardiac rhythm to baseline, so the patient can resume activities of daily living.
    b. Aggressively diagnose and treat life-threatening cardiac dysrhythmias and restore pulmonary wedge pressure.
    c. Closely monitor the patient for accompanying symptoms such as shortness of breath, nausea and vomiting, or indigestion.
    d. Eliminate discomfort by providing pain relief modalities, decrease myocardial oxygen demand, and increase myocardial oxygen supply

70. The ED nurse caring for the patient diagnosed with acute MI gives supplemental oxygen to the patient as ordered. Which medication does the nurse anticipate to give to this patient?
    a. IV nitroglycerin
    b. Beta blocker
    c. IV morphine
    d. Oral aspirin

71. The nurse is caring for the hospitalized patient being treated initially with IV nitroglycerin. What intervention does the nurse include in this patient's care?
    a. Increase the dose rapidly to achieve pain relief.
    b. Assist the patient to the bathroom as needed.
    c. Monitor blood pressure continuously.
    d. Elevate the head of the bed to 90 degrees

72. The patient is currently on oxygen therapy for chest pain. The pulse oximetry is on and signals an abrupt drop from 93% to 89%. What does the nurse do next?
    a. Alert the Rapid Response Team.
    b. Troubleshoot the oxygen setup and the pulse oximeter sensor.
    c. Increase the oxygen flow rate and elevate the head of the bed.
    d. Advise the patient to watch the monitor and take several deep breaths.

73. The home health nurse receives a call from the patient with CAD who reports having new onset of chest pain and shortness of breath. What does the nurse direct the patient to do?
   a. Rest quietly until the nurse can arrive at the house to check the patient.
   b. Chew 325 mg of aspirin and immediately call 911.
   c. Use supplemental home oxygen until symptoms resolve.
   d. Take three nitroglycerin tablets and have family drive the patient to the hospital.

74. The patient is newly diagnosed with cardiovascular disease. What psychosocial reactions does the nurse assess for? *(Select all that apply.)*
   a. Fear
   b. Anxiety
   c. Anger
   d. Suspicion
   e. Denial
   f. Euphoria
   g. Depression

75. Which drug is given within 1 to 2 hours of an MI, if the patient is hemodynamically stable, to help the heart to perform more work without ischemia?
   a. Vasodilators, such as sublingual or spray nitroglycerin (NTG)
   b. Beta-adrenergic blocking agents, such as metoprolol (Lopressor)
   c. Antiplatelet agents, such as clopidogrel (Plavix)
   d. Calcium channel blockers, such as diltiazem (Cardizem)

True or False? *Read the statements about thrombolytic agents used to dissolve thrombi in the coronary arteries and write T for true or F for false in the blanks provided. For statements that are false, correct the statement to make it true.*

_____ 76. Examples of agents are t-PA and reteplase (Retavase) (IV or intracoronary).

_____ 77. Thrombolytic agents are most effective when administered within the first 6 hours of the coronary event.

_____ 78. Streptokinase is the most commonly used thrombolytic agent.

_____ 79. Thrombolytic therapy is indicated for chest pain of duration greater than 1 hour that is unrelieved by other medication.

_____ 80. The nurse must monitor for bleeding by assessing IV site, laboratory values, and neurologic status.

81. The health care provider is considering use of thrombolytic therapy for the patient. What is the criterion for this therapy?
   a. Chest pain of greater than 15 minutes' duration that is unrelieved by nitroglycerin
   b. Indications of transmural ischemia and injury as shown by the ECG
   c. Ventricular dysrhythmias shown on the cardiac monitor
   d. History of chronic, severe, poorly controlled hypertension

82. The patient is being evaluated for thrombolytic therapy. What are contraindications for this procedure? *(Select all that apply.)*
   a. Ischemic stroke within 3 months
   b. Pregnancy
   c. Surgery within the last 10 days
   d. Major trauma in the last 12 months
   e. Intracranial hemorrhage
   f. Malignant intracranial neoplasm
   g. Deep vein thrombosis

83. The patient has received thrombolytic therapy for treatment of acute MI. What are post-administration nursing responsibilities for this treatment? *(Select all that apply.)*
   a. Document the patient's neurologic status.
   b. Observe all IV sites for bleeding and patency.
   c. Monitor WBC count and differential.
   d. Monitor clotting studies.
   e. Monitor hemoglobin and hematocrit.
   f. Test stools, urine, and emesis for occult blood.

84. The patient is receiving beta-blocker therapy for treatment of MI. What does the nurse monitor for in relation to this therapy? *(Select all that apply.)*
   a. Tachycardia
   b. Hypotension
   c. Decreased level of consciousness
   d. Chest discomfort
   e. Increased urinary output

85. The patient is being treated with medication therapy following an acute MI. The nurse questions the order for which type of drug?
   a. Calcium channel blocker
   b. Beta-blocker
   c. Angiotensin-converting enzyme (ACE) inhibitor
   d. Angiotensin receptor blocker (ARB)

86. The patient with angina is taking calcium channel blockers. What does the nurse monitor the patient for?
   a. Wheezes
   b. Hypotension
   c. Bradycardia
   d. Forgetfulness

87. Which diagnostic test is performed after angina or MI to determine cardiac changes that are consistent with ischemia, to evaluate medical interventions, and to determine whether invasive intervention is necessary?
   a. Stress test
   b. ECG
   c. Echocardiography
   d. Chest x-ray

88. The nurse is monitoring the patient who had fibrinolytics and percutaneous transluminal coronary angioplasty (PTCA). What is an indication that the clot has lysed and the artery reperfused?
   a. Abrupt increase of pain or discomfort
   b. Sudden onset of ventricular dysrhythmias
   c. Appearance of ST-segment depression
   d. Obvious T wave inversion

89. The patient has had an MI. The nurse anticipates which type of drug will be prescribed within 48 hours to prevent the development of heart failure?
   a. Calcium channel blockers
   b. ACE inhibitor
   c. Beta blockers
   d. Digoxin

90. The nurse has identified a nursing diagnosis of Activity Intolerance for the patient who had an acute MI. What is the best expected outcome for this patient?
   a. Patient will walk at least 200 feet four times a day without chest discomfort or shortness of breath.
   b. Patient will name three or four activities that will not cause shortness of breath or chest pain.
   c. Nurse will teach the patient to exercise and to take the pulse if symptoms of shortness of breath or pain occur.
   d. Nurse will assist the patient with ADLs until shortness of breath or pain resolves.

91. The patient is in the acute phase (phase 1) of cardiac rehabilitation. Which task is best to delegate to the unlicensed assistive personnel (UAP)?
   a. Assist the patient to ambulate approximately 200 feet three times a day.
   b. Assist the patient with ambulation to the bathroom.
   c. Assess heart rate, blood pressure, respiratory rate, and fatigue with each higher level of activity.
   d. Assist the patient into the bathtub.

92. The patient in the cardiac rehabilitation facility is having difficulty coping with the changes in the her health status. Which statement by the patient is the strongest indicator of ineffective or harmful coping?
   a. "I don't mind going to therapy, but I'm not sure if I'm getting any benefit from it."
   b. "I'll take the pills and just do whatever you want me to do."
   c. "I don't want to go to therapy; I had a bad experience yesterday with the therapist."
   d. "I know I need to talk about going home soon, but could we discuss it later?"

93. The post-MI patient in phase 1 cardiac rehabilitation is encouraged to perform which activity?
    a. Range-of-motion exercises
    b. Modified weight training
    c. Stair climbing
    d. Jogging

94. The nurse is caring for the patient admitted for an IWMI. The patient develops heart block with bradycardia. Because the patient's pulse rate is low and the blood pressure is unstable, which procedure is the nurse prepared to assist with?
    a. Temporary pacemaker
    b. Defibrillation
    c. 16-lead ECG
    d. Percutaneous intervention

95. The nurse is contacted by the cardiac monitoring technician who says the patient is having a dysrhythmia. What does the nurse do next?
    a. Identify the dysrhythmia.
    b. Administer antidysrhythmic medication.
    c. Evaluate for chest pain or discomfort.
    d. Double-check the lead placement.

96. The nurse is evaluating the patient with CAD. What is an expected patient outcome that demonstrates hemodynamic stability?
    a. Blood pressure and pulse within range and adequate for metabolic demands
    b. An increase in urine output
    c. Regular P waves and no abnormal heart sounds
    d. Verbal understanding of risk factors and need for compliance

97. The nurse is assessing the patient at risk for left ventricular failure and inadequate organ perfusion. Which signs and symptoms signal decreased cardiac output? *(Select all that apply.)*
    a. Change in orientation or mental status
    b. Urine output less than 1 mL/kg (2.2 lbs)/hr or less than 30 mL/hr
    c. Hot, dry skin with flushed appearance
    d. Cool, clammy extremities with decreased or absent pulses
    e. Unusual fatigue
    f. Recurrent chest pain

98. The nurse is reviewing medication orders for several cardiac patients. There is an order for beta-adrenergic blocking agent metoprolol XL (Toprol XR) once a day. This drug order is most appropriate for which class of patients according to the Killip classification system?
    a. All classes
    b. Class I only
    c. Class II and III
    d. Class IV only

99. The nurse is caring for the patient with an AWMI. The patient develops tachycardia, hypotension, urine output of 10 mL/hr, cold and clammy skin with poor peripheral pulses, and agitation. What does the nurse suspect in this patient?
    a. Ventricular dysrhythmia
    b. Cardiogenic shock
    c. Post-pericardiotomy syndrome
    d. Acute coronary syndrome

100. The nurse is assessing the cardiac patient and finds a paradoxical pulse, clear lungs, and jugular venous distention that occurs when the patient is in a semi-Fowler's position. What are these findings consistent with?
    a. Right ventricle failure
    b. Unstable angina
    c. CAD
    d. Valvular disease

101. The intensive care nurse is monitoring the patient with a right ventricular MI. The pulmonary artery wedge pressure (PAWP) reading is 30 mm Hg. What does the nurse do next?
    a. Increase the IV fluid rate to 200 mL/hour.
    b. Auscultate the lungs to assess for left-sided heart failure.
    c. Perform an ECG using right-sided precordial leads.
    d. Place the patient in semi-Fowler's position.

102. The patient continues to have chest pain despite compliance with medical therapy. The nurse gives the patient an educational brochure about which diagnostic test?
    a. Left-sided cardiac catheterization with coronary angiogram
    b. PTCA
    c. Coronary artery bypass grafting (CABG)
    d. Stent placement in coronary artery

103. Immediate reperfusion is an invasive intervention that shows some promise for managing which disorder?
    a. Right ventricular failure
    b. Metabolic syndrome
    c. Cardiogenic shock
    d. Acute coronary syndrome

104. The patient is scheduled to have PTCA. The nurse anticipates that an initial dose of which medication will be given before the procedure?
    a. Clopidogrel (Plavix)
    b. Nitroglycerin (Nitrostat)
    c. Isosorbide mononitrate (Imdur)
    d. Carvedilol (Coreg)

105. The patient has angina and is scheduled for PTCA. Based on outcomes of the PTCA, the nurse prepares the patient for immediate transfer to undergo which procedure?
    a. Intra-aortic balloon pump
    b. CABG
    c. Cardiac catheterization
    d. Carotid endarterectomy

106. The nurse is caring for the patient who had PTCA. Which symptom indicates acute closure of the vessel and therefore warrants immediate notification of the health care provider?
    a. Chest pain
    b. Hyperkalemia
    c. Bleeding at the insertion site
    d. Cough and shortness of breath

107. Which patients may be potential candidates for CABG? *(Select all that apply.)*
    a. Patient with angina and greater than 50% occlusion of left main coronary artery that cannot be stented
    b. Patient with unstable angina with moderate vessel disease appropriate for stenting
    c. Patient with valvular disease
    d. Patient with coronary vessels unsuitable for PTCA
    e. Patient with acute MI responding to therapy
    f. Patient with signs of ischemia or impending MI after angiography or PTCA

108. The patient is trying to decide whether to consent to a CABG. What information does the nurse give the patient?
    a. CABG improves the quality of life for most patients.
    b. Most patients are pain-free at 15 years after surgery.
    c. 70% of patients will remain permanently pain-free.
    d. Most patients have a decreased quality of life after 15 years.

109. The patient is having an elective CABG with a minimally invasive surgical technique. What does the nurse include in the preoperative teaching?
    a. Prevention of edema and scarring at the harvest site
    b. Protection and splinting of the chest incision while coughing
    c. Availability of analgesics if needed, but probably unnecessary
    d. Limitation of ambulation for several days after the procedure

110. The patient is having a CABG with the traditional surgical procedure. What does the nurse include in the preoperative teaching? *(Select all that apply.)*
    a. Expect a small 1- to 2-inch incision on the leg.
    b. There will be a sternal incision.
    c. Expect one, two, or three chest tubes.
    d. An indwelling urinary catheter will be placed.
    e. An endotracheal tube will prevent talking.
    f. Sophisticated equipment is used for complications.

111. The intensive care nurse is caring for the patient who has just had a CABG. The nurse notes that the patient has edema. In order to adjust fluid administration, the nurse collects which additional information and then consults the health care provider? *(Select all that apply.)*
    a. Blood pressure
    b. PAWP
    c. Skin turgor
    d. Cardiac output
    e. Blood loss
    f. Urine output

112. A potassium bolus of 80 mEq mixed in 100 mL of IV solution at a rate of 40 mEq/hr is ordered for the patient in the critical care unit. What does the nurse do next?
    a. Contact the health care provider because the order exceeds the recommended amount.
    b. Give the infusion; the order exceeds the recommended amount, but is within acceptable standards of practice for critical care patients.
    c. Contact the health care provider because even though the dosage is acceptable, the rate is too fast.
    d. Consult with the pharmacist because even though the rate is acceptable, the mixture is too concentrated.

113. The intensive care nurse is caring for the patient who has just had a CABG. The patient has a systolic blood pressure of 80 mm Hg. What is the primary concern related to this patient's hypotension?
    a. It is associated with warm cardioplegia.
    b. It may result in the collapse of the graft.
    c. It will result in acute tubular necrosis.
    d. It is related to mechanical ventilation.

114. Following a CABG, the patient has a body temperature below 96.8° F (36° C). What measures (if any) should be used to rewarm the patient?
    a. Infuse warm IV fluids.
    b. Do not rewarm; cold cardioplegia is protective.
    c. Place the patient in a warm fluid bath.
    d. Use lights or thermal blankets.

115. The intensive care nurse is caring for the patient who has just had a CABG. What does the nurse do to assess for postoperative bleeding?
    a. Measure mediastinal and pleural chest tube drainage at least hourly and report drainage amounts over 150 mL/hr to the surgeon.
    b. Measure mediastinal and pleural chest tube drainage at least once a shift and report drainage amounts over 50 mL/hr to the surgeon.
    c. Assess the dressing over the sternal site every 4 hours and reinforce the dressing with sterile gauze as needed.
    d. Assess the donor site every 4 hours and report serous drainage and increasing pain to the surgeon.

116. Following a CABG, the patient in the ICU on a mechanical ventilator suddenly decompensates. The health care provider makes a diagnosis of cardiac tamponade. The nurse prepares the patient for which emergency procedure?
    a. Chest tube
    b. Sternotomy
    c. Pericardiocentesis
    d. Thoracentesis

117. The nurse is assessing the patient who had a CABG. Which finding is a permanent deficit that is associated with an intraoperative stroke?
    a. Decreased level of consciousness that resolves when body temperature is normal
    b. Arousal from anesthesia which takes several hours
    c. Inability to speak clearly and coherently immediately after surgery
    d. Generalized seizure activity

118. The patient reports pain after a CABG. Which statement by the patient suggests that the pain is related to the sternotomy and not anginal in origin?
    a. "The pain goes down my arm or sometimes into my jaw."
    b. "My pain increases when I cough or take a deep breath."
    c. "The nitroglycerin helped to relieve the pain."
    d. "I feel nausea and shortness of breath when the pain occurs."

119. The patient with a CABG is transferred from the ICU to the intermediate care unit. Which activity does the nurse assists the patient with?
    a. Ambulating 25 to 100 feet three times a day as tolerated
    b. Turning the patient every 2 hours for the first 48 hours
    c. Dangling and turning every 2 hours for at least 24 hours
    d. Coughing and deep breathing three times a day

120. The patient had CABG with the radial artery used as a graft. The nurse performs which assessment specific to this patient?
    a. Check the blood pressure every hour on the unaffected arm or use the legs.
    b. Check the fingertips, hand, and arm for sensation and mobility every shift.
    c. Assess hand color, temperature, ulnar/radial pulses, and capillary refill every hour initially.
    d. Note edema, bleeding, and swelling at the donor site which are expected.

121. The patient with a CABG has been diagnosed with mediastinitis. What information does the nurse expect to find in the patient's assessment documentation? *(Select all that apply.)*
    a. Fever continuing beyond the first 4 days after CABG
    b. Bogginess of the sternum
    c. Redness and drainage from suture sites
    d. Decreased white blood cell count
    e. Induration or swelling at the suture sites
    f. Anginal-type chest pain

122. The patient had a CABG with a vein graft. To help prevent collapse of the graft, what assessment does the nurse perform?
    a. Auscultate lung sounds
    b. Monitor for hypotension
    c. Assess for motion and sensation
    d. Observe for generalized hypothermia

123. The nurse is caring for the patient who had a CABG. The nurse pays close attention to which electrolyte levels for this postoperative patient? *(Select all that apply.)*
    a. Sodium
    b. Potassium
    c. Calcium
    d. Magnesium
    e. Phosphorus

124. After a CABG, the postoperative patient suddenly has a decrease in mediastinal drainage, jugular vein distention with clear lung sounds, pulsus paradoxus, and equalizing PAWP and right atrial pressure. What does the nurse suspect these are signs of?
    a. Acute MI
    b. Occlusion at the donor site
    c. Cardiac tamponade
    d. Prinzmetal's angina

125. The nurse coming on duty receives the change of shift report. Which patient is assessed first by the nurse?
    a. Patient with anxiety, nausea, diaphoresis, and shortness of breath
    b. Patient with diabetes mellitus and elevated serum lipid levels
    c. Patient with a friction rub, elevated temperature, and dysrhythmias
    d. Patient with fever, instability of sternum, and increased white blood cell count

126. The nurse is caring for the patient who had a minimally invasive direct coronary artery bypass (MIDCAB). Which sign/symptom prompts the nurse to immediately contact the health care provider?
    a. Acute incisional pain
    b. ST-segment changes in the V leads
    c. Drainage from the chest tubes
    d. Problems with coughing

127. The patient has discrete, proximal, noncalcified lesions of only one or two vessels. Which procedure is most likely to be recommended for this patient?
    a. PTCA
    b. Stress test
    c. Immediate reperfusion
    d. Thrombolytic therapy

128. The nurse is caring for the patient who had a PTCA. Which postoperative interventions are included in the care for this patient? *(Select all that apply.)*
    a. Monitor for acute closure of the vessel.
    b. Observe for bleeding from the insertion site.
    c. Assess for reaction to the dye.
    d. Observe for hypotension, hypokalemia, and dysrhythmias.
    e. Teach about medications such as aspirin and beta blockers or ACE inhibitors.
    f. Instruct about lifestyle changes relating to CAD.

129. Treatment of hypothermia, a common problem after CABG surgery, with warming blankets is necessary because this condition may cause the patient to be at risk for which condition?
    a. Hypotension
    b. Tachycardia
    c. Heart failure
    d. Loss of consciousness

130. Which statement is true about post-pericardiotomy syndrome?
    a. It is a psychological disorder for which the patient needs emotional support.
    b. It is generally mild and self-limiting.
    c. It places the patient at high risk for cardiac tamponade.
    d. It can be prophylactically managed with antibiotics

Matching. *Match the different types of therapy with the correct descriptions.*

Terms

a. Minimally invasive direct coronary artery by-pass (MIDCAB)
b. Endovascular (endoscopic) vessel harvesting (EVH)
c. Transmyocardial laser revascularization
d. Off-pump coronary artery bypass (OPCAB)
e. Robotic heart surgery
f. Telesurgery

Descriptions

_____ 131. Eliminates tremors that can exist with human hands, increases the ability to reach inaccessible sites, and improves depth perception and visual acuity.

_____ 132. Patient has one or two very small incisions in the leg or arm.

_____ 133. Cardiopulmonary bypass (CPB) is not required.

_____ 134. Creates channels that will eventually allow oxygenated blood to flow during diastole from the left ventricle to nourish the muscle.

_____ 135. Procedure in which open heart surgery is performed without the use of a heart-lung bypass machine.

_____ 136. Performing heart procedures over long distances.

CASE STUDY: THE PATIENT WITH ANGINA

Use a separate sheet of paper to answer the questions in this Case Study. Answer guidelines for this Case Study are available on your Evolve website at http://evolve. elsevier.com/Iggy/ in the "Prepare for Class" folder.

A 68-year-old woman arrives in the emergency department stating, "I think I had a heart attack." She states that she had an episode of chest pain that lasted a couple of minutes during her daily 3-mile walk; the pain was relieved by rest. ECG rhythm is normal sinus rhythm. She has no abnormal heart sounds or laboratory values. VS are stable. Po_2 by pulse oximetry is 97% on room air. She is diagnosed with angina.

1. How would this patient's clinical manifestations be different if she had had an MI?

2. What would the nurse explain to the patient about the diagnosis of angina?

3. What teaching would the nurse provide for this patient regarding her diagnosis of angina?

4. What instructions should this patient have received regarding managing her chest pain at home?

5. The patient is seen by a cardiologist who prescribed nitroglycerin tablets, and one aspirin per day. After 6 months, the patient returns to the cardiologist with additional complaints regarding her chest pain. A cardiac catheterization reveals the following results: 50% blockage of the circumflex artery, 60% blockage of the left anterior descending (LAD) artery, and 90% blockage of the right coronary artery. What assessment findings indicate that her angina is now unstable?

6. This patient is a 68-year-old woman. Describe the relationship between older adults, particularly older women, and heart disease.

CASE STUDY: THE PATIENT WITH CORONARY ARTERY DISEASE

Use a separate sheet of paper to answer the questions in this Case Study. Answer guidelines for this Case Study are available on your Evolve website at http://evolve.elsevier.com/Iggy/ in the "Prepare for Class" folder.

The patient is a 40-year-old African-American man with a history of hypertension. He is in for an annual physical and admits that he has experienced chest pain "a time or two" when he takes the stairs at work, so lately he has avoided the stairs. The chest pain subsided once he rested for a few minutes in his office. He smokes one pack of cigarettes per day. He is 5 feet, 8 inches tall and weighs 250 pounds. He takes hydrochlorothiazide and metoprolol (Lopressor) for his hypertension. His last serum cholesterol level was 220 mg/dL, with the HDL 35 mg/dL and LDL 105 mg/dL. His father died of an MI at age 54 and his mother has hypertension. He works 50 hours a week as a lawyer and takes occasional walks on weekends.

1. What are this patient's modifiable risks for CAD? What are his nonmodifiable risks for CAD?

2. What patient education would you provide for this patient?

3. Explain to this patient his risk factors for developing CAD.

41 CHAPTER

Assessment of the Hematologic System

STUDY/REVIEW QUESTIONS

True or False? *Read the statements about blood components and write T for true or F for false in the blanks provided.*

_____ 1. Erythrocytes are the largest proportion of blood cells.

_____ 2. Blood is composed of plasma and cells.

_____ 3. The three major types of plasma proteins are albumin, globulins, and fibrinogen.

_____ 4. Globulins increase the osmotic pressure of the blood, preventing plasma from leaking into the tissues.

_____ 5. Healthy mature RBCs have a life span of about 30 days.

_____ 6. Iron is an essential part of hemoglobin.

_____ 7. The most important feature of hemoglobin is its ability to combine loosely with oxygen.

_____ 8. Erythropoiesis is the selective growth of stem cells into mature erythrocytes.

_____ 9. The liver produces RBC growth factor erythropoietin at the same rate as RBC destruction or loss occurs to maintain a constant normal level of circulating RBCs.

_____ 10. Leukocytes perform actions important for protection through inflammation and immunity.

_____ 11. Platelets are the largest of the blood cells.

_____ 12. Platelets perform most of their functions by aggregation.

_____ 13. The spleen is the site for production of prothrombin and most blood clotting factors.

_____ 14. Vitamin D is the vitamin that plays the most important role in the production of blood clotting factors VII, IX, and X and prothrombin.

_____ 15. After a splenectomy, patients are less able to rid themselves of disease-causing organisms and are at greater risk for infection and sepsis.

True or False? *Read the statements about hemostasis and blood clotting and write T for true or F for false in the blanks provided.*

_____ 16. Platelets normally circulate as individual cell-like structures and do not aggregate until activated.

_____ 17. Platelet plugs are clots that provide complete hemostasis.

_____ 18. Substances that cause platelets to clump include adenosine diphosphate (ADP), calcium, thromboxane A2, and collagen.

_____ 19. The blood clotting cascade is triggered by the formation of a platelet plug.

_____ 20. Extrinsic factors that induce platelet plugs to form are usually the result of changes in blood vessels rather than in the blood.

_____ 21. Fibrin clot formation is the last phase of blood clotting.

_____ 22. Fibrinolysis prevents overenlargement of the fibrin clot.

_____ 23. Fibrinolysis ends by activating plasminogen to plasmin.

_____ 24. Plasmin is a protein that digests fibrin.

_____ 25. A person who has a deficiency of any anti-clotting factor has an increased risk for pulmonary embolism, myocardial infarction, and stroke.

26. The nurse is performing a hematologic assessment in the older adult patient. Which findings does the nurse identify as normal changes in the older adult? *(Select all that apply)*
    a. Progressive loss of body hair
    b. Thickened or discolored nails
    c. Yellowing of the skin
    d. Dryness of the skin
    e. Ecchymosis

27. Which statement about hematologic changes associated with aging is true?
    a. The older adult has increased blood volume.
    b. The older adult has increased levels of plasma proteins.
    c. Platelet counts decrease with age.
    d. Antibody levels and responses are lower and slower in older adults.

28. The nurse is interviewing the patient who reports dizziness and lightheadedness, and bleeding gums every time she brushes her teeth. Which questions does the nurse ask the patient in order to focus in on the problem? *(Select all that apply.)*
    a. "How often do you take aspirin or any other nonsteroidal anti-inflammatory drug?"
    b. "How often do you eat salads or other green leafy vegetables?"
    c. "How much meat do you eat in a week?"
    d. "How much exercise do you get?"
    e. "Does your heart ever seem to pound?"

29. Which drug disrupts platelet action?
    a. Vitamin K (AquaMEPHYTON)
    b. Ibuprofen (Advil)
    c. Methyldopa (Aldomet)
    d. Azathioprine (Imuran)

True or False? *Read the statements and write T for true or F for false in the blanks provided.*

_____ 30. Anticoagulants break down existing clots.

_____ 31. Anticoagulant drugs are classified as thrombin inhibitors, vitamin K antagonists, and indirect factor X inhibitors.

_____ 32. Platelet inhibitors are drugs that either prevent platelets from becoming active or prevent activated platelets from clumping together.

_____ 33. Aspirin inhibits the production of substances that can trigger platelet activation such as thromboxane.

_____ 34. The use of fibrinolytic drugs is limited to 6 hours because the drugs are inactive after this time.

_____ 35. Fibrinolytic drugs are used for the treatment of embolic strokes.

36. Which symptom is the single most common symptom of anemia?
    a. Fatigue
    b. Dizziness
    c. Palpitations
    d. Tinnitus

37. When assessing the patient with darker skin for pallor and cyanosis, which parts of the body does the nurse examine? *(Select all that apply.)*
    a. Palms of the hands
    b. Soles of the feet
    c. Cheek
    d. Oral mucous membranes
    e. Conjunctiva of the eye

38. Severe anemia causes enlargement of which chamber of the heart?
    a. Right atrium
    b. Right ventricle
    c. Left atrium
    d. Left ventricle

39. Complete the chart below about the significance of abnormal findings of the laboratory profile for hematologic assessment.

Test	Significance of Abnormal Findings
Red blood cell (RBC) count	
Hemoglobin (Hgb)	
Hematocrit (Hct)	
Mean cell volume (MCV)	
Mean cell hemoglobin (MCH)	
Mean cell hemoglobin concentration (MCHC)	
White blood cell (WBC) count	
Total iron binding capacity (TIBC)	
Iron (Fe)	
Serum ferritin	
Platelet count	
Hemoglobin electrophoresis	
Direct Coombs' and indirect Coombs' test	
Prothrombin time (PT)	
Bleeding time	
Fibrin degradation products	

40. Which statement is true about tests to measure bleeding and coagulation?
   a. Heparin therapy is monitored using PT levels.
   b. The international normalized ratio (INR) measures the same process as the PTT.
   c. The partial thromboplastin time (PTT) assesses the extrinsic clotting cascade.
   d. Platelet aggregation is tested by mixing the patient's plasma with a substance called ristocetin.

True or False? Read the statements about bone marrow aspiration and biopsy and write T for true or F for false in the blanks provided.

_____ 41. An informed consent is needed for a bone marrow aspiration and biopsy.

_____ 42. The patient should be told that a heavy sensation of pressure and pushing will be felt while the needle is being inserted.

_____ 43. The most common site for bone marrow aspiration and biopsy is the sternum.

_____ 44. Aspirin is commonly used to treat the discomfort often experienced by patients after a bone marrow aspiration and biopsy.

_____ 45. If the iliac crest is used for the bone marrow biopsy or aspiration, the patient should be placed in the prone or side-lying position.

CASE STUDY: HEMATOLOGIC ASSESSMENT

Use a separate sheet of paper to answer the questions in this Case Study. Answer guidelines for this Case Study are available on your Evolve website at http://evolve. elsevier.com/Iggy/ in the "Prepare for Class" folder.

The patient is a 45-year-old woman who is married to a career military officer. Her father was a miner, leading an itinerant life as he worked in uranium mines. She grew up in a western state and remembers playing with other children on slag heaps from the mines. She recalls being ill often as a child and attributes this to being chronically undernourished. The family was often cold during the winter months when there was no money to buy warm clothing or fuel for heat.

Over the past 6 months, the patient has had episodes of epistaxis and prolonged bleeding after having her teeth cleaned by a dental hygienist. She has also noticed that she seems to bruise easily; there are multiple ecchymotic areas on her legs and arms. She reported to the military hospital for a checkup and was referred to a regional civilian hospital for further evaluation. During the admission history, she tells the nurse that she tires easily and often has little energy. Her husband and children are worried about her.

1. What additional data should the nurse elicit from the patient at this time?
2. As part of the diagnostic workup, the patient is scheduled to have blood work drawn for CBC, PT, PTT, INR, and TIBC. What do these laboratory studies measure?
3. The results of the laboratory tests and bone scan indicate that the patient has depressed bone marrow function. The hematologist discusses plans to perform a bone marrow aspiration with her. How does the nurse prepare the patient for this procedure?
4. What is the follow-up care for the patient after a bone marrow aspiration?

42
CHAPTER

Care of Patients with Hematologic Problems

STUDY/REVIEW QUESTIONS

1. The nurse is interviewing the patient who is newly admitted to the unit with a diagnosis of anemia. Which assessment findings does the nurse expect? *(Select all that apply.)*
   a. Dyspnea on exertion
   b. Orthostatic hypotension
   c. Intolerance to cold temperatures
   d. Clublike appearance to the nails
   e. Pallor of the ears
   f. Headache

2. The patient with sickle cell crisis is admitted to the hospital. Which questions does the nurse ask the patient to elicit information about the cause of the current crisis? *(Select all that apply.)*
   a. Ask the patient about recent airplane travel.
   b. Determine the patient's perceived energy level using a scale ranging from 0 to 10.
   c. Review all activities and events during the past 24 hours.
   d. Ask the patient about ability to climb stairs.
   e. Ask the patient about symptoms of infection.

3. The patient is scheduled to undergo laboratory testing to diagnose sickle cell anemia. For which diagnostic test does the nurse provide patient teaching?
   a. Bone marrow biopsy
   b. White blood cell count
   c. MRI
   d. Hemoglobin S

4. The student nurse is caring for the patient with sickle cell crisis. Which action by the student nurse warrants intervention by the supervising nurse?
   a. Keeping the patient's room cold
   b. Using distraction and relaxation techniques
   c. Positioning painful areas of the patient with support
   d. Use of therapeutic touch

5. The patient with vitamin B_{12} deficiency anemia is being discharged home with primary care responsibility being assumed by the family. The nurse has taught the patient and family about dietary modifications to manage this condition. Which statement by the family indicates additional teaching is needed about dietary modification? *(Select all that apply.)*
   a. "Dairy products will be omitted from the diet."
   b. "Dried beans will be a part of the diet."
   c. "Animal protein will be a part of the diet."
   d. "Citrus fruit will be omitted from the diet."
   e. "Nuts will be part of the diet."
   f. "Green leafy vegetables will be omitted from the diet."

6. Which statement is true about the pattern of inheritance for sickle cell disease?
   a. If a patient with sickle cell disease has children, each child will have sickle cell disease.
   b. If a patient with sickle cell trait has children, the children will have sickle cell disease.
   c. If a patient with sickle cell disease has children, each child will inherit one of the two abnormal gene alleles and at least have the sickle cell trait.
   d. If a patient has sickle cell disease, it was the result of an autosomal dominant pattern of inheritance.

7. The nurse is caring for the patient in sickle cell crisis. What is the priority intervention for this patient?
   a. Pain management
   b. Teaching the patient long-term management of the disease
   c. Smoking cessation
   d. Administration of the pneumonia vaccine

8. The nurse's aide is providing care to the patient in sickle cell crisis. Which action by the nurse's aide requires intervention by the supervising nurse?
   a. Elevating the head of the bed to 25 degrees
   b. Keeping the foot of the bed flat
   c. Obtaining the patient's blood pressure with an external cuff
   d. Offering the patient her beverage of choice

9. The patient admitted for sickle cell crisis is being discharged home. Which statement by the patient indicates the need for further post-discharge instruction?
   a. "I will no longer run 2 miles every morning."
   b. "I will visit my friends in Denver."
   c. "I will avoid the sauna at the gym."
   d. "I will not drink alcoholic beverages."

10. When reviewing the procedure for administering intramuscular medications by the Z-track method, which statement by the student nurse indicates that further instruction is needed?
    a. "I will discard the needle used to draw up the medication."
    b. "I will use the ventral gluteal site for the injection."
    c. "I will pull the skin and subcutaneous tissue sideways away from the muscle."
    d. "I will not massage the injection site."

11. The patient with polycythemia vera is being cared for by a nurse's aide. Which action by the nurse's aide requires intervention by the supervising nurse?
    a. Assisting the patient to floss his teeth
    b. Using an electric shaver on the patient
    c. Using a soft-bristled toothbrush on the patient
    d. Assisting the patient to wear support hose

12. The patient with a low white blood cell count is being discharged home. In which situations will the patient be instructed by the nurse to contact his or her health care provider? (Select all that apply.)
    a. For a temperature greater than 100° F (38° C)
    b. If a persistent cough develops with or without sputum
    c. If pus or foul-smelling drainage develops from any open skin area or normal body opening
    d. If a boil or abscess develops
    e. For urine that is cloudy or foul-smelling, or if burning on urination is experienced

13. Which food should the patient with a low white blood cell count be encouraged to eat?
    a. Fresh strawberries
    b. Raw carrots
    c. Pepper
    d. Well-done steak

14. The nurse is caring for the patient with acute leukemia. Which characteristics does the nurse assess the patient for? (Select all that apply.)
    a. Hematuria
    b. Orthostatic hypotension
    c. Bone pain
    d. Joint swelling
    e. Fatigue
    f. Weight gain

15. Which statements are true about ways to prevent lymphoma? (Select all that apply.)
    a. Exposures such as radiation therapy for cancer treatment or heavy radiation exposure increase the risk for lymphoma.
    b. Previous treatment for cancer poses an increased risk for lymphoma.
    c. Genetic factors have not been linked to the development of lymphoma.
    d. Disorders that cause bone marrow hypoplasia increase the risk for developing lymphoma.
    e. Lymphoma is rare, so chances of developing it are slim.

16. Which disorder makes a patient at highest risk for the development of infection?
    a. Sickle cell crisis
    b. Vitamin B_{12} deficiency anemia
    c. Polycythemia vera
    d. Thrombocytopenia

17. Which medication places the patient at risk for infection?
    a. Steroids
    b. Diuretics
    c. ACE inhibitors
    d. Beta blockers

18. The nurse is caring for the patient with thrombocytopenia. Which order does the nurse question?
    a. Test all urine and stool for the presence of occult blood.
    b. Avoid IM injections.
    c. Administer enemas.
    d. Apply ice to areas of trauma.

19. The patient undergoing bone marrow/stem cell transplantation reports severe fatigue. To assist the patient with energy management, what does the nurse encourage the patient to do? *(Select all that apply.)*
    a. Verbalize feelings about limitations.
    b. Monitor nutritional intake to ensure adequate energy resources.
    c. Avoid napping throughout the day.
    d. Limit the number of visitors as appropriate.
    e. Plan activities for periods when the patient has the most energy.
    f. Monitor overall response to self-care activities.

20. The home care nurse is visiting the patient who had a stem cell transplant. Which observation by the nurse requires immediate action?
    a. The patient's grandson is visiting after receiving a MMR vaccine.
    b. The patient bumps his toe on a chair and applies pressure to the toe for 10 minutes.
    c. The patient with a platelet count of 48,000/mm^3 follows platelet precautions.
    d. The patient avoids going grocery shopping in the winter months.

21. The patient has been taught how to care for his central venous catheter at home. Which statements by the patient indicate that further instruction is necessary? *(Select all that apply.)*
    a. "I will flush the catheter with heparin three times a day."
    b. "I will change the Luer-Lok cap on each catheter daily."
    c. "I will tape the catheter to my skin."
    d. "If the catheter lumen breaks or punctures, I will immediately clamp the catheter between myself and the opening."
    e. "I will wash my hands before working with the catheter."

22. The nurse has instructed the patient at risk for bleeding about techniques to manage this condition. Which statements by the patient indicate that teaching has been successful? *(Select all that apply.)*
    a. "I will take a stool softener to prevent straining during a bowel movement."
    b. "I won't take aspirin or aspirin-containing products."
    c. "I won't participate in any contact sports."
    d. "I will report a headache that is not responsive to acetaminophen."
    e. "I will avoid bending over at the waist."
    f. "If I am bumped, I will apply ice to the site for at least 10 minutes."

23. The new registered nurse is giving a blood transfusion to the patient. Which statement by the new nurse indicates the need for action by the supervising nurse?
    a. "I will be sure to complete the red blood cell transfusions within 6 hours of removal from refrigeration."
    b. "I will check the patient verification with another registered nurse."
    c. "I will use normal saline solution to dilute the blood."
    d. "I will remain with the patient for the first 15 to 30 minutes of the infusion."

24. The new registered nurse is identifying the patient for blood transfusion. Which action by the new nurse warrants intervention by the supervising nurse?
    a. Checks the physician's prescription before the blood transfusion.
    b. Determines the patient's identity and whether the hospital identification band name and number are identical to those on the blood component tag.
    c. Uses the patient's room number as a form of identification.
    d. Examines the blood bag tag, the attached tag, and the requisition slip to ensure that the ABO and Rh types are compatible.

25. The patient receiving a stem cell transplant from an identical twin is receiving which type of transplant?
    a. Allogeneic
    b. Syngeneic
    c. Autologous
    d. Human leukocyte antigen (HLA)

26. The patient with hemophilia VIII will most likely receive which component of blood for management of the disease?
    a. Pooled platelets
    b. Fresh frozen plasma
    c. Cryoprecipitate
    d. Washed red blood cells

27. Patients with sickle cell disease are more susceptible to infections, specifically *Streptococcus pneumoniae* and *Haemophilus influenzae*. Which actions help prevent infection? *(Select all that apply.)*
    a. Consistent good handwashing technique
    b. Yearly flu vaccination
    c. Twice-daily oral penicillin
    d. NSAIDs three times a day
    e. Monitoring CBC
    f. Assessment of vital signs at least every 4 hours

Matching: *Match the source with the type of transplant.*

Types
a. Allogeneic
b. Autologous
c. Syngeneic

Sources

_____ 28. From a sibling or HLA match

_____ 29. From an identical twin

_____ 30. From own stem cells

31. The nurse is caring for the patient who has donated bone marrow. In addition to having the aspiration sites monitored, the nurse will anticipate the need for which interventions? *(Select all that apply.)*
    a. Fluid for hydration
    b. Pain management
    c. Possible RBC infusion
    d. Antibiotic therapy
    e. Assessment for complications of anesthesia

32. When caring for the patient after bone marrow stem cell transplantation, when does the nurse expect engraftment (the settling in of stem cells and the start of producing new cells) to occur?
    a. 8 to 12 hours after infusion
    b. 7 days after infusion
    c. 12 to 28 days after infusion
    d. 6 weeks after infusion

33. The patient is at high risk for the development of veno-occlusive disease (VOD). What assessments does the nurse perform for early detection of this disorder? *(Select all that apply.)*
    a. Jaundice
    b. Weight loss
    c. Hepatomegaly
    d. Right upper quadrant abdominal pain
    e. Ascites

Matching: *Match each characteristic with the corresponding disease. Diseases will be used more than once.*

Disease
a. Hodgkin's lymphoma
b. Non-Hodgkin's lymphoma

Characteristics

_____ 34. Pain in lymph nodes brought on or made worse with ingestion of alcohol

_____ 35. One of the most treatable types of cancer

_____ 36. Fevers, drenching night sweats, and unexplained weight loss

_____ 37. Viral infections (Epstein-Barr, HTLV, and HIV) and exposure to chemical agents

_____ 38. Twelve subtypes

_____ 39. Reed-Sternberg cell

_____ 40. Enlarged painless lymph node or nodes

_____ 41. Associated with autoimmune disorders

_____ 42. More common in teens

For questions 43 through 51, indicate whether each characteristic corresponds to autoimmune thrombolytic purpura (ATP) or thrombotic thrombocytopenic purpura (TTP).

_____ 43. Also called idiopathic

_____ 44. Platelets clump

_____ 45. Antibodies directed against own platelets

_____ 46. Inappropriate aggregation of platelets

_____ 47. Women 20 to 40 years of age

_____ 48. Pre-existing autoimmune condition

_____ 49. Plasmapheresis

_____ 50. Immunosuppressive therapy to reduce intensity

_____ 51. Corticosteroids and azathioprine (Imuran)

52. While being interviewed for admission, the patient tells the nurse that he has Christmas disease. What does the nurse documents this as?
    a. Hemophilia A
    b. Hemophilia B
    c. Thrombocytopenia
    d. Sickle cell disease

53. Which characteristics describe patients who have hemophilia? *(Select all that apply.)*
    a. Bleeding more often
    b. Bleeding more rapidly
    c. Bleeding for a longer period
    d. Are not able to form platelet plugs
    e. Exhibit abnormal bleeding in response to any trauma

54. What size of intravenous needle is best for administering a blood transfusion?
    a. 22-gauge needle
    b. 20-gauge needle
    c. 19-gauge needle or larger
    d. Butterfly needle

55. The patient is receiving a blood transfusion. Which solution does the nurse administer with the blood?
    a. Ringer's lactate
    b. Normal saline
    c. Dextrose in water
    d. Dextrose in saline

56. The nurse's aide asks the registered nurse why D_5W is contraindicated when transfusing blood. How does the nurse respond?
    a. "It causes hemolysis of blood cells."
    b. "It dilutes the cells."
    c. "It shrinks the blood cells."
    d. "It causes blood cells to coagulate."

57. The patient is receiving a blood transfusion through a single lumen peripherally inserted central catheter. The patient has two other peripheral IVs: one is capped and the other has $D_5.45$ NS running at a rate of 50 mL/hr. What infusion is acceptable to add to the blood products?
    a. Normal saline
    b. Piggyback of 10 mEq potassium chloride
    c. Total parenteral nutrition
    d. Furosemide (Lasix) 5 mg IV push

58. The nurse realizes that hemolytic reactions to blood transfusions occur most often within the first ____ mL of the infusion.
    a. 5
    b. 50
    c. 100
    d. 150

59. Which type of medication is used for patients receiving a platelet transfusion as a premedication to prevent a reaction?
    a. Demerol and Vistaril
    b. Valium and aspirin
    c. Benadryl and Tylenol
    d. Hydrocortisone and Demerol

60. Complete the chart below to include the characteristics associated with various transfusion reactions.

Transfusion Reactions	Associated Characteristics and Symptoms
Febrile transfusion reactions	
Hemolytic transfusion reactions	
Allergic transfusion reactions	
Bacterial transfusion reactions	
Circulatory overload	
Transfusion-associated graft-versus-host disease (TA-GVHD)	

CASE STUDY: HODGKIN'S AND NON-HODGKIN'S LYMPHOMAS

Use a separate sheet of paper to answer the questions in this Case Study. Answer guidelines for this Case Study are available on your Evolve website at http://evolve. elsevier.com/Iggy/ in the "Prepare for Class" folder.

The nurse is practicing on a unit which specializes in the care of patients with malignant lymphomas. One of the patients is Dan, a 19-year-old college freshman who has been diagnosed with Hodgkin's lymphoma. The other patient is Emily, a 60-year-old woman who has been diagnosed with an indolent non-Hodgkin's lymphoma. Emily tells the nurse, "I know there is nothing that can really be done for me. My sister died of the same thing 16 years ago." Dan appears frightened and confused when the nurse asks him if he has any questions about the treatment plan. Dan tells the nurse, "I have a girlfriend, but we're not that serious, and I'm still young. Will I ever be able to have children?"

1. What are the characteristics of malignant lymphomas and how are they different from leukemia?

2. Compare and contrast the etiology, pathophysiology, and clinical manifestations of Hodgkin's lymphoma and non-Hodgkin's lymphoma.

3. What questions will the nurse ask Emily, and what questions will the nurse ask Dan to elicit more information about possible contributing factors to the development of this disease?

4. When planning care for Dan, what nursing interventions will the nurse focus on to deal with the side effects of therapy?

5. Emily asks the nurse what the doctors mean by saying the cancer is *indolent*. How should the nurse respond?

6. What should the nurse tell Emily about the current treatment of non-Hodgkin's lymphoma?

7. How should the nurse address Dan's concerns about having children?

Assessment of the Nervous System

STUDY/REVIEW QUESTIONS

Matching: Match the cerebral areas with their functions.

Cerebral Areas

a. Motor cortex of the frontal lobe
b. Broca's area
c. Occipital lobe
d. Parietal lobe
e. Limbic lobe
f. Wernicke's area
g. Temporal lobe

Functions

_____ 1. Speech center

_____ 2. Visual center

_____ 3. Initiate voluntary movement

_____ 4. Process language

_____ 5. Spatial perception

_____ 6. Complicated memory patterns

_____ 7. Emotional and visceral patterns

8. Which factor is most likely to depress nerve cell activity in the patient with a neurologic disorder?
   a. Metabolic alkalosis
   b. IV infusion of theophylline
   c. Drinking too much coffee
   d. Low oxygen saturation and hypoxia

9. The patient has sustained trauma affecting Broca's area of the brain. Which intervention does the nurse use to assist the patient to compensate for deficits related to damage in this area?
   a. Obtain an erasable white board and a pen for communication.
   b. Use a picture board to relate the spoken word to a visual picture.
   c. Move into the patient's visual field on the unaffected side.
   d. Put up the side rails and turn on the bed alarm.

10. Which type of stroke or stroke damage is most likely to cause problems with respiratory distress related to neurologic function?
    a. Frontal lobe damage
    b. Thalamic stroke
    c. Affected temporal lobe
    d. Involvement of medulla and pons

11. With what will the patient with a cerebellar dysfunction most likely need assistance?
    a. Orientation to place and time
    b. Buttoning the shirt
    c. Verbal communication
    d. Mood and pain control

12. Identify which substances pass through the blood-brain barrier with a "P" and which are blocked by the barrier with a "B."

    _____ a. Oxygen

    _____ b. Albumin

    _____ c. Most bacteria

    _____ d. Alcohol

    _____ e. Water

    _____ f. Anesthetics

    _____ g. Many antibiotics

    _____ h. Carbon dioxide

Matching: *Match the spinal tract with its function.*

Spinal Tracts

a. Spinothalamic
b. Spinocerebellar
c. Fasciculus gracilis or cuneatus
d. Corticospinal

Functions

_____ 13. Proprioception

_____ 14. Voluntary movement

_____ 15. Carry sensations of pain, temperature, pressure

_____ 16. Vibratory sense

Identify whether each description corresponds to the parasympathetic nervous system (PNS) or the sympathetic nervous system (SNS).

_____ 17. Has cell bodies in the gray matter of the spinal cord from S2 to S4

_____ 18. Lies beside the spinal cord in a chain

_____ 19. Has some sensory function

_____ 20. Is part of cranial nerves III, VII, IX, and X

_____ 21. Causes the heart to pump faster

_____ 22. Constricts pupils

23. The nurse is teaching the older adult patient about medication and healthy lifestyle. Which teaching strategy is the best to use with this patient?
    a. Give limited and simplified information.
    b. Do the teaching late in the afternoon.
    c. Relate the information to recent events.
    d. Allow extra time for teaching and questions.

24. The nurse is caring for the older adult patient who is identified at Risk for Injury related to altered balance and decreased coordination. Which intervention does the nurse employ for this patient?
    a. Instruct the patient to move slowly when changing positions.
    b. Put up all the side rails and place the bed in the lowest position.
    c. Store personal items out of sight and instruct the patient to call for help.
    d. Assign a sitter to stay with the patient and assist as needed.

25. The nurse is obtaining baseline information from the older adult patient at risk for a neurologic disorder about his ability to perform activities of daily living (ADLs). Why does the nurse ask whether the patient is right- or left-handed?
    a. The patient may be somewhat stronger on the dominant side, which is expected.
    b. Effects of a neurologic event will be worse if the nondominant side is involved.
    c. This information is part of any standardized database for patients with neurologic disorders.
    d. The patient should be encouraged to strengthen and rely on the dominant side.

26. The nurse is taking shift report on several patients with changes in functional health patterns. The levels are based on Gordon's Functional Assessment. Which level will require the most assistance during the shift?
    a. Level 0 for toileting
    b. Level I for general mobility
    c. Level II for grooming
    d. Level III for feeding

27. Which statement is included in an assessment of the patient's mental status?
    a. Reports of pain, discomfort, or weakness
    b. Ability to hear and see within normal limits
    c. Appropriateness of clothes to weather conditions
    d. Ability to push and pull against resistance

28. The older adult patient is brought to the clinic by the family who reports that "Dad doesn't seem to be quite like himself." Which behavior is an early sign of a neurologic problem?
    a. Inability to remember a trip that he took last week
    b. Failure to remember his mother's maiden name
    c. Failure to recall where he went to high school
    d. Inability to describe his favorite hobby

29. In assessing the patient's cognitive status and ability to make rational decisions, the nurse asks, "What would you do if you saw a fire in the wastebasket?" The patient replies, "Why? Are you trying to burn me to death?" What is the appropriate nursing diagnosis for this patient?
    a. Disturbed sensory perceptions
    b. Acute confusion
    c. Disturbed thought processes
    d. Impaired memory

30. Which neurologic disorder is most likely to require hourly sensory assessments of the patient?
    a. Parkinson disease
    b. Alzheimer's disease
    c. Guillain-Barré syndrome
    d. Huntington disease

31. Complete the chart below by describing the functions of the listed cranial nerves.

Cranial Nerve	Function
I: Olfactory	
II: Optic	
III: Oculomotor	
IV: Trochlear	
V: Trigeminal	
VI: Abducens	
VII: Facial	
VIII: Vestibulocochlear	
IX: Glossopharyngeal	
X: Vagus	
XI: Accessory	
XII: Hypoglossal	

32. Which sensory assessment technique is correct?
    a. Separate assessments for pain and temperature
    b. Assessment of only the affected or injured side
    c. Assessment of the proximal and distal areas of extremities
    d. Assessment of sharp and dull senses by using a paper clip

33. The nurse is caring for several older adult patients in a long-term care facility. In planning care with consideration for the sensory changes related to aging, which intervention does the nurse implement?
    a. Controls environmental odors because older adults have a heightened sense of smell
    b. Plans simple teaching sessions because of the decline in intellectual ability
    c. Increases the ambient lighting because of the decrease in pupil size
    d. Limits physical contact because the touch sensation increases

34. The nurse is taking an initial history on the patient whose chief complaint is a headache that seems to be associated with blurred vision. The patient also reports several chronic health problems. Which chronic condition is most likely to impact neurologic function?
    a. Hypertension
    b. Obesity
    c. Crohn's disease
    d. Coronary artery disease

35. The older adult patient is admitted into a long-term care facility and the nurse is performing a baseline physical assessment that includes neurologic and sensory function. What is the purpose of the assessment?
    a. Determine a level of function for later comparison
    b. Show the family what problems the older adult has
    c. Gain information on past sensory changes
    d. Determine rehabilitation potential

Matching: *Match each mental and cognitive status assessment question/task to the type of information sought.*

Information Sought
a. Attention span
b. Recent memory
c. Remote memory
d. New memory
e. Language comprehension
f. Cognitive skills

Questions

_____ 36. Repeat three unrelated words.

_____ 37. "What is your birth date?"

_____ 38. Follow simple instructions.

_____ 39. "What health care providers have you seen during the last year?"

_____ 40. Repeat a series of numbers.

_____ 41. "Tell me about your hobbies."

42. The nurse is assessing the sensory functions of the patient with Guillain-Barré syndrome (GBS). The nurse makes a clinical judgment to forgo assessing for light touch discrimination. Why does the nurse make this decision?
    a. The patient's pain and temperature sensations are intact.
    b. Sensory testing is done routinely every 4 hours.
    c. Only patients with spinal trauma require this assessment.
    d. The patient with GBS will be too confused to respond appropriately.

43. The nurse is testing the patient for touch discrimination by touching the patient on both shoulders. What is a normal finding for this assessment?
    a. Pointing to where each shoulder was touched
    b. Moving the shoulders against resistance
    c. Describing the touch as sharp or dull
    d. Sensing touch on the unaffected side

Matching: *Match the component of motor testing with the corresponding test performed.*

Test Component
a. Brainstem integrity
b. Coordination
c. Muscle strength
d. Gait
e. Equilibrium

Test Performed

_____ 44. Patient walks across the room, and returns.

_____ 45. Patient stands, eyes open, feet close together.

_____ 46. Patient holds the arms perpendicular to the body, eyes closed.

_____ 47. Patient grasps and squeezes the nurse's fingers.

_____ 48. With arms out to the side, the patient touches the nose two to three times.

49. The nursing student is performing a neurologic assessment on the patient who sustained a stroke. The nurse observes the student evaluating grip and hand strength only on the affected side. What is the nurse's first action?
    a. Give the student positive feedback for performing the assessment correctly.
    b. Remind the student that strength testing needs to be done bilaterally.
    c. Redo the entire assessment and instruct the student to watch the process.
    d. Suggest to the instructor that the student needs remediation for assessment.

50. The patient is admitted to a rehabilitation center following a stroke that has left him with residual weakness on his left side. The nurse has completed the physical and neurologic assessment. Which documentation note best communicates the patient's progress?
    a. Shows progress and 3+ strength in left leg
    b. Demonstrates 5/5 in left leg and 5/5 in right leg against resistance
    c. Demonstrates 30-degree abduction of left leg
    d. Able to push against resistance with equal power in both legs

51. In assessing the patient's gait and equilibrium, the nurse observes that the patient has Romberg's sign. What is the most appropriate nursing diagnosis associated with this objective data?
    a. Risk for Injury related to dysfunctions in awareness of body position
    b. Activity Intolerance related to decreased muscle strength
    c. Self-Care Deficit in toileting related to inability to ambulate to bathroom
    d. Risk for Impaired Mobility related to unsteady gait

52. Which statement about the Glasgow Coma Scale (GCS) is correct?
    a. It is a thorough neurologic assessment tool.
    b. It establishes a baseline for eye opening and motor and verbal response.
    c. It establishes a baseline cognitive function.
    d. A score of 15 indicates serious neurologic impairment with poor prognosis.

53. The nurse is attempting to assess the coma patient's response to pain. Which technique does the nurse try first?
    a. Gently shake the patient, similar to attempting to wake a sleeping child.
    b. Speak to the patient and call his or her name using a normal tone of voice.
    c. Face the patient and speak loudly and clearly, similar to a hearing-impaired patient.
    d. Apply supraorbital pressure by placing the thumb under the orbital rim.

54. The nurse is assessing response to painful stimuli in the patient. What is the appropriate length of time to apply the stimulus in the comatose patient?
    a. 1 to 2 seconds
    b. 5 to 10 seconds
    c. 20 to 30 seconds
    d. 40 to 60 seconds

55. The nurse is assessing several patients using the GCS. Which factors indicate the most serious neurologic presentation based on the GCS information?
    a. Eye opening to sound, localizes pain, confused conversation
    b. Eye opening to sound, obeys commands, inappropriate words
    c. Eye opening spontaneous, obeys commands, confused conversation
    d. Eye opening to pain, abnormal flexion, incomprehensible sounds

56. The nurse is performing neurologic checks every 4 hours for the patient who sustained a head injury. Which early sign indicates a decline in neurologic status?
    a. Nonreactive, dilated pupils
    b. Change in level of consciousness
    c. Decorticate posturing
    d. Loss of remote memory

57. The student nurse is talking to the patient and family about diagnostic testing. Which statement by the nursing student indicates the need for further study about the understanding of diagnostic procedures?
    a. "You are scheduled for a magnetic resonance imaging (MRI). Do you have a cardiac pacemaker?"
    b. "You are scheduled for a computed tomography (CT) of the head. Are you wearing hairpins?"
    c. "You are to have x-rays of the skull. Are you allergic to iodine?"
    d. "You are to have a cerebral angiography. Do you take medication for diabetes?"

58. Which statement about lumbar puncture is true?
    a. It is indicated for patients with infections at or near the puncture site.
    b. It is done at the T1 to T3 spinal level.
    c. It requires the patient to lie flat for 24 to 48 hours after the procedure.
    d. It is done with the patient in the "fetal" position.

59. The nurse is reviewing the results of a lumbar puncture test. Which cerebrospinal fluid result does the nurse point out to the physician as a significant abnormal finding?
    a. Protein 500-700 mg/100 mL
    b. Cells 0-5 small lymphocytes/mm³
    c. Color straw yellow
    d. Glucose 50 to 75 mg/100 mL

60. The patient is scheduled for an EEG. How does the nurse prepare the patient for this diagnostic test?
    a. Giving a sedative before bedtime
    b. Having the patient drink extra fluids before the test
    c. Keeping the patient NPO after midnight
    d. Keeping the patient awake from 2 AM until the scheduled test time

61. The patient arrives on the unit alert and oriented after undergoing cerebral angiography. The report from the radiology nurse indicates the catheter was inserted into the left femoral artery. For which postprocedural order does the nurse call for clarification?
    a. Keep the left leg straight and immobilized x 2 hours.
    b. Maintain an ice pack and pressure dressing to the insertion site x 2 hours.
    c. IV and oral fluid restrictions for a total of 1000 mL/24 hours.
    d. Neurocirculation checks every 15 minutes x 2 hours; then every hour x 4 hours.

62. The patient is scheduled to have a CT with contrast media and the nurse is reviewing the patient's laboratory results. Which laboratory result could impact the procedure, prompting the nurse to notify the radiology department and the health care provider?
    a. Creatinine level
    b. White blood count
    c. Blood glucose
    d. Urobilinogen level

63. The nurse has instructed the patient and family on information about positron emission tomography (PET). However, the patient is suspected of having early signs of Alzheimer's disease. Which statement by the patient indicates he did not understand the information?
    a. "I may be asked to add or subtract numbers or to remember things during the test."
    b. "I am a little bit nervous by the idea of being blindfolded. Could you tell me about that?"
    c. "They will not give me my insulin shot on the morning of the test."
    d. "I will be asleep during most of the test; I will get a mild medication to help me relax."

64. Which factors are potential contraindications for having an MRI? *(Select all that apply.)*
    a. Cardiac pacemaker
    b. Implanted infusion pump
    c. Ferromagnetic aneurysm clip
    d. Confusion or agitation
    e. Pregnancy
    f. Continuous life support
    h. Recent tattoo

65. The patient is scheduled for a cerebral blood flow evaluation with use of radioactive substance. Which medications does the nurse anticipate the physician will likely withhold from the patient for 24 hours before the test?
    a. Central nervous system depressants and stimulants
    b. Insulin or oral hypoglycemics
    c. Antihypertensives and diuretics
    d. Anticoagulants and antiplatelets

CASE STUDY: NEUROLOGIC ASSESSMENT

Use a separate sheet of paper to answer the questions in this Case Study. Answer guidelines for this Case Study are available on your Evolve website at http://evolve. elsevier.com/Iggy/ in the "Prepare for Class" folder.

The patient is a 48-year-old man, married, and the father of three children. He works as a draftsman, designing decorative iron and other metal products. He is scheduled for a neurologic diagnostic workup. Over the past month, he has noticed that he has had difficulty drawing figures accurately. At times, he has been unable to hold a pencil with sufficient strength to mark the drawing paper. He denies visual changes; however, at times he has difficulty walking without tripping. A lumbar puncture is scheduled following x-rays of the skull and spine.

1. What additional data should the nurse collect initially?

2. Describe the preparation of the patient for the x-ray studies.

3. Identify at least four nursing diagnoses that are appropriate for the patient who is scheduled to have a lumbar puncture.

4. The hospital requires that a consent form be signed by the patient before the lumbar puncture. What is the purpose of this document?

5. The patient asks about complications from the procedure. He asks "Will the test make my symptoms worse? I don't need any more problems right now." How do you reply to the patient?

6. The lumbar puncture is performed and five tubes of cerebrospinal fluid (CSF) are collected. The CSF pressure is 165 cm H_2O. What is the significance of this finding?

7. The physician orders that the specimens be analyzed for cells, protein, and glucose. The laboratory results are:

   Color: straw
   Cells: 7 lymphocytes/mm^3
   RBCs: absent
   Protein: 60 mg/100 mL
   Glucose: 68 mg/100 mL

   Which of the laboratory findings are normal? Which are abnormal?

8. What assessments should the nurse make following the procedure?

9. The patient calls the nurse and says that he has a throbbing headache. What interventions are indicated to help make the patient more comfortable?

CHAPTER 44

Care of Patients with Problems of the Central Nervous System: The Brain

STUDY/REVIEW QUESTIONS

Matching. *Match the current pathophysiology theories with the corresponding type of headache.*

Type of Headache
a. Migraine
b. Cluster headache

Pathophysiology

_____ 1. Blood vessels in the brain overreact to a triggering event

_____ 2. Increase in hypothalamic size

_____ 3. Attributed to vasoreactivity and oxy-hemoglobin desaturation

_____ 4. Spasm in the arteries at the base of the brain

_____ 5. May be caused by hyperexcitability of nerves

_____ 6. Serotonin, a vasoconstrictor, is re-leased

_____ 7. Related to an overactive hypothalamus

_____ 8. A decrease in cerebral blood flow; ce-rebral hypoxia may occur

_____ 9. Prostaglandins, chemicals that cause inflammation and swelling

Matching. *Match each characteristic with the corresponding type of headache.*

Type of Headache
a. Migraine
b. Cluster headache

Characteristics

_____ 10. Familial disorder

_____ 11. Occurs more often in men

_____ 12. Associated with runny nose and ptosis

_____ 13. Has no known cause

_____ 14. May be caused by hyperexcitability of nerves

_____ 15. Patient may walk or rock

_____ 16. May last for several days

_____ 17. Duration limited to 15 to 45 minutes

_____ 18. Occurs at regular intervals with long remission periods

_____ 19. Occurs more often in women

20. The patient arrives at the clinic with a chief complaint of headache. He is irritable and impatient to receive treatment, but he is alert and oriented, his speech is clear, and he is able and willing to answer the nurse's questions. Which questions does the nurse ask to solicit additional relevant information about this patient's headache? *(Select all that apply.)*
    a. "When do the headaches occur?"
    b. "How often do the headaches occur?"
    c. "Why do you have headaches?"
    d. "Did you eat an unusually large meal just before your headache?"
    e. "Do you experience other symptoms with the headache?"
    f. "Have there been any recent changes in your headaches?"

21. The patient with a history of migraine headaches reports his current headache as "my usual throbbing pain, but today it is behind my left eye." Which question does the nurse ask to elicit information about trigger factors?
    a. "Do you have a history of illicit substance abuse?"
    b. "Do you smoke cigars or cigarettes?"
    c. "Are you having any trouble with your vision?"
    d. "Did you drink wine or coffee before the headache occurred?"

22. Which type of medication can be used to prevent migraines?
    a. Lamotrigine (Lamictal)
    b. Metoclopramide (Reglan)
    c. Sumatriptan (Imitrex)
    d. Propranolol (Inderal)

23. During the patient's last visit, the nurse instructed patient about headaches and techniques to manage this condition. Which statement by the patient indicates teaching has been successful?
    a. "I have been keeping track of when my headaches occur."
    b. "My doctor told me that my headaches were not very serious."
    c. "My spouse knows the instructions that you gave me."
    d. "I have not had any headaches since we last talked."

24. Complete the chart below to include the characteristics and symptoms associated with stages of migraine headaches.

Stages of Migraine Headache	Associated Characteristics and Symptoms
Prodrome (or prodromal) phase	
Aura phase (if present)	
Headache phase	
Termination phase	
Postprodrome phase	

25. The patient is prescribed ergotamine with caffeine for migraine headaches. Which statement by the patient indicates the patient is experiencing a side effect of this drug?
    a. "My headache is initially relieved by the medication, but then it returns."
    b. "I seem to be gaining weight since I started taking this medication."
    c. "My headache seems worse in the morning when I take the medication."
    d. "I notice that I bruise more easily and my skin seems fragile and dry."

26. The patient has received a prescription for sumatriptan (Imitrex) for the treatment of migraine headaches. The patient tells the nurse that she elected not to tell the physician about all of her health conditions "because I just wanted treatment for my headaches and I didn't want to go into everything else." What is the nurse's response?
    a. The drug is contraindicated for patients who have glaucoma.
    b. It is necessary to monitor laboratory values such as PT, PTT, and electrolytes.
    c. The drug is contraindicated in actual or suspected ischemic heart disease.
    d. The dosage is calculated by using relevant factors from the health history.

Matching. *Match the type of generalized seizure with its correct definition.*

Types of Generalized Seizures
a. Tonic-clonic
b. Absence
c. Myoclonic
d. Atonic

Definitions

_____ 27. Brief jerking of extremities, singly or in groups

_____ 28. Brief period of staring or loss of consciousness

_____ 29. Rigidity followed by rhythmic jerking

_____ 30. Sudden loss of body tone

31. An elementary school teacher has just been informed that her student's brother has absence seizures. The teacher is fearful that her student may have the same type of seizures and is unsure what to expect. Which signs does the school nurse advise the teacher to look for?
    a. Brief jerking or stiffening of muscles that lasts only a few seconds
    b. Loss of consciousness and rhythmic jerking of extremities
    c. Brief loss of consciousness that may appear as daydreaming or blank staring
    d. "Blackout" that lasts 1 to 3 minutes with lip smacking, patting, or picking at clothes

32. What is the priority nursing diagnosis for atonic (akinetic) seizures?
    a. Risk for Injury related to falls
    b. Ineffective Tissue Perfusion related to neuromuscular dysfunction
    c. Acute Confusion related to postictal state
    d. Activity Intolerance related to atonicity of muscles

33. The patient is scheduled to have several diagnostic tests to verify the medical diagnosis of epilepsy. For which diagnostic tests does the nurse provide patient teaching?
    a. Electrocardiogram (ECG) and positron emission tomography (PET)
    b. Electroencephalogram (EEG) and computed tomography (CT)
    c. Lumbar puncture (LP) and magnetic resonance imaging (MRI)
    d. Complete series of skull x-rays and neuroimaging

34. The nursing student is caring for the patient with partial seizures. Which statement by the student indicates an understanding of partial seizures?
    a. "The patient should be placed in a vest when sitting in a chair."
    b. "There is no medical treatment for partial seizures."
    c. "I should have a padded tongue blade at the bedside."
    d. "The patient may repeatedly pick at the linens."

35. The older adult patient is brought to the emergency department from the local mall after bystanders saw her "having a seizure." The patient is currently responsive to voice, but is lethargic, confused, and unable to give an accurate history. Which aspect of this patient's health history is the most important to verify with the family?
    a. History of acute or chronic respiratory problems
    b. General ability to answer questions accurately
    c. Likelihood of the patient shopping at the mall alone
    d. Patient's doctor's name

36. The patient is treated in the emergency department for status epilepticus and is admitted to the hospital. The physician has ordered seizure precautions. What equipment does the nurse place in the room before the patient's arrival?
    a. Cardiac monitor and a pulse oximeter
    b. Penlight and a neurologic assessment flow sheet
    c. Padded tongue blades and padding for siderails
    d. Oxygen and suction equipment

Matching. *Match each factor with its associated type of meningitis.*

Types of Meningitis
a. Bacterial
b. Viral
c. Fungal

Factors

_____ 37. Condition is usually self-limiting; full recovery is expected.

_____ 38. Manifestations vary according to the state of the immune system.

_____ 39. Cerebrospinal fluid (CSF) is hazy.

_____ 40. No organisms grow from the CSF.

_____ 41. Outbreaks occur in crowded conditions such as dormitories.

42. The nurse is caring for the patient who was admitted for a diagnosis of meningococcal meningitis. Which nursing action is specific to this type of meningitis?
   a. Administer an antifungal agent such as amphotericin B as ordered.
   b. Observe the patient for genital lesions.
   c. Place the patient in isolation per hospital procedure.
   d. Check to see if the patient is HIV positive.

43. The nurse is reviewing the electrolyte values for the patient with bacterial meningitis and notes that the serum sodium is 126 mEq/L. How does the nurse interpret this finding?
   a. Within normal limits considering the diagnosis of bacterial meningitis
   b. Evidence of syndrome of inappropriate antidiuretic hormone (SIADH) which is a complication of bacterial meningitis
   c. A protective measure that causes increased urination and therefore reduces the risk of increased intracranial pressure (ICP)
   d. An early warning sign that the electrolyte imbalances will potentiate an acute myocardial infarction (AMI) or shock

44. The patient with meningitis reports a headache, and the nurse gives the appropriate IV push PRN medication. Several hours later, the patient reports pain in the left hand; the radial pulse is very weak, the hand feels cool, and capillary refill is sluggish compared to the left. What does the nurse suspect is occurring in this patient?
   a. Stroke secondary to increased ICP resulting from meningitis
   b. Sickle cell crisis associated with an increased risk of meningitis
   c. Septic emboli causing vascular compromise which is a complication of meningitis
   d. Local phlebitis from the IV push pain medication that was given for the meningitis headache

45. The patient arrives in the emergency department reporting headache, fever, nausea, and photosensitivity. The patient has been living in close proximity with two people who were diagnosed with meningitis. Which diagnostic test does the nurse anticipate the physician will order to rule out meningitis?
   a. X-rays of the skull
   b. Lumbar puncture
   c. Myelography
   d. Cerebral angiogram

46. The nurse is caring for the patient who has symptoms and risk factors for bacterial meningitis. For which symptom must the nurse alert the physician?
   a. Capillary refill of 3 seconds
   b. Headache with nausea and vomiting
   c. Inability to move eyes laterally
   d. Oral temperature of 101.6° F

47. The nurse is carefully monitoring the patient with a severe case of encephalitis for signs of increased ICP. What vital sign changes are associated with increased ICP?
   a. Tachycardia and shallow, rapid respirations
   b. Increased core temperature and bradycardia
   c. Decreased pulse pressure and tachypnea
   d. Widened pulse pressure and bradycardia

48. The student nurse is caring for the patient with encephalitis. Which action by the student nurse warrants intervention by the supervising nurse?
   a. Performs deep suctioning for copious secretions
   b. Elevates the head of bed to 30 degrees after a lumbar puncture
   c. Turns the patient every 2 hours
   d. Performs a neurologic assessment every 2 hours

49. The older adult patient displays tremors, rigidity, slow movements, and postural instability. Based on the observation of these four cardinal symptoms, which disorder does the nurse suspect?
   a. Alzheimer's disease
   b. Encephalitis
   c. Parkinson disease
   d. Huntington disease

50. Complete the chart below for the characteristics and symptoms associated with each stage of Parkinson disease.

Stages of Parkinson Disease	Associated Characteristics and Symptoms
Stage 1: Initial	
Stage 2: Mild	
Stage 3: Moderate	
Stage 4: Severe disability	
Stage 5: Complete ADLS dependence	

51. During the nurse's assessment of the patient with Parkinson disease, the nurse notes that the patient has masklike facies. What functional assessment does the nurse make after this?
   a. Ability to hear normal voice tones
   b. Ability to chew and swallow
   c. Ability to sense pain in the facial area
   d. Visual acuity

52. The home health nurse is visiting the older adult patient with Stage 1 Parkinson disease. He demonstrates some trembling and weakness in his right hand and arm, and reports he occasionally gets dizzy when he first stands up. The patient is currently living by himself and has no family in the immediate area. What is the priority nursing diagnosis for this patient?
   a. Risk for Self-Care Deficit
   b. Social Isolation
   c. Risk for Falls
   d. Impaired Physical Mobility

53. The patient is on long-term medication therapy for Parkinson disease. What sign indicates that the patient may be having drug toxicity associated with these drugs?
   a. Acute confusion
   b. Tremors and rigidity
   c. Choreiform movements
   d. Seizure activity

54. The patient has moderate Parkinson disease with a nursing diagnosis of Impaired Verbal Communication related to psychomotor deficit. Which nursing intervention is the best to use with this patient?
   a. Speaking clearly and slowly
   b. Watching the patient's lips when he speaks
   c. Giving step-by-step instructions to the patient
   d. Providing visual cues when trying to explain

55. The nurse is assessing the older adult patient who was brought to the clinic by her husband after she went out to do some gardening, but several hours later was spotted walking down the street by a neighbor. She is currently "just like herself," but the patient cannot explain what she was doing or where she was going. Which questions does the nurse ask to assess cognitive changes in this patient? *(Select all that apply.)*
   a. "Have you noticed any forgetfulness, for example misplacing your keys?"
   b. "Has there been any memory loss, such as not remembering a recent conversation?"
   c. "Are there any changes in ability to make judgments, such as taking a medication?"
   d. "Have you noticed any weakness; for example, in the arms or legs?"
   e. "Are there any changes in abilities to do a task like balancing your checkbook?"
   f. "Has there been any incontinence; for example, wetting the bed at night?"

56. The nurse observes the patient with Alzheimer's disease pushing at the food on her tray with her eyeglasses. This is documented as an example of what condition?
    a. Apraxia
    b. Aphasia
    c. Agnosia
    d. Anomia

57. The nurse is assessing the older adult patient with Alzheimer's disease using the Mini Mental State Examination (MMSE). What information about the patient does this exam measure?
    a. Level of intelligence
    b. Functional ability
    c. Severity of the patient's dementia
    d. Alterations in ability to communicate

58. The patient has advanced Alzheimer's disease and is staying in a long-term care facility. Which intervention is the best to use with this patient?
    a. Reality orientation
    b. Cognitive training
    c. Memory training
    d. Validation therapy

59. The patient is experiencing mild memory loss and the patient and family are hoping the nurse can offer suggestions to help stimulate and strengthen the patient's current abilities. What is the nurse's first action?
    a. Show the family how to stimulate the memory by repeating what the patient just said.
    b. Discuss with the family and patient any practical memory problems that are occurring.
    c. Suggest that the patient identify and reminisce about pleasant past experiences.
    d. Provide name tags for the patient, family, and friends for use during group gatherings.

60. The daughter of the older adult patient with Alzheimer's disease has heard that there is a genetic disposition for Alzheimer's, and asks the nurse if there are preventive measures she can take. What does the nurse tell her about the current research on Alzheimer's disease?
    a. There is no evidence that first-degree relatives have an increased risk for this disease.
    b. Eating dark-colored fruits and vegetables has been associated with decreased risk.
    c. Use of NSAIDs such as ibuprofen increases the risk for the disease.
    d. Cessation of all tobacco products has been associated with decreased risk.

61. The patient with mild Alzheimer's disease lives at home with her daughter who is the primary caregiver and who works part-time. Which home safety precaution is appropriate for this patient?
    a. Puzzles and board games are provided for the patient.
    b. A geri-chair with a waist belt is in the patient's bedroom.
    c. The patient is wearing an identification bracelet with the daughter's address.
    d. The patient's medications are carefully organized in the bathroom cabinet.

62. The nurse is caring for several patients with Alzheimer's disease in a long-term care facility. Which task is best to delegate to the nursing assistant?
    a. Give hygienic care to the patient who is currently exhibiting sundowning.
    b. Assist the patient who has incontinence with toileting every 2 hours.
    c. Calm the agitated patient by using soft voice tones and distraction.
    d. Follow the patient and observe for hoarding or rummaging.

CASE STUDY: THE SEIZURE PATIENT

Use a separate sheet of paper to answer the questions in this Case Study. Answer guidelines for this Case Study are available on your Evolve website at http://evolve. elsevier.com/Iggy/ in the "Prepare for Class" folder.

A college student is brought to the emergency department by ambulance. He is alert but confused and uncooperative, and unable to follow simple commands or answer simple questions. His roommate reports, "We were at the library cramming for finals. He just made this really weird sound. Next thing I know he is on the floor shaking and his eyes are rolled back in his head. I turned him on his side. I don't know what is going on with him, but I did call his mother and she said she would meet us here at the hospital." Vital signs are temperature 99° F, pulse 95/min, resp 24/min, BP 140/80.

1. What could the nurse say to the roommate who is most likely to be very stressed by the experience of seeing his friend have a seizure? Why would it be important to calm the roommate and elicit information from him?

2. What should be included in the focused assessment of a patient who has had a seizure?

3. List interventions the nurse would initiate for seizure precautions.

4. Approximately 20 minutes after the patient arrives, he has a repeat seizure. The patient becomes cyanotic and there are copious oral secretions. The tonic-clonic activity lasts approximately 2 minutes. The nurse is at the bedside and immediately intervenes. What interventions does the nurse use?

5. What medications will the physician most likely order for status epilepticus? Describe the nursing implications (administration, side effects, drug level monitoring) for these medications.

6. What are some of the social implications for this young college student who has a new onset of seizures?

7. What should the nurse teach the patient and family about epilepsy?

45 CHAPTER

Care of Patients with Problems of the Central Nervous System: The Spinal Cord

STUDY/REVIEW QUESTIONS

1. The nurse is taking a history on the older adult patient who reports chronic back pain. The nurse seeks to identify if the patient has age-related factors that are contributing to the pain. Which question is the most useful in eliciting this information?
   a. "Have you had any recent falls or have you been in an accident?"
   b. "Do you have a history of osteoarthritis?"
   c. "Do you have a history of diabetes mellitus?"
   d. "Are you having pain that radiates down your leg or into the buttocks?"

2. The nurse is preparing to physically assess the patient's subjective report of paresthesia in the lower extremities. In order to accomplish this assessment, which assessment technique does the nurse use?
   a. Use a Doppler to locate the pedal pulse, the dorsalis pedis pulse, or the popliteal pulse.
   b. Ask the patient to identify sharp and dull sensation by using a paper clip and cotton ball.
   c. Use a reflex hammer to test for deep tendon patellar or Achilles reflexes.
   d. Ask the patient to walk across the room and observe his gait and equilibrium.

3. Which position is therapeutic and comfortable for the patient with lower back pain?
   a. Semi-Fowler's position with a pillow under the knees to keep them flexed
   b. Supine position with arms and legs in a correct anatomical position
   c. Orthopneic position; sitting with trunk slightly forward; arms supported on a pillow
   d. Modified Sims' position with upper arm and leg supported by pillows

4. The patient has been talking to his physician about drugs that could potentially be used in the treatment of his chronic low back pain. Which statement by the patient indicates a need for additional teaching?
   a. "The doctor may prescribe an anti-seizure drug such as oxcarbazepine; therefore, I would need to have blood tests to check my sodium level."
   b. "The doctor may suggest over-the-counter ibuprofen; therefore, I should watch for and report dark or tarry stools."
   c. "The doctor may prescribe an oral steroid such as prednisone; this would be short-term therapy and the dose would gradually taper off."
   d. "The doctor may prescribe hydromorphone and it may cause drowsiness; I should not drive when I take it or drink alcohol."

5. The patient reports back pain described as a continuous, dull, lower back pain, non-radiating (5/10), that increases with certain movements, and has been present for months. The nurse has given the ordered PRN pain medication and a repeat dose is not due for another 2 hours. What is the nurse's first action?
   a. Notify the physician that the prescribed medication is not sufficient.
   b. Give half the dose of the PRN medication now and half the dose in 2 hours.
   c. Reposition the patient and try alternating warm and cold applications.
   d. Wait 2 hours and then give the prescribed PRN pain medication.

6. The patient has just undergone a spinal fusion and a laminectomy and has returned from the operating room. Which assessments are done in the first 24 hours? *(Select all that apply.)*
   a. Take vital signs every 4 hours and assess for fever and hypotension.
   b. Perform a neurologic assessment every 4 hours with attention to movement and sensation.
   c. Monitor intake and output and assess for urinary retention.
   d. Assess for ability and independence in ambulating and moving in bed.
   e. Observe for clear fluid on or around the dressing and test for glucose.

7. The patient has a long history of chronic back pain and has undergone several back surgeries in the past. At this point, the surgeon is recommending a surgical procedure for spine stabilization. Which procedure does the nurse anticipate this patient will need?
   a. Laparoscopic diskectomy
   b. Spinal fusion
   c. Laminectomy
   d. Traditional diskectomy

8. The patient has just undergone a laminectomy and returned from surgery at 1300 hours. At 1530 hours, the nurse is performing the change of shift assessment. Which postoperative finding is reported to the surgeon immediately?
   a. Minimal drainage in the surgical drain after 8 hours
   b. Pain at the operative site
   c. Swelling or bulging at the operative site
   d. Reluctance or refusal to cough and deep-breathe

9. The patient has just undergone spinal fusion surgery and returned from the operating room 12 hours ago. Which task is best to delegate to the nursing assistant?
   a. Log roll the patient every 2 hours.
   b. Help the patient dangle the legs on the evening of surgery.
   c. Assist the patient to put on a brace so he can get out of bed.
   d. Help the patient ambulate to the bathroom as needed.

10. The nurse reviews the discharge and home care instructions with the patient who had back surgery. Which statement by the patient indicates further teaching is needed?
    a. "I will drive myself to my doctor's office next week."
    b. "I will put a piece of plywood under my mattress."
    c. "I will try to increase fruits and vegetables and decrease fat intake."
    d. "I plan to get a new ergonomic chair at work."

11. The patient has had an anterior cervical diskectomy with fusion and has returned from the recovery room. What is the priority assessment?
    a. Assess for the gag reflex and ability to swallow own secretions.
    b. Check for bleeding and drainage at the incision site.
    c. Monitor vital signs and check neurologic status.
    d. Assess for patency of airway and respiratory effort.

12. The patient comes to the emergency department with back pain, but is alert and oriented and is not having any problems breathing. Her husband is very distraught and when the nurse tries to find out what has happened he yells, "Just help her now! Stop asking me these stupid questions!" Why is it important for the nurse to continue trying to obtain information from the husband?
    a. The past medical history and current complaint are part of the legal record.
    b. Engaging the husband will help him to calm down and give him an active role.
    c. Mechanism of injury is important in anticipating potential pathology and damage.
    d. The patient's subjective complaint dictates the focus of the physical examination.

13. The patient is a 65-year-old man who sustained a neck injury during a fall. He has a medical diagnosis of anterior cord syndrome and a nursing diagnosis of Disturbed Sensory Perception. The nurse assesses the patient expecting to observe which type of motor and sensory findings below the level of injury?
    a. No motor functions; no sensation to touch, position, and vibration
    b. Partial motor function; full sense of pain and temperature
    c. Independent movement; no sense of pain or touch
    d. No independent movement; full sense of touch and position

14. The patient with a cervical neck injury is able to spontaneously move the legs when attempting to move himself in bed, but he is not using or moving his arms or hands. What is this observation consistent with?
    a. Anterior cord syndrome
    b. Posterior cord syndrome
    c. Central cord syndrome
    d. Brown-Séquard syndrome

15. The patient involved in a high-speed motor vehicle accident with sustained multiple injuries and active bleeding is transported to the emergency department by ambulance with immobilization devices in place. There is a high probability of cervical spine fracture; the patient has altered mental status and extremities are flaccid. What is the priority assessment for this patient?
    a. Check the mental status using the Glasgow Coma scale.
    b. Assess the respiratory pattern and ensure a patent airway.
    c. Observe for intra-abdominal bleeding and hemorrhage.
    d. Assess for loss of motor function and sensation.

16. The emergency department nurse is assessing and monitoring the patient with a gunshot wound to the middle of the back. Because the patient is at risk for spinal shock, what does the nurse monitor for?
    a. Decreased blood pressure, bradycardia, and flaccid paralysis
    b. Tachycardia and a change in the level of consciousness
    c. Decreased respiratory rate and loss of sensation to pain and touch
    d. Paralytic ileus and loss of bowel and bladder function

17. Which neurologic assessment technique does the nurse use to test the patient for proprioceptive function?
    a. Touch the skin with a clean safety pin and ask whether it is a sharp or dull sensation.
    b. Ask the patient to elevate both arms off the bed and extend wrists and fingers.
    c. Have the patient close the eyes and move the toes up or down; the patient identifies the positions.
    d. Have the patient sit with the legs dangling; use a reflex hammer to test reflex responses.

18. Fill in the chart below with the correct assessment technique for each level of spinal cord injury. The first one has been done for you.

Spinal Cord Level	Assessment
To assess C4-5	Apply downward pressure while the patient shrugs his or her shoulders upward
To assess C5-6	
To assess C7	
To assess C8	
To assess L2-4	
To assess L5	
To assess S1	

Matching. *Match each symptom with its corresponding complication.*

Complications

a. Spinal shock
b. Autonomic dysreflexia

Symptoms

_____ 19. Hypertension

_____ 20. Flaccid paralysis

_____ 21. Hypotension

_____ 22. Severe headache

_____ 23. Loss of reflexes below the injury

_____ 24. Blurred vision

Matching. *Match each physical finding with its corresponding spinal cord lesion.*

Spinal Cord Lesions

a. Anterior cord injury
b. Posterior cord injury
c. Brown-Séquard syndrome

Physical Findings

_____ 25. Motor function is lost on the same side of the body as the injury.

_____ 26. Motor function is lost below the injury.

_____ 27. Motor function remains intact; sensory function is lost.

28. The patient with an upper spinal cord injury is at risk for autonomic dysreflexia. Which nursing diagnosis is the priority for this patient?
    a. Risk for Ineffective Tissue Perfusion, Cerebral
    b. Nausea
    c. Acute Pain, Headache
    d. Impaired Physical Mobility

29. The nurse is caring for the patient with a recent spinal cord injury (SCI). Which intervention does the nurse use to target and prevent the potential SCI complication of autonomic dysreflexia?
    a. Frequently perform passive ROM exercises.
    b. Keep the room warm and control environmental stimuli.
    c. Keep the patient immobilized with neck or back braces.
    d. Monitor urinary output and check for bladder distention.

30. What is a potential adverse outcome of autonomic dysreflexia in the patient with a spinal cord injury?
    a. Heat stroke
    b. Paralytic ileus
    c. Hypertensive crisis
    d. Aspiration and pneumonia

31. After suffering an SCI, the patient develops autonomic dysfunction, including a neurogenic bladder. Which nursing diagnosis is the priority for this condition?
    a. Risk for Infection: urinary tract
    b. Risk for Fluid Volume Deficit: polyuria
    c. Risk for Self-Care Deficit: toileting
    d. Risk for Urinary Incontinence: urge

32. The nurse and the nursing assistant are working together to bathe and reposition the patient who is in a halo fixator device. Which action by the nursing student causes the supervising nurse to intervene?
    a. Uses the log roll technique to clean the patient's back and buttocks
    b. Turns the patient by pulling on the top of the halo device
    c. Positions the patient with the head and neck in alignment
    d. Supports the head and neck area during the repositioning

33. The nurse is caring for several patients with SCIs. Which task is best to delegate to the nursing assistant?
    a. Encourage use of incentive spirometry; evaluate the patient's ability to use it correctly.
    b. Log roll the patient; maintain proper body alignment and place a bedpan for toileting.
    c. Check for skin breakdown under the immobilization devices during bathing.
    d. Insert a Foley catheter and report the amount and color of the urine.

34. The patient with an SCI has paraplegia and paraparesis. The nurse has identified a nursing diagnosis of Impaired Physical Mobility. The nurse assesses the calf area of both legs for swelling, tenderness, redness, or possible complaints of pain. This assessment is specific to the patient's increased risk for which condition?
    a. Contractures of joints
    b. Bone fractures
    c. Pressure ulcers
    d. Deep vein thrombosis

35. The nurse is caring for the patient who has been in a long-term care facility for several months following an SCI. The patient has had issues with urinary retention and subsequent overflow incontinence, and a bladder retraining program was recently initiated. Which is an expected outcome of the training program?
    a. Demonstrates a predictable pattern of voiding
    b. Is able to independently catheterize himself
    c. Pours warm water over perineum to stimulate voiding
    d. Takes bethanechol chloride (Urecholine) 1 hour before voiding

Matching. *Match each medication with its corresponding indication/effect.*

Medications
a. Methylprednisolone
b. Dextran
c. Atropine
d. Dopamine
e. Dantrolene

Indications/Effects
_____ 36. Increases heart rate
_____ 37. Relieves spasticity
_____ 38. Increases capillary blood flow
_____ 39. Reduces inflammation
_____ 40. Regulates blood pressure

41. What does the nurse do to implement bowel and bladder retraining for the patient with an SCI? *(Select all that apply.)*
    a. Ensure the patient gets a sufficient quantity of fluid each day.
    b. Assist the patient in developing a schedule.
    c. Teach the patient about high-fiber foods.
    d. Teach the patient that continence is dependent upon spinal cord healing.
    e. Teach the patient to stimulate voiding by stroking the inner thigh.
    f. Measure bladder residual with a bladder ultrasound device.

42. The patient is an adolescent who is quadriplegic as a result of a diving accident. The nursing assistant reports that the patient started yelling and spitting at her while she was trying to bathe him. He is angry and hostile, stating "Nobody is going to do anything else to me! I'm going to get out of this place!" What is the most appropriate nursing diagnosis for this patient?
    a. Noncompliance
    b. Acute Confusion
    c. Defensive Coping
    d. Hopelessness

43. The nurse is giving home care instructions to the patient who will be discharged with a halo device. What does the nurse instruct the patient to avoid?
    a. Going out in the cold
    b. Swimming or contact sports
    c. Sexual activity
    d. Bathing in the bathtub

44. During the morning assessment of the patient with a spinal cord tumor, the nurse observes decreased sensation in the lower extremities and the linen is smeared with feces and smells of urine. The patient reports low back pain and appears to be having trouble moving his legs. The nurse suspects the tumor to be in which area of the spine?
    a. Upper cervical
    b. Lower cervical
    c. Thoracic
    d. Lumbosacral

45. The patient is hospitalized for a spinal cord tumor and is receiving medication for pain. The patient is having problems with constipation and urinary retention, and in addition, has limited mobility related to site of the tumor. Which task is best to delegate to the nursing assistant?
    a. Measure and record intake and output.
    b. Check for blanching over reddened skin areas.
    c. Report the patient's relief of pain after using PCA morphine.
    d. Manually disimpact fecaliths.

46. The patient reports increased fatigue and stiffness of the extremities. These symptoms have occurred in the past, but resolved and no medical attention was sought. Which question does the nurse ask to assess whether the symptoms may be associated with multiple sclerosis?
    a. "Do you feel unsteady or unbalanced when you walk?"
    b. "Do you have a persistent sensitivity to cold?"
    c. "Do you ever have slurred speech or trouble swallowing?"
    d. "Do you wake at night and then have trouble getting back to sleep?"

47. The patient with multiple sclerosis is prescribed oral prednisone 60 mg daily for 7 days following a course of IV methylprednisolone (Solu-Medrol). Which laboratory abnormality is a side effect of the medication?
    a. Decrease in hematocrit
    b. Decrease in blood glucose
    c. Decrease in serum potassium
    d. Decrease in serum sodium

48. The patient is a woman in her early 30s who has recently been diagnosed with multiple sclerosis. The nurse has taught the patient's husband about the course of the illness and what problems might occur in the future. Which statement by the husband indicates the need for additional teaching?
    a. "She could fall because she may lose her balance and have poor coordination."
    b. "Eventually she will not be able to drive because of vision problems."
    c. "She will probably have a decreased libido and diminished orgasm."
    d. "Later on she could have intermittent short-term memory loss."

49. The patient and family are referred to the nurse for education about amyotrophic lateral sclerosis. What information does the nurse include in the educational session?
    a. It is a progressive disease involving the motor system.
    b. Riluzole (Rilutek) is a specific treatment that reverses symptoms.
    c. Memory loss will occur but it will be very gradual.
    d. Death typically will occur several decades after diagnosis.

50. What early symptoms does the nurse expect to observe in the 50-year-old patient recently diagnosed with amyotrophic lateral sclerosis?
    a. Bowel and bladder incontinence
    b. Tongue atrophy and dysphagia
    c. Blurred vision and headaches
    d. Forgetfulness and decreased attention span

True or False? Read the statements and write T for true or F for false in the blanks provided.

_____ 51. For patients who have back surgery, the nurse should observe the incision site for bleeding and cerebrospinal leakage (clear fluid).

_____ 52. For patients with an SCI, apply immobilization equipment first.

_____ 53. Patients in terminal stages of amyotrophic lateral sclerosis will experience respiratory failure.

_____ 54. Bowel and bladder retraining programs are inappropriate for patients with SCI and spinal diseases.

_____ 55. Interventions to prevent complications associated with immobility include turning, early ambulation or transfers out of bed, and incentive spirometry.

_____ 56. Manifestations of autonomic dysreflexia include severe and rapidly occurring hypotension.

CASE STUDY: THE PATIENT WITH A SPINAL CORD INJURY

Use a separate sheet of paper to answer the questions in this Case Study. Answer guidelines for this Case Study are available on your Evolve website at http://evolve. elsevier.com/Iggy/ in the "Prepare for Class" folder.

The patient is a 23-year-old man who sustained a C7 fracture during a skiing accident. He is being transferred from the medical-surgical unit to the inpatient rehabilitation unit. He has family in the area and they have been supportive throughout his hospital stay. His mother, in particular, has spent many hours at the bedside and expresses a willingness to take him home and continue his care once his hospital and rehab treatment are completed. The patient has lost approximately 18 lbs. during the hospital stay and demonstrates a weak non-productive cough. He had been actively participating with physical therapy and occupational therapy, but he is currently discouraged and withdrawn.

1. Identify at least five nursing diagnoses for this patient and family.
2. Why is this patient at risk for pneumonia and what nursing interventions could be used to help prevent this complication?
3. What are the major complications of prolonged immobility?
4. Identify the major area of education for the patient with an SCI.
5. What are the expected outcomes of a bladder retraining program?
6. What are the essential elements of a bowel retraining program?
7. The nurse assists the patient with SCI with psychosocial adaptation to successful rehabilitation by doing what kinds of interventions?

46 CHAPTER

Care of Patients with Problems of the Peripheral Nervous System

STUDY/REVIEW QUESTIONS

Matching: *Match the terms with the correct definitions.*

Terms

a. Demyelination
b. Parasthesias
c. Hyperesthesia
d. Quadriparesis
e. Ptosis
f. Diplopia
g. Dysphagia
h. Bulbar involvement
i. Eaton-Lambert syndrome
j. Cholinergic crisis
k. Myasthenic crisis
l. Fasciculations
m. Plasmapheresis

Definitions

_____ 1. Overmedication with cholinesterase inhibitors

_____ 2. Weakness in all four extremities

_____ 3. Destruction of myelin between the nodes of Ranvier

_____ 4. Extreme sensitivity to touch

_____ 5. Method to remove antibodies from the plasma to decrease symptoms

_____ 6. Muscles of facial expression, chewing, and speech are affected

_____ 7. Difficulty chewing or swallowing

_____ 8. Double vision

_____ 9. Form of myasthenia; often seen with small cell carcinoma of the lung

_____ 10. Unpleasant sensations such as burning, stinging, and prickly feeling

_____ 11. Undermedication with cholinesterase inhibitors

_____ 12. Muscle twitching

_____ 13. Drooping eyelids

14. The nurse is assessing the patient with a diagnosis of Guillain-Barré syndrome (GBS). Which physical finding is the nurse likely to observe?
    a. Bilateral sluggish pupil response
    b. Sudden onset of weakness in the legs
    c. Muscle atrophy of the legs
    d. Change in level of consciousness

15. During shift report, the nurse hears that the patient with GBS has a decrease in vital capacity that is less than two-thirds of normal, and there is a progressive inability to clear and cough up secretions. The physician has been notified and is coming to evaluate the patient. What intervention is the nurse prepared to implement for this patient?
    a. Frequent oral suctioning
    b. Rigorous chest physiotherapy
    c. Elective intubation
    d. Elective tracheostomy

16. The patient with GBS is identified as having Imbalanced Nutrition, less than body requirements related to inability to swallow safely. A feeding tube is prescribed. How does the nurse monitor this patient's nutritional status?
    a. Checking the patient's skin turgor and urinary output
    b. Giving the prescribed enteral feedings via feeding tube
    c. Weighing the patient three times a week
    d. Reviewing the patient's potassium and sodium levels

17. The patient with GBS has been intubated for respiratory failure. The nurse must suction the patient. In assessing the risk for vagal nerve stimulation, what does the nurse closely monitor the patient for?
    a. Thick secretions
    b. Atrial fibrillation
    c. Cyanosis
    d. Bradycardia

18. The patient is admitted for a probable diagnosis of GBS, but needs additional diagnostic testing for confirmation. Which test does the nurse anticipate will be ordered for this patient?
    a. Electroencephalography (EEG)
    b. Cerebral blood flow (CBF)
    c. Electrocardiogram (ECG)
    d. Electromyography (EMG)

19. The nurse is reviewing the cerebral spinal fluid (CSF) results for the patient with probable GBS. Which abnormal finding is seen in GBS?
    a. Increase in CSF protein level
    b. Increase in CSF glucose level
    c. Cloudy appearance of CSF fluid
    d. Elevation of lymphocyte count in CSF

20. The ambulatory patient has sought treatment for symptoms of GBS within 2 weeks of symptom onset. Which drug therapy is likely preferred for this patient?
    a. Plasmapheresis and immunoglobulin
    b. Plasmapheresis
    c. Immunoglobulin
    d. Corticosteroids

21. The patient is scheduled to receive immunoglobulin therapy. Before administering the medication, the nurse ensures that which laboratory test has been completed?
    a. Serum IgA
    b. Serum IgE
    c. Serum IgD
    d. Serum IgM

True or False? *Read the statements about disorders of GBS and write T for true or F for false in the blanks provided. If the statement is false, correct the statement to make it true.*

_____ 22. Typical clinical manifestations of neuropathy include pain, muscle cramps, and muscle weakness.

_____ 23. Risk factors for GBS include an upper respiratory tract infection or GI illness, and positive antibodies to cytomegalovirus or Epstein-Barr virus (EBV).

_____ 24. In general, GBS is a chronic condition and the subsequent paralysis is permanent.

_____ 25. The most successful treatment of GBS combines plasmapheresis and immunoglobulin.

_____ 26. For a patient with GBS, the nurse assesses the patient's motor (muscle) function every 2 to 4 hours as part of the neurologic assessment.

_____ 27. GBS is the result of a variety of related immune-mediated pathologic processes.

28. The nurse is reviewing the admission and history notes for the patient admitted for GBS. Which medical condition is most likely to be present before the onset of GBS?
   a. Diabetes mellitus
   b. Hyperthyroidism
   c. Peripheral vascular disease
   d. Addison's disease

29. The patient with GBS describes a chronologic progression of motor weakness that started in the legs and then spread to the arms and the upper body. Which type of GBS do these symptoms indicate?
   a. Ascending
   b. Pure motor
   c. Descending
   d. Miller Fisher variant

30. The patient with GBS is in the plateau period. Which intervention is best for the nurse to delegate to the nursing assistant?
   a. Perform passive range of motion every 2 to 4 hours.
   b. Turn the patient every 2 hours and assess for skin breakdown.
   c. Remove the antiembolism stockings every 24 to 48 hours and perform skin care.
   d. Make a communication board for the patient with a list of common requests.

True or False? _Read the statements about myasthenia gravis (MG) and write T for true or F for false in the blanks provided. If the statement is false, correct the statement to make it true._

_____ 31. The Tensilon test can be used to distinguish between a cholinergic crisis and a myasthenic crisis.

_____ 32. MG is characterized by remissions and exacerbations.

_____ 33. For MG, men are affected three times more often than are women.

_____ 34. Evidence suggests a relationship between MG and hyperplasia of the thymus gland.

_____ 35. Although the onset of MG is usually insidious (slow), some instances of fairly rapid development have been caused by infection, emotional upset, pregnancy, or anesthesia.

_____ 36. The patient with MG is deficient in the neurotransmitter serotonin.

37. The nurse is reviewing the biographic data and history for the patient with MG. What does the nurse expect to see included in the patient's records?
   a. Muscle weakness that increases with exertion or as the day wears on
   b. Difficulty sleeping with early morning waking and restlessness
   c. Confusion and disorientation in the late afternoon
   d. Muscle pain and cramps that interfere with activities of daily living

38. Because the most common symptoms of MG are related to involvement of the levator palpebrae or extraocular muscles, which assessment technique does the nurse use?
    a. Use a penlight and check for pupil size and response.
    b. Observe for protrusion of the eyeballs.
    c. Check accommodation by moving the finger toward the patient's nose.
    d. Face the patient and direct him or her to open and close the eyelids.

39. The patient with MG has "bulbar involvement." What is the nurse's priority assessment for this patient?
    a. Presence of pain in the extremities
    b. Loss of bowel and bladder function
    c. Ability to chew and swallow
    d. Quality and volume of the voice

40. The patient with MG and the nurse are having a long discussion about plans for the future. After an extended conversation, what does the nurse anticipate will occur in this patient?
    a. Speech will be slurred and difficult to understand.
    b. Voice may become weaker or exhibit a nasal twang.
    c. Voice quality will become harsh and strident.
    d. Voice will become toneless and affect will be flat.

41. The patient with MG reports having difficulty climbing stairs, lifting heavy objects, and raising arms over the head. What is the pathophysiology of this patient's symptoms due to?
    a. Limb weakness is more often proximal.
    b. Spinal nerves are affected.
    c. Large muscle atrophy is occurring.
    d. Demyelination of neurons is occurring.

42. The nurse is planning activities for the patient with MG. Which factor does the nurse consider to promote self-care, yet prevent excessive fatigue?
    a. Time of day
    b. Severity of symptoms
    c. Medication times
    d. Sleep schedule

43. The patient is suspected of having MG and a Tensilon test has been ordered. What does the nurse do in order to prepare the patient for the test?
    a. Ensure that the patient has a patent IV access.
    b. Draw a blood sample and send it for baseline analysis.
    c. Keep the patient NPO after midnight.
    d. Have the patient void before the beginning of the test.

44. The nurse is caring for the patient recently diagnosed and admitted with MG. During the morning assessment, the nurse notes some abnormal findings. Which symptom does the nurse report to the physician immediately?
    a. Diarrhea
    b. Fatigue
    c. Inability to swallow
    d. Difficulty opening eyelids

45. What is considered a positive diagnostic finding of a Tensilon test?
    a. After the drug is administered, there are no observable changes in muscle strength or tone.
    b. Within 30 to 60 seconds after receiving the drug, there is increased muscle tone that lasts 4 to 5 minutes.
    c. Within 30 minutes of receiving the drug, there is improved muscle strength that lasts for several weeks.
    d. After the drug is first administered, the patient will experience muscle weakness and then return to baseline.

46. Although an adverse reaction to Tensilon is considered rare, which medication should be readily available to give as an antidote in case the patient should experience complications?
    a. Protamine sulfate
    b. Narcan
    c. Atropine sulfate
    d. Regitine

47. The nurse is caring for the patient newly diagnosed with MG. The nurse is vigilant for complications related to both myasthenic crisis and cholinergic crisis. What is the priority nursing assessment for this patient?
    a. Monitor cardiac rate and rhythm.
    b. Assess respiratory status and function.
    c. Monitor fatigue and activity levels.
    d. Perform neurologic checks every 2 to 4 hours.

48. The nurse is performing patient and family teaching about MG medication therapy. What important information does the nurse give during the teaching session?
    a. If a dose of cholinesterase is missed, a double dose is taken the next day.
    b. Antibiotics such as kanamycin synergize cholinesterase inhibitors.
    c. Medications must be taken on an empty stomach with a full glass of water.
    d. Drugs containing morphine or sedatives can increase muscle weakness.

49. The patient with MG develops difficulty coughing. Auscultation of the lungs reveals coarse crackles throughout the lung fields. The nurse identifies the nursing diagnosis of Ineffective Airway Clearance. Which intervention is best for this patient?
    a. Administer oxygen 2 L per nasal cannula.
    b. Perform chest physiotherapy.
    c. Perform endotracheal suction.
    d. Prepare intubation equipment.

50. Complete the chart below by listing characteristics of myasthenic and cholinergic crises and mixed crisis. The first block has been done for you.

Myasthenic Crisis	Cholinergic Crisis	Mixed Crisis
Increased pulse and respiration	Nausea	Apprehension

51. The patient is experiencing acute respiratory failure secondary to MG crisis. Which alternative to mechanical ventilation may this patient benefit from?
    a. Tracheostomy
    b. Bi-level positive airway pressure (Bi-PAP)
    c. IV immunoglobulin therapy (IVIg)
    d. Bronchodilator treatments

52. The nurse has identified the nursing diagnosis of Activity Intolerance for the patient with MG. Which nursing action is best to help this patient avoid excessive fatigue?
    a. Schedule activities before medication administration.
    b. Schedule activities during the late afternoon or early evening.
    c. During periods of maximal strength, provide assistance for ambulation.
    d. Assess the patient's motor strength before and after periods of activity.

53. The nurse is reviewing medication orders for the patient with MG. Which order does the nurse question?
    a. Dosage change in pyridostigmine (Mestinon)
    b. PRN order for Milk of Magnesia
    c. Immediate availability of Tensilon in case of MG crisis
    d. Tapering of corticosteroid treatment

54. The nurse is caring for the patient receiving anticholinesterase drugs for MG. Which symptoms does the nurse immediately report to the physician?
    a. Increasing loss of motor function
    b. Ineffective cough
    c. Dyspnea and confusion
    d. Gastrointestinal side effects

55. During shift report, the nurse learns that the patient with MG deteriorated toward the end of the shift and the physician was called. A Tensilon test indicated that the patient was having a myasthenic crisis. What is the priority nursing diagnosis for this patient?
    a. Risk for Ineffective Breathing Pattern
    b. Risk for Activity Intolerance
    c. Risk for Aspiration
    d. Risk for Autonomic Dysreflexia

56. The patient with MG has been referred to a surgeon for a procedure that may improve the patient's symptoms. Which procedure does the nurse anticipate will be recommended for this patient?
    a. Percutaneous stereotactic rhizotomy
    b. Thymectomy
    c. Resecting severed nerve ends
    d. Partial or complete severance of a nerve

57. The patient with MG experienced a cholinergic crisis. He was intubated and is currently being maintained on a ventilator. He received several 1 mg doses of atropine. What does the nurse closely monitor this patient for?
    a. Increasing muscle weakness
    b. Increased salivation
    c. Ventricular fibrillation
    d. Development of mucous plugs

58. The nurse is performing patient teaching about plasmapheresis. Which statement by the patient indicates understanding of the material?
    a. "Plasmapheresis causes immunosuppression, so I am at risk for infection."
    b. "I will have to be admitted to the hospital for this procedure."
    c. "Two treatments are given over a 2-month period; then I must follow up on a monthly basis."
    d. "The goal of the treatment is to decrease symptoms, but it is not a cure."

59. The nurse is performing teaching for the family of the patient with MG about fatigue and activities of daily living. Which statement by a family member indicates a need for additional teaching?
    a. "Rest is critical because increased fatigue can precipitate a crisis."
    b. "We should do hygienic care for her to avoid undue frustration and fatigue."
    c. "Activities should be done after we give her the medication."
    d. "The physical therapist will be able to recommend some energy-saving devices."

60. The patient with MG is experiencing impaired communication related to weakness of the facial muscles. Which intervention is best in assisting the patient to communicate with the staff and family?
    a. Speak clearly and slowly.
    b. Use short, simple sentences.
    c. Ask "yes" or "no" questions.
    d. Use hand signals.

61. The patient with MG is having difficulty maintaining an adequate intake of food and fluid because of difficulty chewing and swallowing. Which task for this patient is best to delegate to unlicensed assistive personnel (UAP)?
    a. Weigh the patient daily.
    b. Monitor calorie counts.
    c. Ask the patient about food preferences.
    d. Evaluate intake and output.

62. What is the best way for the nurse to protect the patient with MG from corneal abrasions?
    a. Instruct the patient to keep the eyes closed.
    b. Apply an eyepatch to both eyes after breakfast.
    c. Administer artificial tears to keep corneas moist.
    d. Place a clean moist washcloth over the patient's eyes.

63. The patient is receiving a cholinesterase (ChE) inhibitor drug for the treatment of MG. What is a nursing implication for the safe administration of this medication?
    a. Monitor for orthostatic hypotension.
    b. Take the patient's apical pulse prior to administration.
    c. Feed meals 45 to 60 minutes after administration.
    d. Drink at least 8 glasses of water each day.

64. The patient with a thymoma had surgery to relieve symptoms of MG. A single chest tube has been inserted into the patient's anterior mediastinum. The nurse notes that the patient is restless with diminished breath sounds and decreased chest wall expansion. What is the nurse's priority action?
    a. Reposition the patient and perform chest physiotherapy.
    b. Activate the Rapid Response Team.
    c. Suction the patient and tell him to breathe deeply.
    d. Provide oxygen and elevate the head of the bed.

65. Following a thymectomy, what postoperative care does the nurse provide for the patient with MG?
    a. Use of an incentive spirometer once per shift.
    b. Assess for chest pain, dyspnea, hypotension.
    c. Place supine to encourage rest and sleep.
    d. Assist with ambulation every 2 to 3 hours.

66. The nurse is teaching the patient and family about factors that predispose the patient to episodes of exacerbation of MG. Which factors does the nurse mention? *(Select all that apply.)*
    a. Infection
    b. Stress
    c. Change in diet
    d. Any physical exercise
    e. Enemas
    f. Strong cathartics

Completion: Fill in the correct terms to complete the sentences below pertaining to pathophysiology related to peripheral nerve trauma, restless legs syndrome (RLS), trigeminal neuralgia, and Bell's palsy.

67. In peripheral nerve trauma, the most commonly affected sites are the median, _____, and _____ nerves of the arms and the peroneal, _____, and _____ nerves of the legs.

68. After a nerve is transected, the nerve distal to the injury degenerates and retracts within _____ hours.

69. RLS is characterized by leg paresthesias associated with an irresistible _____ _____.

70. Trigeminal neuralgia is usually provoked by minimal stimulation of a _____ _____.

71. In trigeminal neuralgia, _____ and _____ of the teeth, jaw, or ear may be contributing factors.

72. In Bell's palsy, acute maximal paralysis is attained within _____ hours in about half the patients, and within _____ days in almost all patients.

73. The cause of Bell's palsy is believed to be the result of an _____ process.

74. The patient reports that during a game of football, he was tackled and found himself "at the bottom of a pile-up." He reports weakness in the right arm with a burning and tingling sensation in the hand and fingers. How does the nurse assess for movement?
    a. Put the right arm through the normal range of motion.
    b. Ask the patient to flex and extend the elbow.
    c. Defer the first evaluation of movement to the physician.
    d. Ask the patient how much weight he can lift.

75. The nurse is assessing the skin temperature of the patient's right lower extremity. Which technique does the nurse use?
    a. Place a paper strip thermometer on the patient's skin.
    b. Palpate the extremity using the fingertips.
    c. Compare bilateral extremities using the dorsal surface of the hand.
    d. Ask the patient if the skin feels subjectively hotter or colder than usual.

76. The nurse is caring for the patient with peripheral nerve damage to the lower extremity. What does the postoperative positioning and handling of the extremity include?
    a. ROM exercises for the affected limb to maintain mobility
    b. Joint extension to keep the nerve properly aligned
    c. Joint flexion to keep tension off the suture site
    d. Abduction maintained with a wedge pillow

77. The nurse is assessing the arm of the patient with peripheral nerve damage from incorrect use of crutches which occurred several weeks ago. The nurse observes that the arm is reddish-blue and mottled. What does the nurse interpret this finding as evidence of?
    a. Warm phase
    b. Cold phase
    c. Trophic changes
    d. Plateau period

78. The patient has undergone surgical anastomosis of damaged nerve segments. After suturing and surgery is completed, a cast is placed on the extremity to maintain which position?
    a. Neutral anatomical
    b. Flexed
    c. Partial extension
    d. Abducted

79. The nurse is teaching the patient about postsurgical care after repair of a damaged nerve in the arm. Which information does the nurse include?
    a. "You must protect the nerve sutures for a minimum of 2 weeks."
    b. "Physiotherapy will begin immediately within the first or second day after surgery."
    c. "The cast that is applied after surgery will remain in place for 2 to 3 days."
    d. "Discomfort, tingling, or coolness are considered abnormal and should be reported."

80. Which patient has the highest risk factors for RLS?
    a. Obese patient with renal failure
    b. 65-year old woman who routinely jogs
    c. 43-year old man with hypertension
    d. Underweight teenager who smokes

81. The patient is diagnosed with RLS. What non-pharmacologic interventions does the nurse suggest for this patient? *(Select all that apply.)*
    a. Limit caffeine intake
    b. Smoking and alcohol cessation
    c. Avoid strenuous activities 2 to 3 hours before bedtime
    d. Avoid taking naps during the day
    e. Apply ice packs and elevate legs
    f. Walk and perform stretching exercises

82. The patient is prescribed ropinirole (Requip) for RLS. What nursing implication is related to this medication?
    a. Teach the patient to take the medication after meals.
    b. Usual dose is between 50 and 200 mg per day.
    c. Medication should be taken at bedtime.
    d. Medication is contraindicated in Parkinson disease.

Matching: Match each statement to the corresponding condition. Answers can be used more than once.

Conditions
a. Trigeminal neuralgia
b. Facial paralysis (Bell's palsy)

Statements

_____ 83. Pain provoked by stimulation of trigger zone

_____ 84. More common in women

_____ 85. Incidence may be higher in diabetic patients

_____ 86. Thought to be related to brainstem activity

_____ 87. Inflammatory in nature

_____ 88. Taste impaired

_____ 89. Requires protection of the cornea

_____ 90. Arterial compression removed by surgery

_____ 91. 30 to 60 mg daily corticosteroids may be prescribed

_____ 92. Soft diet and frequent small meals encouraged

93. The patient reports "excruciating, sharp, shooting" unilateral facial pain which lasts from seconds to minutes and describes a reluctance to smile, eat, or talk because of fear of precipitating an attack. This patient's description of symptoms is consistent with the symptoms of which disorder?
    a. Peripheral nerve trauma
    b. Trigeminal neuralgia
    c. Bell's palsy
    d. Eaton-Lambert syndrome

94. The patient is diagnosed with trigeminal neuralgia. Which therapy is the first-line choice for this patient?
    a. Antiepileptic such as gabapentin (Neurontin)
    b. Muscle relaxant such as baclofen (Lioresal)
    c. Percutaneous stereotactic rhizotomy
    d. Microvascular decompression

95. The patient has had surgical relocation of the artery to relieve the pain of trigeminal neuralgia. What is included in the postoperative care of this patient? *(Select all that apply.)*
    a. Apply an ice pack to the operative site on the cheek and jaw for 48 hours.
    b. Perform a focused cranial nerve assessment.
    c. Discourage the patient from chewing on the affected side until paresthesias resolve.
    d. Instruct the patient to avoid rubbing the eye on the affected side.
    e. Teach the patient that he may have enhanced pain sensation during dental procedures.
    f. Monitor the patient for headache, cranial nerve dysfunction, and bleeding.

96. The patient is diagnosed with Bell's palsy and the right side of the face is affected. Related to the patient's right eye, which nursing action is best to implement?
    a. Check the pupil size and reaction using a penlight.
    b. Check the patient's visual acuity in both eyes.
    c. Teach the patient to instill artificial tears four times a day.
    d. Teach the patient to prevent eye strain by resting eyes periodically.

CASE STUDY: THE PATIENT WITH GBS

Use a separate sheet of paper to answer the questions in this Case Study. Answer guidelines for this Case Study are available on your Evolve website at http://evolve. elsevier.com/Iggy/ in the "Prepare for Class" folder.

The patient is a 45-year-old construction worker who is admitted for diagnostic testing for possible Guillain-Barré syndrome. The patient reports an abrupt weakness in the legs with a crawling sensation, pain, and tingling in the legs. He complains of a burning sensation that started in the lower trunk area. He states, "I feel a little nervous and scared. Am I having a stroke? Sometimes I feel like I am having trouble taking in a deep breath. Is that just my nerves?" There is history of a recent episode of gastroenteritis, but otherwise reports good general health.

1. List several of the diagnostic tests that this patient is likely to have.
2. Identify and prioritize at least four nursing diagnoses for this patient.
3. Discuss the assessment and monitoring associated for adequate respiratory function for a patient with GBS.
4. The physician orders a plasmapheresis treatment for this patient. Explain the purpose and the procedure to the patient.
5. What are the nursing interventions for the patient undergoing plasmapheresis?

47 CHAPTER

Care of Critically Ill Patients with Neurologic Problems

STUDY/REVIEW QUESTIONS

Matching: *Match each symptom of stroke with the hemisphere most often affected by that symptom. Answers can be used more than once.*

Affected Hemispheres

a. Left
b. Right

Symptoms

_____ 1. Loss of depth perception

_____ 2. Aphasia

_____ 3. Loss of hearing

_____ 4. Cannot recognize faces

_____ 5. Impaired sense of humor

_____ 6. Depression

_____ 7. Denies illness

_____ 8. Frustration and anger

_____ 9. Disoriented to person, place, and time

_____ 10. Poor judgment

11. The nurse is performing a neurologic assessment on the patient. In addition to the level of consciousness (LOC), what is assessed to evaluate cognitive changes that may be occurring? *(Select all that apply.)*
    a. Denial of illness
    b. Proprioceptive dysfunction
    c. Presence of flaccid paralysis
    d. Impairment of memory
    e. Decreased ability to concentrate

12. Following a left hemisphere stroke, the patient has expressive (Broca's) aphasia. Which intervention is best to use when communicating with this patient?
    a. Repeat the names of objects on a routine basis.
    b. Face the patient and speak slowly and clearly.
    c. Obtain a whiteboard with an erasable marker.
    d. Develop a picture board that has objects and activities.

13. The nurse is caring for the patient with right hemisphere damage. The patient demonstrates disorientation to time and place, he has poor depth perception, and demonstrates neglect of the left visual field. Which task is best delegated to the nursing assistant?
    a. Move the patient's bed so that his affected side faces the door.
    b. Teach the patient to wash both sides of his face.
    c. Ensure a safe environment by removing clutter.
    d. Suggest to the family that they bring familiar family pictures.

14. The patient with a right cerebral hemisphere stroke may have safety issues related to which factor?
    a. Poor impulse control
    b. Alexia and agraphia
    c. Loss of language and analytical skills
    d. Slow and cautious behavior

15. The patient is at risk for increased intracranial pressure (ICP) and is receiving oxygen 2 L via nasal cannula. The nurse is reviewing arterial blood gas (ABG) results. Which ABG value is of greatest concern for this patient?
    a. pH 7.32
    b. $Paco_2$ of 60 mm Hg
    c. Pao_2 of 95 mm Hg
    d. HCO_3^- of 28 mEq/L

16. Which statement is true about motor changes in the patient who has had a stroke?
    a. Motor deficit is ipsilateral to the hemisphere affected.
    b. Motor deficit is contralateral to the hemisphere affected.
    c. Bowel and bladder function remain intact.
    d. Flaccid paralysis is not an expected finding and should be reported promptly.

17. The preferred administration time for recombinant tissue plasminogen activator (rtPA [Retavase]) is within how long of stroke symptom onset?
    a. 30 minutes
    b. 3 hours
    c. 6 hours
    d. 24 hours

18. A nursing diagnosis of Risk for Aspiration has been identified for the patient who was admitted for a brain attack. Which intervention is best to delegate to the nursing assistant?
    a. Monitor the patient for and notify the charge nurse of any occurrence of coughing, choking, or difficulty breathing.
    b. Place the patient in a high Fowler's position and slowly feed small spoonfuls of pudding, pausing between each spoonful.
    c. Assess the swallow reflex by placing the index finger and thumb on either side of the Adam's apple.
    d. Give the patient a glass of water before feeding solid foods and have oral suction ready at the bedside.

Matching: *Match each deficit with its corresponding definition.*

Deficits
a. Ptosis
b. Hemianopsia
c. Amaurosis fugax
d. Receptive aphasia
e. Agraphia
f. Alexia
g. Photophobia

Definitions
_____ 19. Inability to comprehend language

_____ 20. Sensitivity to light

_____ 21. Difficulty writing

_____ 22. Blindness in half of the visual field

_____ 23. Blindness in one eye

_____ 24. Difficulty reading

_____ 25. Drooping eyelid

26. The patient is diagnosed with an ischemic stroke. The nursing assistant reports that the patient's vital signs are blood pressure 150/100 mm Hg, pulse 78 beats/min, respiratory rate of 20/min, and temperature of 98.7° F. The patient's blood pressure is normally around 120/80. What action does the nurse take?
    a. Report the blood pressure immediately to the physician because there is a danger of rebleeding.
    b. Ask the nursing assistant to repeat the blood pressure measurement in the other extremity with a manual cuff.
    c. Check the physician's orders to see if the blood pressure is within the acceptable parameters.
    d. Nothing; an elevated blood pressure is necessary for cerebral perfusion.

27. The patient with an ischemic stroke is placed on a cardiac monitor. Which cardiac dysrhythmia places the patient at risk for emboli?
    a. Sinus bradycardia
    b. Atrial fibrillation
    c. Sinus tachycardia
    d. First degree heart block

28. The nurse is caring for the patient receiving medication therapy to prevent a recurrent stroke. Which medication is pharmacologically appropriate for this purpose?
    a. Enteric-coated aspirin (Ecotrin)
    b. Gabapentin (Neurontin)
    c. Recombinant tissue plasminogen activator (Retavase)
    d. Bevacizumab (Avastin)

29. The patient sustained a stroke that affected the right hemisphere of the brain. The patient has visual spatial deficits and deficits of proprioception. After assessing the safety of the patient's home, the home health nurse identifies a nursing diagnosis of Unilateral Neglect. Which environmental feature represents a potential safety problem for this patient?
    a. The handrail that borders the bathtub is on the left-hand side.
    b. The patient's favorite chair faces the front door of the house.
    c. The patient's bedside table is on the right-hand side of the bed.
    d. Family has relocated the patient to a ground-floor bedroom.

30. The patient with a stroke is having some trouble swallowing. Which feeding technique is the safest option to prevent aspiration?
    a. Place a small amount of milk in a cup and offer small sips.
    b. Administer orange juice using a straw.
    c. Give small spoonfuls of custard.
    d. Give tiny bits of finely cut-up chicken breast.

31. Complete the table by identifying the distinguishing features of each type of stroke. Use a separate sheet of paper if necessary.

FEATURE	TYPE OF STROKE		
	Thrombotic	Embolic	Hemorrhagic
Onset			
Evolution			
Contributing Factors			
Duration			

32. The patient received rtPA for the treatment of ischemic stroke and the physician ordered an IV sodium heparin infusion. In relation to the drug therapy, what does the nurse monitor for?
    a. Elevated prothrombin level
    b. Bleeding gums or bruising
    c. Nausea and vomiting
    d. Elevated hematocrit or hemoglobin

33. The nurse is caring for the patient with impaired swallowing. Which intervention does the nurse employ for this patient?
    a. Limit the diet to clear liquids.
    b. Keep the patient on NPO status.
    c. Monitor the patient's weight.
    d. Chat with the patient while the patient eats.

34. The male patient has sustained a stroke and the nurse is planning interventions to help him reestablish urinary continence. What action does the nurse take?
    a. Obtain an order for a Foley catheter.
    b. Offer the urinal to the patient every 6 hours.
    c. Check residual urine with a bladder scanner.
    d. Restrict fluid to 1500 mL/day.

35. The patient with intracranial pressure is to receive IV mannitol (Osmitrol). Which nursing actions are taken concerning this drug? (Select all that apply.)
    a. Draw up the drug through a filtered needle.
    b. Insert a Foley catheter to measure strict urine output.
    c. Monitor serum and urine osmolality on a weekly basis.
    d. Assess for acute renal failure, weakness, or edema.
    e. Administer mannitol through a filter in the IV tubing.
    f. Administer furosemide (Lasix) as an adjunctive therapy.

36. The nurse is talking to the family of the stroke patient about home care measures. Which topics does the nurse include in this discussion? (Select all that apply.)
    a. Need for caregivers to plan for routine respite care and protection of own health
    b. Evaluation for potential safety risks such as throw rugs or slippery floors
    c. Awareness of potential patient frustration associated with communication
    d. Avoidance of independent transfers by the patient because of safety issues
    e. Access to health resources such as publications from the American Heart Association
    f. Referral to hospice and encouragement of family discussion of advance directives

37. Which patients are at increased risk for stroke? (Select all that apply.)
    a. 66-year-old man with diabetes mellitus
    b. 35-year-old healthy woman who uses oral contraceptives
    c. 47-year-old woman who exercises regularly
    d. 35-year-old man with history of multiple transient ischemic attacks
    e. 25-year-old woman with Bell's palsy
    f. 53-year-old man with chronic alcoholism

38. The patient displays signs of increased ICP, confusion, slurred speech, and unilateral weakness in the upper extremity. Which diagnostic test for this patient does the nurse question?
    a. Lumbar puncture (LP)
    b. Computed tomography (CT)
    c. Positron emission tomography (PET)
    d. Magnetic resonance imaging (MRI)

Matching: Match each intervention for the stroke patient to the hemisphere most commonly affected. Answers may be used more than once.

Affected Hemispheres
a.   Right hemisphere
b.   Left hemisphere

Interventions

_____ 39.   Scan side-to-side.

_____ 40.   Place pictures and familiar objects around the patient.

_____ 41.   Approach the patient from the unaffected side.

_____ 42.   Reorient the patient frequently.

_____ 43.   Place objects within the patient's field of vision.

_____ 44.   Establish a structured routine for the patient.

_____ 45.   Teach the patient to wash both sides of body.

_____ 46.   Repeat names of commonly used objects.

47.   The nurse has completed teaching the patient about endarterectomy. Which statement by the patient indicates understanding of the purpose of the procedure?
a.   "The goal is to open the artery enough to establish blood flow."
b.   "The procedure occludes the abnormal artery to prevent bleeding."
c.   "The bulge in the artery is clipped to prevent bleeding."
d.   "The clot is removed to decrease intracranial pressure."

48.   The nurse is caring for the patient with an ischemic stroke. Which position is the patient placed in according to current nursing practice?
a.   Supine with extremities in anatomical position
b.   Head of bed is elevated to 45 degrees
c.   Supine with hips in flexed position
d.   Recovery position

49.   The nurse is caring for the patient at risk for ICP related to ischemic stroke. For what purpose does the nurse place the patient's head in a midline neutral position?
a.   Provide comfort for the patient.
b.   Protect the cervical spine.
c.   Facilitate venous drainage from brain.
d.   Decrease pressure from cerebrospinal fluid.

50.   In planning care for the patient with increased ICP, what does the nurse do to minimize ICP?
a.   Gives the bath, changes the linens, and does passive ROM exercises to hands/fingers, then allows the patient to rest.
b.   Gives the bath, allows the patient to rest, changes the linens, allows the patient to rest, and then performs passive ROM exercises to hands/fingers.
c.   Defers the bath, changes the linens, and does passive ROM exercises to extremities until the danger of increased ICP has passed.
d.   Contacts the physician for specific orders about all activities related to the care of the patient that might cause increased ICP.

51.   The nurse is caring for the patient at risk for increased ICP. Which sign is most likely to be the first indication of increased ICP?
a.   Decline of level of consciousness
b.   Increase in systolic blood pressure
c.   Change in pupil size and response
d.   Abnormal posturing of extremities

Matching: *Match each type of hematoma with its corresponding description.*

Types of Hematomas

a. Epidural hematoma
b. Subdural hematoma
c. Intracranial hemorrhage

Descriptions

_____ 52. Caused by tearing of small vessels within brain tissue

_____ 53. Occurs between the skull and the dura

_____ 54. May present as acute, subacute, or chronic

55. The nurse is caring for the patient admitted with the medical diagnosis of probable epidural hematoma and decreased level of consciousness. During the shift, the patient becomes lucid and is alert and talking. The family reports this is her baseline mental status. What is the nurse's next action?
    a. Stay with the patient and have the charge nurse alert the physician because this is an ominous sign for the patient.
    b. Document the patient's exact behaviors, compare to previous nursing entries, and continue the neurologic assessments every 2 hours.
    c. Point out to the family that the dangerous period has passed, but encourage them to leave so the patient does not become overly fatigued.
    d. Monitor the patient for the next 48 hours to 2 weeks because a subacute condition may be slowly developing.

56. Blood flow to the brain remains fairly constant as a result of which process?
    a. Autostasis
    b. Automobilization
    c. Hemodynamic stasis
    d. Autoregulation

57. The patient has been diagnosed with a large lesion of the parietal lobe and demonstrates loss of sensory function. Which nursing intervention is applicable to this patient?
    a. Play music for the patient for at least 30 minutes each day.
    b. Teach the patient to test the water temperature used for bathing.
    c. Position the patient reclining in bed or in a chair for meals.
    d. Use a picture of the patient's spouse and ask the patient to state the spouse's name.

58. The patient has been diagnosed with subarachnoid hemorrhage. Which drug does the nurse anticipate will be ordered to control cerebral vasospasm?
    a. Nimodipine (Nimotop)
    b. Phenytoin (Dilantin)
    c. Dexamethasone (Decadron)
    d. Clopidogrel (Plavix)

Matching: Match each type of trauma with its corresponding definition.

Types of Trauma
a. Laceration
b. Acceleration
c. Concussion
d. Linear fracture
e. Basilar skull fracture
f. Comminuted fracture
g. Depressed fracture
h. Deceleration
i. Open fracture

Definitions
_____ 59. The head hits a stationary object.
_____ 60. There is a simple, clean break in the skull.
_____ 61. Cortical surface is torn.
_____ 62. The head is in motion.
_____ 63. Bone presses inward into brain tissue.
_____ 64. Cerebrospinal fluid leaks from nose or ears.
_____ 65. There is a direct opening to brain tissue.
_____ 66. Fragments of bone are in brain tissue.
_____ 67. There is a brief loss of consciousness.

68. Which determination must be made first in assessing the patient with traumatic brain injury?
    a. Presence of spinal injury
    b. Whether the patient is hypotensive
    c. Presence of a patent airway
    d. Level of consciousness using the Glasgow Coma Scale

69. Which statement is true about the patient at risk for increased ICP?
    a. The appearance of abnormal posturing occurs only when the patient is not positioned for comfort.
    b. Cushing's reflex, an early sign of increased ICP, consists of severe hypertension, widening pulse pressure, and bradycardia.
    c. Papilledema, edema, and hyperemia of the optic disk are always signs of increased ICP.
    d. Areas of tenderness over the scalp indicate the presence of contrecoup injuries.

70. The nurse is caring for the patient with increased ICP who is on a mechanical ventilator. The patient is awake and agitated, and is attempting to breathe at a different rate than the ventilator setting. Which PRN medication does the nurse administer to the patient?
    a. Midazolam (Versed)
    b. Promethazine (Phenergan)
    c. Naloxone (Narcan)
    d. Pentobarbital sodium (Nembutal)

71. The patient has sustained a traumatic brain injury. Which nursing intervention is best for this patient?
    a. Assess vital signs every 8 hours.
    b. Position to avoid extreme flexion.
    c. Increase fluid intake for the first 48 hours.
    d. Administer glucocorticoids.

72. The nurse is caring for the patient with a relatively minor head injury after a bump to the head. The nurse has the greatest concern about which symptom?
    a. Headache
    b. Nausea and vomiting
    c. Unequal pupils
    d. Dizziness

73. Which statement is true about respiratory problems in the patient with a major head injury?
    a. Atelectasis and pneumonia can be prevented by proper pulmonary hygiene.
    b. Suctioning should be avoided because of the increase in ICP.
    c. Neurologic pulmonary edema occurs frequently.
    d. The patient should avoid breathing deeply because of increased ICP.

74. Which Glasgow Coma Scale (GCS) data set indicates the most severe injury for a patient with traumatic brain injury and loss of consciousness (LOC)?
    a. GCS of 13 with LOC of 15 minutes
    b. GCS of 9 with LOC of 30 minutes
    c. GCS of 12 with LOC of 3 hours
    d. GCS of 8 with LOC of 6.5 hours

75. The nurse is assessing the patient who was struck in the head several times with a bat. There is a clear fluid that appears to be leaking from the nose. What action does the nurse take?
    a. Hand the patient a tissue and ask him to gently blow the nose; observe the nasal discharge for blood clots.
    b. Immediately report the finding to the physician and document the observation in the nursing notes.
    c. Place a drop of the fluid on a white absorbent background and look for a yellow halo.
    d. Allow the patient to wipe his nose, but no other action is needed; he has most likely been crying.

76. Which statement is true for the patient with a basilar skull fracture?
    a. There is potential for hemorrhage caused by damage to the internal carotid artery.
    b. There is an increased risk for loss of functional abilities such as toileting.
    c. There is an increased risk for cytotoxic or cellular edema with loss of consciousness.
    d. There is potential for decorticate or decerebrate posturing with loss of motor function.

77. The patient is admitted for a closed head injury from a fall down the stairs. The patient has no history of respiratory disease and no apparent respiratory distress, but the physician orders oxygen 2 L via nasal cannula. What does the nurse do next?
    a. Check the pulse oximetry and apply the oxygen if the saturation level drops below 90%.
    b. Call the physician to discontinue the order because it is unnecessary.
    c. Deliver the oxygen as ordered because hypoxemia may precipitate increased ICP.
    d. Apply the nasal cannula as ordered and gradually wean the patient off the oxygen when the LOC improves.

78. The nurse is conducting a presentation to a group of students on the prevention of head injuries. Which statement by a student indicates a need for additional teaching?
    a. "Drinking, driving, and speeding contribute to the risk for injury."
    b. "Males are more likely to sustain head injury compared to females."
    c. "Young people are less likely to get injured because of faster reflexes."
    d. "Following game rules and not 'goofing around' can prevent injuries."

79. The nurse is taking a history on the teenager who was involved in a motor vehicle accident with friends. The patient has an obvious contusion of the forehead, seems confused, and is laughing loudly and yelling, "Stella! Stella!" What is the best question for the nurse to ask the patient's friends?
    a. "Where and why did the accident occur?"
    b. "How can we notify the family for consent for treatment?"
    c. "Was the patient using drugs or alcohol prior to the accident?"
    d. "Who is Stella and why is the patient calling for her?"

80. The provider has prescribed barbiturate coma therapy for the patient with increased ICP. Which complication does the nurse monitor for?
    a. Decreased LOC
    b. Reduced gastric motility
    c. Decreased respiratory rate
    d. Reduced Glasgow Coma Scale score

81. The nurse is performing discharge teaching for the family and patient who has had prolonged hospitalization and rehabilitation therapy for severe craniocerebral trauma after a motorcycle accident. What elements of instruction does the nurse include? *(Select all that apply.)*
    a. Review seizure precautions.
    b. Stimulate the patient with frequent changes in the environment.
    c. Develop a routine of activities with consistency and structure.
    d. Attend follow-up appointments with therapists.
    e. Encourage the family to seek respite care if needed.
    f. Encourage the patient to wear a helmet when riding.

82. The patient has sustained a major head injury and the nurse is assessing the patient's neurologic status every 2 hours. What early sign of increased ICP does the nurse monitor for?
    a. Change in the LOC
    b. Cheyne-Stokes respirations
    c. Severe hypertension with widened pulse pressure (Cushing's reflex)
    d. Dilated and nonreactive pupils

83. The nurse is giving discharge instructions to the mother of a child who bumped her head on a table. Which statement by the mother indicates an understanding of the instructions?
    a. "I should not allow her to fall asleep."
    b. "She may have nausea or headache for the first 24 hours."
    c. "She should gently blow her nose and I'll observe for bleeding."
    d. "She can run and play as she usually does."

84. The nurse is caring for the intubated patient with increased ICP. If the patient needs to be suctioned, which nursing action does the nurse take to avoid further aggravating the increased ICP?
    a. Manually hyperventilate with 100% oxygen before passing the catheter.
    b. Maintain strict sterile technique when performing endotracheal suctioning.
    c. Perform oral suctioning frequently, but do not perform endotracheal suctioning.
    d. Obtain an order for an arterial blood gas before suctioning the patient.

Matching: *Match each key feature of brain tumors with their most likely tumor site. Answers may be used more than once.*

Tumor Sites
a. Cerebral tumor
b. Brainstem tumor

Features of Brain Tumors
_____ 85. Vomiting unrelated to food intake
_____ 86. Hemiparesis
_____ 87. Facial pain or weakness
_____ 88. Nystagmus
_____ 89. Seizures
_____ 90. Headache
_____ 91. Hoarseness
_____ 92. Aphasia
_____ 93. Ataxia
_____ 94. Hearing loss

95. The nurse is caring for the patient with a brain tumor. Which drug therapy does the nurse anticipate this patient will receive?
    a. Glucocorticosteroids for edema
    b. NSAIDs for pain
    c. Insulin for diabetes insipidus
    d. Ticlopidine hydrochloride (Ticlid) for platelet adhesiveness

96. Which statement is true about gamma knife therapy for brain tumors?
    a. It is used for easily reached tumors.
    b. It is noninvasive and has few complications.
    c. It is administered under general anesthesia.
    d. It replaces conventional radiation therapy.

97. The patient is scheduled for a craniotomy. What does the nurse tell the patient and family about the procedure?
    a. The head will not need to be shaved at the surgical site.
    b. There is a coma state for up to several days after surgery.
    c. Drainage of cerebrospinal fluid after surgery is normal; bloody drainage is not.
    d. The family will need to remind the patient of their names and relationships.

98. The patient has had an infratentorial craniotomy. Which position does the nurse use for this patient?
    a. High-Fowler's position, turned to the operative side
    b. Head of bed at 30 degrees, turned to the nonoperative side
    c. Flat in bed, turned to the operative side
    d. Flat in bed, may turn to either side

99. The nurse is performing discharge teaching for the patient who underwent a craniotomy for a brain tumor. What instruction does the nurse include? *(Select all that apply.)*
    a. Suggestions to make the environment safe, such as removing scatter rugs
    b. Reminders that seizures could occur frequently for the first several months
    c. Information about drugs such as dose, administration, and side effects
    d. Directions about how and when to contact emergency services or the physician
    e. Advice about which over-the-counter products are safe to use
    f. Referral to a resource such as the American Brain Tumor Association

100. The nurse is providing education for the patient with a brain tumor. What educational elements does the nurse include?
    a. Instructions to avoid physical activity
    b. Instructions to avoid over-the-counter drugs
    c. Advice that seizures will occur in the immediate postoperative period
    d. Information about dietary changes to prevent recurrence of the tumor

101. The patient who had a craniotomy develops the postoperative complication of syndrome of inappropriate antidiuretic hormone (SIADH). The patient's sodium level is 126 mEq/L and the serum osmolality is decreased. In light of this development, which physician order does the nurse question?
    a. Encourage oral fluids
    b. Normal saline IV at 150 mL/hr
    c. Strict intake and output
    d. Daily weights

102. The nurse is assisting the patient who had a large brain tumor removed to get positioned in bed. Which recommended position does the nurse place the patient in?
    a. Operative side to protect the unaffected side of the brain
    b. Flat and repositioned on either side to decrease tension on the incision
    c. Elevate the head of bed 30 degrees to promote venous drainage
    d. Nonoperative side to prevent displacement of the cranial contents by gravity

103. The patient is admitted to the critical care unit after a craniotomy to debulk a grade 3 astrocytoma. Which nursing diagnosis is the priority?
    a. Risk for Infection
    b. Disturbed Thought Processes
    c. Decreased Intracranial Adaptive Capacity
    d. Impaired Physical Mobility

104. The nurse observes that the patient who had surgery for a benign hemangioblastoma has bilateral periorbital edema and ecchymosis. Because this patient's care is based on the general principles of caring for the patient with a craniotomy, what is the nurse's first action?
    a. Immediately inform the surgeon.
    b. Apply cold compresses.
    c. Check the pupillary response.
    d. Perform a full neurologic assessment.

105. Which statement is true about increased ICP in the surgical patient?
    a. It is a minor postoperative complication.
    b. Diuretics such as furosemide may be given to decrease it.
    c. Cerebral edema usually subsides within 72 hours.
    d. If not contraindicated, the head of bed should be placed at 30 degrees.

106. The nurse is teaching the patient who will receive the disc-shaped Gliadel wafer as part of the treatment for a brain tumor. Which statement by the patient indicates understanding of how the wafer works?
    a. "I'll place the wafer under my tongue and allow it to dissolve."
    b. "The wafer will be taped to my chest and the drug will be absorbed."
    c. "The wafer will be placed directly into the cavity during the surgery."
    d. "The wafer is to be dissolved in water and taken with meals."

107. Which organism is commonly involved in opportunistic central nervous system infections for patients with AIDS?
    a. Streptococcus
    b. Enterobacter
    c. *Haemophilus influenzae*
    d. Toxoplasmosis

108. The nurse who is providing postoperative care for the patient who had a craniotomy immediately notifies the surgeon for which assessment finding?
    a. Drainage in the Jackson Pratt container of 45 mL/8 hours
    b. Intracranial pressure of 15 mm Hg
    c. Pco$_2$ level of 35 mm Hg
    d. Serum sodium of 117 mEq/L

109. What is most likely to be included in the history of the patient with a brain abscess?
    a. Family history of Huntington disease
    b. History of HIV/AIDS
    c. History of osteoarthritis
    d. Vaccination against influenza

110. The patient is admitted for diagnostic testing for probable encapsulated brain abscess and risk for increased ICP. Which statement about diagnostic testing for this patient is true?
    a. WBCs may be normal, even if an infection is present.
    b. Blood cultures are the only cultures likely to grow the causative organism.
    c. MRI is useful late in the course of the disease to identify permanent lesions.
    d. The first test performed is a lumbar puncture to determine if the cerebrospinal fluid is cloudy.

111. The patient has an abscess caused by anaerobic bacteria. Which drug does the nurse expect to be ordered for this patient?
    a. Nafcillin sodium (Nafcil)
    b. Fluconazole (Diflucan)
    c. Metronidazole (Flagyl)
    d. Penicillin G benzathine (Bicillin)

CASE STUDY: THE PATIENT WITH HEAD INJURY

Use a separate sheet of paper to answer the questions in this Case Study. Answer guidelines for this Case Study are available on your Evolve website at http://evolve. elsevier.com/Iggy/ in the "Prepare for Class" folder.

The patient is a 68-year-old man who sustained a head injury after falling in the bathroom. He arrives in the emergency department (ED) cheerful, alert, and oriented to person. On physical exam, he has a large hematoma on his left forehead. His wife was present during the incident. Admission vital signs are blood pressure 170/92 mm Hg, pulse 92 beats/min, respirations 14/min, and temperature 98.7° F.

1. Why is it important to determine the circumstances of the fall for this patient?

2. Discuss the importance of obtaining baseline behavior and information from the wife.

3. The ED physician orders computed tomography (CT) of the brain for the patient. What is the purpose of this test and what are the nursing responsibilities in preparing the patient for this procedure?

4. Because the patient is at risk for increased ICP, explain how the patient should be positioned and moved in bed.

5. The CT and other diagnostic results are negative and the patient is diagnosed with a minor head injury and contusion to the right extremity. He is discharged to home. Review the patient teaching instructions that should be given to the patient and his wife.

6. The wife appears unwilling to take her husband home and she states that she doesn't understand the discharge instructions. What can the nurse do in this situation?

48 CHAPTER

Assessment of the Eye and Vision

STUDY/REVIEW QUESTIONS

1. Which statement about the optic disk is true?
   a. Nerve fibers and photoreceptor cells are contained in this depressed area on the retina.
   b. It is the clear layer that forms the external coat on the front of the eye.
   c. It is sometimes called the blind spot.
   d. It forms a circular, convex structure behind the iris.

2. Light waves pass through each of the eye structures listed below to reach the retina. Place them in sequence using the numbers 1 through 5, with number 1 being the outermost structure, ending at the retina.

   _____ a. Vitreous humor

   _____ b. Aqueous humor

   _____ c. Lens

   _____ d. Cornea

   _____ e. Retina

3. The patient's intraocular pressure has increased. Which fluids in the eye does this affect? (*Select all that apply.*)
   a. Blood
   b. Vitreous humor
   c. Vitreous body
   d. Aqueous humor
   e. Fovea centralis
   f. Ciliary body

4. Which muscle is responsible for pulling the eye upward?
   a. Inferior oblique
   b. Lateral rectus
   c. Medial rectus
   d. Superior oblique

Matching. Match each cranial nerve with its function.

Nerves
a. Cranial nerve II (optic)
b. Cranial nerve III (oculomotor)
c. Cranial nerve V (trigeminal)
d. Cranial nerve VII (facial)

Functions

_____ 5. Corneal reflex

_____ 6. Visual acuity

_____ 7. Eyelid closure

_____ 8. Eyelid muscle movements

9. What is astigmatism caused by?
   a. Eye over-refracting light
   b. Eye not refracting enough light
   c. Normal aging process
   d. Unevenly curved surfaces of the eye

Matching. Match each description with the corresponding name for the eye change associated with aging.

Eye Changes
a. Sunken eyes
b. Decreased ability to accommodate
c. Astigmatism
d. Arcus senilis
e. Loss of night vision

Descriptions

_____ 10. Opaque, bluish white ring on the outer aspect of the cornea

_____ 11. Decreased ability of iris to dilate

_____ 12. Loss of subcutaneous fat, skin elasticity, and muscle tone

_____ 13. Flattened cornea, resulting in irregular curvature

_____ 14. Loss of lens elasticity

15. The 29-year-old patient has told the nurse that he spends a great deal of time in the sun. In preparing a teaching plan for the patient, what information about protecting vision does the nurse include? *(Select all that apply.)*.
   a. Wear sunglasses to filter UV light.
   b. Unprotected UV light exposure increases the risk for cataracts.
   c. Melanoma is the most common eye malignancy in adulthood.
   d. UV light exposure is only a concern with sunlight.
   e. Manifestations of melanoma of the eye will be readily apparent.

16. The patient is 45 years old with diabetes mellitus. Which information about vision protection does the nurse include in the teaching plan? *(Select all that apply.)*
   a. Wash hands before touching the eyes.
   b. Monitor blood glucose levels closely.
   c. Contact the health care provider immediately if eye infection is suspected.
   d. Do not share eye drops with others.
   e. Twice-yearly eye examinations are recommended for routing care with diabetes mellitus.

17. In the chart below, write a brief answer for why it is important to address each area of health history with your patient when assessing the eyes.

Health History	Reason for Obtaining Information
Family history and genetic risk	
Current medical systemic diseases	
Types of sports activities in which patient participates	
All medications	

18. Which statement about the pupil of the eye is true?
    a. The patient with myopia has smaller pupils.
    b. Normal pupil size is between 1 and 3 mm.
    c. Pupils are larger in older adults.
    d. Anisocoria is normal in 5% of the population.

19. The patient reports not being able to see objects in his peripheral vision. Which tests are used to evaluate this symptom? *(Select all that apply.)*
    a. Jaeger card
    b. Visual field testing
    c. Confrontation test
    d. Six cardinal positions of gaze
    e. Cover-uncover test

20. The patient who works in a machine shop has a suspected metal foreign body in the eye. Which test is contraindicated for this patient?
    a. Corneal staining
    b. CT scan
    c. MRI
    d. Ultrasonography

Matching. Match each physical finding with the corresponding related technique.

Techniques
a. Ishihara chart
b. Confrontation
c. Corneal light reflex
d. Snellen chart
e. Six cardinal positions of gaze

Physical Findings
_____ 21. Color blindness
_____ 22. Visual acuity
_____ 23. Peripheral vision
_____ 24. Eye muscle imbalance
_____ 25. Eye muscle weakness, nerve dysfunction

26. When preparing the patient for a fluorescein angiography, which statements are included in the nurse's teaching plan? *(Select all that apply.)*
    a. Intravenous access will be necessary.
    b. Sunlight must be avoided for 2 days.
    c. Urine voided after the test will be bright orange.
    d. Fluids are limited for the first 24 hours after the procedure.
    e. The skin may temporarily have a yellow or green hue for a few hours after the procedure.
    f. Mydriatic drops will be instilled 1 hour before the procedure.

27. Which are correct procedures for instilling ophthalmic drops in the patient's eyes? *(Select all that apply.)*
    a. Check the name, strength, and expiration date of the solution.
    b. Have the patient tilt the head backward and look down.
    c. Release drops into the conjunctival pocket.
    d. Avoid contaminating the tip of the bottle.
    e. After instilling the drop, have the patient close the eyes tightly.

28. Which statement about tonometry is true?
    a. Tonometry readings are indicated for all patients 55 years of age and older.
    b. Tonometry is used to measure intraocular pressure.
    c. Adults with a family history of glaucoma should be checked monthly.
    d. Intraocular pressure stays constant throughout the day.

29. Which procedures are correct for using the ophthalmoscope? *(Select all that apply.)*
    a. The nurse comes toward the patient's eye from 6 inches away.
    b. The nurse comes toward the patient to the side of the patient's line of vision.
    c. When examining the right eye, the nurse holds the ophthalmoscope in the left hand.
    d. The nurse stands on the same side as the eye being examined.
    e. The test should be done in a brightly lit room to enhance visibility.
    f. The nurse should observe for the presence of the red reflex, which should be seen in the pupil.

Matching. *Match the assessment findings to the structures observed by ophthalmoscopy. Answers may be used more than once.*

Structures
a. Red reflex
b. Optic disk
c. Optic blood vessels
d. Fundus
e. Macula

Assessment Findings

_____ 30. Bleeding

_____ 31. Nicking at arteriovenous crossings

_____ 32. Presence or absence

_____ 33. Tears or holes

_____ 34. Margins

_____ 35. Presence of blood vessels

_____ 36. Light reflection

_____ 37. Lesions

_____ 38. Kinks or tangles

_____ 41. The lacrimal gland is located in the inner canthus and secretes tears over the eye surface.

_____ 42. Exophthalmos is the sunken appearance of the eye.

_____ 43. A vision acuity of 20/70 means that the patient is able to see at 70 feet what a "healthy eye" can see at 20 feet.

True or False? *Read each statement and write T for true or F for false in the blanks provided. If the statement is false, rewrite the statement to make it true.*

_____ 39. Presence of the arcus senilis is a change of aging that affects vision.

_____ 40. The fovea centralis is the point in the macula where the vision is the most acute.

44. Which assessment findings of the eye are normal? *(Select all that apply.)*
    a. Presbyopia in a 45-year-old woman
    b. Ptosis of the eyelids
    c. Yellow sclera with small pigmented dots in a dark-skinned person
    d. Pupil constriction in response to accommodation
    e. Pupil constriction within 2 seconds in response to light
    f. Nystagmus in the far lateral gaze
    g. Consensual pupil response

Matching. Match each diagnostic test with its purpose.

Tests
a. Corneal staining
b. Slit-lamp examination
c. Jaeger card
d. Radioisotope scanning
e. MRI
f. CT

Purpose

_____ 45. Magnifies anterior eye structures, abnormalities of cornea, lens, aqueous humor

_____ 46. View of eyes, bony structures around eyes, extraocular muscles; contrast often used

_____ 47. Contraindicated with the presence of metal

_____ 48. Topical dye into conjunctival sac, outlines irregularities of cornea

_____ 49. Locates tumors or lesions; patient is not radioactive after procedure

_____ 50. Used to test near vision

Care of Patients with Eye and Vision Problems

CHAPTER 49

STUDY/REVIEW QUESTIONS

Matching. *Match each eyelid disorder with its corresponding description.*

Disorders

a. Ectropion
b. Blepharitis
c. Hordeolum
d. Chalazion
e. Entropion

Descriptions

_____ 1. Eyelid margin inflammation

_____ 2. Sweat gland infection at the lash/lid margin

_____ 3. Inflammation of a sebaceous gland of the eyelid

_____ 4. The turning inward of the eyelid

_____ 5. The turning outward and sagging of the eyelid

6. Which statements about an entropion are true? *(Select all that apply.)*
    a. Pain and tearing may be present.
    b. The orbicular muscle can be surgically tightened for correction.
    c. Entropion can be caused by eyelid spasms.
    d. The patient lacks sufficient tears to wash adequately over the eye.
    e. Entropion rarely occurs with older adults.

7. Which factors are causes of keratoconjunctivitis sicca? *(Select all that apply.)*
    a. Use of antihistamines
    b. Lacrimal gland malfunction
    c. Multiple sclerosis
    d. Cranial nerve VII malfunction
    e. Vision enhancement surgery

8. Which statement about keratoconjunctivitis sicca and its management is true?
    a. Use of antihistamines can stimulate tear production.
    b. Warm, moist compresses help restore moisture to the eye.
    c. Artificial tears can be used as often as necessary.
    d. Care must be taken to avoid transferring contamination from one eye to the other.

9. The patient has been diagnosed with trachoma. Which nursing intervention is the focus of this patient's care?
    a. Pain control
    b. Nutrition
    c. Infection control
    d. Loss of visual function

10. Bacterial conjunctivitis is associated with which signs/symptoms? *(Select all that apply.)*
   a. Significant ocular discharge
   b. Tearing
   c. Itching
   d. Blurred vision
   e. Mild conjunctival edema
   f. Formation of scales and granulations on the eyelids

11. What are the nursing care priorities for the patient who is a corneal donor? *(Select all that apply.)*
   a. Instill saline solution into the eyes.
   b. Instill antibiotic drops into the eyes.
   c. Raise the head of the bed to 30 degrees.
   d. Close the eyes and apply an ice pack to the eyes.
   e. Contact the patient's family regarding tissue donation.

12. The patient is scheduled for a keratoplasty. What are the possible complications from this procedure? *(Select all that apply.)*
   a. Bleeding
   b. Graft rejection
   c. Infection
   d. Pain
   e. Photosensitivity

13. Which statement about postoperative care for the patient who has had a keratoplasty is true?
   a. The patient should lie on the operative side to reduce intraocular pressure.
   b. The patient's eye will be covered for 1 week with the initial dressing and shield.
   c. The patient should wear the patch at night for the first month after surgery.
   d. The head of the bed must be elevated 15 degrees.

True or False? Read the statements about cataracts and write T for true or F for false in the blanks provided. For those statements that are false, rewrite the statement to make it true.

_____ 14. Age-related cataract formation is associated with pain and eye redness.

_____ 15. Early manifestations of cataracts include slightly blurred vision and decreased color perception.

_____ 16. A cataract is an opacity of the lens that distorts the image projected onto the retina.

_____ 17. Cataracts develop in both eyes at the same rate.

_____ 18. Cataracts may be present at birth.

19. The patient has had cataract surgery and is ready to go home. In the discharge education prepared by the nurse, which activities will the nurse tell the patient to avoid?

20. Which signs and symptoms should the patient who has had cataract surgery report to the physician? *(Select all that apply.)*
   a. Pain with nausea and vomiting
   b. Decreased vision
   c. Significant swelling or bruising
   d. Increasing redness of eyes
   e. Photophobia

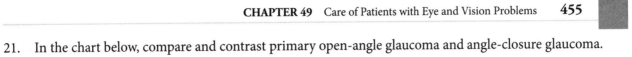

21. In the chart below, compare and contrast primary open-angle glaucoma and angle-closure glaucoma.

	Primary Open-Angle Glaucoma	**Angle-Closure Glaucoma**
Prevalence		
Symptoms		
Onset		
Physical examination		
Tonometry reading		

22. Drug therapy for glaucoma focuses on reducing increased ocular pressure through what two mechanisms?

    a. _____

    b. _____

23. Compare the medications used for glaucoma by completing the chart below.

Drug	**Classification**	**Action**	**Nursing Implication**
Timolol			
Pilocarpine			
Latanoprost			

24. Which factors may be a cause of blood leakage into the vitreous humor? *(Select all that apply.)*
    a. Hypertension
    b. Aging
    c. Cataract surgery
    d. Glaucoma
    e. Traumatic injury

25. Which statement about uveitis is correct?
    a. Anterior uveitis is also known as retinitis.
    b. Posterior uveitis is an inflammation of the iris.
    c. Symptoms include seeing a red haze or series of floaters.
    d. Steroid drops are given hourly to prevent adhesion of the iris to the cornea and lens.

26. Which conditions are associated with posterior uveitis? *(Select all that apply.)*
    a. Tuberculosis
    b. Syphilis
    c. Herpes zoster
    d. Rheumatoid arthritis
    e. Toxoplasmosis
    f. Allergies

27. Which nursing interventions are included for the patient with uveitis?
    a. Patching the affected eye
    b. Offering aspirin and opioids for increased pain
    c. Darkening the room
    d. Instructing the patient to drive only when necessary

28. Which factors are related to dry age-related macular degeneration? *(Select all that apply.)*
    a. Gradual blockage of retinal capillaries
    b. Retinal cells in the macula become ischemic and necrotic
    c. Progresses more rapidly in smokers
    d. Fluid and blood collect under the macula
    e. Eventual loss of all central vision

Matching. *Match the retinal dysfunctions with the correct definitions.*

Retinal Dysfunctions
a. Retinal detachment
b. Retinal tear
c. Retinal hole

Definitions

_____ 29. Separation of the retina from the epithelium

_____ 30. Jagged, irregular break in the retina

_____ 31. Hole in the retina caused by trauma or aging

32. Which statement about retinal detachment is true?
    a. Onset is usually sudden and painful.
    b. Patients may notice loss of peripheral vision.
    c. Patients may suddenly see bright flashes of light.
    d. Hyperopia is directly associated with its occurrence.

33. The patient has a retinal tear that must be closed or sealed. Which procedures may the ophthalmologist use to do this? *(Select all that apply.)*
    a. IV Veteporfin
    b. Laser therapy
    c. Cryotherapy
    d. Patch on the eye and rest
    e. Diathermy

34. After a scleral buckling procedure involving a gas bubble insertion, the patient is placed in which position?
    a. High Fowler's
    b. Supine with head to nonoperative side
    c. Prone with head turned so that the operative eye is facing up
    d. Trendelenburg position

35. What activities should the patient avoid after a scleral buckling procedure?

36. Which sign/symptom is the most common early clinical manifestation of retinitis pigmentosa?
    a. Cataracts
    b. Night blindness
    c. Headache
    d. Vitamin A deficiency

Matching. Match the refractive errors with their definitions.

Refractive Errors
a. Myopia
b. Astigmatism
c. Presbyopia
d. Hyperopia

Definitions

_____ 37. Short eye length causes images to be focused behind the retina.

_____ 38. Curve of the cornea is not even.

_____ 39. Images are bent and fall in front of the retina.

_____ 40. This condition usually appears in people in their 30s and 40s.

41. Complete the chart comparing the surgical management for the treatment of refractive errors.

	Radial Keratotomy (RK)	Photorefractive Keratotomy (PRK)	Laser-in-situ Keratomileusis (LASIK)
Indication			
Procedure			
Postoperative Recovery			

42. The 10-year-old patient was hit in the left eye with a baseball. There is discoloration around the eye. Which treatment does the nurse expect to give for this patient?
    a. Eye patch to rest the eye
    b. Surgical repair of injury
    c. Ice to area
    d. Bedrest in semi-Fowler's position

43. Cycloplegic eye drops may be used with which traumatic disorder of the eye?
    a. Foreign body in eye
    b. Periorbital ecchymosis
    c. Hyphema
    d. Contusion

44. Which traumatic injury of the eye is the most likely to cause loss of vision in the injured eye?
    a. Hyphema
    b. Contusion
    c. Laceration
    d. Penetration injury of eye

45. What is the most common intraocular malignant tumor in adults? _____

46. Which visual acuity test result classifies a person as blind, even if they are wearing corrective lenses?
    a. 20/50
    b. 20/100
    c. 20/150
    d. 20/200

47. What may patients who have lost their sight experience? *(Select all that apply.)*
    a. Hopelessness
    b. Grieving
    c. Anger
    d. Immobility
    e. Fear

48. What is the priority intervention to include in the nurse's teaching plan for the patient with impaired vision?
    a. Self-care
    b. Communication
    c. Mobility
    d. Safety

49. The nurse is teaching the patient about self-medication with eyedrops for glaucoma. Which intervention does the nurse suggest the patient do to prevent systemic absorption of the medication?
    a. Wait 10 to 15 minutes between applications of different eye drops
    b. Punctal occlusion
    c. Place all eye medications in one eye, then the other
    d. Blink rapidly after instilling drops

50. What time frame does the nurse use when instilling more than one ophthalmic drug to the patient?
    a. 20 to 30 minutes
    b. 1 hour
    c. 10 to 15 minutes
    d. There is no need to wait to administer subsequent drops

CASE STUDY: THE PATIENT WITH EYE AND VISION PROBLEMS

Use a separate sheet of paper to answer the questions in this Case Study. Answer guidelines for this Case Study are available on your Evolve website at http://evolve. elsevier.com/Iggy/ in the "Prepare for Class" folder.

A 45-year-old woman has come into the ophthalmology office for an annual eye examination. She has had progressive myopia and astigmatism since age 11 years. In addition to her job as a high school physical education teacher, she also plays in local recreation league volleyball teams and plays tennis with friends. She wears eyeglasses that also correct for beginning presbyopia and has satisfactory correction. This year, the physician notes that she has a very small hole in the retina of her left eye, but no treatment is indicated for now. However, the physician does recommend that she stop playing tennis and volleyball at this time.

1. What is the probable cause of this retinal hole? Why did the physician recommend that she stop these activities?

2. Later, the patient works in her yard trimming hedges with an electric clipper. Despite wearing her eyeglasses, a branch whips backward and strikes her in the left eye. She immediately sees bright flashes of light, and at first notes that it seems as if a curtain or shadow is pulled over her eye. What should the patient do?

3. Upon ophthalmoscopic examination, the physician sees gray bulges in the retina that quiver. A tear is seen at the lateral edge of retina. What is the probable diagnosis? Be specific.

4. The patient is scheduled for immediate surgery. Describe the type and purpose of the surgery needed for this condition.

5. Postoperatively, the patient has an eye patch and shield over her left eye. She is now fully awake and wants to use the bathroom. She also is reporting severe nausea. What should the nurse do?

6. The patient tells the nurse that she is looking forward to going home because she wants to be able to work outside in her garden for relaxation. What instructions should the nurse give to the patient about her activity, diet, and postoperative care?

50 CHAPTER

Assessment of the Ear and Hearing

STUDY/REVIEW QUESTIONS

1. Which is the spiral organ of hearing?
   a. Cochlea
   b. Semicircular canal
   c. Pinna
   d. Stapes

2. Which cranial nerve is stimulated by vibrations, aiding the sense of hearing?
   a. V
   b. VI
   c. VIII
   d. IX

Matching. Match each ear structure with the corresponding locations. Answers may be used more than once.

Locations
a. External ear
b. Middle ear
c. Inner ear

Structures
_____ 3. Mastoid process
_____ 4. Incus
_____ 5. Stapes
_____ 6. Cochlea
_____ 7. Tympanic membrane
_____ 8. Organ of Corti
_____ 9. Malleus

10. Identify the events in sequential order, using the numbers 1 through 6, that lead to the sense of hearing.
    _____ a. Sound waves are transferred to the malleus.
    _____ b. Sound waves are transferred to the incus and the stapes.
    _____ c. Vibrations are transmitted to the cochlea.
    _____ d. Neural impulses are conducted by the auditory nerve.
    _____ e. Sound waves strike the mastoid and the movable tympanic membrane.
    _____ f. Sound is processed and interpreted by the brain.

11. Which are changes in the ear that are related to aging? *(Select all that apply.)*
    a. Tympanic membrane may appear dull and retracted.
    b. Pinna becomes shorter and thickened.
    c. Cerumen-producing glands decrease in number and function.
    d. Bony ossicles have decreased movement.
    e. Hearing of high-frequency sound increases.

Matching. *Match the following terms with their definitions.*

Terms

a. Decibel
b. Masking
c. Vestibular hearing loss
d. Otosclerosis
e. Sensorineural

Definitions

_____ 12. Relating to the functions of the ear needed for the sense of balance and position

_____ 13. A unit of sound for expressing loudness

_____ 14. Formation of spongy bone around structures of the middle and inner ear

_____ 15. The process of hiding a specific sound from one ear while the other ear is tested

_____ 16. Hearing loss resulting from neural defects

17. A sensorineural hearing loss results from impairment of which structure?
    a. Fused bony ossicles
    b. First cranial nerve
    c. Seventh cranial nerve
    d. Eighth cranial nerve

18. The adult patient is having problems with hearing. Which of the patient's medications listed are ototoxic? *(Select all that apply.)*
    a. Ibuprofen (Motrin)
    b. Digoxin (Lanoxin)
    c. Furosemide (Lasix)
    d. Levothyroxine (Synthroid)
    e. Aspirin
    f. Gentamicin (Garamycin)

19. Which statement about otoscopic assessment is true?
    a. The patient's head should be tilted slightly toward the nurse for support.
    b. The nurse holds the otoscope upside down, like a large pen.
    c. The pinna is pulled down and back.
    d. The internal canal is visualized while the speculum is slowly inserted.

20. In otoscopic assessment, what does a normal tympanic membrane look like? *(Select all that apply.)*
    a. Slightly convex in nature
    b. Pink to deep-red color
    c. Mobile pars tensa
    d. Opaque or pearly gray
    e. Always intact

21. Which structure is seen through a normal tympanic membrane?
    a. Utricle
    b. Pars flaccida
    c. Umbo
    d. Cochlea

22. Which is the more sensitive test of hearing, air conduction or bone conduction?

    _____

Matching. Match the hearing test terms with their correct definitions.

Hearing Tests
a. Voice test
b. Electronystagmography (ENG)
c. Dix-Hallpike test
d. Audiometry
e. Watch test
f. Weber tuning fork test

Definitions

_____ 23. Measurement of hearing acuity

_____ 24. Test for hearing of high-frequency sounds

_____ 25. Used to differentiate between conductive and sensorineural hearing losses

_____ 26. Test for detecting central and peripheral disease of the vestibular system

_____ 27. Tests for vertigo

_____ 28. A simple acuity test

29. Which statement about the Weber tuning fork test is correct?
    a. The preferred site for testing is above the upper lip over the teeth.
    b. Ask the patient in which ear the sound is louder.
    c. Proper handling of the fork includes grasping the upper part of the fork for stability.
    d. Lateralization is a normal result.

30. Which statements are true regarding the Rinne tuning fork test? (*Select all that apply.*)
    a. The test assists in differentiating hearing by air conduction and bone conduction.
    b. The test involves timed responses.
    c. The vibrating fork stem is placed on the patient's mastoid process.
    d. Sound is normally heard longer by bone conduction than by air conduction.
    e. Ask the patient in which ear the sound is heard loudest.

31. What is the measurement of hearing acuity?
    a. Frequency
    b. Audiometry
    c. Threshold
    d. Intensity

32. What is defined as the lowest level of intensity at which pure tones and speech are heard by a patient about 50% of the time?
    a. Frequency
    b. Audiometry
    c. Threshold
    d. Intensity

33. What is defined as the highness or lowness of tones (expressed in Hertz)?
    a. Frequency
    b. Audiometry
    c. Threshold
    d. Intensity

34. Which is a contraindication for the patient having ENG?
    a. Fasting for the past 24 hours
    b. Previous ENG
    c. Prostheses
    d. Pacemaker

35. What does speech discrimination testing determine?
    a. Ability to hear sounds
    b. Ability to understand speech
    c. Ability to receive speech
    d. Ability to hear sounds at varying intensity

36. Tympanometry is helpful in distinguishing which disorder?
    a. Middle ear infections
    b. Outer ear infections
    c. Furuncles
    d. Indurated lesions on the pinna

37. What is the normal response to caloric testing?
    a. Vertigo and nystagmus within 20 to 30 seconds
    b. Vertigo and nystagmus immediately
    c. Vertigo and nystagmus within 5 minutes
    d. Nystagmus with no vertigo

38. What does using a gentle puff of air when examining the external ear canal with an otoscope assess for?
    a. Presence of infection
    b. Pain
    c. Mobility of the eardrum
    d. Eardrum patency

Matching. *Match the type of hearing loss with its definition.*

Types of Loss
a. Sensorineural hearing loss
b. Conductive hearing loss
c. Mixed conductive-sensorineural hearing loss

Definitions

_____ 39. Profound hearing loss

_____ 40. Results from a defect in the cochlea, eighth cranial nerve, or the brain

_____ 41. Results from any physical obstruction of sound wave transmission

51 CHAPTER

Care of Patients with Ear and Hearing Problems

STUDY/REVIEW QUESTIONS

1. Which treatments are used for external otitis? *(Select all that apply.)*
   a. Application of heat
   b. Oral analgesics
   c. Topical antibiotics
   d. Myringotomy
   e. Bedrest

2. What are the most common organisms associated with external otitis? *(Select all that apply.)*
   a. *E. coli*
   b. Aspergillus
   c. *Pseudomonas aeruginosa*
   d. *Staphylococcus aureus*
   e. Streptococcus

3. Which condition caused by trauma results in the calcification and hardening of the pinna?
   a. Atresia
   b. Flower ear
   c. Hard ear
   d. Boxer's ear

4. Which statement about necrotizing or malignant external otitis is true?
   a. It is the most virulent form of external otitis.
   b. There is a low mortality rate related to complicating disorders.
   c. It can destroy cranial nerve V.
   d. It is a very common problem among younger adults.

5. The adult patient has external otitis. After the inflammation resolves, which actions should the patient *avoid*?
   a. Using earplugs while swimming
   b. Dropping diluted alcohol in the ear to prevent recurrence
   c. Using cotton-tipped applicators to dry the ears thoroughly after bathing
   d. Using analgesics for pain relief

6. A furuncle may be caused by which factor?
   a. Self-limiting viral infection
   b. Congenital malformation
   c. Bacterial infection of a hair follicle
   d. Bacterial infection of the structures of the inner ear

7. Ear irrigation fluid would be *least* likely to stimulate the vestibular sense at what temperature?
   a. 78° F
   b. 98° F
   c. 110° F
   d. 120° F

8. The adult patient has otitis media. What does the nurse expect the patient's chief complaint to be?
   a. Ear pain
   b. Rhinitis
   c. Drainage from the ear canal
   d. Itchiness in the ear canal

9. The patient has been diagnosed with perichondritis. What is the most likely cause of the infection for this patient?
   a. Recent ear piercing
   b. Recent sun exposure
   c. Previous diagnosis of otitis media
   d. Previous treatment of otitis externa

10. The adult patient with a history of otitis media states that his left ear pain is better. Now the patient has noticed some pus with blood in the affected ear. What does the nurse suspect has happened?
    a. Antibiotics have been successful in treating the infection.
    b. The eardrum has perforated.
    c. The condition has worsened.
    d. The ear has been permanently damaged.

11. Which steps are a correct part of the procedure for instilling eardrops? *(Select all that apply.)*
    a. Irrigate the ear if the membrane is not intact.
    b. Place the bottle of eardrops in a bowl of warm water for 5 minutes.
    c. Tilt the patient's head in the opposite direction of the affected ear.
    d. Use sterile gloves during the procedure.
    e. Check medication labels to ensure correct dosage and time.
    f. Pack the opening of the ear with a cotton ball.

12. The adult patient has wax in the left ear. When irrigating his ear, the nurse uses which amount of fluid?
    a. 50 to 70 mL
    b. 90 to 120 mL
    c. 125 to 140 mL
    d. 150 to 170 mL

13. The nurse stops irrigating the ear if the patient reports which symptom?
    a. Headache
    b. Nausea
    c. Tingling sensation
    d. Fatigue

14. What are the nurse's instructions to the patient after a myringotomy? *(Select all that apply.)*
    a. Report an excessive drainage to your physician.
    b. Restrict hair washing for 1 week.
    c. Use a straw for drinking liquids.
    d. Do not change the ear dressing until the next office visit.
    e. Blow the nose gently, one side at a time, with the mouth open.

15. Mastoiditis is an inflammation of which structure?
    a. Bones in the middle ear
    b. Temporal bone behind the ear
    c. Sixth and seventh cranial nerves
    d. Labyrinth structure

16. Which statements about tinnitus are true? *(Select all that apply.)*
    a. It is one of the most common complaints of patients with hearing disorders.
    b. Diagnostic tests cannot confirm the disorder.
    c. This disorder does not have observable characteristics.
    d. Tinnitus can lead to particularly disturbing emotional consequences.
    e. Treatment may include music during sleeping hours.

17. Tinnitus may be caused by which factors? *(Select all that apply.)*
    a. Repeated otitis media
    b. Otosclerosis
    c. Continuous exposure to loud noise
    d. Medications
    e. Ménière's disease

18. The patient reports an odd sensation of "whirling in space." Based on the patient's description, is this patient experiencing vertigo or dizziness? _____

19. Ménière's disease is associated with which condition? *(Select all that apply.)*
    a. Viral or bacterial infection
    b. Allergic reactions
    c. Biochemical disturbances
    d. Genetic and familial traits
    e. Long-term stress

20. The adult patient has been diagnosed with Ménière's disease. Which points does the nurse include in the teaching plan for this patient? *(Select all that apply.)*
    a. Make slow head movements.
    b. Reduce the intake of salt.
    c. Stop smoking.
    d. Take aspirin every 4 hours.
    e. Avoid alcohol and caffeine.

21. Which phrase defines an acoustic neuroma?
    a. Tumor that is benign and rarely causes a problem
    b. Malignant tumor that metastasizes quickly
    c. Benign tumor that can be neurologically damaging
    d. Benign tumor of cranial nerve VI

22. Which factors may be causes of conductive hearing loss? *(Select all that apply.)*
    a. Obstruction of external ear
    b. Obstruction of inner ear
    c. Perforation of eardrum
    d. Otosclerosis from previous middle ear surgery
    e. Prolonged exposure to loud noise

23. Which factor may be a cause of sensorineural hearing loss?
    a. Ototoxic drugs
    b. Inflammatory process
    c. Bulging eardrum
    d. Tumor of the ear canal

True or False? *Read the statement and write T for true or F for false in the blank provided. If the statement is false, rewrite the statement to make it true.*

_____ 24. Presbycusis is a common cause of sensorineural hearing loss associated with aging.

25. What percentage of the population of patients 65 to 75 years of age suffers hearing loss?
    a. 10%
    b. 25%
    c. 35%
    d. 50%

26. Which action could prevent ear trauma?
    a. Holding the nose when sneezing to reduce pressure.
    b. Not using small objects to clean the external ear canal
    c. Occluding one nostril when blowing the nose
    d. Not washing the external ear and canal

27. Which is a part of the nursing education for a patient beginning hearing aid use? *(Select all that apply.)*
    a. Avoid excessive wetting of the hearing aid.
    b. Turn off the hearing aid when not in use.
    c. Avoid exposing the hearing aid to extreme temperatures.
    d. Adjust volume to the lowest setting that allows hearing.
    e. Avoid hairspray and cosmetics coming in contact with the hearing aid.

28. Which statements are true about tympanoplasty reconstruction of the middle ear? *(Select all that apply.)*
    a. The goal of a tympanoplasty is to improve hearing after conductive hearing loss.
    b. Hearing loss after surgery is usually normal but temporary.
    c. Local anesthesia is preferred over general anesthesia.
    d. Activity is permitted after 6 hours of bedrest.
    e. Postoperative coughing and deep breathing will be modified to eliminate forceful coughing.

29. Which points are included in the nurse's discharge teaching plan for the patient after ear surgery? *(Select all that apply.)*
    a. Avoid drinking through a straw.
    b. Avoid rapid head movements for 2 months.
    c. Report excessive ear drainage to the physician.
    d. Do not change the ear dressing for 1 to 2 weeks.
    e. Avoid straining with bowel movements.

30. What should the patient who is having a stapedectomy be told about the procedure? *(Select all that apply.)*
    a. Hearing is initially worse after surgery.
    b. Success rate is high.
    c. There is a risk of total hearing loss on the affected side.
    d. Hearing is improved immediately after surgery.
    e. Facial nerve damage is a possible complication of the surgery.

31. Which methods are best for communicating with a hearing-impaired patient? *(Select all that apply.)*
    a. Speak as loudly as possible to the patient.
    b. Assume that the patient is unable to read and do not attempt written messages.
    c. Position yourself directly in front of the patient.
    d. Make sure room is well-lit.
    e. Try not to distract the patient with hand motions.

Matching. *Match each term with its definition.*

Terms
a. Ototoxic
b. Vertigo
c. Cauliflower or boxer's ear
d. Atresia
e. External otitis
f. Dizziness
g. Presbycusis
h. Otitis media
i. Barotrauma

Definitions

_____ 32. Calcification and hardening of the auricle that occurs as a result of trauma and subsequent hematoma

_____ 33. Swimmer's ear

_____ 34. Complete absence of the auditory canal

_____ 35. Damage to the middle ear due to extreme pressure changes

_____ 36. Has three forms: acute, chronic, and serous

_____ 37. Disturbed sense of a person's proper position in space

_____ 38. A sensation of whirling or turning in space

_____ 39. Hearing loss that occurs with aging

_____ 40. Term that describes drugs that damage inner-ear structures

41. Which statement(s) about hearing loss is/are true? *(Select all that apply.)*
    a. Hearing loss is always gradual.
    b. The ability to hear high-frequency, soft consonants (such as *s, sh, f, th, ch*) sounds is lost first.
    c. Tinnitus rarely accompanies hearing loss.
    d. Vertigo may be present with hearing loss.
    e. Patients often state that they cannot understand specific words.

True or False? *Read the statements about otitis and write T for true or F for false in the blanks provided. For those statements that are false, rewrite the statement to make it true.*

_____ 42. For external otitis, topical antibiotics and steroid therapies are most effective in decreasing inflammation and pain.

_____ 43. Cerumen is the most common cause of an impacted ear canal.

_____ 44. Irrigation is indicated for eardrum perforation or otitis media.

_____ 45. Insects in the ear canal are best removed while still alive, if possible.

_____ 46. Anyone can easily remove earwax using a small curette or cerumen spoon.

_____ 47. Topical antibiotics are not used to treat otitis media.

_____ 48. A myringotomy may be used to drain fluids and ease inner-ear pain.

_____ 49. Tinnitus, or ringing in the ears, is a common disorder that rarely causes problems.

CASE STUDY: OTOSCLEROSIS

Use a separate sheet of paper to answer the questions in this Case Study. Answer guidelines for this Case Study are available on your Evolve website at http://evolve. elsevier.com/Iggy/ in the "Prepare for Class" folder.

The 53-year-old patient is visiting the ENT clinic today. She has had progressive hearing loss since her late 20s. Her ability to hear is better with her right ear, and she has been using bilateral hearing aids for the past 5 years. After being evaluated, it is determined that she has otosclerosis. She discusses options with her physician and the decision is made for her to have a stapedectomy of the left ear.

1. Why is the procedure done on the left ear rather than the right ear?

2. Develop a preoperative teaching-learning plan for this patient. What should the nurse discuss about the hearing aids?

3. Discuss alternative ways for the patient to cope with her reduced hearing ability until the surgery is performed.

4. Postoperatively, the patient is nauseated and states that "things are spinning" when she tries to sit up. Her postoperative orders include meclizine (Antivert) and droperidol (Inapsine). What interventions are implemented for patient safety? What side effects should the nurse monitor for while the patient is receiving these medications?

5. Following removal of the external dressing, the patient becomes upset and begins to cry. She states, "I don't notice any difference; in fact, I think it's worse! Now I can't hear anything with my right ear!" What is the probable cause of her hearing loss? What can the nurse say to the patient to assist her at this time?

52 Assessment of the Musculoskeletal System

CHAPTER

STUDY/REVIEW QUESTIONS

1. Complete the chart below to identify types of bones and examples of each type. The first box has been done for you.

Type of Bone	Example
1. Long bones	Femur
2.	
3.	
4.	
5.	

2. Which ethnic group has the *least* risk for developing osteoporosis?
   a. African American
   b. European American
   c. Asian American
   d. Hispanic American

3. The patient has a family history of osteoporosis but currently denies pain or dysfunction. To plan health promotion interventions related to this finding, what does the nurse do?
   a. Ask the patient's age and assess for weight loss.
   b. Assess the dietary intake of calcium.
   c. Assess for kyphoscoliosis or other deformities.
   d. Assess for occult fractures of the long bones.

Matching. *Match each of the following musculoskeletal terms with the corresponding descriptions.*

Terms
a. Cancellous
b. Cortex
c. Diaphysis
d. Epiphysis
e. Haversian system
f. Osteoblast
g. Osteoclast
h. Osteocyte
i. Periosteum
j. Trabeculae
k. Volkmann's canal

Descriptions
_____ 4. Living bone cells
_____ 5. Shaft of a long bone
_____ 6. Outer layer of bone tissue
_____ 7. Longitudinal canal network containing microscopic blood vessels
_____ 8. End of a long bone
_____ 9. Spongy inner layer of bone
_____ 10. Network connecting bone marrow vessels to outer bone covering
_____ 11. Bone-forming cells
_____ 12. Bone tissue containing marrow
_____ 13. Highly vascular bone covering
_____ 14. Bone-destroying cells

15. Based on bone physiology and the dynamic process of bone formation and resorption, which group has the greatest risk for bone injury?
    a. Older adult men regardless of exercise habits
    b. Young adults who exercise frequently
    c. Older adult women regardless of exercise habits
    d. Children who never or very rarely exercise

16. The patient is at risk for a parathyroid hormone (PTH) imbalance related to a recent surgical procedure. Based on this information, which blood level must the nurse monitor in the patient?
    a. Blood glucose
    b. Serum calcium
    c. Serum potassium
    d. Serum magnesium

17. Which vitamin plays a key role in bone health?
    a. Vitamin A
    b. Vitamin B
    c. Vitamin D
    d. Vitamin E

18. The nurse is caring for the adult patient with a recent increase in growth hormone and acromegaly. In assessing this patient, what does the nurse expect to find?
    a. Bone and soft-tissue deformities
    b. Pain that increases when flexing joints
    c. Unusually tall height for ethnic background
    d. Marked lateral curvature of the spine

True or False? *Read the statements and write T for true or F for false in the blanks provided. If a statement is false, correct it to make it true.*

_____ 19. The knee is considered to be a "ball-and-socket" joint.

_____ 20. The elbow is considered to be a "hinge" joint.

_____ 21. Pivot joints allow for flexion and extension only.

_____ 22. Biaxial joints allow for gliding movement such as that of the wrist.

_____ 23. Condylar joints allow for flexion and extension only.

24. The patient is an athletic young adult man who broke his leg during a sports accident. The cast, which has been in place for several weeks, is being removed for the first time and the patient is stunned by the appearance of his leg. What is the nurse's best response to this patient's surprise?
    a. "Don't worry; it looks crusty and withered, but the strength and function are normal."
    b. "The cast compresses the tissue, but your leg will look normal in a couple of days."
    c. "Let's just wash off the dead skin and you will see that it is not as bad as it seems."
    d. "Without regular exercise muscles atrophy; strength can be restored with use."

25. The 55-year-old woman with a small frame is aware of her increased risk for osteoporosis and loss of bone mass, although she currently reports no pain or loss of function. She asks the nurse to recommend a good type of exercise to counteract the risk. What does the nurse suggest?
    a. Swimming
    b. Deep breathing and isometric exercise
    c. Walking with arm weights
    d. Golfing

26. The patient has osteoarthritis that affects the most common joints. In doing a functional assessment of this patient, the home health nurse anticipates the patient is most likely to have problems with which activity?
    a. Going up and down the stairs
    b. Buttoning a shirt
    c. Lifting more than 15 pounds
    d. Getting an arm into a coat sleeve

Matching. _Match each of the following musculoskeletal terms with their corresponding definitions._

Terms
a. Atrophy
b. Bursa
c. Cartilage
d. Fascia
e. Fasciculi
f. Ligament
g. Synovium
h. Synovial fluid
i. Tendon

Definitions

_____ 27. Membrane that secretes a lubricating fluid

_____ 28. Decrease in size and number of muscle fibers

_____ 29. Small sacs lined with synovial membrane

_____ 30. Band of tough, fibrous tissue attaching muscle to bone

_____ 31. Bundles of muscle fibers

_____ 32. Lubricates joints

_____ 33. Band of tough, fibrous tissue attaching bone to bone

_____ 34. Fibrous tissue surrounding muscle

_____ 35. Collagen fibers at bone ends

True or False? *Read the statements and write T for true or F for false in the blanks provided. If a statement is false, correct it to make it true.*

_____ 36. As one ages, bone density often increases.

_____ 37. As one ages, synovial joint cartilage regenerates.

_____ 38. Degenerative joint disease, muscle atrophy, slowed movement, and decreased strength are common changes in the musculoskeletal system of the older adult.

39. Which group has the greatest risk for trauma resulting in injuries to muscles and bones?
    a. Older adult men related to occupational injuries
    b. Young men related to motor vehicle accidents
    c. Young women related to sports injuries
    d. Children who are not supervised during play

40. The patient is a construction worker in his early 30s who was treated with oral antibiotics after stepping on a nail. The wound does not appear to be responding to antibiotic treatment as expected, despite the patient's compliance. The nurse suspects the patient may have a family history of which disorder?
    a. Renal disease
    b. Heart disease
    c. Skin or bone cancer
    d. Diabetes mellitus

41. The patient is recovering from a long bone fracture. Which lifestyle choice decreases the vitamins and nutrients required for bone and tissue growth?
    a. Smoking cigarettes
    b. Vegetarian diet
    c. Excessive alcohol consumption
    d. Excessive caffeine consumption

42. While observing the patient performing range-of-motion (ROM) exercises, the nurse notes the patient can move the leg outward from the side of the body. How does the nurse identify this movement?
    a. Flexion
    b. Extension
    c. Adduction
    d. Abduction

43. Which instrument is used to assess joint ROM?
    a. Odometer
    b. Ergometer
    c. Goniometer
    d. Spectrometer

44. Which assessment finding of the musculoskeletal system indicates an abnormality?
    a. Symmetry in the upper extremities and equal muscle mass
    b. Gait balance and a smooth and regular stride
    c. Flexion, extension, and rotation of the neck
    d. Opposition of three of four fingers to the thumb

45. Which factor is primarily responsible for regulating serum calcium levels?
    a. Calcitonin
    b. Vitamin D
    c. Glucocorticoids
    d. Growth hormone

46. The nurse is reviewing the laboratory results for the patient with severe diarrhea and hypocalcemia. What does the nurse find is present in bone and serum in inverse proportion to calcium?
    a. Estrogen
    b. Phosphorus
    c. Thyroxine
    d. Insulin

47. Which laboratory result may indicate bone or liver damage, such as metastatic cancer of the bone?
    a. Serum calcium 9.5 mg/dL
    b. Serum calcium 8.2 mg/dL
    c. Lactate dehydrogenase (LDH) 185 units/L
    d. Alkaline phosphatase 140 units/L

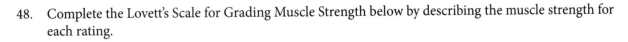

48. Complete the Lovett's Scale for Grading Muscle Strength below by describing the muscle strength for each rating.

Rating	Description
5	
4	
3	
2	
1	
0	

49. The patient reports pain in the left lower ankle. Which questions does the nurse ask to elicit relevant information about this patient's musculoskeletal problem? *(Select all that apply.)*
    a. "Do you have adequate calcium and vitamin D intake?"
    b. "What seems to make the pain worse?"
    c. "What measures seem to help alleviate the symptoms?"
    d. "What did your family doctor tell you?"
    e. "When did your pain start?"
    f. "Do you have a history of diabetes mellitus?"

50. The nurse is assessing the patient's posture and gait, and notes that the patient shifts his shoulders from side to side while walking. How is this finding considered?
    a. Abnormality in the swing phase, called a *lurch*
    b. Abnormality in the stance phase, called an *antalgic gait*
    c. Normal and automatic gait
    d. Limp or other type of asymmetric body movement

51. In assessing the patient's functional ability and ROM, the patient is unable to actively move a joint through the expected ROM. Which technique does the nurse use to assess joint mobility?
    a. The patient relaxes the muscles in the extremity, then moves the joint through the fullest motion possible.
    b. The nurse holds the part with one hand above and one hand below the joint to be evaluated, and allows passive ROM to evaluate joint mobility.
    c. The patient moves the joints while the nurse applies gentle resistance.
    d. The patient moves the joint to the best of ability while the nurse palpates for crepitus.

52. The nurse is assessing the patient who is obese, especially in the abdominal area. What is the most common musculoskeletal assessment finding in this patient?
    a. Scoliosis
    b. Crepitus
    c. Lordosis
    d. Kyphosis

53. What activity does the nurse ask the patient to perform when assessing ROM in the patient's hands?
    a. Wave the hand as though waving good-bye.
    b. Grip the nurse's hand as hard as possible.
    c. Rapidly move the hands into the palm-up and palm-down positions.
    d. Make a fist and then appose each finger to the thumb.

54. The patient has an effusion of the right knee. Which assessment finding does the nurse expect to see in this patient?
    a. Limitations in movement and accompanying pain
    b. Obvious appearance of genu valgum
    c. Crepitus and difficulty weight bearing
    d. Obvious redness and skin breakdown

55. Which orthopedic conditions will require the patient to have a neurovascular assessment performed at least every 4 hours? *(Select all that apply.)*
    a. Presence of a cast
    b. Crush injury to the forearm
    c. Multiple rib fractures
    d. Femoral angiogram assessment
    e. Recent hip surgery

56. The nurse is reviewing laboratory results for the patient who was involved in an accident. There is no evidence of fracture or bone damage, but multiple soft tissue injuries were sustained. Which muscle enzymes are expected to be elevated because of the injuries? *(Select all that apply.)*
    a. Creatine kinase (CK)
    b. Aspartate aminotransferase (AST)
    c. Alkaline phosphatase (ALP)
    d. Lactic dehydrogenase (LDH)
    e. Aldolase (ALD)

57. The patient who is currently on anticoagulant therapy is advised to undergo diagnostic testing for musculoskeletal weakness. Which diagnostic test is contraindicated because of the therapy?
    a. Electromyography
    b. Computed tomography
    c. Xeroradiography
    d. Magnetic resonance imaging

Matching. *Match the substances related to the musculoskeletal system with their functions.*

Substances
a. Glucocorticoids
b. Calcitonin
c. Vitamin D
d. Parathyroid hormone
e. Growth hormone

Functions

_____ 58. Promotes absorption of calcium and phosphorus from the small intestine

_____ 59. Responsible for increasing bone length

_____ 60. If serum calcium levels are increased above normal, this hormone decreases serum calcium levels by inhibiting bone resorption and increasing renal excretion of calcium and phosphorus

_____ 61. Regulate protein metabolism

_____ 62. If serum calcium levels are lowered, this hormone stimulates bone to promote osteoclastic activity and release calcium into the blood, thus raising serum calcium levels

True or False? *Read the statements and write T for true or F for false in the blanks provided. If a statement is false, correct it to make it true.*

_____ 63. African-American women have denser bones than African-American men.

_____ 64. Caucasian women are more likely, out of all groups, to have osteoporosis and fractures.

_____ 65. Lactose-intolerant people need to obtain calcium from other sources, such as yogurt and cheese.

66. **Crossword Puzzle.** Complete the puzzle by answering the questions related to physical assessment of the musculoskeletal system.

Across

1. Genu _____, also called bowlegged
3. Assess the stance phase and the swing phase
4. Assess by asking the patient to perform activities of daily living

Down

1. Genu _____, also called knock-kneed
2. A lateral curve in the spine found upon inspection when the patient flexes forward from the hips

Matching. Match each of the following radiographic examinations and diagnostic tests with the corresponding definitions.

Radiographic Examinations

a. Tomography
b. Xeroradiography
c. Myelography
d. Arthrography
e. Computed tomography (CT)
f. Bone biopsy
g. Muscle biopsy
h. Electromyography (EMG)
i. Arthroscopy
j. Bone scan
k. Gallium/thallium scan
l. Magnetic resonance imaging (MRI)
m. Ultrasonography

Definitions

_____ 67. A more sensitive and specific isotope scan used to detect bone problems. Can be used to examine the brain, liver, and breast tissue when disease is suspected.

_____ 68. Used to detect musculoskeletal problems, particularly in the vertebral column. Can produce three-dimensional images. Can be done with or without contrast.

_____ 69. Helpful in detailing the musculoskeletal system because it produces planes, or slices, for focus and blurs the images of other structures.

_____ 70. Invasive test that may confirm the presence of infection or neoplasm of the bone.

_____ 71. Margins and edges are clearly seen because this test highlights the contrast between structures.

_____ 72. A contrast medium or dye is injected into the subarachnoid space of the spine. The vertebral column, intervertebral disks, spinal nerve roots, and blood vessels all can be visualized.

_____ 73. Used for the diagnosis of atrophy (as in muscular dystrophy) and inflammation (as in polymyositis).

_____ 74. A fiberoptic tube is inserted into a joint (usually the knee or shoulder) for direct visualization. Procedures such as synovial biopsy or repair of traumatic injury may also be done.

_____ 75. Radioactive material is injected for visualization of the entire skeletal system. This test is used to detect tumors, arthritis, osteomyelitis, vertebral compression fractures, osteoporosis, and unexplained bone pain.

_____ 76. A test that uses sound waves to produce an image of the tissue. This test may be used to visualize osteomyelitis, soft-tissue disorders (such as masses and fluid accumulation), and traumatic injuries.

_____ 77. An image is produced through the interaction of magnetic fields, radio waves, and atomic nuclei showing hydrogen density. This test is particularly useful in identifying problems with muscles, tendons, and ligaments.

_____ 78. An x-ray study of a joint after contrast medium (air or solution) is injected to enhance visualization. Most commonly done on the knee and shoulder joints.

_____ 79. Used to determine the electrical potential of an individual muscle, and usually accompanied by nerve conduction studies. Used to diagnose neuromuscular, lower motor neuron, and peripheral nerve disorders.

CASE STUDY: THE PATIENT WITH MUSCULOSKELETAL INJURY

Use a separate sheet of paper to answer the questions in this Case Study. Answer guidelines for this Case Study are available on your Evolve website at http://evolve.elsevier.com/Iggy/ in the "Prepare for Class" folder.

The patient with a 5-year history of osteoarthritis comes to the clinic with severe intermittent left knee pain. She describes the pain as starting yesterday in her foot and moving up her shin to her knee. At the time, she was gardening in her yard and was walking to the curb to put out the trash when the pain suddenly stopped her. She says that the pain is a burning pain "like nothing I've ever had before," and rates it as between an 8 or 9 on a 10-point scale. She says that she hobbled up to her house, put an ice pack on her knee, and rested for the remainder of the evening after taking Tylenol. The ice helped at first, but her knee throbbed all night; this morning the pain has resumed even though she has tried to stay off of her leg. On assessment, the left knee appears slightly swollen, pain increases with movement, and she is unable to fully bear weight on it. Skin is intact, no redness, warm to the touch; capillary refill less than 3 seconds.

1. From the scenario, find the answers to these questions:
   a. When did the pain start?
   b. What factors caused the pain or made it worse?
   c. What has been the course of the pain?
   d. What are the clinical manifestations?
   e. What was the description of the pain?
   f. Were there any functional problems?
   g. What measures were tried to reduce pain? Were those methods successful?

2. Describe the physical assessment that should be conducted for this patient.

3. The physician orders an arthroscopy for surgical repair. Explain the procedure in terms that the patient will understand.

4. Identify at least three nursing diagnoses that are appropriate for this patient in the post-procedure period.

Care of Patients with Musculoskeletal Problems

CHAPTER 53

STUDY/REVIEW QUESTIONS

Matching. Match each musculoskeletal disorder with its corresponding risk factor.

Musculoskeletal Disorder

a. Osteoporosis
b. Osteomalacia
c. Paget's disease

Risk Factor

_____ 1. Older adults, vitamin D deficiency, insufficient exposure to sunlight

_____ 2. Possibly a result of latent viral infection

_____ 3. Female, white, menopausal, thin, lean, immobilization

Matching. Match the patient data with the musculoskeletal disorders they are primarily associated with. Answers may be used more than once.

Musculoskeletal Disorder

a. Osteoporosis
b. Osteomalacia
c. Paget's disease

Subjective Patient Data

_____ 4. Apathy or lethargy

_____ 5. Loss of height

_____ 6. Muscle cramps

_____ 7. Smokes cigarettes

_____ 8. Back pain relieved by rest

_____ 9. Bone pain worsened by walking

_____ 10. Vitamin D deficiency

_____ 11. Sedentary lifestyle

_____ 12. Muscle weakness in the pelvic girdle area

_____ 13. Drinks eight cups of coffee per day

_____ 14. Urinary or renal stones

_____ 15. Muscle weakness in legs

_____ 16. First indication may be a fracture

Matching. Match the objective patient data with the musculoskeletal disorders they are primarily associated with. Answers may be used more than once.

Musculoskeletal Disorders

a. Osteoporosis
b. Osteomalacia
c. Paget's disease

Objective Patient Data

_____ 17. Unsteady gait

_____ 18. Hip flexion contractures

_____ 19. Flushed, warm skin

_____ 20. Vertebral fracture

_____ 21. Bone tenderness over rib cage

_____ 22. Kyphosis

_____ 23. Long bone bowing

_____ 24. Discomfort on vertebral palpation

_____ 25. Soft skull

26. The nurse is reviewing T-scores for a 68-year-old woman. The patient has a T-score of –2.5. How does the nurse interpret this data?
    a. The patient has osteopenia.
    b. The patient has osteoporosis.
    c. This is a normal score for the patient's age.
    d. There is osteoblastic activity.

27. Which patient is at risk for regional osteoporosis?
    a. Patient who has been in a long leg cast for 10 weeks
    b. Patient on long-term corticosteroid therapy
    c. Patient with a history of hyperparathyroidism
    d. Menopausal patient

28. Which patients are at risk for osteoporosis because of nutritional issues? *(Select all that apply.)*
    a. Older adult female patient who likes to drink a lot of coffee
    b. Patient who has had gastric bypass surgery for obesity
    c. Patient who is on the high-protein Atkins diet
    d. Patient who prefers to drink diluted powdered milk
    e. Patient who drinks two diet sodas per day
    f. Patient with chronic alcoholism

29. The nurse is assessing the older adult patient at risk for osteoporosis. Which task can be delegated to the unlicensed assistive personnel (UAP)?
    a. Inspect the vertebral column.
    b. Take height and weight measurements.
    c. Compare observations to previous findings.
    d. Ask if the patient is shorter or has gained or lost weight.

30. The patient with osteoporosis moves slowly and carefully with voluntarily restriction of movement. The lower thoracic area is tender on palpation. How does the nurse interpret this assessment data?
    a. Vertebral compression fracture
    b. Kyphosis of the dorsal spine
    c. Osteopenia related to immobility
    d. Increased osteoblastic activity

31. The home health nurse is visiting the older adult patient with osteoporosis and severe kyphosis. When the nurse asks about activities she has been doing, the patient replies, "I used to be very active and beautiful when I was younger." What is the nurse's best response?
    a. "You are still very beautiful."
    b. "Activity can help to prevent fractures and complications."
    c. "Tell me what you used to do."
    d. "Do you need information about age-appropriate exercises?"

32. The patient is scheduled to have a dual x-ray absorptiometry (DXA). What information does the nurse give to the patient about preparing for the test?
    a. "Leave metallic objects such as jewelry, coins, and belt buckles at home."
    b. "Have someone come with you to drive you home after the test."
    c. "You will be asked to give a urine specimen prior to the test."
    d. "Bring a comfortable loose nightgown without buttons or snaps."

33. The patient is lactose intolerant and would like suggestions about food sources that supply adequate calcium and vitamin D. In addition to a generally well-balanced diet, what foods does the nurse suggest?
    a. Fresh apples and pears
    b. Whole-wheat bread
    c. Fortified soy or rice products
    d. Prune or cranberry juice

34. The patient has been advised by the health care provider that exercising may help prevent osteoporosis. Which exercise does the nurse recommend to the patient?
    a. Swimming 10 to 15 laps three to five times a week
    b. Running for 20 minutes four times a week
    c. Bowling for 60 minutes three times a week
    d. Walking for 30 minutes three to five times a week

Matching. Match each precaution and/or side effect to the appropriate drug therapy.

Drug Therapies
a. Calcitonin
b. Vitamin D
c. Estrogen
d. Calcium
e. Selective estrogen receptor modulators (SERMs)
f. Bisphosphonates (BPs)

Precautions/Side Effects
_____ 35. Esophagitis and esophageal ulcers
_____ 36. Hypercalcemia; can cause serious damage to the urinary system
_____ 37. Low doses prescribed due to potentially serious side effects, such as endometrial or breast cancer
_____ 38. May cause nasal mucosal irritation when given intranasally
_____ 39. Should not be given to women with a history of venous thromboembolism
_____ 40. Hypercalcemia and hyperphosphatemia

41. The nurse is reviewing the prescriptions for the patient receiving drug therapy for the prevention of osteoporosis. The patient also has hypertension. Which prescription order does the nurse question?
    a. Calcium supplements
    b. Hormone replacement therapy
    c. Alendronate (Fosamax)
    d. Raloxifene (Evista)

42. The nurse is helping the health care provider in determining if the patient is a candidate for IV biphosphonate therapy, such as zoledronic acid (Reclast). Which factor dissuades the use of this therapy?
    a. History of venous thromboembolism
    b. History of previous fractures
    c. History of cancer
    d. Recent dental assessment

43. The patient is taking an oral biphosphonate. What information does the nurse include in the patient teaching?
    a. Take the oral drug early in the morning with 8 ounces of water.
    b. Rest in a supine position for at least 15 minutes after taking the drug.
    c. Chest discomfort is an expected side effect that should eventually subside.
    d. Chew the tablets well and take adequate amounts of water.

44. The patient is prescribed calcitonin for treatment of Paget's disease. What does the nurse advise the patient to do?
    a. Avoid eating salmon because calcitonin is derived from salmon.
    b. Alternate nares to prevent nasal mucosal irritation.
    c. Take a drug holiday after 1 year of therapy.
    d. Store the drug in a cool, dry, dark place.

45. The patient reports pain in the lower legs and pelvis which is aggravated by activity and worse at night. The nurse observes muscle weakness which appears to be causing a waddling and unsteady gait. What additional information supports the likelihood of osteomalacia in this patient?
    a. Recent immigration from a country where famine is common
    b. Taking hormone replacement therapy for a prolonged time
    c. Unable to perform a prescribed exercise regimen
    d. History of recent vertebroplasty for osteoporosis

46. An x-ray shows the presence of radiolucent bands (Looser's lines or zones) in the patient. What is this diagnostic finding specific for?
    a. Osteoporosis
    b. Osteomalacia
    c. Paget's disease
    d. Osteomyelitis

47. The nurse is assessing the patient who reports moderate bone pain in the hip and has a family history of Paget's disease. In performing a musculoskeletal assessment, the nurse pays particular attention to which element?
    a. Size and shape of the skull
    b. Long-bone bowing in the legs
    c. Asymmetrical deformity of the extremities
    d. Loose teeth and difficulty chewing

48. The patient with Paget's disease has complications related to bony enlargements of the skull. Which complication is potentially the most serious and life-threatening?
    a. Basilar complications with compression on the cranial nerves
    b. Platybasia, or basilar invagination with brainstem manifestations
    c. Blockage of cerebrospinal fluid (CSF), resulting in hydrocephalus
    d. Pressure from an enlarged temporal bone leading to deafness and vertigo

49. The patient with Paget's disease comes to the clinic for evaluation. Which symptom reported by the patient alerts the nurse to the possibility of osteogenic sarcoma?
    a. Change in hearing
    b. Warmth and redness of the joints
    c. Changes in balance and gait
    d. Severe bone pain

50. The patient with Paget's disease has a kidney problem associated with an increased serum calcium. What is the nursing priority for this patient?
    a. Encourage the patient to increase fluids, unless contraindicated.
    b. Encourage moderate consumption of milk and dairy products.
    c. Assist the patient to problem-solve incontinence issues.
    d. Direct the UAP to measure and record all urine output.

51. The patient is having diagnostic testing to determine the probability of Paget's disease. If the disease is present, which laboratory result does the nurse expect to see?
    a. Slightly decreased serum calcium level
    b. Increased serum alkaline phosphatase (ALP)
    c. Decreased pyridinium (PYD)
    d. Absence of osteocalcin

52. The patient with Paget's disease has been prescribed drug therapy. The nurse prepares patient teaching information for which medication as a first line therapy?
    a. Calcitonin
    b. Ibuprofen (Motrin)
    c. Plicamycin (Mithracin)
    d. Risedronate (Actonel)

53. The patient is admitted for acute osteomyelitis of the left lower leg. What does the nurse expect to find documented in the patient's admitting assessment?
    a. Temperature greater than 101° F; swelling, tenderness, erythema, and warmth of area
    b. Ulceration resulting with sinus tract formation, localized pain, and drainage
    c. Pain is aching, poorly described, deep, and worsened by pressure and weight bearing
    d. Shortening of the extremity with pain during weight bearing or palpation

54. The nurse is caring for the patient with osteomyelitis. Which laboratory results are of primary concern for this disorder?
    a. Bone-specific alkaline phosphatase and osteocalcin
    b. Serum calcium level and alkaline phosphatase
    c. White blood cell count and erythrocyte sedimentation rate
    d. Thyroid function tests and uric acid levels

55. Which patient is mostly likely to be a candidate for hyperbaric oxygen therapy?
    a. Patient with chronic, unremitting osteomyelitis
    b. Patient with an advanced case of Paget's disease
    c. Patient with osteomalacia related to poverty
    d. Patient with osteoporosis and recurrent fractures

56. The patient comes to the emergency department (ED) after accidentally puncturing his hand with an automatic nail gun. Which disorder is this patient primarily at risk for?
    a. Osteoporosis
    b. Osteomyelitis
    c. Osteomalacia
    d. Dupuytren's contracture

57. The nurse is caring for the patient with acute osteomyelitis. What assessment findings typically accompany this medical diagnosis? *(Select all that apply.)*
    a. Fever; temperature usually above 101° F
    b. Sinus tract formation
    c. Erythema of the affected area
    d. Swelling around the affected area
    e. Decreased peripheral pulses

58. The nurse is teaching the patient about antibiotic therapy for osteomyelitis. What information does the nurse give to the patient?
    a. Single-agent therapy is the most effective treatment for acute infections.
    b. Chronic osteomyelitis may require 1 month of antibiotic therapy.
    c. Patients usually remain hospitalized to complete the full course of antibiotic therapy.
    d. The infected wound may be irrigated with one or more types of antibiotic solutions.

True or False? *Write T for true or F for false in the blanks provided. If the statement is false, rewrite the statement to make it true.*

_____ 59. Osteosarcoma is the most common type of primary malignant bone tumor.

_____ 60. Ewing's sarcoma is the most malignant of all the bone tumors.

_____ 61. Ewing's sarcoma rarely extends into the soft tissue.

_____ 62. Patients with chondrosarcoma typically verbalize sudden swelling and constant, severe, throbbing pain.

_____ 63. Fibrosarcoma clinically presents slowly and without specific symptoms.

Matching. *Match the radiographic findings with their associated types of bone tumor growths. Answers may be used more than once.*

Types of Bone Tumor
a.   Benign
b.   Malignant

Radiographic Findings

_____ 64. Poor margination

_____ 65. Intact cortices

_____ 66. Bone destruction

_____ 67. Cortical breakthrough

_____ 68. Smooth uniform periosteal bone

_____ 69. Irregular new periosteal bone

_____ 70. Sharp margins

71. Which assessment finding in the patient who has undergone a bone graft for a tumor does the nurse report to the health care provider immediately?
   a. Extremity distal to the operative site is warm and pink.
   b. Cast over the operative site is cool to the touch.
   c. Delayed capillary refill presents in digits distal to the site.
   d. Pain is present in the operative extremity.

72. The patient with a bone tumor is grieving and anxious. The nurse includes which psychosocial interventions? *(Select all that apply.)*
   a. Allow the patient to verbalize feelings.
   b. Offer to call the patient's spiritual or religious adviser.
   c. Prepare the patient for death.
   d. Share stories of personal losses.
   e. Redirect the patient to more cheerful topics.
   f. Listen attentively while the patient talks.

73. The patient had a microvascular bone transfer on the left leg. What does nursing care for this patient include?
   a. Frequent neurovascular assessments
   b. Gently massaging the affected extremity
   c. Maintaining the leg in a 30-degree flexed position
   d. Reassuring the patient that some pain and tingling are expected

74. The nurse is reviewing the x-ray report of the patient being evaluated for bone pain. The report includes: poor demonstration of bone margins, bone destruction, irregular periosteal new bone, and breakthrough of the cortical layer. The nurse interprets this report as consistent with which disorder?
   a. Malignant bone tumor such as osteosarcoma
   b. Benign bone tumor such as osteochondroma
   c. Advanced Paget's disease
   d. Osteomalacia with osteoporosis

75. The patient with bone sarcoma had surgery to salvage an upper limb. The nurse has identified the nursing diagnosis of Impaired Physical Mobility related to musculoskeletal impairment. Which intervention does the nurse perform in the early postoperative period?
    a. Encourage the patient to use the opposite hand to achieve forward flexion and abduction of the affected shoulder.
    b. Encourage the patient to emphasize strengthening the quadriceps muscles by using passive and active motion.
    c. Instruct the UAP to completely perform hygiene for the patient until the patient expresses readiness to do self-care.
    d. Evaluate the patient's and family's readiness to use the continuous passive motion machine in the home setting.

76. The patient with bone cancer has had the right lower leg surgically removed. The patient has been brave and uncomplaining, but the nurse recognizes that the patient is likely to experience grieving. What is the nurse's most important role?
    a. Act as a patient advocate to promote the physician-patient relationship.
    b. Encourage the patient to talk to the family and complete an advance directive.
    c. Be an active listener and encourage the patient and family to verbalize feelings.
    d. Help the patient and family cope with and resolve grief and loss issues.

Matching. *Match each term related to bone tumors with its corresponding definition.*

Bone Tumors
a. Chondrogenic
b. Fibrogenic
c. Osteogenic
d. Sarcoma
e. Secondary tumor

Definitions
_____ 77. Tumor arising from bone.
_____ 78. Malignant tumor metastasizing to bone.
_____ 79. Tumor arising from cartilage.
_____ 80. Tumor arising from fibrous tissue.
_____ 81. Malignant bone tumor arising from underlying tissue.

Matching. *Match each type of benign tumor with its most common location.*

Types of Benign Tumors
a. Chondroma
b. Giant cell tumor
c. Osteochondroma

Most Common Locations
_____ 82. Hands and feet
_____ 83. Femur and tibia
_____ 84. Often spreads to lungs

Matching. *Match each type of malignant bone tumor with the associated signs and symptoms.*

Types of Malignant Bone Tumors
a. Chondrosarcoma
b. Ewing's sarcoma
c. Fibrosarcoma
d. Osteosarcoma

Signs and Symptoms
_____ 85. Local tenderness in lower extremity long bones
_____ 86. Short-term pain and swelling in distal femur
_____ 87. Long-term dull pain near proximal femur
_____ 88. Pain and swelling in lower pelvis

89. The patient, who is a long-distance runner, reports severe pain in the arch of the foot, especially when getting out of bed and with weight bearing. What does the nurse suspect in this patient?
    a. Morton's neuroma
    b. Plantar fasciitis
    c. Hammertoe
    d. Hallux valgus deformity

90. The nurse is assessing the older Caucasian man and notes there are flexion contractures of the fourth or and fifth fingers. The patient reports that he had a similar problem on the other hand and had a fasciectomy which improved the function. What is this condition known as?
    a. Dupuytren's contracture
    b. Ganglion cyst
    c. Bunion
    d. Plantar digital neuritis

91. The patient is diagnosed with plantar fasciitis. What instruction does the nurse give to the patient about self-care for this condition?
    a. Use rest, elevation, and warm packs.
    b. Perform gentle jogging exercises.
    c. Strap the foot to maintain the arch.
    d. Wear loose or open shoes, such as sandals.

Matching. *Match the characteristics to the hand disorders they are primarily associated with. Answers may be used more than once.*

Hand Disorders
a. Ganglion
b. Dupuytren's contracture

Characteristics

_____ 92. Usually occurs in older Caucasian men

_____ 93. Round, cyst-like lesion

_____ 94. Can be bilateral

_____ 95. Progressive palmar flexion deformity

_____ 96. Joint discomfort after strain

_____ 97. Cause unknown

_____ 98. Fourth and fifth digits affected

_____ 99. Painless on palpation

_____ 100. Familial tendency common

_____ 101. Function becomes impaired; surgical release is required

_____ 102. Most likely to develop in people between 15 and 50 years of age

Matching. Match each characteristic to the foot disorder it is primarily associated with. Answers may be used more than once.

Foot Disorders

a.   Hallux valgus
b.   Hammertoe
c.   Morton's neuroma
d.   Bunion
e.   Plantar fasciitis

Characteristics

_____ 103. Dorsiflexion of any metatarsophalan-geal joint with plantar flexion of the adjacent proximal interphalangeal joint

_____ 104. Small tumor in a digital nerve of the foot

_____ 105. Great toe deviates laterally

_____ 106. Acute pain; burning sensation in the web space

_____ 107. First metatarsal head becomes en-larged

_____ 108. Pain in the arch of the foot, especially when getting out of bed

_____ 109. Can occur as a result of poorly fitted shoes

_____ 110. Corns may develop on the dorsal side of the toe

_____ 111. Insertion of wires or screws for fixa-tion

_____ 112. Removal of the bony overgrowth and bursa

_____ 113. May be seen in athletes, especially runners

_____ 114. Inflammation of the plantar fascia

115. The nurse is assessing the patient with a spinal deformity. Which technique does the nurse use to accomplish inspection of the spine?
  a.   Observe the patient from the front and back while standing and during forward flexion from the hips.
  b.   Observe the patient in a sitting and stand-ing position and ask the patient to walk around the room.
  c.   Ask the patient to remove the clothes from the waist up and then view the visible cur-vature of the spine.
  d.   Look at the patient's back while the patient moves in different positions: touching toes, lateral bending, twisting.

116. The adult patient is advised to have surgical correction for scoliosis, but is reluctant be-cause the patient is concerned about missing too much work. The nurse tells the patient that most people who undergo the surgery are able to return to work in how many weeks?
  a.   1
  b.   2
  c.   3
  d.   6

117. The nurse is caring for the patient with muscular dystrophy. Although all body systems can be affected, the nurse is alert and carefully assesses for which major problem?
    a. Renal failure
    b. Cardiac failure
    c. Muscle weakness
    d. Respiratory failure

True or False? *Read the statements about scoliosis and write T for true or F for false in the blanks provided. If a statement is false, correct the statement it to make it true.*

_____ 118. Scoliosis is a C- or S-shaped lateral curvature of the vertebral spine.

_____ 119. The abnormal curvature can cause low back pain.

_____ 120. Curvature of greater than 50 degrees results in an unstable spine.

_____ 121. Children are typically screened for scoliosis before starting school.

_____ 122. Structural scoliosis results from a cause outside the spine itself, such as a leg length discrepancy.

_____ 123. Methods of treatment for adults are the same as for children.

CASE STUDY: THE PATIENT WITH OSTEOPOROSIS

Use a separate sheet of paper to answer the questions in this Case Study. Answer guidelines for this Case Study are available on your Evolve website at http://evolve. elsevier.com/Iggy/ in the "Prepare for Class" folder.

A 67-year-old postmenopausal woman has come to the clinic reporting lower backache. She states that this pain is interfering with her sleep. She gets together weekly with her friends to play cards, and lately has had to cancel. She says she is afraid her back will give out on her and she will fall. She states that the pain is interfering with her social life and other daily activities and that the episodes are becoming unbearable so she has decided to seek treatment.

1. Identify six questions that the nurse would ask the patient while performing the assessment.

2. During the assessment, the nurse discovers that the patient does not take estrogen. What are contraindications or precautions if the physician decides to place her on estrogen replacement therapy?

3. The patient says that she does not like milk and rarely drinks it. How could she increase her calcium intake?

4. The health care provider suspects osteoporosis. What test is most likely to be ordered and what should the nurse tell the patient about the test?

5. The patient is given a prescription for alendronate (Fosamax). What should the nurse tell her before she begins therapy with this drug?

6. Determine appropriate measures to relieve this patient's back pain.

7. The patient states that she does not exercise. She says that the most exercise she gets is going up and down a few stairs to get to and from her car. What advice could the nurse give her in regard to exercise?

Care of Patients with Musculoskeletal Trauma

CHAPTER 54

STUDY/REVIEW QUESTIONS

Matching. *Match each of the following terms related to the fracture healing process with its definition.*

Terms
a. Callus
b. Granulation
c. Hematoma
d. Remodeling

Definitions

_____ 1. Mass of clotted blood at fracture site

_____ 2. Process of bone building and resorption

_____ 3. Vascular and cellular proliferation

_____ 4. Nonbony union at fracture site

5. The nurse is caring for several patients on an orthopedic trauma unit. Which conditions have a high risk for development of acute compartment syndrome? *(Select all that apply.)*
   a. Lower legs caught between the bumpers of two cars
   b. Massive infiltration of IV fluid into forearm
   c. Bivalve cast on the lower leg
   d. Multiple insect bites to lower legs
   e. Daily use of oral contraceptives
   f. Severe burns to the upper extremities

6. The patient has a fracture of the right wrist. What is an early sign that indicates this patient may be having a complication?
   a. Patient loses ability to wiggle fingers without pain.
   b. Fingers are cold and pale; capillary refill is sluggish.
   c. Pain is severe and seems out of proportion to injury.
   d. Patient reports a subjective numbness and tingling.

7. The nurse is assessing the patient for severe pain in the right wrist after falling off a step stool. How does the nurse assess this patient's motor function?
   a. Performing passive range of motion for the wrist
   b. Asking the patient to move the fingers
   c. Having the patient flex and extend the elbow
   d. Instructing the patient to rotate the wrist

8. The patient in traction reports severe pain from a muscle spasm. What is the nurse's priority action?
   a. Assess the patient's body alignment.
   b. Give the patient a PRN pain medication.
   c. Notify the health care provider.
   d. Remove some of the weights.

9. The nurse is reviewing the orders for the patient who was admitted for 23-hour observation of a leg fracture. A cast is in place. Which order does the nurse question?
   a. Elevate lower leg above the level of the heart.
   b. Perform neuro-circ checks every 8 hours.
   c. Apply ice pack for 24 hours.
   d. Provide regular diet as tolerated.

10. The patient with a leg cast denies pain; toes are pink; capillary refill is brisk and toes move freely; the leg is elevated with an ice pack. Six hours later, the patient reports worsening pain unrelieved by medication. The patient's toes are cool and capillary refill is sluggish. What does the nurse suspect is occurring with this patient?
    a. Crush syndrome
    b. Fat embolism syndrome
    c. Acute compartment syndrome
    d. Fasciitis

11. The older adult sustained injury to the lower legs after being trapped underneath a fallen bookcase. Because this patient is at high risk for crush syndrome, which laboratory values will the nurse specifically monitor?
    a. Serum potassium level and myoglobin in urine
    b. White cell count and red cells in the urine
    c. Prothrombin level and serum lipase level
    d. Platelet count and serum calcium level

12. The older adult has been admitted with a hip fracture. Approximately 20 hours post-injury, the patient develops a symptom recognized as an early sign of fat embolism syndrome. Which symptom is the patient displaying?
    a. Severe respiratory distress
    b. Significantly increased pulse rate
    c. Change in mental status
    d. Petechiae rash over the neck

13. Which behavior represents an increased risk for deep vein thrombosis?
    a. Taking an overseas airplane trip
    b. Recently running in a marathon
    c. Losing weight by crash dieting
    d. Noncompliance with asthma medication

14. Indicate the numeric sequence of bone healing from the beginning using the numbers 1 through 5.
    _____ a. Callus formation
    _____ b. Bone remodeling
    _____ c. Hematoma formation
    _____ d. Osteoblastic proliferation
    _____ e. Hematoma to granulation tissue

15. The student nurse is assessing the patient with a probable fractured tibia-fibula. What assessment technique used by the student nurse causes the supervising nurse to intervene?
    a. Inspects the fracture site for swelling or deformity.
    b. Instructs the patient to wiggle the toes.
    c. Assesses the bilateral dorsalis pedis pulse.
    d. Pushes on the leg to elicit pain response.

16. The nurse is caring for several orthopedic patients who are in different types of traction. What should the nurse do in assessing the traction equipment? *(Select all that apply.)*
    a. Inspect all ropes, knots, and pulleys once every 24 hours.
    b. Inspect ropes and knots for fraying or loosening every 8 to 12 hours.
    c. Check the amount of weight being used against the prescribed weight.
    d. Observe the traction equipment for proper functioning.
    e. Check if the ropes have been changed or cleaned within the past 48 hours.

17. The patient was put into traction at 0800 hours. Hourly neuro-circ checks were ordered for the first 24 hours and then every 4 hours thereafter. At what time can the nursing staff start performing the every 4 hour checks?
    a. 2000 hours same day
    b. 0000 hours next day
    c. 0800 hours next day
    d. 1200 hours next day

18. The nurse is educating the patient who will have external fixation for treatment of a compound tibial fracture. What information does the nurse include in the teaching session?
    a. "The device allows for early ambulation."
    b. "There is some danger of blood loss, but no danger of infection."
    c. "The device is a substitute therapy for a cast."
    d. "The advantage of the device is rapid bone healing."

19. The nurse is helping to evaluate several patients to determine candidacy for the Ilizaroz external fixation device. Which patient is the best candidate?
    a. Older woman who lives alone with a fracture of nonunion
    b. Child with a congenital bone deformity whose mother is a licensed practical nurse
    c. Teenager with an open fracture and bone loss of the left lower leg
    d. Middle-aged man with a new comminuted fracture of the dominant forearm

20. The older adult patient has a fractured humerus. The physician is considering the use of electrical bone stimulation and asks the nurse to take a medical history on the patient. Which specific condition, which is a contraindication for this therapy, does the nurse ask the patient about?
    a. Seizures
    b. Cardiac pacemaker
    c. Stroke
    d. Peripheral nerve damage

21. The patient is prescribed low-intensity pulsed ultrasound treatments for a very slow healing fracture of the right lower leg. What instructions does the nurse give this patient related to the treatment?
    a. Test for pregnancy before the therapy and use birth control until treatment is complete.
    b. The treatment is experimental, but there are no known adverse effects.
    c. The device is implanted directly into the fracture site and there is no external apparatus.
    d. Expect to dedicate approximately 20 minutes a day for one treatment.

22. The nursing student is assisting with the care of the patient with musculoskeletal pain related to soft tissue injury and bone disruption. The student sees that the patient has a PRN order for pain medication. What does the student do first in order to decide when to give the pain medication?
    a. Ask the physician to clarify the order for specific parameters.
    b. Check with the primary nurse or the charge nurse for advice.
    c. Ask the patient about types of activities that increase the pain.
    d. Ask the instructor for help in interpreting the order.

23. The patient is receiving scheduled and PRN narcotics for severe pain related to a musculoskeletal injury. The nurse finds that the patient's abdomen is distended and bowel sounds are hypoactive. Because the nurse suspects that the patient is having a medication side effect, which question does the nurse ask the patient?
    a. "Are you having nausea and vomiting?"
    b. "When was your last bowel movement?"
    c. "Does your abdomen hurt?"
    d. "Are you having diarrhea or loose stool?"

Matching. *Match each description to its corresponding type of fracture.*

Types of Fracture
a. Pathologic (spontaneous)
b. Incomplete
c. Open (compound)

Descriptions

_____ 24. The adult patient was riding his four-wheeler on a country road late one evening. He suddenly saw several cows in the middle of the road. He turned sharply to avoid hitting them and spun out of control. His four-wheeler landed on top of him. His lower leg is obviously broken; it is bleeding and bone fragments are protruding from the skin.

_____ 25. One afternoon in her classroom, a schoolteacher slipped on some chalk that had fallen from the blackboard. She did not fall far and seemed to be all right. With the help of a student she was able to walk to the office. The secretary drove her to the emergency department (ED).

_____ 26. The adult female patient has osteoporosis. She plays cards often with her friends. One morning she was opening her car door while on her way to play cards when she fell suddenly. She said it felt as though her "leg gave way" and caused her to fall.

27. The nurse is caring for the patient with an open fracture. Which intervention does the nurse perform in order to prevent infection of the fracture?
   a. Use strict aseptic technique for dressing changes and wound irrigations.
   b. Use clean techniques for dressing changes and wound irrigations.
   c. Place the patient in contact isolation and wear sterile gloves.
   d. Place the patient in reverse isolation and perform scrupulous hand hygiene.

28. The nurse must adjust a pair of crutches to properly fit the patient. Which description illustrates correct crutch adjustment?
   a. Axilla rests lightly on the top of the crutch when the crutch is moved forward.
   b. Patient can easily use the crutch without subjective complaints.
   c. Elbow is flexed no more than 30 degrees when the palm is on the handle.
   d. Adult patient is of average height and the crutches are medium-sized.

29. The older patient's family is trying to find an appropriate cane for the patient to use because of chronic pain in the right ankle. The nurse instructs the family to purchase which type of cane?
    a. One with the top being parallel to the greater trochanter of the femur
    b. One that creates about 45 degrees of flexion of the elbow
    c. One that is based on the patient's weight to provide adequate support
    d. One that has padding on the handle grip to ensure safety

30. The nurse is caring for the patient who has been immobilized for 10 days. The nurse recognizes that the patient is now at risk for a negative nitrogen balance. Which intervention is best to address this risk?
    a. Obtain a laboratory order for a nitrogen balance test.
    b. Offer high-protein nutritional drinks.
    c. Obtain an order for supplemental oxygen.
    d. Perform or delegate range-of-motion (ROM) exercises.

31. The older patient with a lower leg fracture is having difficulty performing the weight-bearing exercises. Based on fracture pathophysiology and the patient's abilities, which condition could the patient develop?
    a. Osteomyelitis
    b. Internal derangement
    c. Neuroma
    d. Anemia

32. The nurse case manager is making a home visit to assist an older patient with a hip fracture. During the home visit, the nurse reviews home environment safety. Which observation indicates a need for additional teaching?
    a. Patient's bed has been moved to the ground floor level.
    b. There are handle bars around the toilet and tub.
    c. Floors are clean and shiny and covered with throw rugs.
    d. Patient's walker is close to the patient's bedside.

33. The patient has a scapular injury after being kicked by a horse. With this type of injury, it is important to assess for signs and symptoms of which condition?
    a. Cardiac tamponade
    b. Pneumothorax
    c. Aneurysm
    d. Pulmonary edema

Matching. Match each fracture complication with its corresponding description.

Fracture Complications
a. Delayed union
b. Fat embolism
c. Crush syndrome
d. Osteomyelitis
e. Avascular necrosis
f. Nonunion

Descriptions
_____ 34. Disrupted blood supply to the bone, resulting in the death of bone tissue
_____ 35. Bone infection
_____ 36. Fat globules released from the yellow bone marrow into the bloodstream
_____ 37. Incomplete fracture healing
_____ 38. External crush injury that compresses one or more compartments in the leg, arm, or pelvis
_____ 39. Lack of fracture healing

40. The patient who tripped and fell down several stairs reports having heard a popping sound and fears that she has broken her ankle. How does the nurse initially assess for fracture in this patient?
    a. Measuring the circumference of the distal leg
    b. Gently moving the ankle through the full range of motion
    c. Inspecting for crepitus and skin color
    d. Observing for deformity or misalignment

41. The nurse is assessing the patient with an injury to the shoulder and upper arm after being thrown from a horse. What is the best position for this patient's assessment?
    a. Supine so that the extremity can be elevated
    b. Low Fowler's on an exam table for patient comfort
    c. Sitting to observe for shoulder droop
    d. Slow ambulation to observe for natural arm movement

42. The nurse is caring for the patient with skeletal pins that have been placed for traction. What does the nurse expect to see in the first 48 hours?
    a. Clear fluid drainage weeping from the pin insertion site
    b. Some bloody drainage, but very minimal
    c. Swelling at the site with tenderness to gentle touch
    d. Dressings around the pin sites to be dry and intact

43. The adult patient has been involved in a motor vehicle accident. The nurse is preparing to insert a urinary catheter, but sees blood oozing from the urethra. What does the nurse do next?
    a. Insert an adult-sized catheter because the need for accurate I&O is essential.
    b. Obtain the smallest catheter possible to minimize tissue trauma.
    c. Use the largest catheter possible because of the likelihood of blood clots.
    d. Delay catheterization because of possible urethral tear and inform the physician.

44. The patient with a hip fracture is at risk for avascular necrosis (AVN) because of long-term corticosteroid therapy. Which diagnostic test does the nurse prepare the patient for to determine if AVN is occurring?
    a. Magnetic resonance imaging
    b. Doppler ultrasonography
    c. McMurray test
    d. Transcutaneous electrical nerve stimulation

45. The patient has a fracture of the femur. As the healing progresses, which laboratory results does the nurse expect to see?
    a. Decrease in hematocrit and hemoglobin
    b. Decrease in erythrocyte sedimentation rate
    c. Increase in serum calcium and phosphorus levels
    d. Increase in potassium and magnesium levels

46. The unlicensed assistive personnel (UAP) is assisting the orthopedic physician to cut a window in the patient's cast. What does the nurse instruct the UAP to do?
    a. Check the pulse that is accessed after the window is cut.
    b. Clean up and dispose of all casting debris.
    c. Inform the patient that the procedure is painless.
    d. Save the plaster piece that was cut so it can be taped in place.

47. The nurse is caring for the patient in Buck's traction. Which task is best to delegate to the UAP (with supervision)?
    a. Turning and repositioning
    b. Inspecting heels and sacral area
    c. Asking the patient about muscle spasms
    d. Adjusting the weights on the apparatus

48. The nurse is instructing the teenage patient with a tibia-fibula fracture that was treated with internal fixation and a long leg cast. He is anxious to know when the cast will be removed so that he can resume football practice. Which statement by the patient indicates a need for additional teaching?
    a. "There's a possibility that the cast could be removed in 4 weeks."
    b. "The plates and screws reduce the length of time I'll be in the cast."
    c. "The cast could remain in place as long as 6 weeks."
    d. "I'll use crutches for 2 weeks and then the cast will be removed."

49. The patient was an unrestrained driver involved in a motor vehicle accident who sustained a 5th rib fracture. As the patient is being assessed, what is the nurse's major concern?
    a. Pain that increases with inspiration
    b. Muffled heart sounds
    c. Widespread bruising over the chest
    d. Crepitus over the 5th rib

50. Complete the chart below by indicating assessment techniques and normal findings for patients with musculoskeletal injuries. The first block has been done for you.

	Assessment Technique	**Normal Findings**
Skin Color	Inspect the area distal to the injury.	No change in pigmentation compared with other parts of the body.
Skin Temperature		
Movement		
Sensation		
Pulses		
Capillary Refill		
Pain		

51. Place the steps in the correct order for emergency care of the patient with fracture using the numbers 1 through 6.

    _____ a. Cover the affected area with a dressing (preferably sterile).

    _____ b. Check the neurovascular status of the area distal to the extremity: temperature, color, sensation, movement, and capillary refill. Compare affected and unaffected limbs.

    _____ c. Remove the patient's clothing (cut if necessary) to inspect the affected area while supporting the injured area above and below the injury. Do not remove shoes because this can cause increased trauma.

    _____ d. Apply direct pressure on the area if there is bleeding and pressure over the proximal artery nearest the fracture.

    _____ e. Immobilize the extremity by splinting; include joints above and below the fracture site. Recheck circulation after splinting.

    _____ f. Put the patient in a supine position; keep warm.

52. According to the patient's chart, there is a family history of osteoporosis. In order to plan interventions related to this finding, what action does the nurse take?
    a. Ask the patient's age and assess for weight loss.
    b. Review the patient's dietary intake of calcium.
    c. Assess the patient for kyphoscoliosis or other deformities.
    d. Assess the patient for occult fractures of the long bones.

53. The nurse's neighbor comes running over because her husband "cut his finger off with a power saw." After calling for help, what is the priority action when the nurse gets to the neighbor's house?
    a. Examine the amputation site.
    b. Assess for airway or breathing problems.
    c. Elevate the hand above the heart.
    d. Assess the severed finger.

54. An excited group of teenagers brings a friend to the ED who severed a finger while playing sports. The bleeding from the site is well controlled and the patient is alert and stable. What does the nurse do with the severed finger?
    a. Place it directly into a bag of ice and then put the bag into a refrigerator.
    b. Wrap it in moist sterile gauze and ensure that it stays with the patient.
    c. Wrap it in a dry gauze, place it in a waterproof bag, and put the bag in ice water.
    d. Carefully clean it with sterile saline, then place it in a sterile container.

55. Which nursing intervention is best to prevent increased pain in the patient experiencing phantom limb pain?
    a. Handle the residual limb carefully when assessing the site or changing the dressing.
    b. Advise the patient that the sensation is temporary and will diminish over time.
    c. Remind the patient that the part is not really there, so the pain is not real.
    d. Encourage the patient to mourn the loss of the body part and express grief.

56. The young patient had a great toe amputated because of severe injury. The patient is depressed and withdrawn after the physician tells him that the amputation will affect balance and gait. What is the nurse's best response?
    a. "The physical therapy department can help you with exercises for balance and gait."
    b. "Let me get your parents and we can talk about rehabilitation programs."
    c. "When the doctor was explaining things to you, what were you thinking about?"
    d. "How have you usually handled stressful situations in the past?"

57. The patient is a middle-aged man with a history of uncontrolled diabetes. His right foot is a dark brownish-purple color and there is no palpable dorsalis pedis or posterior tibial pulse. The nurse prepares the patient for which diagnostic test?
    a. X-ray of the foot and ankle
    b. Doppler ultrasound
    c. Electromyelogram
    d. Arthrogram

58. The nurse is caring for the patient with phantom limb pain. Which order for pain medication does the nurse question?
    a. IV infusion of calcitonin (Calcimar)
    b. Oral gabapentin (Neurontin)
    c. IV opioid analgesics
    d. Oral antispasmodic

59. The patient injured a lower extremity and has been placed in a running traction. What instructions does the nurse give to the UAP?
    a. Support the weights when turning the patient every 2 hours.
    b. Apply countertraction before moving the patient.
    c. Defer hygienic care and moving the patient until traction is removed.
    d. Moving the patient or the bed during care can alter the countertraction.

60. The patient is in circumferential traction. The nurse removes the belt and inspects the skin at least once every how many hours?
    a. 2
    b. 4
    c. 8
    d. 12

61. The nurse is caring for the patient with an above-the-knee amputation (AKA). In order to prevent hip flexion contractures, how does the nurse position the patient?
    a. Supine position with the residual limb elevated on a pillow
    b. Prone position every 3 to 4 hours for 20- to 30-minute periods
    c. Supine position with an abduction pillow placed between the legs
    d. Head of the bed elevated 30 degrees with assurance that the bandage is wrapped around the limb

62. The nurse applies bandages to the patient's residual limb in order to help shape and shrink the limb for a prosthesis. What is the proper technique for the nurse to use?
    a. Reapply the bandages every 8 hours or more often if they become loose.
    b. Use a proximal to distal direction when wrapping.
    c. Use a soft and flexible bandage material and pad the area with gauze.
    d. Use a figure-eight wrapping method to prevent restriction of blood flow.

Matching. *Match each definition to its corresponding type of traction.*

Types of Traction
a. Plaster traction
b. Brace traction
c. Skin traction
d. Circumferential traction
e. Skeletal traction

Definitions

_____ 63. Involves the use of a fabric fastener boot (Bucks), belt, or halter, which is secured around a body part

_____ 64. Pins, wires, tongs, or screws surgically inserted directly into bone

_____ 65. Combines skeletal traction and a plaster cast

_____ 66. Exerts a pull for correction of alignment deformities

_____ 67. Uses a belt around the body

68. The older patient is discharged to home following an orthopedic injury. Which mobilization device is usually preferred for older patients?
    a. Crutches
    b. Cane
    c. Walker
    d. Wheelchair

69. The nurse is interviewing the older adult with a history of osteoporosis who reports falling and catching her weight on her outstretched dominant hand. This patient is most likely to have sustained what type of fracture?
    a. Carpal scaphoid bone
    b. Phalanges fracture
    c. Humeral fracture
    d. Colle's wrist fracture

70. Which factor carries the greatest risk for hip fracture?
    a. Decreased visual acuity
    b. Joint stiffness
    c. Osteoporosis
    d. Cardiac drug regimen

71. The older adult patient is taken to the ED and diagnosed with a hip fracture after being found lying on the floor of his home. The patient lives alone and is in an extremely debilitated condition. What treatment option is best for this patient?
    a. Open reduction with internal fixation
    b. Bedrest and Buck's traction
    c. External fixation with pin placement
    d. Plaster casting and immobilization

72. The nurse is caring for the patient with open reduction and internal fixation (ORIF) for a hip fracture. Because the patient is at risk for hip dislocation, the nurse ensures that the hip is maintained in which position?
    a. Adduction
    b. Anatomically neutral
    c. Abduction
    d. Extended

73. The patient reports dramatic changes in color and temperature of the skin over the left foot with intense burning pain, sensitive skin, excessive sweating, and edema. The physician makes a preliminary medical diagnosis of complex regional pain syndrome. What is the priority nursing diagnosis?
    a. Knowledge Deficit
    b. Impaired Skin Integrity
    c. Acute Pain
    d. Impaired Tissue Perfusion

74. The patient is admitted to the same-day surgery unit following a meniscectomy. What does postoperative care for this patient include? *(Select all that apply.)*
    a. Perform neurovascular checks every hour for the first few hours and then every 4 hours.
    b. Check the surgical dressing for bleeding
    c. Monitor vital signs.
    d. Strict I&O.
    e. Teach about signs and symptoms of infection.
    f. NPO until fully awake.

75. Following a meniscectomy, the nurse assists the patient to immediately start performing which exercises?
    a. Range-of-motion exercises to both legs
    b. Straight leg raises on both legs
    c. Flexion and extension of knees
    d. Flexion and extension of ankles

76. The patient arrives in the ED reporting pain and immobility of the right shoulder. The patient reports a history of recurrent dislocations of the same shoulder. The nurse observes for which other signs and symptoms that are associated with a dislocation injury? *(Select all that apply.)*
    a. Alteration in contour of the joint
    b. Deviation in length of the extremity
    c. Muscle atrophy
    d. Mottled skin discoloration
    e. Rotation of the extremity

True or False? *Read the following statements and write T for true or F for false in the blanks provided. If a statement is false, correct it to make it true.*

_____ 77. The lateral meniscus is more likely to tear than the medial meniscus.

_____ 78. When the anterior cruciate ligament (ACL) is torn, the person may feel a "snap."

_____ 79. Complete healing of knee ligaments after surgery only takes 3 to 4 weeks.

_____ 80. Rupture of the Achilles tendon is common in older adults.

_____ 81. Dislocation is most common in the hip, shoulder, knee, and fingers.

_____ 82. A strain is excessive stretching of a ligament.

_____ 83. Management of a strain usually involves cold and heat applications.

_____ 84. Sprains are usually precipitated by twisting motions from a fall or sports injury.

_____ 85. Patients with a torn rotator cuff have shoulder pain and cannot initiate or maintain adduction of the arm at the shoulder (drop arm test).

86. The physician tells the patient that she has a mild first-degree sprain to the ankle. What instructions does the nurse give to the patient about the treatment for the injury? *(Select all that apply.)*
    a. Rest.
    b. Apply ice for the first 4 to 6 hours.
    c. Apply a compression bandage for a few days to reduce swelling and provide joint support.
    d. Elevate the foot.
    e. Perform range-of-motion exercises every 4 hours.

87. The patient is informed by the physician that he must have a plaster cast applied to the lower extremity. What does the nurse teach the patient about the procedure before the cast is applied?
    a. "Plaster will be applied directly to the skin surface."
    b. "The cast material will feel hot at first, but will quickly become cool."
    c. "The cast will be dry within 2 to 3 hours after application."
    d. "The plaster is a durable, waterproof material that protects the skin."

88. The nurse is caring for the patient with a plaster splint applied to the ankle. The patient received oral pain medication at 0900. At 1100, the patient reports that the pain is getting worse, not better. What is the nurse's priority action?
    a. Give the patient IV pain medication.
    b. Reposition the extremity on a pillow and place an ice pack.
    c. Assess the pulses and skin temperature distal to the splint.
    d. Call the physician to report the patient's increasing pain.

89. The patient had a cast applied to the leg several days ago. He returns to the clinic because the "edge of the cast is falling apart and rubbing my skin." How can the nurse or the orthopedic technician intervene?
    a. Cut a cast window.
    b. Change the cast.
    c. Bivalve the cast.
    d. Petal the cast.

90. The nurse is providing teaching for the patient with a forearm cast. What information does the nurse give to the patient?
    a. "The hand should be elevated above the shoulder when resting."
    b. "Use an ice pack for the first 6 to 8 hours, and cover the pack with a towel to absorb condensation."
    c. "The sling should distribute the weight over a large area of the shoulders and trunk."
    d. "Limit movement of the fingers or wrist joints to prevent pain."

91. The nurse and nursing student are assisting the patient with a new hip spica cast to transfer from the stretcher to the bed. What does the nurse advise the student to do?
    a. Delay the transfer until the cast is dry.
    b. Assist the patient to log roll from the stretcher to the bed.
    c. Keep the affected leg elevated during the transfer.
    d. Handle the cast with the flat palmar surface of the hand.

Matching. Match each term related to musculoskeletal injuries with its corresponding definition.

Types of Injury
a. Dislocation
b. Sprain
c. Strain
d. Subluxation

Definitions

_____ 92. Partial joint surface separation

_____ 93. Injury to ligament

_____ 94. Joint surfaces not approximated

_____ 95. Excessive stretching of muscle or tendon

96. The patient with a lower extremity injury is being treated by external fixation. What nursing assessment is of particular concern in the care of this patient with this type of system?
    a. Maintaining a 30-degree flexed position of the knee
    b. Measuring the weights used for counter-traction
    c. Observing the patient's abilities to adjust the clickers
    d. Observing the points of entry of the pins and wires

97. The nurse's older neighbor has slipped and fallen and reports pain to the left forearm. There is also a small abrasion over the area. Place the steps for first responder care in the correct order using the numbers 1 through 6.

    _____ a. Applies a splint that extends below the wrist and above the elbow

    _____ b. Inspects the extremity for swelling and deformity

    _____ c. Palpates for pulse and questions about sensation

    _____ d. Places a sterile gauze loosely over the abrasion to protect from further contamination

    _____ e. Assesses for motor function

    _____ f. Reevaluates neurovascular function after immobilization

98. The nurse is caring for the patient who had a kyphoplasty. What does postoperative care for this patient include? *(Select all that apply.)*
    a. Place the patient in a flat supine position for 8 hours.
    b. Monitor and record vital signs.
    c. Perform frequent neurologic assessments.
    d. Apply a warm pack to the puncture site if needed to relieve pain.
    e. Assess the patient's pain level and compare it to the preoperative level.
    f. Give opioid analgesics as needed.
    g. Monitor for bleeding at the puncture site.

99. The patient in a body cast reports nausea, vomiting, and epigastric pain. The nurse notifies the physician for orders. Which intervention is the most conservative, and therefore the first thing to try, to address this patient's symptoms?
    a. Insert a nasogastric tube and attach to low wall suction.
    b. Cut a window over the abdominal area of the cast.
    c. Obtain an order for an x-ray to diagnose a paralytic ileus.
    d. Administer PRN antiemetic and PRN pain medication.

100. The patient with a long leg cast that was applied in the ED is being admitted to the orthopedic unit. Which task is best for the nurse to delegate to the UAP?
    a. Obtain a fracture pan and use caution to prevent spillage on the cast.
    b. Obtain several plastic covered pillows for elevation of the leg.
    c. Check flexion/extension and color of the toes.
    d. Turn the patient every 4 to 6 hours to allow the cast to dry.

CASE STUDY: THE PATIENT WITH TRAUMATIC AMPUTATION

Use a separate sheet of paper to answer the questions in this Case Study. Answer guidelines for this Case Study are available on your Evolve website at http://evolve. elsevier.com/Iggy/ in the "Prepare for Class" folder.

A 25-year-old carpenter comes running into the ED with a blood-soaked rag over his right hand. He states that while working on a house he was building, he sawed off his right index finger. He has the finger in his pocket. The nurse puts on gloves and applies pressure with sterile gauze to the amputated area. The nurse discovers during the assessment that he has a history of depression and takes medication for it. The nurse identifies during the assessment that he has no significant medical history other than depression.

1. Identify the type of amputation that would be considered for this patient.
2. Identify the top nursing priority in dealing with the patient's amputated finger.
3. What should the nurse do with the patient's finger?
4. Identify two appropriate nursing diagnoses for this patient.
5. Identify the type of shock for which this patient is at risk.
6. Considering this patient's history, what recommendations would you make?

CASE STUDY: THE PATIENT WITH FRACTURE

Use a separate sheet of paper to answer the questions in this Case Study. Answer guidelines for this Case Study are available on your Evolve website at http://evolve. elsevier.com/Iggy/ in the "Prepare for Class" folder.

The 20-year-old patient was admitted with fractures of the right tibia and fibula after a fall. She has a long leg cast that was applied this morning. The physician has ordered bedrest for now until her condition stabilizes.

1. What is the priority for assessment during this time?

2. Later that evening, as the nurse performs an assessment, the patient states that the cast seems "too tight." It was difficult, but not impossible, for the nurse to insert one finger between the top of the cast and the patient's skin. Is this a concern, and what actions, if any, should the nurse take at this time?

3. A few days later, the patient is allowed to get out of bed with crutches. The crutches have been delivered, but the physical therapist has not yet been in to see the patient. The patient states, "I can't wait any longer. Let me try walking with those crutches—I'm sure I can do it because I've played with my brother's crutches before." Should the nurse let her walk with the crutches? Why or why not?

4. What type of gait will she be taught to use while crutch-walking?

5. The patient has been discharged, and has received instructions for cast care. One week later, she calls the office and asks, "Can I get a new cast? This one smells moldy or musty, and it's getting uncomfortable." What does the nurse suspect? When she comes to the office to have it checked, what further assessments should be done?

6. The patient is fearful when she sees the cast saw. What should the nurse tell her?

55 CHAPTER

Assessment of the Gastrointestinal System

STUDY/REVIEW QUESTIONS

Matching. *Match the terms associated with the GI system with their corresponding definitions.*

Terms

a. Bile
b. Chyme
c. Duodenum
d. Elimination
e. Esophagus
f. Gallbladder
g. Kupffer cells
h. Jejunum
i. Sphincter of Oddi
j. Liver
k. Lobule
l. Mouth
m. Intrinsic factor
n. Pancreas
o. Mastication
p. Saliva
q. Secretin
r. Stomach
s. Submucosa
t. Villi

Definitions

_____ 1. Organ with both exocrine and endocrine functions

_____ 2. Muscle that surrounds the ampulla of Vater

_____ 3. Finger-like projections into the small intestine

_____ 4. Oral secretion that softens food

_____ 5. Thick, liquid mass of partially digested food

_____ 6. Temporary reservoir for food

_____ 7. Intestinal hormone that inhibits acid secretion and decreases gastric motility

_____ 8. Epithelial cell layer lining the GI tract

_____ 9. Process of expelling feces

_____ 10. Central part of small intestine

_____ 11. Chewing

_____ 12. Conduit for food from mouth to stomach

_____ 13. First 10 inches of small intestine

_____ 14. A substance that facilitates the absorption of vitamin B_{12}

_____ 15. Functional unit of liver

_____ 16. Liver secretion essential to fat emulsification

_____ 17. Largest abdominal organ with numerous functions

_____ 18. Organ that concentrates and stores bile

_____ 19. Phagocytic cells found in the liver that are part of the body's reticuloendothelial system

_____ 20. Beginning pathway for digestion

21. Which drugs predispose the patient to peptic ulcer disease and GI bleeding? *(Select all that apply.)*
    a. Nonsteroidal anti-inflammatory drugs
    b. Steroids
    c. Aspirin
    d. Lasix
    e. Digitalis

True or False? *Read the statements and write T for true or F for false in the blanks provided.*

_____ 22. About 80% to 90% of African-American people are lactose intolerant.

_____ 23. *Anorexia* is the term used for self-inflicted vomiting after eating.

_____ 24. *Dyspepsia* refers to indigestion or heartburn associated with eating.

_____ 25. Familial adenomatous polyposis (FAP) is an inherited autosomal dominant disorder that predisposes the patient to colon cancer.

26. The nurse is caring for the patient with abdominal pain. While assessing the patient, which questions will the nurse ask the patient? *(Select all that apply.)*
    a. "Is the pain burning, gnawing, or stabbing?"
    b. "Can you point to where you feel the pain?"
    c. "Does your skin feel itchy?"
    d. "When did you first notice the pain?"
    e. "Does the pain spread anywhere?"

27. Indicate the usual sequence that the abdominal examination occurs using the numbers 1 through 4.

    _____ a. Right lower quadrant (RLQ)

    _____ b. Left lower quadrant (LLQ)

    _____ c. Left upper quadrant (LUQ)

    _____ d. Right upper quadrant (RUQ)

28. Indicate the correct sequence of examination techniques for abdominal assessment using the numbers 1 through 4.

    _____ a. Inspection

    _____ b. Percussion

    _____ c. Palpation

    _____ d. Auscultation

29. The nurse is performing an abdominal assessment on the patient. For which finding does the nurse alert the physician?
    a. Cullen's sign
    b. Borborygmus
    c. Blumberg's sign
    d. Bulging, pulsating mass

Matching. *Match the terms with the correct descriptions.*

Terms
a. Cullen's sign
b. Bruits
c. Tympanic
d. Blumberg's sign

Descriptions

_____ 30. Areas of pain that also show rebound tenderness

_____ 31. High pitched, loud, musical sound of an air-filled intestine

_____ 32. "Swooshing" sounds

_____ 33. The presence of ecchymoses around the umbilicus

34. Complete the chart below regarding the significance of each assessment finding.

Assessment	Significance
Fruity-smelling breath	
Asymmetry in the upper quadrants of the abdomen	
Asymmetry in the lower quadrants of the abdomen	
Cullen's sign	
Bruit heard over the abdominal aorta	
Diminished or absent bowel sounds	
Loud, gurgling bowel sounds	

35. What will laboratory values for the patient with liver disease most likely show? *(Select all that apply.)*
    a. Decreased prothrombin time
    b. Increased AST and ALT
    c. Increased albumin levels
    d. Decreased ammonia levels
    e. Increased unconjugated bilirubin

36. Laboratory values for the patient with acute pancreatitis may show decreased levels of which factor?
    a. Calcium
    b. Serum amylase
    c. Serum lipase
    d. Urine amylase

Matching. *Match the diagnostic studies with their corresponding descriptions.*

Diagnostic Studies

a. Esophagogastroduodenoscopy (EGD)
b. Upper GI radiographic series
c. Small bowel series (SBFT)
d. Barium enema
e. Percutaneous transhepatic cholangiography
f. Gallbladder radiographic series
g. Intravenous cholangiography
h. Endoscopic retrograde cholangiopancreatography (ERCP)
i. Enteroscopy

Descriptions

_____ 37. Visualization of the small intestine.

_____ 38. X-ray study of the gallbladder and biliary ducts. IV injection of contrast material is given and films are taken at 20-minute intervals for 1 hour (or until the biliary ducts are visualized).

_____ 39. Visualization of the esophagus, stomach, and duodenum.

_____ 40. Visual radiographic examination of the liver, gallbladder, bile ducts, and pancreas to identify the cause and location of an obstruction.

_____ 41. A radiographic visualization of the large intestine; usually ordered for the patient with blood or mucus in the stool or a change in bowel habits.

_____ 42. Visualization of the gallbladder after oral ingestion of radiopaque, iodine-based contrast medium. The day before the test, the patient eats a fat-free or low-fat meal and takes six radiopaque iodine tablets approximately 2 hours after the meal. Patient is NPO from midnight on the night before the test.

_____ 43. X-ray study of the biliary duct system using instillation of an iodinated dye into the liver.

_____ 44. Visualization from the oral part of the pharynx to the duodenojejunal junction. Used to detect disorders of structure or function of the esophagus, stomach, or duodenum.

_____ 45. An extension of the upper GI series; this test continues to trace the barium through the small intestine, up to and including the ileocecal junction, to detect disorders of the jejunum or ileum.

Matching. Match the endoscopic procedures to the appropriate follow-up care.

Endoscopic Procedures

a. Esophagogastroduodenoscopy (EGD)
b. Endoscopic retrograde cholangiopancreatography (ERCP)
c. Colonoscopy
d. Proctosigmoidoscopy

Follow-Up Care

_____ 46. The patient is informed that mild gas pain and flatulence may be experienced as a result of air instilled into the rectum during the examination. If a biopsy specimen is obtained, a small amount of bleeding may be observed.

_____ 47. Vital signs must be checked every 15 minutes until the patient is stable. Siderails are kept up until sedation wears off. Observe for signs of perforation or hemorrhage. The nurse instructs the patient that a feeling of "fullness," cramping, and passage of flatus can be expected for several hours after the test. A small amount of blood may be in the first stool after the test if a biopsy specimen is taken or a polypectomy is performed. Excessive bleeding should be reported immediately.

_____ 48. Vital signs are assessed frequently until the patient is stable. Observe for cholangitis, perforation, sepsis, and pancreatitis (these problems may not occur immediately after the procedure and may take several hours to 2 days to develop). The patient is instructed to report abdominal pain, fever, nausea, or vomiting that fails to resolve. The patient is on NPO status until the gag reflex returns.

_____ 49. Vitals checked frequently (usually every 30 minutes) and siderails are up until sedation wears off. Patient remains NPO until the gag reflex returns. Monitor for signs of perforation such as pain, bleeding, or fever. Patient is instructed not to drive for 12 hours after the test. A hoarse voice and sore throat may persist for several days; throat lozenges may be used to relieve the discomfort.

CASE STUDY: THE PATIENT WITH UPPER GI PAIN

Use a separate sheet of paper to answer the questions in this Case Study. Answer guidelines for this Case Study are available on your Evolve website at http://evolve. elsevier.com/Iggy/ in the "Prepare for Class" folder.

The patient is an 87-year-old woman who is admitted to a medical nursing unit from a local nursing home. She had surgery for abdominal adhesions 4 weeks ago and is now passing blood-streaked stools. She also reports that her stomach hurts, especially during the night. "It feels like someone is burning a hole inside me." The patient states that she lives alone in an apartment building for retirees. Last week, a close friend and neighbor visited her at the nursing home and reported news of deaths of two mutual friends who were residents of the apartment building.

1. What additional data should the nurse collect for a thorough GI system assessment of the patient?

2. The patient is scheduled to have an upper GI and small bowel series the next day. What does the nurse do to prepare her for these diagnostic studies?

3. The patient is unable to tolerate the barium solution, becomes nauseated, and vomits. Her physician orders that an EGD be done. What additional preparation is needed before this procedure can be performed on the patient?

4. Following the EGD, the patient is returned to her room by stretcher. The nurse assists her to transfer to bed. What position should the patient be assisted to assume? What assessments should the nurse initially perform? Why?

5. While the nurse is assessing her, the patient asks for some water to drink. What should the nurse do?

56
CHAPTER

Care of Patients with Oral Cavity Problems

STUDY/REVIEW QUESTIONS

1. What statement is true about the *Candida albicans* form of stomatitis?
   a. It is common type of primary stomatitis.
   b. *Candida albicans* is a bacterial infection.
   c. This infection is uncommon in patients who are immunocompromised.
   d. Patients on steroid therapy often experience this infection.

2. The nurse has provided teaching to the patient on ways to prevent the recurrence of aphthous ulcers. Which statement by the patient indicates teaching has been effective?
   a. "I will avoid gluten in my diet."
   b. "Potatoes have nothing to do with the development of the ulcers."
   c. "I will continue to eat peanut butter and jelly sandwiches."
   d. "It doesn't matter what types of foods I eat as long as I brush my teeth after every meal."

3. When caring for the patient with stomatitis, what is it most important for the nurse to assess?
   a. Nutritional status
   b. Level of pain
   c. Self-care abilities
   d. Airway status

4. The nurse is performing an oral assessment on the patient and notes white plaque-like lesions on the tongue, palate, pharynx, and buccal mucosa. When the patches are wiped away, the underlying surface is red and sore. What disorder does the nurse suspect the patient has?
   a. Leukoplakia
   b. *Candida albicans*
   c. Erythroplakia
   d. Kaposi's sarcoma

5. The nurse's aide is providing care to the patient with stomatitis. Which intervention by the nurse's aide illustrates correct care for this patient?
   a. Using a hard-bristled toothbrush to thoroughly clean the oral cavity
   b. Rinsing the mouth with a commercial mouthwash
   c. Using a warm saline, hydrogen peroxide, or sodium bicarbonate solution to rinse the mouth
   d. Rinsing the mouth frequently with cold tap water and vinegar solution

6. What is the drug of choice for the treatment of a fungal mouth infection?
   a. Nystatin (Mycostatin)
   b. Acyclovir (Zovirax)
   c. Minocycline
   d. Benzocaine (Kenalog in Orabase)

7. Which statement by the student nurse indicates the need for a better understanding of the care of patients with oral cavity problems?
   a. "I will use lemon-glycerin swabs to clean the patient's mouth."
   b. "The patient should eat a soft, bland diet."
   c. "Dentures should be removed."
   d. "Gauze may be used for oral care."

Matching. Match the types of oral cavity tumors with their corresponding descriptions.

Oral Cavity Tumors
a. Leukoplakia
b. Erythroplakia
c. Squamous cell carcinoma
d. Basal cell carcinoma
e. Kaposi's sarcoma

Descriptions

_____ 8. Painless, raised purple nodule or plaque on the hard palate

_____ 9. Red, raised, eroded areas on the lips, tongue, buccal mucosa, and oropharynx

_____ 10. Thickened, white, firmly attached patches in the oral mucosa, lips, or tongue

_____ 11. Raised scab, primarily on the lips; evolves to an ulcer with a raised pearly border

_____ 12. Red, velvety lesion on the tongue, palate, floor of the mouth, or mandibular mucosa

13. The patient is scheduled for multiple tests to evaluate an oral tumor. The patient asks the nurse which of the tests is the best to determine if the tumor is cancerous. How does the nurse respond?
    a. "All of the tests need to be looked at together because no one test can tell if you have cancer."
    b. "Magnetic resonance imaging is the only diagnostic test that will need to be done."
    c. "Biopsy is the definitive method for diagnosing oral cancer."
    d. "An aqueous solution of toluidine blue 1% can be applied to the oral lesion. If the lesion is malignant it will not absorb the solution; however, the preparation stains the normal tissue."

14. What is the priority nursing diagnosis for patients with oral cancer?
    a. Imbalanced Nutrition: Less Than Body Requirements related to inability to ingest food
    b. Impaired Swallowing related to oral cavity or oropharyngeal abnormalities
    c. Disturbed Body Image related to surgery
    d. Risk for Ineffective Airway Clearance related to obstructed airway by the tumor, edema, or secretions

15. During an assessment of the patient with an oral tumor, the nurse notes that the patient develops stridor. What functional assessment is *not* a priority for the nurse to complete?
    a. Ability to speak
    b. Gag reflex
    c. Quality of respirations
    d. Pain rating

Matching. Match the operative procedures with their correct definitions.

Procedures

a. Radical neck dissection
b. Glossectomy
c. Mandibulectomy
d. Commando procedure

Descriptions

_____ 16. Excision of a segment of the mandible with the oral lesion

_____ 17. Tongue removal

_____ 18. Jaw removal

_____ 19. Removal of all cervical lymph nodes on the affected side, along with cranial nerve XI, the internal jugular vein, and the sternocleidomastoid muscle

20. After the patient has undergone a radical neck dissection, what is the priority nursing intervention?
    a. Manage the patient's pain.
    b. Maintain fluid and electrolyte balance.
    c. Maintain the patient's airway.
    d. Enhance the patient's ability to communicate.

21. Which intervention prevents or minimizes the risk factors in patients at risk for aspiration?
    a. Request medications in pill form.
    b. Avoid liquids or use a thickening agent.
    c. Position the patient upright at 30 degrees.
    d. Keep the head of bed elevated 10 to 15 minutes after eating.

True or False? *Read the statements about oral cancer and write T for true or F for false in the blanks provided.*

_____ 22. Acute effects of radiation therapy include treatment-related mucositis, stomatitis, and alteration in taste.

_____ 23. The term *xerostomia* refers to excessive mouth dryness.

_____ 24. Fatigue is an uncommon side effect of radiation therapy.

_____ 25. Taste sensation usually returns several weeks after completion of radiation therapy.

_____ 26. Saliva production is greatly reduced as a consequence of radiation.

27. The nurse's aide is caring for the patient undergoing radiation therapy to the neck. Which action by the nurse's aide requires intervention by the supervising nurse?
    a. Using powder on the patient's neck
    b. Shaving the patient with an electric razor
    c. Avoiding use of alcohol-based aftershave lotion
    d. Using gentle nondeodorant soap to wash the patient

28. The patient with which condition or disorder is at lowest risk for the development of acute sialoadenitis?
    a. Sjögren's syndrome
    b. HIV infection
    c. Anemia
    d. Phenothiazine use

29. When assessing the patient with a salivary gland tumor, the nurse pays particular attention to the facial nerve. Which request by the nurse is *least* likely to determine if the tumor has affected the facial nerve?
    a. "Puff out your cheeks."
    b. "Wrinkle your nose."
    c. "Cough."
    d. "Raise your eyebrows."

30. The nurse has taught the patient with acute sialoadenitis to use sialagogues to stimulate saliva. The patient demonstrates teaching has been effective when the patient states he will eat which food?
    a. Oranges
    b. Apples
    c. Bananas
    d. Bread

CASE STUDY: THE PATIENT WITH AN ORAL TUMOR

Use a separate sheet of paper to answer the questions in this Case Study. Answer guidelines for this Case Study are available on your Evolve website at http://evolve. elsevier.com/Iggy/ in the "Prepare for Class" folder.

The patient is admitted to the surgical unit for a radical neck dissection. He has a painless raised purple nodule on the hard palate. The lesion is large and the patient states, "I feel like there is something back there that makes it hard for me to breathe." His vital signs are temperature 102.2° F, pulse 98, blood pressure 138/90, respiratory rate 22. The patient has a CBC which indicates a Hgb of 18 g/dL, Hct 47%, and a WBC count of 18,000/mm^3. When reviewing the notes, the nurse reads that he had testing with an aqueous solution of toluidine blue 1% before his admission.

1. Based on the description of the tumor, what kind of tumor does the nurse identify the tumor as most likely being?

2. What effect does the nurse expect for the toluidine solution if the tumor is malignant?

3. The patient is diagnosed with Kaposi's sarcoma. After this diagnosis, the nurse anticipates that the patient will most likely be tested for what other disease?

4. Based on the patient's assessment and laboratory results, what should the nurse anticipate as priority nursing interventions for the patient at this time?

5. The patient undergoes a radical neck dissection. Describe the nursing care for patients after this procedure.

57 CHAPTER

Care of Patients with Esophageal Problems

STUDY/REVIEW QUESTIONS

1. Which physiologic factor contributes to gastroesophageal reflux disease (GERD)?
    a. Accelerated gastric emptying
    b. Irritation from refluxate
    c. Competent lower esophageal sphincter
    d. Increased esophageal clearance

2. Which statement is true about Barrett's epithelium in the patient with GERD?
    a. While the body heals, a different type of cell forms on the lower part of the esophagus.
    b. This new tissue is less resistant to acid so it must be taken care of.
    c. Barrett's epithelium is resistant to the development of cancer.
    d. Esophageal strictures are less likely to occur with this type of epithelium.

True or False? Read the statements and write T for true or F for false in the blanks provided.

_____ 3. GERD is the most common upper GI disorder in the United States.

_____ 4. Overweight and obese patients are at an increased risk for GERD.

_____ 5. GERD does not occur in children.

Matching. Match each of the following GERD-associated conditions with their corresponding definitions.

GERD-Associated Conditions
a. Dyspepsia
b. Regurgitation
c. Water brash
d. Dysphagia
e. Odynophagia
f. Flatulence
g. Globus
h. Eructation
i. Pyrosis

Definitions

_____ 6. Pain described as a substernal or retrosternal burning sensation that tends to move up and down the chest in a wavelike fashion

_____ 7. Difficulty swallowing

_____ 8. Occurrence of warm fluid traveling up the throat with a sour or bitter taste

_____ 9. Painful swallowing

_____ 10. Reflex salivary hypersecretion in response to reflux

_____ 11. Gas

_____ 12. Belching

_____ 13. Feeling of something in the back of the throat

_____ 14. Retrosternal burning

15. The patient is scheduled to have several diagnostic tests to verify the medical diagnosis of GERD. Which diagnostic test is the most accurate method of diagnosing this disorder?
    a. Esophagogastroduodenoscopy (EGD)
    b. 24-hour ambulatory pH monitoring
    c. Esophageal manometry
    d. Motility testing

16. The nurse has provided teaching to the patient with GERD. Which statement by the patient indicates the teaching has been effective?
    a. "I will eat three meals a day."
    b. "I won't snack for 1 hour before I go to bed."
    c. "I won't nap for 30 minutes after eating dinner."
    d. "I won't lift heavy objects."

17. The patient is on nizatidine (Axid) therapy for the treatment of GERD. Which sign indicates that the patient may be having an adverse effect associated with this drug?
    a. Dysrhythmia
    b. Constipation
    c. Diarrhea
    d. Headache

18. The patient who has been prescribed metoclopramide (Reglan) is being discharged home. Which statement by the patient indicates a need for further discharge teaching by the nurse?
    a. "I will take the drug after meals."
    b. "I am using this drug to increase the rate at which my stomach empties."
    c. "I will call the health care provider if I have any ataxia."
    d. "I will inform the doctor if I start to have any hallucinations."

19. Which statement is true about the drug rabeprazole (Aciphex) for treatment of GERD?
    a. It is rapidly released into the body after it is administered.
    b. The tablets are large and may be crushed if the patient has difficulty swallowing them.
    c. It is a histamine receptor antagonist.
    d. Patients who use this drug should be instructed to wear sunscreen.

20. The patient has returned to the unit after a Stretta procedure for GERD. Which action by the student nurse requires the supervising nurse to intervene?
    a. The patient is offered clear liquids in the early post-procedure period.
    b. The patient's routine 81 mg of aspirin is held.
    c. A proton pump inhibitor is administered.
    d. A nasogastric tube is prepared for insertion.

21. Which lifestyle adjustment may the patient have to make to best control GERD?
    a. Sleep in the Trendelenburg position.
    b. Attain and maintain ideal body weight.
    c. Wear snug-fitting belts and waistbands.
    d. Engage in strenuous exercise such as weightlifting.

True or False? *Read the statements about hiatal hernia and write T for true or F for false in the blanks provided.*

_____ 22. Hiatal hernias are also called *diaphragmatic hernias*.

_____ 23. The primary symptoms of sliding hiatal hernias are associated with reflux.

_____ 24. Symptoms resulting from hiatal hernia typically improve after a meal or when the patient is in a supine position.

_____ 25. The barium swallow study with fluoroscopy is the most specific diagnostic test for identifying hiatal hernia.

26. Which statements will the nurse include when providing health teaching for the patient with hiatal hernia? *(Select all that apply.)*
    a. "Elevate the head of your bed at least 6 inches for sleeping at night."
    b. "Remain in the upright position for several hours after eating."
    c. "Avoid straining or excessive vigorous exercise."
    d. "Avoid wearing clothing that is tight around the abdomen."
    e. "Avoid eating in the late evening."

27. The nurse has provided postoperative teaching for the patient who underwent a laparoscopic Nissen fundoplication (LNF). Which statement by the patient indicates a need for additional teaching?
    a. "I will walk every day."
    b. "I'll discontinue the antireflux drugs."
    c. "I will report a fever above 101° F."
    d. "I'll remove the gauze dressing 2 days after surgery and shower."

28. What is the primary focus of care after conventional surgery for hiatal hernia?
    a. Prevention of respiratory complications
    b. Pain management
    c. Management of fluid balance
    d. Teaching the patient self-care activities

True or False? Read the statements about the patient who has had a fundoplication procedure and write T for true or F for false in the blanks provided.

_____ 29. The nurse elevates the head of the patient's bed 10 degrees to lower the diaphragm and facilitate lung expansion.

_____ 30. Incentive spirometry and deep breathing are routinely used after surgery to maintain patency of the airways.

_____ 31. Nasogastric drainage is initially dark brown with old blood but should become normal yellowish-green within the first 8 hours after surgery.

_____ 32. The nurse explains to the patient that meals consumed will need to be much larger and less frequent than before.

_____ 33. The nurse teaches the patient to avoid drinking carbonated beverages, eating gas-producing foods, chewing gum, and drinking with a straw.

_____ 34. The patient is taught to inspect the healing incision daily. The nurse explains that if swelling, redness, tenderness, discharge, or fever occur, the patient should not worry because these are all common responses to the procedure.

35. After esophageal dilation of the patient, which intervention does the nurse perform?
    a. Monitors the patient for subcutaneous emphysema, hemoptysis, fever, and signs of perforation
    b. Encourages the patient to consume a small meal immediately after the procedure
    c. Massages the patient's shoulder when he or she complains of shoulder pain
    d. Teaches the patient to swallow any oral secretions that accumulate

36. The patient comes to the clinic reporting difficulty swallowing, weight loss, and painful swallowing as well as vomiting and persistent hiccups. Which disorder does the nurse suspect?
    a. Hiatal hernia
    b. Esophageal tumor
    c. GERD
    d. Achalasia

True or False? Read the statements and write T for true or F for false in the blanks provided.

_____ 37. More than half of esophageal cancers metastasize.

_____ 38. The two primary risk factors associated with the development of squamous cell carcinoma of the esophagus are tobacco use and heavy alcohol intake.

_____ 39. Barrett's esophagus ultimately becomes cancerous.

_____ 40. The definitive diagnosis of esophageal cancer is made by esophageal ultrasound with fine needle aspiration to examine the tumor tissue.

41. Nonsurgical treatment options for cancer of the esophagus can include which therapies? *(Select all that apply.)*
    a. Swallowing therapy
    b. Chemoradiation
    c. Targeted therapies
    d. Photodynamic therapy
    e. Endoscopic therapies

CASE STUDY: THE PATIENT WITH AN ESOPHAGEAL PROBLEM

Use a separate sheet of paper to answer the questions in this Case Study. Answer guidelines for this Case Study are available on your Evolve website at http://evolve. elsevier.com/Iggy/ in the "Prepare for Class" folder.

The 53-year-old man comes to the clinic reporting heartburn. He describes the pain as a substernal burning sensation that tends to move up and down the chest in a wavelike fashion.

1. What other questions should the nurse ask the patient at this time? What are the possible causes of this substernal burning?

2. The patient is ordered to have 24-hour ambulatory pH monitoring. What patient teaching concerning this test should the nurse provide?

3. The patient is diagnosed with GERD. What patient and family health promotion modifications to control reflux should the nurse include in the teaching?

4. The patient is ordered the following medications for treatment of GERD: Mylanta 30 mL orally between meals and PRN throughout the day and at bedtime; nizatidine (Axid) 150 mg orally twice a day; metoclopramide (Reglan) 10 mg orally three times a day; and esomeprazole (Nexium) 30 mg orally daily. For each drug, identify what type it is, the purpose, and nursing interventions associated with administering the drug.

Type of Drug	Purpose	Nursing Interventions
Mylanta		
Nizatidine (Axid)		
Metoclopramide (Reglan)		
Esomeprazole (Nexium)		

58 CHAPTER

Care of Patients with Stomach Disorders

STUDY/REVIEW QUESTIONS

True or False? *Read each statement and write T for true and F for false in the blanks provided.*

_____ 1. The pathologic changes of gastritis include vascular congestion, edema, acute inflammatory cell infiltration, and degenerative changes in the superficial epithelium of the stomach lining.

_____ 2. The diagnosis of gastritis is made solely on clinical symptoms.

_____ 3. A complication of chronic gastritis is pernicious anemia.

_____ 4. The onset of infection with *Helicobacter pylori* can result in acute gastritis.

_____ 5. Long-term use of acetaminophen (Tylenol) creates a high risk for acute gastritis.

_____ 6. Atrophic gastritis is a type of chronic gastritis that is seen most often in older adults.

7. The nurse is teaching the patient about health promotion and maintenance to prevent gastritis. Which information does the nurse include? *(Select all that apply.)*
    a. "A balanced diet can help prevent gastritis."
    b. "To prevent gastritis, you should limit your intake of salt."
    c. "If you stop smoking, there is less of a chance that you will develop gastritis."
    d. "Yoga has been found to be effective in preventing gastritis."
    e. "Although regular exercise is good for you, it has not been found to have an effect on the prevention of gastritis."

8. The patient with chronic gastritis is being admitted. Which sign/symptom does the nurse identify as being associated with this patient's condition?
    a. Pernicious anemia
    b. Gastric hemorrhage
    c. Hematemesis
    d. Dyspepsia

9. When teaching the patient about pernicious anemia, which statement does the nurse include?
    a. "Patients with pernicious anemia are not able to digest fats."
    b. "Pernicious anemia results in a deficiency of vitamin B_{12}."
    c. "All patients with gastrointestinal bleeding will eventually develop pernicious anemia."
    d. "Oral iron supplements are an effective treatment for pernicious anemia."

10. The patient comes to the emergency department (ED) reporting rapid onset of epigastric pain with nausea and vomiting. The patient says the pain is worse than any heartburn he has had, and that he has not had an appetite for the past day. What does the nurse suspect this patient has?
    a. Peritonitis
    b. *H. pylori* infection
    c. Duodenal ulcer
    d. Acute gastritis

11. Which diagnostic test is the gold standard for diagnosing gastritis?
    a. Esophagogastroduodenoscopy (EGD)
    c. CT scan
    d. Upper GI series
    e. Cholangiogram

12. The nurse is teaching the patient about ranitidine (Zantac) prescribed for gastritis. Which statement by the patient indicates effective teaching by the nurse?
    a. "The drug will heal the areas of my stomach that are sore."
    b. "This drug will block the secretions of my stomach."
    c. "Zantac will make the inside of my stomach not as acidy as it is now."
    d. "This pill will kill the bacterial infection I have in my stomach."

13. The patient with acute gastritis is receiving treatment to block and buffer gastric acid secretions to relieve pain. Which drug does the nurse identify as an antisecretory agent (proton-pump inhibitor)?
    a. Sucralfate (Carafate)
    b. Ranitidine (Zantac)
    c. Mylanta
    d. Omeprazole (Prilosec)

14. The nursing student caring for the patient with a duodenal ulcer is about to administer a prostaglandin analogue. Which statement about this medication is true?
    a. A significant adverse effect of this drug is uterine contraction.
    b. Prostaglandin analogues are most effective in the treatment of gastric ulcers.
    c. These drugs help prevent stress-induced ulcers.
    d. Prostaglandin analogues work by coating the stomach with a protective prostaglandin barrier.

15. The nurse is teaching the patient being discharged home about taking prescribed medications that include sucralfate (Carafate). Which statements by the patient indicate teaching has been effective? (Select all that apply.)
    a. "The main side effect of sucralfate is diarrhea."
    b. "I will take sucralfate with meals."
    c. "I will take sucralfate along with the antacid medication I take."
    d. "Sucralfate works to heal my ulcer."
    e. "One of the many things sucralfate does is to stop acid secretion in my stomach."

True or False? Read each statement and write T for true and F for false in the blanks provided.

_____ 16. *Peptic ulcer* is the term used to describe both gastric and duodenal ulcers.

_____ 17. Prostaglandins increase the stomach's resistance to ulceration.

_____ 18. Cushing's ulcer is a type of stress ulcer commonly seen in patients with extensive burns.

_____ 19. IV famotidine (Pepcid) or pantoprazole (Protonix) are often prescribed to prevent stress ulcers.

_____ 20. Hematemesis usually indicates bleeding at or below the duodenojejunal junction.

_____ 21. COX-2 inhibitors such as celecoxib (Celebrex) are less likely to cause mucosal damage to the stomach as compared to nonsteroidal anti-inflammatory drugs (NSAIDs).

Matching. Match the drugs used to treat peptic ulcer disease with their corresponding nursing interventions.

Drugs
a. Magnesium hydroxide (Maalox)
b. Aluminum hydroxide (Amphogel)
c. Esomeprazole (Nexium)
d. Misoprostol (Cytotec)

Interventions

_____ 22. Assess the patient for hepatic problems because he or she will need to take a lower dose of this drug.

_____ 23. Observe the patient for the side effect of diarrhea.

_____ 24. Useful for patients to protect against NSAID-induced ulcers.

_____ 25. Observe the patient for the side effect of constipation.

26. Which statement about the use of antacids in the treatment of gastric ulcers is true?
    a. Antacids should be administered with meals.
    b. The patient should take calcium carbonate (Tums) if they still have pain after taking their usual antacid.
    c. The patient should take antacid on an empty stomach.
    d. Avoid using antacids with phenytoin (Dilantin).

27. The patient with peptic ulcer disease is receiving Maalox. Which actions does the nurse take in regards to administering this medication? *(Select all that apply.)*
    a. Give the medication 2 hours after the patient's meal.
    b. Do not give other drugs within 1 to 2 hours of antacids.
    c. Assess the patient for a history of renal disease before giving Maalox.
    d. Assess the patient for a history of heart failure before giving Maalox.
    e. Observe the patient for the side effect of diarrhea.

28. The nurse has provided instruction for the patient prescribed sucralfate (Carafate) to treat a gastric ulcer. Which statement by the patient indicates that teaching has been effective?
    a. "This drug will stop the secretion of acid in my stomach."
    b. "I will take this drug on an empty stomach."
    c. "I will not be able to take ranitidine (Zantac) with this drug."
    d. "The main side effect of this drug that I can expect is diarrhea."

29. The patient is admitted with an upper GI bleed. Which finding does the nurse expect to assess in the patient?
    a. Decreased pulse
    b. Increased hemoglobin and hematocrit
    c. Syncope
    d. Increased blood pressure

30. The patient develops an active upper GI bleed. Which actions does the nurse take in caring for this patient? *(Select all that apply.)*
    a. Provide oxygen.
    b. Start 1 or 2 large-bore IV lines.
    c. Prepare to infuse 0.9% normal saline solution or lactated Ringer's solution.
    d. Monitor serum electrolytes.
    e. Prepare for nasogastric (NG) tube insertion.

31. When performing an assessment on the patient with an active upper GI bleed, which conditions does the nurse identify as common causes of upper GI bleeding? *(Select all that apply.)*
    a. Esophageal cancer
    b. Esophageal varices
    c. Duodenal ulcer
    d. Gastritis
    e. Gastric cancer

32. The licensed practical nurse (LPN) is caring for the patient with an NG tube. The supervising nursing intervenes when the LPN attempts to perform which action?
    a. Lubricate the tube with a petroleum-based product.
    b. Measure the length of the tube to be passed from the bridge of the nose to the earlobe to the xiphoid process.
    c. Ask the patient to swallow while the tube is being passed.
    d. Obtain a sample of gastric contents by aspirating with a 50 mL catheter-tipped syringe.

33. The student nurse is performing a gastric lavage on the patient with an active upper GI bleed. Which action by the student requires intervention by the supervising nurse?
    a. Using an ice-cold solution to lavage the stomach.
    b. Instilling the lavage solution in volumes of 200 to 300 mL.
    c. Continuing the lavage until the solution returned is clear or light pink without clots.
    d. Positioning the patient on his left side during the procedure.

34. Which drug is the drug of choice for aggressive acid suppression to prevent rebleeding in the patient with a gastric bleed?
    a. Ranitidine (Zantac)
    b. Omeprazole (Prilosec)
    c. Ocetreotide (Sandostatin)
    d. Pantoprazole (Protonix)

True or False? *Read each statement and write T for true and F for false in the blanks provided.*

_____ 35. Gastrinomas are a common finding in patients with Zollinger-Ellison syndrome (ZES).

_____ 36. Steatorrhea is an excessive amount of fat in the feces.

_____ 37. Almost half of the patients with Zollinger-Ellison syndrome have constipation.

_____ 38. Patients with Zollinger-Ellison syndrome usually also have infection with *H. pylori*.

_____ 39. Infection with *H. pylori* is the largest risk factor for gastric cancer.

_____ 40. Asians and Asian Americans are at an especially high risk for the development of gastric cancer.

41. The nurse is caring for several patients with gastric and duodenal ulcers. Which differential features of gastric ulcers compared to duodenal ulcers does the nurse identify? *(Select all that apply.)*
    a. Normal secretion or hyposecretion
    b. Relieved by ingestion of food
    c. Hematemesis more common
    d. No gastritis present
    e. Most often, the patient has type O blood

42. The nurse is performing a physical assessment on the patient admitted to the unit with gastric cancer. Which findings indicate signs of distant metastasis? *(Select all that apply.)*
    a. Cullen's sign
    b. Virchow's nodes
    c. Blumer's shelf
    d. "Sister Mary Joseph nodes"
    e. Krunkenberg's tumor

43. The nurse is assessing the patient who has had a total gastrectomy and notes bright red blood in the NG and abdominal distention. What does the nurse do next?
    a. Irrigate the NG tube.
    b. Reposition the NG tube.
    c. Inform the surgeon of these findings.
    d. Remove the NG tube.

True or False? *Read each statement and write T for true and F for false in the blanks provided.*

_____ 44. *Dumping syndrome* is a term that refers to a group of vasomotor symptoms that occur after eating.

_____ 45. Late dumping syndrome is caused by a release of an excessive amount of insulin.

_____ 46. To manage dumping syndrome, the patient needs to eliminate liquid ingested with meals.

_____ 47. Patients with dumping syndrome are instructed to eat a diet that is high in carbohydrates and low in fat and low in protein.

_____ 48. After gastric resection, patients should be assessed for the development of atrophic glossitis which occurs secondary to vitamin B_{12} deficiency.

49. The nurse is teaching the patient with dumping syndrome about diet. Which statement by the patient indicates that teaching has been effective?
    a. "I will use sugar-free gelatin with caution."
    b. "I will avoid rice in my diet."
    c. "Meat in my diet will consist of a total of 4 ounces a day."
    d. "I will limit fluids with my meals to 8 ounces."

50. Which statement about general principles of diet therapy for patients with dumping syndrome is true?
    a. Patients with dumping syndrome should have liquids between meals only.
    b. Patients with dumping syndrome should be encouraged to eat a diet high in roughage.
    c. Patients with dumping syndrome should eat a high-carbohydrate diet.
    d. The diet for a patient with dumping syndrome must be low in fat and protein.

CASE STUDY: THE PATIENT WITH A GASTRIC ULCER

Use a separate sheet of paper to answer the questions in this Case Study. Answer guidelines for this Case Study are available on your Evolve website at http://evolve. elsevier.com/Iggy/ in the "Prepare for Class" folder.

A patient with a history of arthritis has been admitted with a possible diagnosis of peptic ulcer disease. The patient states that she takes ibuprofen to treat the arthritis pain instead of the medication that was prescribed for her. The patient says, "I told my doctor I wasn't going to take expensive drugs that will do more harm to me than good. The ibuprofen works just fine." After a diagnosis of peptic ulcer disease is confirmed, the health care provider prescribes misoprostol (Cytotec). On the day of discharge, the nurse enters the patient's room and finds her in bed spitting bright red blood. After the bleeding is controlled, the patient is discharged home.

1. The patient asks, "Why do people keep talking about an infection that I might have in my stomach?" How should the nurse respond?
2. What, if any, effect has the ibuprofen played in the development of the peptic ulcer?
3. Why has misoprostol (Cytotec) been prescribed for this patient?
4. What complication is likely happening to the patient and what actions should the nurse take?
5. What considerations should the nurse take into account when providing community-based care for this patient?

59 CHAPTER

Care of Patients with Noninflammatory Intestinal Disorders

STUDY/REVIEW QUESTIONS

True or False? *Read each statement and write T for true and F for false in the blanks provided.*

_____ 1. Irritable bowel syndrome (IBS) is a functional GI disorder characterized by chronic or recurrent diarrhea, constipation, and/or abdominal pain and bloating.

_____ 2. No actual pathophysiologic changes occur in IBS.

_____ 3. Symptoms of IBS typically begin in late adulthood.

_____ 4. IBS is the most common digestive disorder seen in clinical practice.

_____ 5. The characteristic symptoms of IBS are known as the *Manning criteria*.

_____ 6. The most common symptom of IBS is pain in the right lower quadrant of the abdomen.

_____ 7. Management of IBS includes a low-fiber diet.

_____ 8. A newer group of drugs used to manage IBS are the muscarinic (M3)-receptor antagonists which act by inhibiting intestinal motility.

9. Which drug is the drug of choice for the treatment of IBS when pain is the predominant symptom?
   a. Amitriptyline (Elavil)
   b. Muscarinic (M_3)-receptor antagonists
   c. Loperamide (Imodium)
   d. Psyllium hydrophilic mucilloid (Metamucil)

10. The nurse is teaching the patient with IBS about complementary and alternative therapies for the disease. Which patient statements indicate that teaching has been effective? *(Select all that apply.)*
   a. "Hypnotherapy may help decrease symptoms."
   b. "I should exercise regularly to help manage the disease."
   c. "Peppermint oil has been used to expel gas and relax spastic intestinal muscles."
   d. "Aloe can be used to ease constipation."
   e. "Ginger can be used for abdominal discomfort and to expel gas."

Matching. Match each type of hernia with its appropriate description.

Hernia Types
a. Femoral
b. Incarcerated
c. Indirect inguinal
d. Reducible
e. Strangulated
f. Umbilical
g. Ventral

Descriptions

_____ 11. Contents of the sac can be replaced into the abdominal cavity by gentle pressure.

_____ 12. A plug of fat in the femoral canal enlarges and eventually pulls the peritoneum and often the urinary bladder into the sac.

_____ 13. Acquired as a result of increased intra-abdominal pressure.

_____ 14. Sac formed from the peritoneum that contains a portion of the intestine omentum. Hernia pushes downward at an angle into the inguinal canal.

_____ 15. Cannot be replaced back into the abdominal cavity.

_____ 16. Blood supply to the herniated bowel segment is cut off.

_____ 17. Occurs at the site of a previous surgical incision.

18. The nurse is performing an abdominal assessment on the patient suspected of having an abdominal hernia. The nurse auscultates the abdomen and determines the absence of bowel sounds. What does the nurse suspect in this patient?
    a. Peritonitis
    b. IBS
    c. Obstruction and strangulation
    d. Low intra-abdominal pressure

19. What does nursing care for the patient who uses a truss for a hernia include?
    a. Using a surgical binder to hold the truss in place
    b. Removing the truss only for bathing
    c. Applying the truss before the hernia has been reduced
    d. Applying powder to the skin under the truss daily

20. Which activity does the nurse tell the patient to avoid after surgery for a hernia repair?
    a. Ambulating
    b. Turning
    c. Coughing
    d. Deep breathing

21. What do postoperative measures for the male patient who has had an inguinal herniorrhaphy include?
    a. Applying a warm pack to the scrotum
    b. Elevating the scrotum on a pillow
    c. Encouraging use of a bedpan to void
    d. Decreasing fluid intake to decrease bladder emptying

True or False? Read the statements about colorectal cancer (CRC) and write T for true and F for false in the blanks provided.

_____ 22. CRC is one of the most prevalent malignancies in the United States.

_____ 23. To reduce the risk of CRC, diets should be low in fat, low in refined carbohydrates, and high in fiber.

_____ 24. The most common signs of CRC are rectal bleeding, anemia, and a change in stool.

_____ 25. Hematochezia is the passage of red blood via the rectum.

_____ 26. Hemoglobin and hematocrit values are usually increased as a result of the intermittent bleeding associated with the tumor.

_____ 27. A negative test result for occult blood in the stool confirms bleeding in the GI tract.

_____ 28. Colonoscopy with biopsy is the definitive test for the diagnosis of CRC.

_____ 29. Carcinoembryonic antigen (CEA), an oncofetal antigen, is elevated in many people with CRC.

30. After colostomy surgery, which intervention does the nurse employ?
    a. Cover the stoma with a dry, sterile dressing.
    b. Apply a pouch system as soon as possible.
    c. Make a hole in the pouch for gas to escape.
    d. Watch for the colostomy to start functioning on day 1.

31. Which discharge instruction does the nurse include for the patient after abdominoperitoneal (AP) resection?
    a. "Use a soft pillow to sit on whenever you sit down."
    b. "Lie on your back when you are resting in bed."
    c. "Use a rubber doughnut device for sitting on when in the car."
    d. "Sit in a chair for at least 4 consecutive hours a day."

32. The nurse immediately reports to the surgeon all but which sign/symptom related to a colostomy?
    a. Liquid stool immediately postoperatively
    b. Unusual bleeding
    c. Signs of ischemia and necrosis
    d. Mucocutaneous separation

33. Which statement about the care of the patient with a colostomy is correct?
    a. A healthy stoma should be dry.
    b. The stoma should protrude about 2 inches from the abdominal wall.
    c. When palpating the stoma, it should feel firm.
    d. A slight amount of edema is normal in the initial postoperative period.

34. The nurse is teaching the patient about what to expect after a descending colon colostomy. The nurse tells the patient to expect the stool to have what kind of form?
    a. Similar to that of stool expelled from the rectum
    b. Thick and paste-like
    c. Thin and gelatin-like
    d. Watery

35. Which sign/symptom is the patient who had an AP resection instructed to report to the health care provider immediately?
    a. Serosanguineous drainage from the wound
    b. Sensations of having a bowel movement
    c. Constant perineal odor and pain
    d. Occasional perineal pain and itching

36. The nurse is teaching the patient about colostomy care. Which information does the nurse include in the teaching plan?
    a. The stoma will enlarge within 6 to 8 weeks of surgery.
    b. Use a moisturizing soap to cleanse the area around the stoma.
    c. Place the colostomy bag on the skin when the skin sealant is still damp.
    d. An antifungal cream or powder can be used if a fungal rash develops.

37. The patient with a colostomy may safely include which food item in the diet?
    a. Burritos
    b. Chicken noodle soup
    c. Cabbage
    d. Carbonated beverages

38. The nurse is teaching the patient about how to control gas and odor from a colostomy. Which information does the nurse include?
    a. Do not chew gum.
    b. Place an aspirin in the colostomy.
    c. Do not consume buttermilk.
    d. Do not eat parsley.

True or False? Read each statement and write T for true and F for false in the blanks provided.

_____ 39. Crohn's disease can cause a mechanical obstruction.

_____ 40. Nonmechanical obstruction is also known as *paralytic ileus* or *adynamic ileus.*

_____ 41. Hypovolemia is a common complication of intestinal obstruction.

_____ 42. An obstruction high in the small intestine often results in metabolic acidosis.

_____ 43. Intussusception is twisting of the intestine.

_____ 44. Volvulus is telescoping of a segment of the intestine within itself.

_____ 45. Hypokalemia is the most common electrolyte disturbance that predisposes the patient to intestinal obstruction.

_____ 46. Obstipation is the term which refers to no passage of stool.

47. Which key feature does the nurse most likely find when performing a physical assessment on the patient with a small-bowel obstruction?
    a. Visible peristaltic waves in the upper and middle abdomen
    b. Minimal or no vomiting
    c. No major fluid and electrolyte imbalances
    d. Metabolic acidosis

48. What does care of the patient with a nasogastric (NG) tube require? *(Select all that apply.)*
    a. Assessment of proper placement at least every 4 hours
    b. Cleansing of the nose with the same type of skin protectant used for ostomy skin care before applying the NG tube securing device
    c. Confirmation of NG tube placement by x-ray if it is repositioned
    d. Aspiration of contents of the NG tube and irrigation of the tube with 30 mL of normal saline every 4 hours
    e. Questioning the patient about the passage of flatus

49. What does nursing care of the patient with intestinal obstruction who reports discomfort in the early diagnostic period consist of?
    a. Administration of opioid analgesics
    b. Placing the patient in a semi-Fowler's position
    c. Providing the patient with fluids
    d. Offering the patient semi-soft foods

50. Which NG tube is connected to low intermittent suction?
    a. Salem sump
    b. Levin
    c. Anderson
    d. Carney

51. Which interventions apply to patients with Fluid Volume Deficit related to an intestinal obstruction?
    a. Provide frequent mouth care with lemon glycerin swabs.
    b. Offer ice chips to suck on before surgery.
    c. Offer a small glass of water.
    d. Assess for edema from third spacing.

52. Which observation of the patient with an intestinal obstruction does the nurse report immediately?
    a. Urinary output of 1000 mL in an 8-hour period
    b. The patient's request for something to drink
    c. Abdominal pain changing from colicky to constant discomfort
    d. The patient who is changing positions frequently

53. Which discharge information does the nurse include for the patient who has had an intestinal obstruction caused by fecal impaction?
    a. Encourage the patient to report abdominal distention, nausea or vomiting, and constipation.
    b. Provide the patient a written description of a low-fiber diet.
    c. Remind the patient to limit activity.
    d. Remind the patient to decrease fluid intake.

True or False? *Read each statement and write T for true and F for false in the blanks provided.*

_____ 54. The spleen is the most commonly injured organ in blunt abdominal trauma.

_____ 55. The liver is the most commonly injured organ in blunt and penetrating trauma.

_____ 56. Once the ABCs of the patient with abdominal trauma have been stabilized, the nurse focuses on risks of hemorrhage, shock, and peritonitis.

_____ 57. Ecchymoses in the distribution of a lap seat belt should be reported to the health care provider immediately because the bowel may be injured.

_____ 58. Ecchymoses on either flank is known as *Cullen's sign.*

_____ 59. Turner's sign may indicate retroperitoneal bleeding into the abdominal wall.

60. The patient with abdominal trauma has a positive Ballance's sign. What does the nurse suspects in the patient?
    a. Ruptured spleen
    b. Lacerated liver
    c. Infarcted bowel
    d. Pelvic fracture

61. Emergency care of the patient with abdominal trauma includes which interventions? *(Select all that apply.)*
    a. Insertion of at least two large-bore IV catheters in the lower extremities
    b. Type and cross-matching of four to eight units of blood
    c. Measurement of arterial blood gases
    d. Continuous hemodynamic monitoring
    e. Insertion of a Foley catheter

62. Which statement about intra-abdominal pressure (IAP) monitoring is correct?
    a. The normal IAP for adults is 15 to 20 mm Hg.
    b. Patients with high IAP have bradycardia.
    c. High IAP leads to increased afterload and decreased preload.
    d. Patients with high IAP are hypertensive.

True or False? *Read each statement and write T for true and F for false in the blanks provided.*

_____ 63. Most polyps are benign.

_____ 64. Pedunculated polyps are stalk-like; a thin stem attaches them to the intestinal wall.

_____ 65. Polyps can cause gross rectal bleeding, intestinal obstruction, or intussusception.

_____ 66. Hemorrhoids are unnaturally swollen or distended veins in the anorectal region.

_____ 67. Hemorrhoids are precancerous growths.

_____ 68. Decreased fluid intake can cause hemorrhoids.

_____ 69. Prevention of constipation is the most important preventive measure for hemorrhoids.

70. Which intervention is contraindicated in the nonsurgical management of hemorrhoids?
    a. Diets low in fiber and fluids
    b. Dibucaine (Nupercainal) ointment
    c. Warm sitz baths three or four times a day
    d. Cleansing the anal area with moistened cleaning tissues

71. Which statement by the patient indicates an understanding of surgical management of hemorrhoids?
    a. "It will take 10 to 14 days for the rubber band used on the hemorrhoid to fall off."
    b. "Urinary retention is a complication of surgical resection of the hemorrhoid."
    c. "After surgery, I will need to eat a low-fiber, low-fluid diet."
    d. "Stool softeners and laxatives are avoided after hemorrhoid surgery."

True or False? *Read each statement and write T for true and F for false in the blanks provided.*

_____ 72. Deficiencies of bile salts can lead to malabsorption of fats and fat-soluble vitamins.

_____ 73. Pancreatic enzymes are necessary for absorption of vitamin B_{12}.

_____ 74. Gastric surgery is one of the most common causes of malabsorption and maldigestion.

_____ 75. Constipation is a classic symptom of malabsorption.

_____ 76. The Schilling test measures urinary excretion of vitamin B_{12} for diagnosis of pernicious anemia and a variety of other malabsorption syndromes.

77. Which drug is used to treat tropical sprue?
    a. Bentyl
    b. Lomotil
    c. Steroids
    d. Bactrim

CASE STUDY: THE PATIENT WITH A BOWEL OBSTRUCTION

Use a separate sheet of paper to answer the questions in this Case Study. Answer guidelines for this Case Study are available on your Evolve website at http://evolve.elsevier.com/Iggy/ in the "Prepare for Class" folder.

A 47-year-old man comes to the emergency department reporting acute upper to mid-abdominal, sporadic pain and cramping. Upon assessment, the nurse observes abdominal distention and high-pitched bowel sounds. The physician has ordered flat plate and upright abdominal x-rays that show distention of loops of intestine, with fluid and gas in the small intestine in conjunction with absence of gas in the colon. The physician has diagnosed a bowel obstruction.

1. Based on the findings, identify which type of bowel obstruction this patient most likely has.
2. What other signs and symptoms would the nurse observe for in this patient?
3. Identify the most likely interventions for this patient based on his type of bowel obstruction.
4. It is found that the patient has a small fecal impaction. What should the patient be taught to avoid this complication from occurring in the future?

60
CHAPTER

Care of Patients with Inflammatory Intestinal Disorders

STUDY/REVIEW QUESTIONS

True or False? *Read the statements and write T for true or F for false in the blanks provided.*

_____ 1. Appendicitis is the most common cause of right lower quadrant pain.

_____ 2. The initial obstruction of the appendix is usually a result of fecaliths.

_____ 3. The diagnosis of appendicitis is difficult to establish in the older adult because symptoms of pain and tenderness may not be as pronounced in this age group, resulting in increased risk for perforation, peritonitis, and mortality.

_____ 4. Classically, appendicitis presents with cramp-like pain in the right lower quadrant.

_____ 5. McBurney's point is the area in the left lower quadrant between the anterior iliac crest and the umbilicus.

_____ 6. Laboratory findings do not establish the diagnosis of appendicitis.

7. The nurse is caring for the patient with acute appendicitis. Which interventions will the nurse perform? *(Select all that apply.)*
   a. Maintain the patient on NPO status.
   b. Administer IV fluids as prescribed.
   c. Apply warm compresses to the right lower abdominal quadrant.
   d. Maintain the patient in the supine position.
   e. Administer laxatives.

8. The patient has been diagnosed with acute appendicitis. Based on this diagnosis, which intervention does the nurse perform?
   a. Start a bowel cleansing program.
   b. Prepare the patient for surgery.
   c. Apply a heating pad to the lower abdomen.
   d. Assess the patient's knowledge about dietary modifications.

9. The nurse on the surgical unit is expecting to admit the patient who has had an appendectomy with abscess. What does the nurse anticipate care for this patient will include? *(Select all that apply.)*
   a. Clear liquids
   b. Wound drains
   c. IV antibiotics
   d. Nonsteroidal anti-inflammatory drugs (NSAIDs) for pain control
   e. Bedrest for 24 hours

True or False? *Read the statements and write T for true or F for false in the blanks provided.*

_____ 10. Peritonitis is caused by contamination of the peritoneal cavity by bacteria or chemicals.

_____ 11. Continuous ambulatory peritoneal dialysis (CAPD) can cause peritonitis.

_____ 12. White blood cell counts are often decreased with peritonitis.

_____ 13. Abdominal wall rigidity is a classic finding in patients with peritonitis.

14. The fluid shift that occurs in peritonitis may result in which of the following?
    a. Intracellular fluid moving into the peritoneal cavity
    b. Significant increase in circulatory volume
    c. Eventual renal failure and electrolyte imbalance
    d. Increased bowel motility caused by increased fluid volume

15. The respiratory problems that may accompany peritonitis are a result of which factor?
    a. Associated pain interfering with ventilation
    b. Decreased pressure against the diaphragm
    c. Fluid shifts to the thoracic cavity
    d. Decreased oxygen demands related to the infectious process

16. Which nursing intervention is part of nonsurgical management for the patient with peritonitis?
    a. Monitor weekly weight and intake and output.
    b. Insert a nasogastric tube to decompress the stomach.
    c. Order a breakfast tray when the patient is hungry.
    d. Administer NSAIDs for pain.

17. What are the cardinal signs of peritonitis?
    a. Fever and headache
    b. Dizziness and vomiting
    c. Abdominal pain and tenderness
    d. Nausea and loss of appetite

18. The nurse is instructing the patient about home care after an exploratory laparotomy for peritonitis. Which statement by the patient indicates that teaching has been effective?
    a. "It is normal for the incision site to be warm."
    b. "I will stop taking the antibiotics if diarrhea develops."
    c. "I will call the health care provider for a temperature greater than 101° F."
    d. "I will resume activity with my bowling league this week for exercise."

True or False? *Read the statements and write T for true or F for false in the blanks provided.*

_____ 19. Gastroenteritis is an increase in the frequency and water content of stools or vomiting as a result of inflammation of the mucous membranes of the stomach and intestinal tract.

_____ 20. *E. coli* can release enterotoxin which results in diarrhea.

_____ 21. *Shigella* and *Campylobacter* will attach themselves to the mucosal epithelium and penetrate it, resulting in destruction of the intestinal villi and malabsorption.

_____ 22. The Norwalk virus infection can occur year-round and affects adults and children.

23. The nurse is assessing the patient with viral gastroenteritis. Which symptom is the nurse most concerned about?
    a. Orthostatic blood pressure changes
    b. Poor skin turgor
    c. Dry mucous membranes
    d. Rebound tenderness

24. What is the priority nursing concern for the patient with gastroenteritis?
    a. Nutrition therapy
    b. Fluid replacement
    c. Skin care
    d. Drug therapy

25. As part of the routine treatment plan for the patient with bacterial gastroenteritis, which drugs does the nurse anticipate the patient will be prescribed? *(Select all that apply.)*
    a. Anticholinergics
    b. Antiemetics
    c. Antiperistaltic drugs
    d. Antibiotics
    e. Bismuth subsalicylate (Pepto-Bismol)

26. The nurse is caring for the patient with gastroenteritis who has frequent stools. Which task is best to delegate to the nursing assistant?
    a. Teach the patient to avoid toilet paper and harsh soaps.
    b. Assist the patient with a sitz bath.
    c. Use a warm washcloth to remove stool from the skin.
    d. Dry the skin with absorbent cotton.

27. Identify whether each characteristic pertains to Crohn's disease (CD) or ulcerative colitis (UC).

    _____ a. Begins in the rectum and proceeds in a continuous manner toward the cecum

    _____ b. Fistulas commonly develop

    _____ c. Infrequent need for surgery

    _____ d. Five to six soft, loose stools per day that are non-bloody

    _____ e. Increased risk of colon cancer

    _____ f. Some patients experience extraintestinal manifestations such as migratory polyarthritis, ankylosing spondylitis, and erythema nodosum

    _____ g. Cobblestone appearance to the internal intestine

28. The patient is suspected to have UC. Which definitive diagnostic test does the nurse expect the patient to undergo in order to confirm the diagnosis?
    a. Colonoscopy
    b. C-reactive protein
    c. Albumin levels
    d. Erythrocyte sedimentation rate

29. What is the priority nursing diagnosis for the patient with UC?
    a. Imbalanced Nutrition: Less than Body Requirements related to inability to absorb food due to biologic factors
    b. Diarrhea related to inflammation of the bowel mucosa
    c. Activity Intolerance related to generalized weakness
    d. Disturbed Body Image related to biophysical factors and possible surgery

30. The patient is prescribed sulfasalazine (Azulfidine) for the treatment of UC. Which patient statement indicates the patient is experiencing a side effect of this drug?
    a. "My skin is turning a yellow color."
    b. "My knees hurt."
    c. "My stomach hurts when I take this pill."
    d. "I wake up at night sweating sometimes."

31. Which statement is true about the medical treatment of UC?
    a. Infliximab (Remicade) is approved as a first-line therapy.
    b. Immunomodulators are not thought to be effective; however, in combination with steroids, they may offer a synergistic effect.
    c. When a therapeutic level of glucocorticoids is reached, the dosage of the drug stays the same to maintain the therapeutic effect.
    d. The method of action for the aminosalicylates is interruption of the pain pathway.

32. The patient with UC who has had a Kock's ileostomy is being discharged home. The nurse has provided discharge teaching. Which statements by the patient indicate the teaching has been effective? *(Select all that apply.)*
    a. "I will avoid caffeinated beverages."
    b. "I will call the health care provider if I have a fever over 101° F."
    c. "I will change the adhesive for the appliance daily."
    d. "I know the pouch needs emptying when I feel pain in that area."
    e. "I will call the health care provider if I feel like my heart is beating fast."

Matching. *Match each type of surgical procedure with its description.*

Procedures

a. Total colectomy with ileoanal anastamosis
b. Ileoanal reservoir
c. Ileostomy
d. Total proctocolectomy with a permanent ileostomy
e. Colectomy
f. Kock's ileostomy

Descriptions

_____ 33. Procedure in which a loop of the ileum is placed through the abdominal wall

_____ 34. Surgical removal of the colon

_____ 35. Removal of the colon, rectum, and anus with surgical closure of the anus

_____ 36. Intra-abdominal pouch or reservoir from the terminal ileum is constructed by the surgeon where stool is stored via a nipple-like valve in the pouch until the patient drains it by using a catheter

_____ 37. Surgical removal of the colon and rectum with suturing of the ileum into the anal canal or small cuff of rectum

_____ 38. "J pouch"

39. Which statement is true about drug therapy for CD?
    a. Budesonide (Entocort EC) is a rapid-release compound that delivers low local glucocorticoid concentrations to the terminal ileum for patients with CD.
    b. Methotrexate (Rheumatrex) is contraindicated in the treatment of CD.
    c. Metronidazole (Flagyl) has been helpful in patients with fistulas and CD.
    d. Adalimumab (Humira) is a glucocorticoid approved for the treatment of CD.

40. The patient with CD has a fistula. Which assessment by the nurse should be reported immediately to the health care provider?
    a. Weight loss of 2 pounds in one day
    b. Abdominal pain
    c. Diarrhea
    d. Decreased urinary output

41. What is the priority nursing care for the patient with CD?
    a. Adequate nutrition and fluid and electrolyte balance
    b. Pain relief
    c. Health care management
    d. Management of altered bowel elimination

True or False? *Write T for true or F for false in the blanks provided.*

_____ 42. Diverticulitis is the inflammation of one or more diverticula.

_____ 43. Diverticulitis is the presence of many abnormal pouch-like herniations in the wall of the intestine.

_____ 44. Diets high in cereal fiber that cause more bulky stool have been implicated in the formation of diverticula.

_____ 45. The patient with diverticulosis usually has no symptoms.

_____ 46. Diverticulitis is found in one-half of adults over age 60 years.

_____ 47. The patient with diverticulitis usually goes through a barium enema procedure in the acute phase of the illness to confirm the diagnosis.

48. Which drug is often used in older patients for pain management of moderate to severe diverticulitis?
    a. Meperidine hydrochloride (Demerol)
    b. Acetaminophen (Tylenol)
    c. ASA (aspirin)
    d. MsO_4 (morphine)

49. Which statement about diverticular disease is true?
    a. Most diverticula occur in the sigmoid colon.
    b. Diverticula are uncomfortable even when not inflamed.
    c. High-fiber diets contribute to diverticula occurrence.
    d. Diverticula form where intestinal wall muscles are weak.

50. Which is a preventive measure for diverticular disease?
    a. Excluding whole-grain breads from the diet
    b. Avoiding fresh apples, broccoli, and lettuce
    c. Taking bulk agents such as psyllium hydrophilic mucilloid
    d. Taking routine anticholinergics to reduce bowel spasms

51. Which type of stoma will the patient with diverticulitis most likely have postoperatively?
    a. Ileostomy
    b. Kock's pouch
    c. Colostomy
    d. Cecostomy

Matching. Match each anorectal problem with its corresponding description.

Anorectal Problem
a. Anal fissure
b. Anal fistula
c. Anorectal abscess

Description
_____ 52. Duct obstruction and infection

_____ 53. Perianal laceration, superficial erosion

_____ 54. Communicating tract

55. The nurse is providing teaching for the patient with an anal fissure as a complication of CD. Which statement by the patient indicates the need for further teaching?
    a. "I will use warm sitz baths."
    b. "A diet that is low in bulk-producing agents is best for me."
    c. "I will use opiate suppositories if spasms are severe."
    d. "Topical anti-inflammatory agents will help if I am uncomfortable."

Matching. Match the parasitic infection with its appropriate description.

Parasitic Infections

a. *Entamoeba histolytica*
b. *Cryptosporidium*
c. *Giardia lamblia*

Descriptions

_____ 56. A protozoal parasite that causes superficial invasion, destruction, and inflammation of the mucosa in the small intestine. It is a well recognized problem in travelers, campers and immunosuppressed patients.

_____ 57. This condition is also known as *amebiasis.*

_____ 58. This infection is manifested by diarrhea and occurs most commonly in immunosuppressed patients, particularly those with human immunodeficiency virus (HIV).

59. Which statements does the nurse include while providing discharge instructions for the patient with giardiasis? *(Select all that apply.)*
   a. "Avoid contact with stool from dogs and beavers."
   b. "All household and sexual partners should have stool examinations for parasites."
   c. "Treatment will most likely consist of metronidazole."
   d. "The infection can be transmitted to others until the amebicides kill the parasites."
   e. "Stools are examined 6 days after treatment to assess for eradication."

Matching. Match the helminthic infestations with their appropriate descriptions.

Helminthic Infestations

a. Enterobiasis (pinworm infection)
b. Trichinosis
c. Hookworms
d. Tapeworm

Descriptions

_____ 60. Patients with symptoms of this disease receive iron therapy and a diet high in protein and vitamins for at least 3 months after anemia is corrected.

_____ 61. The most common helminthic infection in the U.S. Manifestations of infection include intense perianal pruritus (especially at night), vaginitis, insomnia, and restlessness.

_____ 62. This organism is usually transmitted to people who ingest undercooked pork or pork products.

_____ 63. Generally patients with this infection either have no symptoms or occasional GI upset, such as nausea, diarrhea, or abdominal pain.

True or False? Read the statements and write T for true or F for false in the blanks provided.

_____ 64. Food poisoning is communicable from person to person.

_____ 65. The incubation period for food poisoning is shorter than gastroenteritis.

_____ 66. Food poisoning can be differentiated from gastroenteritis by obtaining a thorough history of common food intake in patients who have common symptoms of acute diarrhea, nausea, and vomiting.

_____ 67. Patients may be carriers of the salmonellosis bacterium for up to 1 year.

_____ 68. Botulism is a paralytic disease resulting from an ingestion of toxin in a food contaminated with *Clostridium botulinum*. Botulism occurs most often with home-canned foods.

_____ 69. Staphylococcal infections occur most commonly with the slow cooling of food after it is cooked.

CASE STUDY: THE PATIENT WITH DIVERTICULITIS

Use a separate sheet of paper to answer the questions in this Case Study. Answer guidelines for this Case Study are available on your Evolve website at http://evolve. elsevier.com/Iggy/ in the "Prepare for Class" folder.

An 18-year-old body-builder has just come into the office reporting left lower quadrant abdominal pain, temperature of 100.8° F, constipation, and blood-streaked stool. On examination of the abdomen, the nurse observes slight distention and tenderness on palpation, especially in the left lower quadrant. This patient has an elevated white blood cell count and his stool for occult blood is positive. Diverticulitis is diagnosed.

1. Identify key findings noted in the examination and indicate the significance.

2. The patient says, "Oh, I'll just go home and take a laxative or an enema and I'll be fine." Explain why these should be avoided.

3. Nonsurgical management has been selected for this patient, and he may return home after receiving special instructions. Identify a key factor, based on your assessment, on which the nurse would need to instruct him.

4. What community-based care will the nurse incorporate for the care of this patient?

61 CHAPTER

Care of Patients with Liver Problems

STUDY/REVIEW QUESTIONS

True or False? Read each statement and write T for true or F for false in the blanks provided.

_____ 1. Cirrhosis is extensive, irreversible scarring of the liver, usually caused by a chronic reaction to hepatic inflammation and necrosis.

_____ 2. The most common causes for cirrhosis in the United States are alcoholic liver disease and hepatitis C.

_____ 3. Laennec's cirrhosis is caused by viral hepatitis and exposure to drugs or chemicals.

_____ 4. Ascites is the accumulation of free fluid within the peritoneal cavity caused by increased hydrostatic pressure from portal hypertension.

_____ 5. Massive ascites may cause renal vasoconstriction, triggering the renin-angiotensin system resulting in sodium and water loss.

_____ 6. Esophageal varices occur when fragile, thin-walled esophageal veins become distended from increased pressure.

_____ 7. *Melena* is the term that refers to black, tarry stools.

_____ 8. Patients with cirrhosis are susceptible to bleeding and easy bruising because they are lacking in factors II, VII, IX, and X.

_____ 9. Hepatorenal syndrome is often the cause of death in patients with cirrhosis.

_____ 10. Cirrhosis has a rapid onset with severe and specific early manifestations.

11. When admitting the patient with cirrhosis, the nurse assesses for which conditions as possible complications of the disease? *(Select all that apply.)*
    a. Ascites
    b. Bleeding esophageal varices
    c. Hepatorenal syndrome
    d. Coagulation defects
    e. Portal hypertensive gastropathy

12. Patients with cirrhosis are susceptible to bleeding and easy bruising because there is a decrease in the production of bile in the liver preventing the absorption of which vitamin?
    a. A
    b. D
    c. E
    d. K

13. The nurse identifies which laboratory value as the usual indication of hepatic encephalopathy?
    a. Elevated sodium level
    b. Elevated ammonia level
    c. Increased blood urea nitrogen (BUN)
    d. Increased clotting time

Matching. Match the terms to their correct definitions.

Terms

a. Pruritus
b. Petechiae
c. Gynecomastia
d. Icterus
e. Spider angiomas
f. Palmar erythema
g. Melena
h. Ecchymosis
i. Fector hepaticus
j. Asterixis

Definitions

_____ 14. Nonrhythmic extensions and flexions in the wrists and fingers

_____ 15. Itching

_____ 16. Warm, bright red palms

_____ 17. Fruity or musty breath odor

_____ 18. Enlarged breasts

_____ 19. Blood in the stool

_____ 20. Vascular lesions with a red center and radiating branches

_____ 21. Large purple, blue, or yellow bruises

_____ 22. Yellowing of the sclera

_____ 23. Round, pinpoint, red-purple lesions

24. Which elevated laboratory test results indicate hepatic cell destruction? *(Select all that apply.)*
    a. Serum aspartate aminotransferase (AST)
    b. Serum alanine aminotransferase (ALT)
    c. Lactate dehydrogenase (LDH)
    d. Serum total bilirubin
    e. Urine urobilinogen
    f. International Normalized Ratio (INR)

25. The patient is scheduled for a procedure to place a stent in the biliary tract. For which procedure does the nurse provide patient teaching?
    a. Esophagogastroduodenoscopy (EGD)
    b. Endoscopic retrograde cholangiopancreatography (ERCP)
    c. Upper GI series
    d. Cholangiogram

26. When caring for the patient with cirrhosis who has pruritus, the nurse delegates which task to the unlicensed assistive personnel (UAP)?
    a. Assessment of open skin areas from scratching
    b. Use of warm water for bathing
    c. Use of lotion to soothe the skin
    d. Temperature control of the room to maintain a warm environment

27. The nurse is teaching the patient with cirrhosis about nutrition therapy. Which statement by the patient indicates teaching has been effective?
    a. "I will only use table salt with my dinner meal."
    b. "I will read the sodium content labels on all food and beverages."
    c. "I will avoid the use of vinegar."
    d. "I will not take vitamin supplements."

28. When preparing the patient for paracentesis, what does the nurse do? *(Select all that apply.)*
    a. Ask the patient to void before the procedure.
    b. Place the patient in the supine position.
    c. Weigh the patient before the procedure.
    d. Obtain the patient's heart rate.
    e. Assess the patient's respiratory rate.
    f. Obtain the patient's blood pressure.

29. While a paracentesis is being performed, the patient develops hypotension and tachycardia. What does the nurse suspect the patient is developing?
    a. Shock from fluid shifts
    b. Spontaneous bacterial peritonitis
    c. Anaphylactic reaction
    d. Intra-abdominal bleeding

30. The student nurse is caring for the patient with cirrhosis. Which action by the student nurse causes the supervising nurse to intervene?
    a. Uses a straight-edge razor to shave the patient
    b. Monitors for orthostatic changes of blood pressure
    c. Avoids intramuscular injections
    d. Uses a toothette for oral care

31. The nurse who is assessing the patient with portal-systemic encephalopathy finds that the patient has fector hepaticus, a positive Babinski's sign, and seizures, but no asterixis. The nurse identifies the patient as being in which stage of portal-systemic encephalopathy?
    a. Stage I prodromal
    b. Stage II impending
    c. Stage III stuporous
    d. Stage IV comatose

True or False? *Read the statements about esophageal varices and write T for true or F for false in the blanks provided.*

_____ 32. All patients with cirrhosis should be screened for esophageal varices by endoscopy to detect them early before they bleed.

_____ 33. Bleeding esophageal varices are a medical emergency.

_____ 34. Propranolol (Inderal) or nadolol (Corgard) with or without a nitrate is usually prescribed to prevent esophageal varices from bleeding.

_____ 35. IV octreotide is the mainstay for acute hemorrhage due to esophageal varices in the United States.

_____ 36. Esophagogastric balloon tamponade is rarely used today because it is difficult to use, uncomfortable for the patient, and prone to dangerous complications.

37. The nurse is teaching the patient with cirrhosis about lactulose therapy. Which statement by the patient indicates the teaching has been effective?
    a. "This therapy will promote the removal of ammonia in my stool."
    b. "Constipation is a frequent side effect of this therapy."
    c. "I will know the therapy is working when I am less itchy."
    d. "The drug tastes bitter and is watery."

38. How is neomycin sulfate (Mycifradin) used to treat patients with cirrhosis?
    a. It treats the current infection the patient has.
    b. It prevents future infections of the liver.
    c. It restores normal function to the liver cells.
    d. It destroys the normal flora of the bowel, diminishing protein breakdown and decreasing the rate of ammonia production.

True or False? *Read the statements about the different types of hepatitis and write T for true or F for false in the blanks provided.*

_____ 39. Bacterial hepatitis is the most common type of hepatitis.

_____ 40. Hepatitis A is spread via the fecal-oral route.

_____ 41. Hepatitis B can be transmitted by unprotected sexual intercourse with an infected partner.

_____ 42. Hepatitis carriers have chronic obvious signs of hepatitis B.

_____ 43. Hepatitis C is transmitted by casual contact or intimate household contact.

_____ 44. Hepatitis D only occurs with hepatitis B to cause viral replication.

_____ 45. Hepatitis E is transmitted via the fecal-oral route.

46. When teaching a group of adult patients measures for preventing hepatitis A (HAV), which information does the nurse include? *(Select all that apply.)*
   a. Perform proper handwashing, especially after handling shellfish.
   b. Receive immune globulin within 14 days if exposed to the virus.
   c. Receive the HAV vaccine before traveling to Mexico or the Caribbean.
   d. Receive the vaccine if living in a college dormitory.
   e. Receive the vaccine if working in a long-term care facility.

47. Which people are in need for immunization against hepatitis B (HBV)? *(Select all that apply.)*
   a. People who have unprotected sex with more than one partner.
   b. Men who have sex with men.
   c. People with any chronic liver disease.
   d. Firefighters.
   e. Police officers.

True or False? *Read the statements about hepatitis and write T for true or F for false in the blanks provided.*

_____ 48. Needle sticks are the major source of hepatitis B transmission in health care workers.

_____ 49. The hepatitis B vaccine is administered in a series of two injections.

_____ 50. Hepatitis B vaccine also prevents hepatitis E.

_____ 51. If a health care worker is exposed to hepatitis A, immunoglobulin (Ig) should be administered immediately.

_____ 52. All cases of hepatitis should be reported to the health department.

_____ 53. A person who has a history of being infected with hepatitis may never donate blood, body organs, or other body tissue.

_____ 54. A person with viral hepatitis can no longer transmit the disease once the jaundice is resolved.

_____ 55. Patients with hepatitis should eat small frequent meals with a high-carbohydrate, moderate-fat, and moderate-protein content.

_____ 56. People who have been vaccinated against HBV have a positive HBsAb because they also have immunity to the disease.

57. Which laboratory test result indicates permanent immunity to hepatitis A?
   a. Immunoglobulin G (IgG) antibodies
   b. Immunoglobulin M (IgM) antibodies
   c. A positive enzyme-linked immunosorbent assay (ELISA)
   d. The presence of anti-HAV antibodies

58. Which drug is used to destroy the hepatitis B virus in patients with chronic disease and to increase immunity?
   a. Lamivudine (Epivir-HBV)
   b. Entecavir (Baraclude)
   c. Telbivudine (Tyzeka)
   d. Pegylated interferon alpha-2b (Peg-Intron)

59. Which conditions place the patient at high risk for the development of fatty liver (steatosis)? *(Select all that apply.)*
   a. Hypertension
   b. Diabetes mellitus
   c. Obesity
   d. Elevated lipid profile
   e. Alcohol abuse

60. In performing an assessment on the patient with liver trauma, what does the nurse expect to find? *(Select all that apply.)*
   a. Positive Kehr's sign
   b. Guarding of the abdomen
   c. Abdominal distention
   d. Bradypnea
   e. Dry skin

True or False? *Read each statement about liver cancer and write T for true or F for false in the blanks provided.*

_____ 61. Liver cancer is most often seen in regions of Asia and the Mediterranean.

_____ 62. Risk factors for the development of liver cancer include use of anabolic steroids, androgens, or estrogens.

_____ 63. Alpha-fetoprotein (AFP) is a tumor marker for cancers of the liver.

_____ 64. Chemotherapy is the treatment of choice for cancer of the liver.

True or False? _Read each statement about liver transplantation and write T for true or F for false in the blanks provided._

_____ 65. Liver transplantation may be used for the patient with a primary liver tumor.

_____ 66. Patients with advanced cardiac disease are not considered candidates for liver transplantation.

_____ 67. The donor liver is able to be stored in a solution for up to 12 hours before transplantation to the recipient occurs.

_____ 68. The success of all transplantation has greatly improved since the introduction of cyclosporin, an immunosuppressant drug.

_____ 69. Transplant rejection is treated aggressively with immunosuppressive medication.

_____ 70. Clinical manifestations of organ rejection may include tachycardia, fever, right upper quadrant or flank pain, decreased bile pigment and volume, and increasing jaundice.

CASE STUDY: THE PATIENT WITH CIRRHOSIS AND ESOPHAGEAL BLEEDING

Use a separate sheet of paper to answer the questions in this Case Study. Answer guidelines for this Case Study are available on your Evolve website at http://evolve. elsevier.com/Iggy/ in the "Prepare for Class" folder.

A recently retired locomotive engineer is looking forward to his retirement so he and his wife "can finally enjoy" their lives together. He states he feels he has maintained sobriety quite well, but occasionally "sneaks a little drink now and then." Unfortunately, his cirrhotic liver has never fully recovered from 25 years of fairly heavy drinking. Although he has been diagnosed with Laennec's cirrhosis, the patient has not been compliant with follow-up visits to his health care provider. Periodically, and through the years, he still has symptoms of residual effects. For the past several days, he states he has been coughing on and off. His wife states that this morning he coughed up "bright red blood" and that is why she made him come to the hospital. As for now, he is not coughing or bleeding but has been admitted for observation. The nurse notes that he is jaundiced, has gynecomastia, and has multiple ecchymotic areas on his body. The site for the maintenance IV has fresh bloodstains noted on the dressing. As the nurse is doing rounds, his wife comes out of his room hysterical; the nurse enters his room and observes blood all over his gown and bed linens. He appears terrified.

1. What does the nurse suspect has happened? How could this have been prevented?

2. The nurse notifies the physician. What does the nurse anticipate treatment will include? What is an older treatment for bleeding esophageal varices and why is it rarely used today?

Continued

CASE STUDY: THE PATIENT WITH CIRRHOSIS AND ESOPHAGEAL BLEEDING *(Cont'd)*

3. The patient is discharged back to the unit after some time in the intensive care unit where his bleeding esophageal varices were controlled. The patient is ordered neomycin sulfate (Mycifradin) and lactulose. The patient asks the nurse, "Why is my body so changed? I have yellow skin, my chest looks like a woman's, and everywhere I look there are bruises. Even my IV seems to be leaking." How should the nurse answer these questions?

4. The patient's wife asks the nurse if her husband has an infection. She says, "The other nurse told me my husband is getting neomycin. I had that once for an infection I had. Where is my husband's infection?" How should the nurse respond?

5. What are the nursing interventions associated with lactulose therapy?

62 CHAPTER

Care of Patients with Problems of the Biliary System and Pancreas

STUDY/REVIEW QUESTIONS

1. The patient is admitted to the unit with obstructive jaundice. Which sign/symptom does the nurse expect to find upon assessment of the patient?
   a. Pruritus
   b. Pale urine in increased amounts
   c. Pink discoloration of sclera
   d. Dark, tarry stools

2. The daughter of the patient with cholelithiasis has heard that there is a genetic disposition for cholelithiasis. The daughter asks the nurse if there are preventive measures she can take. How does the nurse respond?
   a. "There is no evidence that first-degree relatives have an increased risk for this disease."
   b. "Cholecystitis is seen more frequently in patients who are underweight."
   c. "Drugs such as estrogen have been associated with increased risk for cholecystitis."
   d. "Patients with diabetes mellitus are at increased risk for cholecystitis."

3. Which patient is at low risk for the development of gallbladder disorders?
   a. Patient with sickle cell anemia
   b. Patient who is Mexican American
   c. Patient who is 30 years old and male
   d. Patient with a history of prolonged parenteral nutrition

4. The nurse on a medical-surgical unit is caring for several patients with acute cholecystitis. Which task is best to delegate to the nursing assistant?
   a. Obtain the patients' vital signs.
   b. Ask the patients if any foods are not tolerated.
   c. Ask the patients to describe what measures relieve the abdominal pain.
   d. Ask the patients to describe their daily activity or exercise routines.

Matching. *Match each term with its correct definition.*

Terms
a. Flatulence
b. Dyspepsia
c. Eructation
d. Biliary colic
e. Prostration
f. Murphy's sign
g. Blumberg's sign
h. Steatorrhea

Definitions
_____ 5. Pain that increases with deep inspiration with right subcostal palpation
_____ 6. Belching
_____ 7. Gas
_____ 8. Severe pain that is produced by obstruction of the cystic duct of the gallbladder
_____ 9. Indigestion
_____ 10. Extreme exhaustion
_____ 11. Assessment for rebound tenderness on deep palpation
_____ 12. Fatty stools

13. The patient is scheduled for tests to verify the medical diagnosis of cholecystitis. For which diagnostic test does the nurse provide patient teaching?
    a. Extracorporeal shock wave lithotripsy (ESWL)
    b. Ultrasonography of the right upper quadrant
    c. Endoscopic retrograde cholangiopancreatography (ERCP)
    d. Serum level of aspartate aminotransferase (AST)

14. Which type of drug is used to treat acute biliary pain?
    a. Acetaminophen (Tylenol)
    b. NSAIDs (Ibuprofen)
    c. Meperidine (Demerol)
    d. Opioids (Morphine)

15. The nurse is administering meperidine (Demerol) to a 78-year-old patient for pain management. Which assessment finding indicates the patient is experiencing a side effect of this drug?
    a. Seizure
    b. Cardiac dysrhythmia
    c. Low urinary output
    d. Jaundice

16. The nurse is caring for an older adult patient with acute biliary pain. Which drug order does the nurse question?
    a. Ketorolac (Toradol, Acular)
    b. Dicyclomine (Bentyl, Lomine)
    c. Morphine
    d. Hydromorphone (Dilaudid)

17. Which factor renders a patient the least likely to benefit from ESWL for the treatment of gallstones?
    a. Height 5 feet 10 inches, 170 lbs.
    b. Pigment-based stones
    c. Good gallbladder function
    d. Small gallstones

True or False? Read the statements about cholecystectomy and write T for true or F for false in the blanks provided.

_____ 18. Laparoscopic cholecystectomy is considered the "gold standard" and is performed far more often than the traditional open approach.

_____ 19. Removing the gallbladder with the laparoscopic technique reduces the risk of wound complications.

_____ 20. Patients who have their gallbladder removed by the laparoscopic technique should be taught the importance of early ambulation to promote absorption of carbon dioxide.

_____ 21. Use of open surgical approach (abdominal laparotomy) has greatly declined during past 15 years.

_____ 22. Examples of patients who have the open surgical approach (abdominal laparotomy) include those with chronic lung disease or heart failure who cannot tolerate the oxygen used in the laparoscopic procedure.

23. Which statement about the care of the patient with a T-tube after a cholecystectomy is true?
    a. The patient is maintained in the prone position.
    b. When the patient is allowed to eat, the T-tube is clamped continuously.
    c. The T-tube is irrigated every hour for the first 72 hours.
    d. Avoid raising the drainage system above the level of the gallbladder.

Matching. Match each definition with the associated procedure.

Procedures
a.   Cholecystectomy
b.   Cholecystotomy
c.   Choledocholithotomy
d.   Choledochoscopy
e.   ESWL

Definitions
_____ 24.   Powerful shock waves shatter gall-stones

_____ 25.   Incision into common bile duct for stone removal

_____ 26.   Removal of gallbladder

_____ 27.   Direct visualization of biliary tract

_____ 28.   Opening into the gallbladder

29.   The nurse is evaluating electrolyte values for the patient with acute pancreatitis and notes that the serum calcium is 6.8 mEq/L. How does the nurse interpret this finding?
   a.   Within normal limits considering the diagnosis of acute pancreatitis
   b.   The result of the body not being able to use bound calcium
   c.   A protective measure that will reduce the risk of complications
   d.   Full compensation of the parathyroid gland

Matching. Match each complication of pancreatitis with its pathophysiology.

Complications
a.   Acute renal failure
b.   Paralytic (adynamic) ileus
c.   Acute respiratory distress syndrome (ARDS)
d.   Disseminated intravascular coagulation (DIC)

Pathophysiology
_____ 30.   Disruption of alveolar-capillary membrane results in edema

_____ 31.   Hypovolemia

_____ 32.   Consumption of clotting factors and microthrombi formation

_____ 33.   Peritoneal irritation and seepage of pancreatic enzymes into the abdominal cavity

True or False? Read the statements about acute pancreatitis and write T for true or F for false in the blanks provided.

_____ 34.   Patients with pancreatitis often have Turner's sign which is a gray-blue discoloration of the abdomen and periumbilical area.

_____ 35.   The pain of acute pancreatitis is often described as intense, boring, and continuous.

_____ 36.   Typically, a patient is diagnosed with acute pancreatitis after presenting with severe abdominal pain in the mid-epigastric area or left upper quadrant.

_____ 37. Abdominal pain is the prominent symptom of pancreatitis.

_____ 38. Anticholinergics are given to increase vagal stimulation, motility, and pancreatic flow.

_____ 39. Pain management for acute pancreatitis should begin with rapid infusion of opioids by means of patient-controlled analgesia (PCA).

_____ 40. Helping the patient to assume a supine position decreases the abdominal pain of pancreatitis.

_____ 41. Surgical intervention for acute pancreatitis is usually not indicated.

_____ 42. Patients in the early stages of acute pancreatitis are usually maintained on NPO status.

43. What is the priority nursing diagnosis for acute pancreatitis?
   a. Risk for Deficient Fluid Volume related to abnormal and normal routines
   b. Nausea related to pancreatic disease
   c. Risk for Infection related to necrotic pancreatic tissue
   d. Acute Pain related to biologic and injury agents

44. Which diagnostic test is the most accurate in verifying a diagnosis of acute pancreatitis?
   a. Trypsin
   b. Lipase
   c. Alkaline phosphatase
   d. Alanine aminotransferase

45. The patient with acute pancreatitis is at risk for the development of paralytic (adynamic) ileus. Which action provides the nurse with the best indication of bowel function?
   a. Observing contents of the nasogastric drainage
   b. Auscultation of bowel sounds
   c. Asking the patient if he or she has passed flatus or had a stool
   d. Obtaining a computed tomography (CT) scan of the abdomen with contrast medium

46. Which drug is contraindicated for the patient with paralytic ileus?
   a. Ranitidine (Zantac)
   b. Cefuroxime (Zinacef)
   c. Papaverine (Pavabid)
   d. Dicyclomine (Bentyl)

47. The nurse has instructed the patient in the recovery phase of acute pancreatitis about diet therapy. Which statement by the patient indicates that teaching has been successful?
   a. "I will eat the usual three meals a day that I am used to."
   b. "I am eating tacos for my first meal back home."
   c. "I will avoid eating chocolate."
   d. "I will limit the amount of protein in my diet."

48. The nursing student is caring for the patient with chronic pancreatitis who is receiving pancreatic enzyme replacement therapy. Which statement by the student indicates the need for further study concerning this therapy?
   a. "The enzymes will be administered with meals."
   b. "The patient will take the drugs with a glass of water."
   c. "If the patient has difficulty swallowing the enzyme preparation, I will mix it with foods containing protein."
   d. "The effectiveness of pancreatic enzyme treatment is monitored by the frequency and fat content of stools."

True or False? _Read the statements about pancreatic cancer and write T for true or F for false in the blanks provided._

_____ 49. Venous thromboembolism is a common complication of pancreatic cancer.

_____ 50. Pancreatic cancer often presents in a slow and vague manner.

_____ 51. The most common concern of the patient with pancreatic cancer is pain.

_____ 52. There are no specific blood tests to diagnose pancreatic cancer.

_____ 53. Chemotherapy is the treatment of choice for pancreatic cancer.

_____ 54. The position of choice for the patient after a Whipple procedure is semi-Fowler's.

CASE STUDY: THE PATIENT WITH PANCREATIC CANCER

Use a separate sheet of paper to answer the questions in this Case Study. Answer guidelines for this Case Study are available on your Evolve website at http://evolve. elsevier.com/Iggy/ in the "Prepare for Class" folder.

A patient is admitted to the medical surgical unit with jaundice, abdominal pain, and reports fatigue over the past several weeks. The patient states that he has been losing weight but didn't think too much of it because he hadn't had much of an appetite due to some nausea and vomiting as well as some dull abdominal pain. On physical assessment the nurse's findings include splenomegaly, ascites, and a tender, warm, enlarged right calf. The patient rates his pain at this time as an 8 on a scale of 0 to 10. The patient's family is very concerned. His adult daughter states, "The doctor doesn't even know what is wrong with Dad. Why don't they just do an x-ray of his stomach to find out the problem?" Pancreatic cancer is suspected.

1. What is the most likely cause of the patient's tender, warm, and enlarged right calf?

2. What is the most likely cause of the patient's jaundice, ascites, and splenomegaly?

3. What can the nurse tell the patient's daughter about the diagnostic tests for pancreatic cancer?

4. A diagnosis of pancreatic cancer is confirmed. The patient is scheduled to undergo a Whipple procedure. What preoperative teaching should the nurse include?

5. When caring for the patient postoperatively, what should nursing care include?

6. The patient's daughter wishes to care for her father at home. She works full time as a waitress and is a single parent of two small children. The physician has told the patient and his daughter that he has a short time to live because of the advanced state of the disease. What should nursing care for this family include?

63 CHAPTER

Care of Patients with Malnutrition and Obesity

STUDY/REVIEW QUESTIONS

True or False? *Read each statement and write T for true and F for false in the blanks provided.*

_____ 1. Body proteins are used for energy when calorie energy is inadequate.

_____ 2. A lacto-vegetarian eats milk, cheese, and dairy foods but avoids meats, fish, poultry, and eggs.

_____ 3. A vegan eats only foods of plant origin.

_____ 4. People with lactose intolerance have difficulty digesting meat.

_____ 5. Every patient needs a complete nutritional assessment.

6. Which signs/symptoms in the older adult can be an indication of "failure to thrive?" *(Select all that apply.)*
   a. Weakness
   b. Slow walking speed
   c. Low physical activity
   d. Unintentional weight loss
   e. Exhaustion

7. The nurse is providing teaching for a group of older adults about the risk factors for malnutrition. What factors does the nurse emphasize in the teaching plan? *(Select all that apply.)*
   a. Poor dental health
   b. Hypersecretion of saliva
   c. Depression
   d. Fatigue
   e. Lack of transportation

8. The patient is malnourished. What is the priority nursing intervention?
   a. Determine the patient's food preferences.
   b. Provide the patient with high-calorie, high-protein food.
   c. Weigh the patient.
   d. Offer the patient snacks.

9. The nurse is caring for three patients who have undergone bariatric surgery. Which activity is most appropriate for the nurse to delegate to the unlicensed assistive personnel (UAP)?
   a. Give analgesics about 1 hour before mealtimes.
   b. Document the percentage of food eaten at mealtimes.
   c. Assess the patient's food preferences.
   d. Teach the family methods to feed the patient who is unable to feed him- or herself.

10. After the UAP tells the nurse that the older patient will not eat her dinner, the nurse enters the patient's room to assess the situation. Which factors likely contribute to the patient's lack of desire to eat? *(Select all that apply.)*
    a. An emesis basin is on the bedside table.
    b. The volume of the television is loud.
    c. The food is cold.
    d. The cleaning lady is in the room disinfecting the bathroom.
    e. The patient's roommate has two adults and three children visiting.

11. The nurse is teaching the male patient about the 2005 Dietary Guidelines for Americans. Which statement by the patient indicates a need for additional teaching?
    a. "I'll limit consumption of alcohol to two drinks a day."
    b. "I'll consume at least 6 cups of milk products a day."
    c. "I'll consume 3 or more ounce-equivalents of whole-grain products per day."
    d. "I'll limit added sugar and salt in my diet."

Matching. *Match each nutritional deficiency with its appropriate sign/symptom.*

Nutritional Deficiency
a. Zinc
b. Vitamin A
c. Riboflavin
d. Vitamin C
e. Niacin
f. Protein
g. Vitamin D
h. Thiamine
i. Selenium

Signs/Symptoms

_____ 12. Hepatomegaly

_____ 13. Osteomalacia, bone pain, rickets

_____ 14. Xerosis of conjunctiva

_____ 15. Alopecia

_____ 16. Swollen, bleeding gums

_____ 17. Fissured tongue

_____ 18. Magenta tongue

_____ 19. Confabulation

_____ 20. Cardiomyopathy

True or False? *Read the statements about anthropometric measurements and write T for true or F for false in the blanks provided.*

_____ 21. The nurse must obtain accurate measurements, because patients who report their own measurements tend to underestimate height and overestimate weight.

_____ 22. Patients should be measured and weighed while wearing minimal clothing and no shoes.

_____ 23. In determining height, the patient should stand erect and look straight ahead, with the heels apart and the arms forward.

_____ 24. For patients who cannot stand erect, a sliding-blade knee height caliper should be used if available.

_____ 25. Ambulatory patients should be weighed using an upright balance-bean scale.

_____ 26. The preferred time to weigh patients daily is immediately before dinner.

_____ 27. Weight is the most reliable indicator of fluid gain or loss.

_____ 28. An involuntary weight loss of 10% at any time significantly affects nutritional status.

_____ 29. The body mass index is a measure of nutritional status that depends on frame size.

_____ 30. Skin fold measurements estimate body fat.

True or False? *Read each statement and write T for true or F for false in the blanks provided.*

_____ 31.   Marasmus is a lack of protein quantity and quality in the presence of adequate calories.

_____ 32.   Kwashiorkor is generally a calorie malnutrition in which body fat and protein are wasted.

_____ 33.   Patients who are malnourished often have a decreased vital capacity.

_____ 34.   *Cachexia* is the term used to describe muscle wasting with prolonged malnutrition.

35.   The patient is severely malnourished. The nurse assesses for which potential complications of malnourishment? *(Select all that apply.)*
a.   Poor wound healing
b.   Intolerance to heat
c.   Infection
d.   Lethargy
e.   Edema

Matching. *Match the laboratory test values with their indications of nutritional status.*

Laboratory Tests
a.   Cholesterol
b.   Total lymphocyte count (TLC)
c.   Serum albumin
d.   Prealbumin
e.   Hemoglobin
f.   Hematocrit

Indications

_____ 36.   Low levels may indicate anemia, recent hemorrhage, or hemodilution caused by fluid retention.

_____ 37.   Low levels may reflect anemia, hemorrhage, excessive fluid, renal disease, or cirrhosis.

_____ 38.   Reflects nutritional status a few weeks before testing.

_____ 39.   More sensitive indicator of protein deficiency because of its short half-life of 2 days.

_____ 40.   Values are typically low with malabsorption, liver disease, pernicious anemia, terminal stages of cancer, or sepsis.

_____ 41.   Used to assess immune function.

42.   Which medication is the drug of choice to increase appetite in those patients who have cachexia, acquired immune deficiency syndrome (AIDS), or unexplained weight loss?
a.   Cyproheptadine (Periactin)
b.   Megestrol acetate (Megace)
c.   Zinc
d.   Vitamin C

43.   Total enteral nutrition (TEN) is contraindicated for which patient?
a.   Older adult receiving chemotherapy
b.   Patient who has had a stroke and has dysphagia
c.   Patient who has had extensive jaw and mouth surgery
d.   Patient with intestinal obstruction that has progressed to diffuse peritonitis

Matching. *Match the types of feedings to their descriptions.*

Types of Feeding
a. Bolus feeding tube
b. Continuous feeding tube
c. Cycle feeding tube

Descriptions

_____ 44. Small amounts are continually infused over a specified time.

_____ 45. Infusion is stopped for a specified time.

_____ 46. Intermittent feeding of a specified amount at specified times.

True or False? *Read each statement about tube feeding care and maintenance and write T for true or F for false in the blanks provided.*

_____ 47. The initial placement of a nasogastric or nasoduodenal feeding tube should be confirmed by x-ray study.

_____ 48. Auscultation of gastric air flow via the nasoduodenal feeding tube is the current preferred method for rechecking placement after an x-ray.

_____ 49. A jejunostomy tube should be rotated 360 degrees each day and the tube should be checked for in-and-out play of about 0.5 cm.

_____ 50. Residual volume of the tube feeding should be checked every 12 hours.

_____ 51. The feeding bag and tubing should be changed every 12 hours.

_____ 52. To prevent aspiration, the head of the patient's bed should be elevated at least 30 degrees.

53. The patient is receiving a tube feeding. Which action by the UAP requires intervention by the supervising nurse?
a. Weighing the patient
b. Placing food coloring in the tube feeding to assess for aspiration
c. Discarding any unused open cans of feeding solution after 24 hours
d. Monitoring the patient for the development of diarrhea

54. Which statement about the patient with a tube feeding indicates best practice for patient safety and quality care?
a. If the tube becomes clogged, use 30 mL of water for flushing, while applying gentle pressure with a 50 mL piston syringe.
b. Use cranberry juice to flush the tube if it is clogged.
c. When administering medications, use cold water to dissolve the drug before administering it.
d. Administer drugs down the feeding tube without flushing first, but flush the feeding tube after the drug is given.

55. The patient in a starvation state has been started on enteral feedings. The nurse assesses the patient and finds shallow respirations, weakness, acute confusion, and oozing from the IV site. What does the nurse suspect is happening in this patient?
a. Septicemia
b. Hypoglycemia
c. Aspiration
d. Refeeding syndrome

56. Which statement describes the correct method of testing the pH of GI contents at the bedside?
a. The tube is in the stomach if the pH reading is 8.0.
b. Before aspirating the GI contents, flush the tube with 10 mL of air.
c. If the patient takes certain medications such as H_2 blockers, the pH of the stomach is usually 2.0.
d. Wait at least 1 hour after drug administration before assessing the pH of GI contents.

57. When caring for the patient receiving fat emulsions, which adverse reactions can occur with this therapy as identified by the nurse? *(Select all that apply.)*
    a. Dyspnea
    b. Back pain
    c. Fever
    d. Flushing
    e. Phlebitis

58. When administering total parenteral nutrition (TPN), what does the nurse do?
    a. Administer TPN via the gravity drip method.
    b. Administer TPN via a peripheral IV.
    c. Monitor the patient's blood glucose levels.
    d. Use clean technique when changing the tubing.

59. The nurse is assessing the patient receiving TPN at 100 mL/hour. The TPN solution has 50 mL left in the bag. The nurse looks for the next bag of TPN but it is not on the unit. When the pharmacy is called, the nurse is told it will take at least 1 hour for the next bag of TPN solution to be delivered. What does the nurse do?
    a. Call the health care provider.
    b. Administer 10% dextrose/water (D/W) until the TPN is available.
    c. Prepare to treat the patient for hyperglycemia.
    d. Cap the TPN line until the next TPN solution is available.

Matching. Match the terms related to obesity with their definitions.

Terms
a. Obesity
b. Overweight
c. Morbid obesity

Definitions

_____ 60. Weight that has a severely negative effect on health.

_____ 61. Excessive amount of body fat when compared to lean body mass.

_____ 62. Increase in body weight for height as compared to a standard.

True or False? Read each statement and write T for true or F for false in the blanks provided.

_____ 63. Obesity is not just one disease, but rather many conditions with varying causes.

_____ 64. Obesity is the second-leading cause of preventable deaths in the United States.

_____ 65. Waist circumference is a stronger predictor of coronary artery disease than is body mass index (BMI).

_____ 66. Once an adolescent is overweight, he or she is likely to remain overweight.

_____ 67. Waist to hip ratio (WHR) is a strong predictor of colon cancer.

68. The nurse is performing an admission assessment on the morbidly obese patient. Which common complications of obesity does the nurse assess for? *(Select all that apply.)*
    a. Type 1 diabetes mellitus
    b. Metabolic syndrome
    c. Urinary incontinence
    d. Gout
    e. Early osteoarthritis

69. Which prescribed drugs can contribute to weight gain when they are taken on a long-term basis? *(Select all that apply.)*
    a. Estrogens
    b. Acetaminophen
    c. Corticosteroids
    d. NSAIDs
    e. Antiepileptics

70. Which drug is the most commonly used ano-rectic drug for the long-term treatment of obesity?
    a. Phentermine (Adipex-p)
    b. Diethylpropion (Tenuate)
    c. Orlistat (Xenical)
    d. Sibustramine (Meridia)

71. The nurse is caring for the patient after bariatric surgery. What is the immediate nursing priority for this patient?
    a. Nutritional intake
    b. Pain management
    c. Prevention of infection
    d. Airway management

72. The patient comes to the clinic after having bariatric surgery and says, "After I eat, I feel really funny. My heart races, I feel nauseated, and my abdomen cramps up. I even have diarrhea." What does the nurse suspect is happening with this patient?
    a. Hyperglycemia
    b. Intestinal obstruction
    c. Peritonitis
    d. Dumping syndrome

CASE STUDY: THE PATIENT WITH OBESITY

Use a separate sheet of paper to answer the questions in this Case Study. Answer guidelines for this Case Study are available on your Evolve website at http://evolve.elsevier.com/Iggy/ in the "Prepare for Class" folder.

The patient is 100% above ideal body weight and has been diagnosed with morbid obesity. The patient tells the nurse, "I've always been big; my family is big and so am I. What's so wrong about being a plus size? Can being overweight really cause problems for me?" The patient has tried to lose weight by following fad diets such as the Hollywood diet. The patient did initially lose some weight, but gained it back plus more. The patient has also tried an over-the-counter medication to help with weight loss called orlistat (Xenical). The patient stopped taking the drug because he had loose stools, abdominal cramps, and nausea while taking it. The patient decides to undergo gastric bypass surgery.

1. The patient asks the nurse, "What is wrong with me that I am this heavy?" How should the nurse explain the pathophysiology of obesity?
2. How should the nurse respond to the patient's question about complications of obesity?
3. Why has dieting by the patient not been effective?
4. Why did the patient have side effects while using orlistat (Xenical)?
5. Describe preoperative nursing care for the patient undergoing gastric bypass surgery.
6. What is the most common complication that the nurse must assess the patient for postoperatively?

64 Assessment of the Endocrine System

CHAPTER

STUDY/REVIEW QUESTIONS

1. Which glands are part of the endocrine system? *(Select all that apply.)*
   a. Thyroid
   b. Occipital
   c. Parathyroid
   d. Adrenal
   e. Pituitary

2. Which is the name of the substance secreted by the glands in question #1 above?
   a. Vasoactive amines
   b. Chemotaxins
   c. Hormones
   d. Cytotoxins

3. Which mechanism is used to transport the substance produced by the endocrine glands to their target tissue?
   a. Lymph system
   b. Bloodstream
   c. Direct seeding
   d. Gastrointestinal system

Matching. Match each hormone with its corresponding gland. Answers may be used more than once.

Glands
a. Anterior pituitary
b. Posterior pituitary
c. Adrenal cortex
d. Adrenal medulla
e. Thyroid gland
f. Alpha cells—islets of Langerhans
g. Beta cells—islets of Langerhans
h. Delta cells—islets of Langerhans
i. Parathyroid
j. Ovaries
k. Testes
l. Hypothalamus

Hormones
_____ 4. Somatostatin
_____ 5. Thyrocalcitonin (calcitonin)
_____ 6. Cortisol
_____ 7. Epinephrine and norepinephrine
_____ 8. Corticotropin-releasing hormone (CRH)
_____ 9. Growth hormone
_____ 10. Glucagon
_____ 11. Parathyroid hormone (PTH)
_____ 12. Aldosterone
_____ 13. Triiodothyronine (T_3)
_____ 14. Estrogen
_____ 15. Insulin
_____ 16. Testosterone
_____ 17. Antidiuretic hormone (ADH)
_____ 18. Oxytocin
_____ 19. Thyroxin (T_4)
_____ 20. Thyroid-stimulating hormone (TSH)
_____ 21. Adrenocorticotropic hormone (ACTH)

22. The target tissue for ADH is which organ?
    a. Hypothalamus
    b. Thyroid
    c. Ovary
    d. Kidney

True or False? *Read the statements about hormones and the endocrine system and write T for true or F for false in the blanks provided. If the statement is false, correct the statement to make it true.*

_____ 23. Usually, low concentration of hormone is all that is needed to have an effect on the body.

_____ 24. When hormones are secreted, the duration of effect is long.

_____ 25. Hormones must be bound to a plasma protein in order to be connected with a receptor site.

_____ 26. All hormones are stored in significant amounts so that response can be immediate.

_____ 27. All hormones must be able to attach themselves to a receptor site in order to be used by the body.

_____ 28. Most hormones are "recycled" after use through reuptake by the secreting gland.

_____ 29. Homeostasis involves the endocrine system working together with the nervous system for good hormone function.

_____ 30. Tropic hormones have another endocrine gland as their target tissue.

_____ 31. There are specific normal levels of each of the hormones.

_____ 32. More than one hormone can be stimulated before the target tissue is affected.

_____ 33. Only the hypothalamus has releasing and inhibiting factors that affect specific hormone production.

34. Which hormone is directly suppressed when circulating levels of cortisol are above normal?
    a. CRH
    b. ADH
    c. ACTH
    d. Growth hormone–releasing hormone (GH-RH)

35. The release of epinephrine into the bloodstream is an example of which endocrine process?
    a. "Lock and key" manner
    b. Neuroendocrine regulation
    c. Positive feedback mechanism
    d. Stimulus-response theory

36. Identify the hormones that are secreted for each of the endocrine glands listed below.

Endocrine Gland	Principal Hormones Secreted
a. Hypothalamus	
b. Anterior pituitary	
c. Posterior pituitary	
d. Thyroid	
e. Parathyroid	
f. Adrenal cortex	
g. Pancreas	
h. Ovaries	
i. Testes	

37. Which statement about the pituitary gland is correct?
    a. The main role of the posterior pituitary is to secrete tropic hormones.
    b. The posterior pituitary gland stores hormones produced by the hypothalamus.
    c. The anterior pituitary is connected to the thalamus gland.
    d. The anterior pituitary releases stored hormones produced by the hypothalamus.

38. The anterior pituitary gland secretes tropic hormones in response to which hormones from the hypothalamus?
    a. Releasing hormones
    b. Target tissue hormones
    c. Growth hormones
    d. Demand hormones

39. Which statement about pituitary hormones is correct?
    a. ACTH acts on the adrenal medulla.
    b. Follicle-stimulating hormone (FSH) stimulates sperm production in men.
    c. Growth hormone promotes protein catabolism.
    d. Vasopressin decreases systolic blood pressure.

40. Which statement about the gonads is correct?
    a. Ovaries and testes develop from the same embryonic tissue.
    b. The function of the hormones begins at birth in low, undetectable levels.
    c. The placenta secretes testosterone for the development of male external genitalia.
    d. External genitalia maturation is stimulated by gonadotropins in late adolescence.

41. Which statement about the adrenal glands is correct?
    a. The cortex secretes androgens in men and women.
    b. Catecholamines are secreted from the cortex.
    c. Glucocorticoids are secreted by the medulla.
    d. The medulla secretes hormones essential for life.

42. Which is the major function of the hormones produced by the adrenal cortex?
    a. "Fight or flight" response
    b. Control of glucose, sodium, and water
    c. Regulation of cell growth
    d. Calcium and stress regulation

True or False? *Read the statements about the hormone cortisol secreted by the adrenal cortex and write T for true or F for false in the blanks provided. If the statement is false, correct the statement to make it true.*

_____ 43. It affects only carbohydrate metabolism.

_____ 44. It is needed for other physiologic processes, such as secretion of insulin, to occur.

_____ 45. It is regulated by ACTH from the posterior pituitary and CRH.

_____ 46. Peaks occur late in the day, with lowest points 12 hours after each peak.

_____ 47. Stress causes an increase in the production of cortisol from the adrenal cortex.

_____ 48. Cortisol has an effect on the body's immune function.

49. Which assessment findings does the nurse monitor in response to catecholamines released by the adrenal medulla? *(Select all that apply.)*
   a. Increased heart rate related to vasoconstriction
   b. Increased blood pressure related to vasoconstriction
   c. Increased perspiration
   d. Constriction of pupils
   e. Increased blood glucose in response to glycogenolysis

True or False? *Read the statements about the thyroid gland and its hormones and write T for true or F for false in the blanks provided. If the statement is false, correct the statement to make it true.*

_____ 50. The gland is located posteriorly in the neck directly below the cricoid cartilage.

_____ 51. Thyroid hormone production depends on sufficient iodine and potassium intake.

_____ 52. The gland has four distinct lobes joined by a thin isthmus.

_____ 53. Oxygen consumption decreases in response to thyroid hormones.

54. Which hormone responds to a low serum calcium by increasing bone resorption?
   a. PTH
   b. T_4
   c. T_3
   d. Calcitonin

55. Which hormone responds to elevated serum calcium by decreasing bone resorption?
   a. PTH
   b. T_4
   c. T_3
   d. Calcitonin

56. Which statements about T_3 and T_4 hormones are correct? *(Select all that apply.)*
   a. The basal metabolic rate is affected.
   b. Hypothalamus is stimulated by cold and stress to secrete thyrotropin-releasing hormone (TRH).
   c. These hormones need intake of protein and iodine for production.
   d. Circulating hormone in the blood directly affects the production of TSH.
   e. T_3 and T_4 increase oxygen use in tissues.

57. Which are the target organs of PTH in the regulation of calcium and phosphorus? *(Select all that apply.)*
   a. Stomach
   b. Kidney
   c. Bone
   d. Intestinal tract
   e. Thyroid gland

58. Which statement about the pancreas is correct?
    a. Endocrine functions of the pancreas include secretion of digestive enzymes.
    b. Exocrine functions of the pancreas include secretion of glucagon and insulin.
    c. The islets of Langerhans are the only source of somatostatin secretion.
    d. Somatostatin inhibits pancreatic secretion of glucagon and insulin.

59. Which statement about glucagon secretion is correct?
    a. It is stimulated by an increase in blood glucose levels.
    b. It is stimulated by a decrease in amino acid levels.
    c. It exerts its primary effect on the pancreas.
    d. It acts to increase blood glucose levels.

60. Which statement about insulin secretion is correct?
    a. Insulin levels drop sharply following the ingestion of a meal.
    b. Insulin is stimulated primarily by fat ingestion.
    c. Basal levels are secreted continuously.
    d. Insulin promotes glycogenolysis and gluconeogenesis.

61. In addition to the pancreas that secretes insulin, which gland secretes hormones that affect protein, carbohydrate, and fat metabolism?
    a. Posterior pituitary
    b. Thyroid
    c. Ovaries
    d. Parathyroid

62. The bloodstream delivers glucose to the cells for energy production. Which hormones control the cells' use of glucose?
    a. T_4
    b. Growth hormone
    c. Adrenal steroids
    d. Insulin

63. Which disease involves a disorder of the islets of Langerhans?
    a. Diabetes insipidus
    b. Diabetes mellitus
    c. Addison's disease
    d. Cushing's disease

64. Which endocrine tissues are most commonly found to have reduced function as a result of aging? *(Select all that apply.)*
    a. Hypothalamus
    b. Ovaries
    c. Testes
    d. Pancreas
    e. Thyroid gland

65. Which statement about age-related changes in older adults and the endocrine system is true?
    a. All hormone levels are elevated.
    b. Thyroid hormone levels decrease.
    c. Adrenal glands enlarge.
    d. The thyroid gland enlarges.

Matching. *Match the physiologic changes noted with the decreased function of glands due to aging.*

Glands
a. Thyroid
b. Pancreas
c. Ovary
d. Posterior pituitary gland

Physiologic Changes

_____ 66. Osteoporosis, decreased production of estrogen

_____ 67. Decreased sensitivity of peripheral tissues to the effects of insulin

_____ 68. Decreased concentrating ability of the kidneys

_____ 69. Decreased metabolic rate

70. The older adult reports a lack of energy and not being able to do the usual daily activities without several naps during the day. Which problem may these symptoms indicate that is often seen in the older adult?
    a. Hypothyroidism
    b. Hyperparathyroidism
    c. Overproduction of cortisol
    d. Underproduction of glucagon

71. The nurse is performing a physical assessment of the patient's endocrine system. Which gland can be palpated?
    a. Pancreas
    b. Thyroid
    c. Adrenal glands
    d. Parathyroid

72. Which statement about performing a physical assessment of the thyroid gland is correct?
    a. The thyroid gland is easily palpated in all patients.
    b. The patient is instructed to swallow to aid palpation.
    c. The anterior approach is preferred for thyroid palpation.
    d. The thumbs are used to palpate the thyroid lobes.

73. Which are diagnostic methods to measure patient hormone levels? *(Select all that apply.)*
    a. Stimulation testing
    b. Suppression testing
    c. 24-hour urine testing
    d. Chromographic assay
    e. Needle biopsy

74. What is the correct nursing action before beginning a 24-hour urine collection for endocrine studies?
    a. Place each voided specimen in a separate collection container.
    b. Check whether any preservatives are needed in the collection container.
    c. Start the collection with the first voided urine.
    d. Weigh the patient before beginning the collection.

75. Which instructions are included when teaching the patient about urine collection for endocrine studies? *(Select all that apply.)*
    a. Fast before starting the urine collection.
    b. Measure the urine in mL rather than ounces.
    c. Empty the bladder completely, then start timing.
    d. Time the test for exactly 24 hours.
    e. Notify the laboratory of all medications you are taking.
    f. Empty the bladder at the end of the time period and keep that specimen.

76. Which are the types of radiographic tests that may be used for an endocrine assessment? *(Select all that apply.)*
    a. Ultrasonography
    b. Skull x-ray
    c. Chest x-ray
    d. Magnetic resonance imaging (MRI)
    e. Computed tomography (CT)

77. The patient is suspected of having a pituitary tumor. Which radiographic test aids in determining this diagnosis?
    a. Skull x-rays
    b. CT/MRI
    c. Angiography
    d. Ultrasound

78. After an ultrasound of the thyroid gland, which diagnostic tests determine the need for surgical intervention?
    a. CT scan
    b. MRI
    c. Angiography
    d. Needle biopsy

79. The nursing diagnosis of Risk for Falls related to the effect of pathologic fractures as a result of bone demineralization is pertinent to which endocrine problem?
    a. Underproduction of PTH
    b. Overproduction of PTH
    c. Underproduction of thyroid hormone
    d. Overproduction of thyroid hormone

65 CHAPTER

Care of Patients with Pituitary and Adrenal Gland Problems

STUDY/REVIEW QUESTIONS

1. Complete the table below.

Dysfunction	Cause	Result
Primary pituitary dysfunction		
Secondary pituitary dysfunction		

2. Which are hormones produced and secreted by the anterior pituitary gland? *(Select all that apply.)*
    a. Growth hormone (GH; somatotropin)
    b. Prolactin (PRL)
    c. Thyrotropin (thyroid-stimulating hormone [TSH])
    d. Serotonin (5-HT)
    e. Gonadotropins (follicle-stimulating hormone [FSH] and luteinizing hormone [LH])
    f. Epinephrine (EPI)

3. A malfunctioning posterior pituitary gland can result in which disorders? *(Select all that apply.)*
    a. Hypothyroidism
    b. Altered sexual function
    c. Diabetes insipidus
    d. Growth retardation
    e. Syndrome of inappropriate antidiuretic hormone (SIADH)

4. A malfunctioning anterior pituitary gland can result in which disorders? *(Select all that apply.)*
    a. Pituitary hypofunction
    b. Pituitary hyperfunction
    c. Diabetes insipidus
    d. Hypothyroidism
    e. Osteoporosis

5. The assessment findings of the male patient with anterior pituitary tumor include reports of changes in secondary sex characteristics, such as episodes of impotence and decreased libido. The nurse explains to the patient that these findings are a result of overproduction of which hormone?
    a. Gonadotropins inhibiting PRL.
    b. Thyroid hormone inhibiting PRL.
    c. PRL inhibiting secretion of gonadotropins.
    d. Steroids inhibiting production of sex hormones.

6. The patient with PRL-secreting tumor is likely to be treated with which medication?
   a. Dopamine agonists
   b. Vasopressin
   c. Steroids
   d. Growth hormone

7. The patient is prescribed bromocriptine mesylate (Parlodel). Which information does the nurse teach the patient?
   a. Get up slowly from a lying position.
   b. Take medication on an empty stomach.
   c. Take daily for purposes of raising GH levels to reduce symptom of acromegaly.
   d. Begin therapy with a maintenance level dose.

8. Patients diagnosed with an anterior pituitary tumor can have symptoms of acromegaly or gigantism. These symptoms are a result of overproduction of which hormone?
   a. ACTH
   b. PRL
   c. Gonadotropins
   d. GH

9. The nurse is performing an assessment of the adult patient with new-onset acromegaly. What does the nurse expect to find?
   a. Extremely long arms and legs
   b. Thickened, oily facial skin
   c. Changes in menses with infertility
   d. Rough, extremely dry skin

10. Acromegaly and gigantism are both caused by overproduction of which anterior pituitary hormone?
    a. PRL
    b. ACTH
    c. GH
    d. FSH

11. When analyzing laboratory values, the nurse expects to find which value as a direct result of overproduction of GH?
    a. Hyperglycemia
    b. Hyperphosphatemia
    c. Hypocalcemia
    d. Hypercalcemia

12. In caring for the patient with hyperpituitarism, which symptoms does the nurse expect the patient to report? *(Select all that apply.)*
    a. Joint pain
    b. Visual disturbances
    c. Changes in menstruation
    d. Decreased libido
    e. Headache

13. A deficiency of which anterior pituitary hormones is considered life-threatening? *(Select all that apply.)*
    a. GH
    b. Melanocyte-stimulating hormone (MSH)
    c. PRL
    d. TSH
    e. ACTH

14. Which statement about the etiology of hypopituitarism is correct?
    a. Secondary dysfunction can result from radiation treatment to the pituitary gland.
    b. Primary dysfunction can result from infection or a brain tumor.
    c. Infarction following systemic shock results in secondary hypopituitarism.
    d. Severe malnutrition and body fat depletion can depress pituitary gland function.

15. Which statement about hormone replacement therapy for hypopituitarism is correct?
    a. Once manifestations of hypofunction are corrected, treatment is no longer needed.
    b. The most effective route of androgen replacement is the oral route.
    c. Testosterone replacement therapy is contraindicated in men with prostate cancer.
    d. Clomiphene citrate (Clomid) is used to suppress ovulation in women.

16. The female patient has been prescribed hormone replacement therapy. What does the nurse instruct the patient to do regarding this therapy?
    a. Report any recurrence of symptoms, such as decreased libido, between injections.
    b. Monitor blood pressure at least weekly for potential hypotension.
    c. Treat leg pain, especially in the calves, with gentle muscle stretching.
    d. Take measures to reduce risk for hypertension and thrombosis.

17. The patient suspected of having abnormal pituitary function has a circulating GH level of 9 ng/mL 1 hour after receiving 100 g of oral glucose. What does the nurse suspect in this patient?
    a. Anterior pituitary hypofunction
    b. Posterior pituitary hypofunction
    c. Anterior pituitary hyperfunction
    d. Posterior pituitary hyperfunction

18. The patient is recovering from a transsphenoidal hypophysectomy. What postoperative nursing interventions apply to this patient? *(Select all that apply.)*
    a. Vigorous coughing and deep-breathing exercises
    b. Instructing on the use of a soft-bristled toothbrush for brushing the teeth
    c. Strict monitoring of fluid balance
    d. Hourly neurologic checks for first 24 hours
    e. Instructing the patient to alert the nurse regarding postnasal drip

19. Following a hypophysectomy, the patient requires instruction on hormone replacement for which hormones? *(Select all that apply.)*
    a. Cortisol
    b. Thyroid
    c. Gonadal
    d. Vasopressin
    e. PRL

20. After a hypophysectomy, home care monitoring by the nurse includes assessing which factors? *(Select all that apply.)*
    a. Hypoglycemia
    b. Bowel habits
    c. Possible leakage of cerebrospinal fluid (CSF)
    d. 24-hour intake of fluids and urine output
    e. 24-hour diet recall
    f. Activity level

21. Postoperative care for the patient who has had a transsphenoidal hypophysectomy includes which intervention?
    a. Encouraging coughing and deep breathing to decrease pulmonary complications
    b. Testing nasal drainage for glucose to determine whether it contains CSF
    c. Keeping the bed flat to decrease central CSF leakage
    d. Assisting the patient with brushing the teeth to reduce risk of infection

22. A postoperative "halo sign" is indicative of which condition?
    a. Worsening neurologic status of the patient
    b. Drainage of CSF from the patient's nose
    c. Onset of postoperative infection
    d. Onset of postoperative visual disturbance

23. The patient with a hypophysectomy can postoperatively experience transient diabetes insipidus. Which manifestation alerts the nurse to this problem?
    a. Output much greater than intake
    b. Change in mental status indicating confusion
    c. Laboratory results indicating hyponatremia
    d. Nonpitting edema

24. The action of ADH influences normal kidney function by stimulating which mechanism?
    a. Glomerulus to control the filtration rate
    b. Proximal nephron tubules to reabsorb water
    c. Distal nephron tubules and collecting ducts to reabsorb water
    d. Constriction of glomerular capillaries to prevent loss of protein in urine

25. What is the disorder that results from a deficiency of vasopressin (ADH) from the posterior pituitary gland called?
    a. SIADH
    b. Diabetes insipidus
    c. Cushing's syndrome
    d. Addison's disease

True or False? *Read the statements about diabetes insipidus and write T for true or F for false in the blanks provided. If the statement is false, correct the statement to make it true.*

_____ 26. Because the fluid lost is isotonic, the patient's plasma osmolality remains normal.

_____ 27. The primary indication of diabetes insipidus is the patient's decreased urinary output and thirst.

_____ 28. The primary complications of diabetes insipidus are hypovolemia and shock.

_____ 29. A diagnostic test for diabetes insipidus is urine specific gravity greater than 1.005.

_____ 30. Urine output of greater than 4 L/24 hours is the first diagnostic indication of diabetes insipidus.

31. What does the nurse instruct patients with permanent diabetes insipidus to do?
    a. Continue vasopressin therapy until symptoms disappear.
    b. Monitor for recurrence of polydipsia and polyuria.
    c. Monitor and record weight twice a week.
    d. Check urine specific gravity three times a week.

32. The patient uses desmopressin acetate metered dose spray as a replacement hormone for ADH. Which is an indication for another dose? *(Select all that apply.)*
    a. Excessive urination
    b. Specific gravity of 1.003
    c. Dark, concentrated urine
    d. Edema in the legs
    e. Decreased urination

33. The patient is undergoing a dehydration test for diabetes insipidus. Which statements regarding this test are correct? *(Select all that apply.)*
    a. Teach the patient that fluid restriction must be maintained for accurate results.
    b. Administer a normal water load followed by infusion of hypertonic saline.
    c. Measure urine output, specific gravity, and osmolality hourly.
    d. Five units of aqueous vasopressin are given for this test.
    e. Weigh the patient hourly.

34. Which oral medication is *not* used to treat mild diabetes insipidus?
    a. Chlorpropamide (Diabinese)
    b. Indomethacin (Indocin)
    c. Lithium (Eskalith)
    d. Lypressin (Diapid)

35. Upon taking a history, which patients are associated with the development of SIADH?
    a. 27-year-old patient on high-dose steroids
    b. 47-year-old hospitalized adult patient with acute renal failure
    c. 58-year-old with metastatic lung or breast cancer
    d. Older adult with history of a stroke within the last year

36. In the chart below, compare diabetes insipidus with the SIADH.

	Cause	Evidence
Diabetes insipidus		
SIADH		

37. Which statement about the pathophysiology of SIADH is correct?
    a. ADH secretion is inhibited in the presence of low plasma osmolality.
    b. Water retention results in dilutional hyponatremia and expanded extracellular fluid (ECF) volume.
    c. The glomerulus is unable to increase its filtration rate to reduce the excess plasma volume.
    d. Renin and aldosterone are released and help to decrease the loss of urinary sodium.

38. Which statement about the etiology and incidence of SIADH is correct?
    a. Malignant cells act on the posterior pituitary gland to decrease ADH release.
    b. Demeclocycline may be used to treat SIADH.
    c. Ectopic ADH production can result from benign gastrointestinal polyps.
    d. SIADH that results from vasopressin overdose in diabetes insipidus is irreversible.

39. The effect of increased ADH in the blood results in which effect on the kidney?
    a. Urine concentration tends to decrease.
    b. Glomerular filtration tends to decrease.
    c. Tubular reabsorption of water increases.
    d. Tubular reabsorption of sodium increases.

40. In SIADH as a result of water retention from excess ADH, which laboratory value does the nurse expect to find? *(Select all that apply.)*
    a. Increased urine osmolality (increased sodium in urine)
    b. Elevated serum sodium level
    c. Increased specific gravity (concentrated urine)
    d. Decreased serum osmolarity
    e. Decreased urine specific gravity

41. Which nursing intervention is the priority for the patient with SIADH?
    a. Restrict fluid intake.
    b. Monitor neurologic status at least every 2 hours.
    c. Offer ice chips frequently to ease discomfort of dry mouth.
    d. Monitor urine tests for decreased sodium levels and low specific gravity.

42. Which type of IV fluid does the nurse use to treat the patient with SIADH?
    a. D_5 1/2 normal saline
    b. D_5W
    c. 3% normal saline
    d. Normal saline

43. In addition to IV fluids, the patient is on a fluid restriction as low as 500 to 600 mL/24 hours. Indicate the serum and urine results that demonstrate effectiveness of this treatment by writing *increases* or *decreases* for each item below.

    a. Urine specific gravity results _____

    b. Serum sodium results _____

    c. Urine output _____

44. Which statement about pheochromocytoma is correct?
    a. It is most often malignant.
    b. It is a catecholamine-producing tumor.
    c. It is found only in the adrenal medulla.
    d. It is manifested by hypotension.

45. The patient in the emergency department is diagnosed with possible pheochromocytoma. What is the priority nursing intervention for this patient?
    a. Monitor the patient's intake and output and urine specific gravity.
    b. Monitor blood pressure for severe hypertension.
    c. Monitor blood pressure for severe hypotension.
    d. Administer medication to increase cardiac output.

46. The nurse expects to perform which diagnostic test for pheochromocytoma?
    a. 24-hour urine collection for sodium, potassium, and glucose
    b. Catecholamine stimulation test
    c. Administration of beta-adrenergic blocking agent and monitor results
    d. 24-hour urine collection for vanillylmandelic acid (VMA)

47. Which intervention applies to the patient with pheochromocytoma?
    a. Assist to sit in a chair for blood pressure monitoring.
    b. Instruct not to smoke or drink coffee.
    c. Encourage to maintain an active exercise schedule including activity such as running.
    d. Encourage one glass of red wine nightly to promote rest.

48. Which intervention is contraindicated for the patient with pheochromocytoma?
    a. Monitoring blood pressure
    b. Palpating the abdomen
    c. Collecting 24-hour urine specimens
    d. Instructing the patient to limit activity

49. Which diuretic is ordered by the physician to treat hyperaldosteronism?
    a. Furosemide (Lasix)
    b. Ethacrynic acid (Edecrin)
    c. Bumetanide (Bumex)
    d. Spironolactone (Aldactone)

50. Which statement about hyperaldosteronism is correct?
    a. Painful "charley horses" are common from hyperkalemia.
    b. It occurs more often in men than in women.
    c. It is a common cause of hypertension in the population.
    d. Hypokalemia and hypertension are the main issues.

51. When diagnosed with Cushing's syndrome, the manifestations are most likely related to an excess production of which hormone?
    a. Insulin from the pancreas
    b. ADH from posterior pituitary gland
    c. PRL from anterior pituitary gland
    d. Cortisol from the adrenal cortex

52. What is the most common cause of endogenous hypercortisolism, or Cushing's syndrome?
    a. Pituitary hypoplasia
    b. Insufficient ACTH production
    c. Adrenocortical hormone deficiency
    d. Hyperplasia of the adrenal cortex

53. Which are physical findings of Cushing's syndrome? *(Select all that apply.)*
    a. "Moon-faced" appearance
    b. Decreased amount of body hair
    c. Barrel chest
    d. Truncal obesity
    e. Coarse facial features
    f. Thin, easily damaged skin
    g. Excessive sweating
    h. Extremity muscle wasting

54. When assessing the patient with Cushing's syndrome, what does the nurse expect to find?
    a. Signs of dehydration
    b. Facial flushing
    c. Hypertension
    d. Muscle hypertrophy

55. Which laboratory findings does the nurse expect to find with Cushing's syndrome? *(Select all that apply.)*
    a. Decreased serum sodium
    b. Increased serum glucose
    c. Increased serum sodium
    d. Increased serum potassium
    e. Decreased serum potassium

56. The female patient with Cushing's syndrome expresses concern about the changes in her general appearance. The nurse determines a nursing diagnosis of Disturbed Body Image. What is the desired outcome for this patient?
    a. To verbalize an understanding that treatment will reverse many of the problems
    b. To ventilate about the frustration of these lifelong physical changes
    c. To verbalize ways to cope with the changes such as joining a support group or changing style of dress
    d. To achieve a personal desired level of sexual functioning

Matching. Match each drug with its corresponding clinical use for hypercortisolism.

Drugs
a. Mitotane (Lysodren)
b. Aminoglutethimide (Cytadren)
c. Cyproheptadine (Periactin)

Clinical Uses
_____ 57. Adrenal cytotoxic agent used for inoperable adrenal tumors
_____ 58. Interferes with ACTH production
_____ 59. Adrenal enzyme inhibitor that decreases cortisol production

60. The patient is scheduled for bilateral adrenalectomy. Before surgery, steroids are to be given. Which is the reasoning behind the administration of this drug?
    a. To promote glycogen storage by the liver for body energy reserves
    b. To compensate for sudden lack of adrenal hormones following surgery
    c. To increase the body's inflammatory response to promote scar formation
    d. To enhance urinary excretion of salt and water following surgery

61. The nurse is teaching the patient being discharged after bilateral adrenalectomy. What medication information does the nurse emphasize in the teaching plan?
    a. The dosage of steroid replacement drugs will be consistent throughout the patient's lifetime.
    b. The steroid drugs should be taken in the evening so as not to interfere with sleep.
    c. The patient should take the drugs on an empty stomach.
    d. The patient should learn how to give himself an intramuscular injection of hydrocortisone.

62. Which statement about the patient with hyperaldosteronism after a successful unilateral adrenalectomy is correct?
    a. The low-sodium diet must be continued postoperatively.
    b. Glucocorticoid replacement therapy is temporary.
    c. Spironolactone (Aldactone) must be taken for life.
    d. Additional measures are needed to control hypertension.

63. Which are causes for decreased production of adrenocortical steroids? *(Select all that apply.)*
    a. Inadequate secretion of ACTH
    b. Dysfunction of hypothalamic-pituitary control mechanism
    c. Adrenal gland dysfunction
    d. Cancer
    e. AIDS

64. Which patient is at risk for developing secondary adrenal insufficiency?
    a. Patient who suddenly stops taking high-dose steroid therapy
    b. Patient who tapers the dosages of steroid therapy
    c. Patient deficient in ADH
    d. Patient with an adrenal tumor causing excessive secretion of ACTH

65. An ACTH stimulation test is the most definitive test for which disorder?
    a. Adrenal insufficiency
    b. Cushing's syndrome
    c. Pheochromocytoma
    d. Acromegaly

66. Which interventions are necessary for the patient with acute adrenal insufficiency (Addisonian crisis)? *(Select all that apply.)*
    a. IV infusion of normal saline
    b. IV infusion of 3% saline
    c. Hourly glucose monitoring
    d. Insulin administration
    e. IV potassium therapy

67. The patient in the emergency department who reports lethargy, muscle weakness, nausea, vomiting, and weight loss over the past weeks is diagnosed with Addisonian crisis (acute adrenal insufficiency). Which drugs does the nurse expect to administer to this patient?
    a. Beta blocker to control the hypertension and dysrhythmias
    b. Solu-Cortef IV along with IM injections of hydrocortisone
    c. IV fluids of D_5NS with KCl added for dehydration
    d. Spironolactone (Aldactone) to promote diuresis

68. The nurse determines that the administration of hydrocortisone for Addisonian crisis is effective when which assessment is made?
    a. Increased urine output
    b. No signs of pitting edema
    c. Weight gain
    d. Lethargy improving; patient alert and oriented

69. Complete the chart below by comparing the clinical findings in adrenal insufficiency with those in Cushing's syndrome. Write *increase* or *decrease* in each box.

Clinical Finding	Adrenal Insufficiency	Cushing's Syndrome
a. Serum sodium level		
b. Serum potassium level		
c. ECF volume		
d. Blood pressure		
e. Serum glucose level		
f. Cortisol level		

70. Which nursing intervention is a preventive measure for adrenocortical insufficiency?
    a. Maintaining diuretic therapy
    b. Instructing the patient on salt restriction
    c. Reducing high-dose glucocorticoid therapy quickly
    d. Reducing high-dose glucocorticoid doses gradually

71. The patient on prolonged cortisone therapy is instructed to observe for and report signs of which sign/symptom?
    a. Anuria and hypoglycemia
    b. Weight gain and moon face
    c. Anorexia and muscle twitches
    d. Hypotension and fluid loss

CASE STUDY: THE PATIENT WITH DIABETES INSIPIDUS

Use a separate sheet of paper to answer the questions in this Case Study. Answer guidelines for this Case Study are available on your Evolve website at http://evolve. elsevier.com/Iggy/ in the "Prepare for Class" folder.

A 22-year-old man has been admitted to the emergency department after his girlfriend found him lying on the floor of their apartment. He had fallen off a ladder 2 days ago but "seemed fine," according to the girlfriend, even though he had hit his head slightly when he fell. He never lost consciousness. He has a few abrasions on his arms, face, and legs, and is drowsy but arousable. His girlfriend states that yesterday he started "going to the bathroom nonstop" and he drank "everything in sight" because he was so thirsty. A magnetic resonance imaging (MRI) scan reveals a small intracerebral hemorrhage, and he is admitted to the intensive care unit with the diagnosis of head trauma and diabetes insipidus.

1. What physical and laboratory findings led to the diagnosis of diabetes insipidus?

2. The physician is considering whether this patient is a candidate for the fluid deprivation and hypertonic saline tests to confirm the diagnosis of diabetes insipidus. How is this determined?

3. Identify potential nursing diagnoses for this patient based on the above data.

4. Identify nursing measures that would assist the patient to maintain an adequate fluid balance. State the rationale for these measures.

5. The physician initially orders aqueous vasopressin (Pitressin) 10 units IM every 3 to 4 hours as indicated. How does the nurse determine when to give the medication?

66 CHAPTER

Care of Patients with Problems of the Thyroid and Parathyroid Glands

STUDY/REVIEW QUESTIONS

1. The nurse is performing a physical examination of the patient's thyroid gland. Precautions are taken in performing the correct technique because palpation can result in which occurrence?
   a. Damage to the esophagus causing gastric reflux
   b. Obstruction of the carotid arteries causing a stroke
   c. Pressure on the trachea and laryngeal nerve causing hoarseness
   d. Exacerbation of symptoms by releasing additional thyroid hormone

Matching. *Differentiate the general assessment findings by matching them with the corresponding type of thyroid deficiency. Answers will be used more than once.*

Thyroid Deficiencies
a. Hyperthyroidism
b. Hypothyroidism

Assessment Findings
_____ 2. Weight loss with increased appetite
_____ 3. Constipation
_____ 4. Increased heart rate, palpitations
_____ 5. Photophobia
_____ 6. Manic behavior
_____ 7. Decreased libido
_____ 8. Dyspnea with or without exertion
_____ 9. Insomnia
_____ 10. Cold intolerance
_____ 11. Increased stools
_____ 12. Corneal ulcers
_____ 13. Fatigue, increased sleeping
_____ 14. Irritability
_____ 15. Impaired memory
_____ 16. Fine, soft, silky body hair
_____ 17. Facial puffiness
_____ 18. Increased libido
_____ 19. Heat intolerance, warm skin
_____ 20. Weight gain
_____ 21. Dry, coarse, brittle hair
_____ 22. Diaphoresis
_____ 23. Tremors

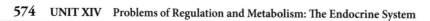

24. Which factor is the hallmark assessment finding that signifies hyperthyroidism?
    a. Weight loss
    b. Increased libido
    c. Heat intolerance
    d. Diarrhea

25. Which factor is a main assessment finding that signifies hypothyroidism?
    a. Irritability
    b. Cold intolerance
    c. Constipation
    d. Fatigue

26. Which sign/symptom is one of the first indicators of hyperthyroidism that is often noticed by the patient?
    a. Eyelid or globe lag
    b. Vision changes or tiring of the eyes
    c. Protruding eyes
    d. Photophobia

27. Which laboratory result is consistent with a diagnosis of hyperthyroidism?
    a. Decreased serum triiodothyronine (T_3) and thyroxine (T_4) levels
    b. Elevated serum thyrotropin-releasing hormone (TRH) level
    c. Decreased radioactive iodine uptake
    d. Increased serum T_3 and T_4

28. The laboratory results for the 53-year-old patient indicate a low T_3 level and elevated TSH. What do these results indicate?
    a. Hyperthyroidism
    b. Hypothyroidism
    c. Malfunctioning pituitary gland
    d. Normal laboratory values for this age

29. The clinical manifestation resulting from an increase in thyroid hormone production is known as which condition?
    a. Thyrotoxicosis
    b. Euthyroid function
    c. Graves' disease
    d. Hypermetabolism

30. What is the most common cause of hyperthyroidism?
    a. Radiation to thyroid
    b. Graves' disease
    c. Thyroid cancer
    d. Thyroiditis

31. The nurse is examining the patient with a goiter and notes that the mass is not visible with the neck in the normal position, but the goiter can be palpated and moves up when the patient swallows. What grade does the nurse classify this goiter as?
    a. 0
    b. 1
    c. 2
    d. 3

Matching. *Match the assessment finding associated with hyperthyroidism and Graves' disease with the correct name.*

Names
a. Globe lag
b. Pretibial myxedema
c. Eyelid retraction
d. Exophthalmos
e. Goiter

Assessment Findings

_____ 32. Enlargement of the thyroid gland, noticeable swelling of the neck

_____ 33. Dry, waxy swelling of the front surfaces of the lower legs

_____ 34. Abnormal protrusion of the eyes

_____ 35. Upper eyelid fails to descend when the patient gazes downward

_____ 36. Upper eyelid pulls back faster than the eyeball when the patient gazes upward

True or False? *Read the statements about hypothyroidism and hyperthyroidism and write T for true or F for false in the blanks provided. If the statement is false, correct the statement to make it true.*

_____ 37. Exophthalmos only occurs in hyperthyroidism resulting from Graves' disease.

_____ 38. Graves' disease is hereditary.

_____ 39. A decreased metabolic rate results in TSH binding to thyroid cells, causing an enlarged thyroid.

_____ 40. Hypothyroidism can occur anytime throughout the life span.

_____ 41. Hypothyroidism and hyperthyroidism occur more frequently in women than men.

_____ 42. Simple goiter associated with hypothyroidism is usually due to insufficient iodine intake.

_____ 43. Hashimoto's disease is a type of hypothyroidism.

_____ 44. The effect of antithyroid medication can be delayed due to storage and release of large amounts of thyroid hormone.

_____ 45. Hypothyroidism causes elevated systolic pressure, wide pulse pressure, tachycardia, and dysrhythmias.

_____ 46. Thyroid storm following surgical intervention for hyperthyroidism is rare because of pretreatment with medications.

_____ 47. Euthyroid is defined as near-normal thyroid function.

_____ 48. Radiation precautions are required with treatment of ^{131}I for hyperthyroidism.

_____ 49. Nonsurgical treatment is the preferred treatment for hyperthyroidism.

50. Laboratory findings of elevated T_3 and T_4, decreased TSH, and high thyrotropin receptor antibody titer indicate which condition?
   a. Multinodular goiter
   b. Hyperthyroidism related to overmedication
   c. Pituitary tumor suppressing TSH
   d. Graves' disease

Matching. Match the cause of hyperthyroidism with its mechanism.

Causes

a. Thyroid carcinoma
b. Thyroiditis (radiation-induced)
c. Graves' disease
d. Toxic multinodular goiter
e. Pituitary hyperthyroidism

Mechanisms

_____ 51. Autoimmune disease; antibodies bind to TSH receptors and keep them activated, increasing the size of the gland and increasing the production of thyroid hormones.

_____ 52. Uncommon; usually occurs with large follicular carcinomas.

_____ 53. T_3 and T_4 secretion increased before destruction of gland. Hyperthyroid state usually transient.

_____ 54. Multiple thyroid nodules resulting in thyroid hyperfunction.

_____ 55. Pituitary adenoma resulting in excessive TSH secretion.

56. After a visit to the physician's office, the patient is diagnosed with general thyroid enlargement and elevated thyroid hormone level. This is an indication of which condition?
   a. Hyperthyroidism and goiter
   b. Hypothyroidism and goiter
   c. Nodules on the parathyroid gland
   d. Thyroid or parathyroid cancer

57. Which condition is a life-threatening emergency and serious complication of untreated or poorly treated hypothyroidism?
   a. Endemic goiter
   b. Myxedema coma
   c. Toxic multinodular goiter
   d. Thyroiditis

58. The patient with exophthalmos from hyperthyroidism reports dry eyes, especially in the morning. The nurse teaches the patient to perform which intervention to help correct this problem?
   a. Wear sunglasses at all times when outside in the bright sun.
   b. Use cool compresses to the eye four times a day.
   c. Tape the eyes closed with nonallergenic tape.
   d. There is nothing that can be done to relieve this problem.

59. Which factors are considered to be triggers for thyroid storm? *(Select all that apply.)*
   a. Infection
   b. Cold temperatures
   c. Vigorous palpation of a goiter
   d. Pregnancy
   e. Extremely warm temperatures

60. The patient has the following assessment findings: elevated TSH level, low T_3 and T_4 level, difficulty with memory, lethargy, and muscle stiffness. These are clinical manifestations of which disorder?
   a. Hypothyroidism
   b. Hyperthyroidism
   c. Hypoparathyroidism
   d. Hyperparathyroidism

61. The patient has been prescribed thyroid hormone for treatment of hypothyroidism. Within what time frame does the patient expect improvement in mental awareness with this treatment?
   a. A few days
   b. 2 weeks
   c. 1 month
   d. 3 months

62. Which factors are assessment findings indicative of thyroid storm? *(Select all that apply.)*
    a. Abdominal pain and nausea
    b. Hypothermia
    c. Fever
    d. Tachycardia
    e. Elevated systolic blood pressure
    f. Bradycardia

63. Management of the patient with hyperthyroidism focuses on which goals? *(Select all that apply.)*
    a. Blocking the effects of excessive thyroid secretion
    b. Treating the signs and symptoms the patient experiences
    c. Establishing euthyroid function
    d. Preventing spread of the disease
    e. Maintaining an environment of reduced stimulation

Matching. *Match each characteristic with its corresponding intervention for hyperthyroidism. Answers may be used more than once. Choose all answers that apply to each characteristic.*

Interventions for Hyperthyroidism
a. Antithyroid drug Tapazole
b. Antithyroid drug PTU
c. Iodine preparations
d. Lithium carbonate
e. Beta-blocking agents (Inderal)
f. Radioactive iodine (^{131}I)
g. Subtotal thyroidectomy
h. Total thyroidectomy
i. Dexamethasone

Characteristics

_____ 64. Discontinued if sore throat, fever, headache, or skin eruptions occur

_____ 65. Use includes preoperative treatment to obtain euthyroid

_____ 66. Action decreases the production of thyroid hormone

_____ 67. Works to control symptoms related to sympathetic nervous system of tachycardia, palpations, anxiety, and diaphoresis

_____ 68. Requires lifelong thyroid replacement

_____ 69. Limited use due to side effects

_____ 70. Taken with food

_____ 71. Monitor for hypothyroidism over time

_____ 72. Contraindicated in pregnancy; crosses placental barrier

_____ 73. Administered around the clock

_____ 74. May require antithyroid medication for up to 8 weeks past treatment

_____ 75. Acts to decrease blood flow to reduce hormone production with results in 2 to 6 weeks

_____ 76. Works by damaging thyroid gland

_____ 77. Removal of all of the thyroid gland

_____ 78. Instruct the patient to avoid crowds and sick people due to reduced immune response

_____ 79. Treatment for thyroid cancer

80. Which are preoperative instructions for the patient having thyroid surgery? *(Select all that apply.)*
    a. Teach postoperative restrictions such as no coughing and deep-breathing exercises to prevent strain on the suture line.
    b. Teach the moving and turning technique of manually supporting the head and avoiding neck extension to minimize strain on the suture line.
    c. Inform the patient that hoarseness for a few days after surgery is usually the result of a breathing tube (endotracheal tube) used during surgery but will be monitored with respiration and weakness of voice.
    d. Humidification of air may be helpful to promote expectoration of secretions. Suctioning may also be used.
    e. Clarify any questions regarding placement of incision, complications, and postoperative care.
    f. A supine position and lying flat will be maintained postoperatively to avoid strain on suture line.
    g. Teach the patient to report immediately any respiratory difficulty, tingling around the lips or fingers, or muscular twitching.
    h. A drain may be present in the incision. All drainage and dressings will be monitored closely for 24 hours.

81. The nurse is preparing for the patient to return from thyroid surgery. What priority equipment does the nurse ensure is immediately available? *(Select all that apply.)*
    a. Tracheostomy equipment
    b. Calcium gluconate or calcium chloride for IV administration
    c. Humidified oxygen
    d. Suction equipment
    e. Sandbags

82. After a thyroidectomy, the patient reports tingling around the mouth and muscle twitching. Which complication do these assessment findings indicate to the nurse?
    a. Hemorrhage
    b. Respiratory distress
    c. Thyroid storm
    d. Hypocalcemia, parathyroid gland injury

83. The nurse assesses the patient post-thyroidectomy for laryngeal nerve damage. Which findings indicate this complication? *(Select all that apply.)*
    a. Dyspnea
    b. Sore throat
    c. Hoarseness
    d. Weak voice
    e. Dry cough

84. After hospitalization for myxedema, the patient is prescribed thyroid replacement medication. Which statement by the patient demonstrates a correct understanding of this therapy?
    a. "I'll be taking this medication until my symptoms are completely resolved."
    b. "I'll be taking thyroid medication for the rest of my life."
    c. "Now that I'm feeling better, no changes in my medication will be necessary."
    d. "I'm taking this medication to prevent symptoms of an overactive thyroid gland."

Matching. *Match each characteristic with its corresponding thyroid disorder. Answers may be used more than once.*

Thyroid Disorders
a. Thyroiditis
b. Hashimoto's disease
c. Acute thyroiditis
d. Subacute thyroiditis

Characteristics

_____ 85. Defined as inflammation of the thyroid gland

_____ 86. "Chronic thyroiditis"

_____ 87. Common in age range 30s to 50s

_____ 88. Caused by viral infection of thyroid gland after an upper respiratory infection

_____ 89. Bacterial infection of thyroid gland

_____ 90. Subtotal thyroidectomy is a form of treatment

_____ 91. Treated with antibiotics

_____ 92. Treated with thyroid replacement hormone

_____ 93. Diagnosed by circulating antithyroid antibodies and needle biopsy

94. Serum calcium levels are maintained by which hormone?
a. Cortisol
b. Calcium
c. Antidiuretic hormone (ADH)
d. Parathyroid hormone (PTH)

Matching. *Match each hormone with its corresponding effect on serum calcium levels.*

Effects
a. Raises levels
b. Lowers levels

Hormones
_____ 95. PTH production
_____ 96. Calcitonin production

97. Bone changes in the older adult are often seen with endocrine dysfunction and increased secretion of which substance?
a. PTH
b. Calcitonin
c. Insulin
d. Testosterone

98. In addition to regulation of calcium levels, PTH and calcitonin regulate the circulating blood levels of which substance?
a. Potassium
b. Sodium
c. Phosphate
d. Chloride

99. The patient has a positive Trousseau's or Chvostek's sign resulting from hypoparathyroidism. What condition does this assessment finding indicate?
a. Hypercalcemia
b. Hypocalcemia
c. Hyperphosphatemia
d. Hypophosphatemia

100. Which food does the nurse instruct the patient with hypoparathyroidism to avoid?
a. Canned vegetables
b. Fresh fruit
c. Red meat
d. Milk

101. The patient with continuous spasms of the muscles is diagnosed with hypoparathyroidism. The muscle spasms are a clinical manifestation of which condition?
    a. Nerve damage
    b. Seizures
    c. Tetany
    d. Decreased potassium

Matching. *Match the parathyroid disorders with their causes. Answers will be used more than once.*

Parathyroid Disorders
a.   Hypoparathyroidism
b.   Hyperparathyroidism

Causes
_____ 102. Chronic renal disease
_____ 103. Vitamin D deficiency
_____ 104. Removal of the thyroid gland
_____ 105. Neck trauma
_____ 106. Carcinoma of the lung, kidney, or GI tract producing PTH-like substance
_____ 107. Parathyroidectomy

108. When interpreting laboratory values, what does the nurse expect to find in relation to hypoparathyroidism and hyperparathyroidism? Indicate *increase* or *decrease* in the adult normal range for each laboratory test listed below.

Laboratory Test	Hyperparathyroidism	Hypoparathyroidism
a. Serum calcium		
b. Serum phosphate		
c. Serum PTH		

109. The patient has hyperparathyroidism and high levels of serum calcium. Which initial treatment does the nurse prepare to administer to the patient?
    a. Force fluids (intravenous or oral) and administer Lasix
    b. Calcitonin
    c. Oral phosphates
    d. Mithramycin

110. Which are assessment findings of hypocalcemia? *(Select all that apply.)*
    a. Numbness and tingling around the mouth
    b. Muscle cramping
    c. Mental status changes including irritability
    d. Fever
    e. Tachycardia

111. Which medication therapies does the nurse expect patients with hypoparathyroidism to receive? *(Select all that apply.)*
    a. Calcium chloride
    b. Calcium gluconate
    c. Calcitrol
    d. Magnesium sulfate
    e. Ergocalciferol

112. Discharge planning for the patient with chronic hypoparathyroidism include which instructions? *(Select all that apply.)*
    a. Prescribed medications must be taken for the patient's entire life.
    b. Eat foods low in vitamin D and high in phosphorus.
    c. Eat foods high in calcium but low in phosphorus.
    d. After several weeks, medications can be discontinued.
    e. Kidney stones are no longer a risk to the patient.

113. In older adults, assessment findings of fatigue, altered thought processes, dry skin, and constipation are often mistaken for signs of aging rather than assessment findings for which endocrine disorder?
    a. Hyperthyroidism
    b. Hypothyroidism
    c. Hyperparathyroidism
    d. Hypoparathyroidism

114. Which conditions may precipitate myxedema coma? *(Select all that apply.)*
    a. Rapid withdrawal of thyroid medication
    b. Vitamin D deficiency
    c. Untreated hypothyroidism
    d. Surgery
    e. Excessive exposure to iodine

CASE STUDY: THE PATIENT WITH ENDOCRINE PROBLEMS

Use a separate sheet of paper to answer the questions in this Case Study. Answer guidelines for this Case Study are available on your Evolve website at http://evolve. elsevier.com/Iggy/ in the "Prepare for Class" folder.

The nurse is caring for a 41-year-old woman who is the mother of two small children. She states that she has felt "nervous and tired" for approximately 1 month. Today she has had a sudden onset of breathlessness with cardiac palpitations. She states "I have not been feeling well for about a month, but when I felt breathless I thought I should be checked out." Upon further questioning the nurse finds that the woman also has had a loss of weight of approximately 30 lbs., frequent loose stools, loss of hair on the scalp, and a feeling of "burning up."

1. What findings would the nurse expect to see on physical examination of this patient?

2. What laboratory tests would the nurse expect to be ordered for this patient? What abnormalities could be expected for these laboratory tests?

3. Identify four nursing diagnoses for this patient.

4. What nonsurgical interventions would the nurse expect to be ordered for this patient?

5. If surgical intervention is necessary, what preoperative care would the nurse anticipate?

6. If surgical intervention is employed, identify the appropriate postoperative care for this patient.

7. Identify complications of the surgical procedure that the nurse should remain alert for.

Care of Patients with Diabetes Mellitus

CHAPTER 67

STUDY/REVIEW QUESTIONS

Matching. Match the descriptions with the corresponding type of diabetes. Answers may be used more than once.

Types of Diabetes
a. Type 1
b. Type 2
c. Gestational

Descriptions

_____ 1. Diagnosis based on results of 100G glucose tolerance test.

_____ 2. Cells have a reduced ability to respond to insulin.

_____ 3. Autoimmune process is causing beta cell destruction.

_____ 4. Carbohydrate intolerance is first recognized during pregnancy.

_____ 5. Most who suffer with this type of diabetes are obese adults.

_____ 6. Usually abrupt onset of thirst and weight loss.

7. Which statement is true about insulin?
   a. It is secreted by alpha cells in the islets of Langerhans.
   b. It is a catabolic hormone that builds up glucagon reserves.
   c. It is necessary for glucose transport across cell membranes.
   d. It is stored in muscles and converted to fat for storage.

8. Why is glucose vital to the body's cells?
   a. It is used to build cell membranes.
   b. It is used by cells to produce energy.
   c. It affects the process of protein metabolism.
   d. It provides nutrients for genetic material.

Matching. Match the terms with their correct definitions.

Terms
a. Polydipsia
b. Polyphagia
c. Polyuria

Definitions

_____ 9. Frequent urination

_____ 10. Frequent fluid intake

_____ 11. Frequent eating

12. Which individual is at greatest risk for developing type 2 diabetes mellitus?
    a. 25-year-old African-American woman
    b. 36-year-old African-American man
    c. 56-year-old Hispanic woman
    d. 40-year-old Hispanic man

13. Which of the following four laboratory findings is most indicative of diabetes mellitus?
    a. Fasting blood glucose = 80 mg/dL
    b. 2-hour postprandial blood glucose = 110 mg/dL
    c. 1-hour glucose tolerance blood glucose = 110 mg/dL
    d. 2-hour glucose tolerance blood glucose = 210 mg/dL

14. Untreated hyperglycemia results in which condition?
    a. Respiratory acidosis
    b. Metabolic alkalosis
    c. Respiratory alkalosis
    d. Metabolic acidosis

15. What is the respiratory pattern of the patient with untreated hyperglycemia?
    a. Rapid and shallow (tachypneic)
    b. Deep and labored (Cheyne-Stokes respiration)
    c. Rapid and deep (Kussmaul respiration)
    d. Shallow and labored (Biot respiration)

16. Which electrolyte is most affected by hyperglycemia?
    a. Sodium
    b. Chloride
    c. Potassium
    d. Magnesium

17. Which complications of diabetes mellitus are considered emergencies? *(Select all that apply.)*
    a. Diabetic ketoacidosis (DKA)
    b. Hypoglycemia
    c. Diabetic retinopathy
    d. Hyperglycemic-hyperosmolar state (HHS)
    e. Diabetic neuropathy

18. In determining if the patient is hypoglycemic, the nurse looks for which characteristics in addition to checking the patient's blood glucose? *(Select all that apply.)*
    a. Nausea
    b. Hunger
    c. Irritability
    d. Palpitations
    e. Profuse perspiration
    f. Rapid deep respirations

19. Which factors differentiate DKA from HHS? *(Select all that apply.)*
    a. Level of hyperglycemia
    b. Amount of ketones produced
    c. Potassium levels
    d. Amount of volume depletion
    e. Dosage of insulin needed

20. The patient is admitted with a blood glucose level of 900 mg/dL. IV fluids and insulin are administered. Two hours after treatment is initiated, the blood glucose level is 400 mg/dL. Which complication is the patient most at risk for developing?
    a. Hypoglycemia
    b. Pulmonary embolus
    c. Renal shutdown
    d. Pulmonary edema

21. What type of insulin is used in the emergency treatment of DKA and hyperglycemic-hyperosmolar nonketotic syndrome (HHNS)?
    a. NPH
    b. Lente
    c. Regular
    d. Protamine zinc

22. Early treatment of DKA and HHNS includes IV administration of which fluid?
    a. Glucagon
    b. Potassium
    c. Bicarbonate
    d. Normal saline

23. Glucagon is used primarily to treat the patient with which disorder?
    a. DKA
    b. Idiosyncratic reaction to insulin
    c. Severe hypoglycemia
    d. HHNS

24. Why is glucagon given in a dextrose solution?
    a. Dextrose promotes more storage of glucose in the liver.
    b. Dextrose stimulates the pancreas to produce more insulin.
    c. Dextrose increases blood sugar levels at a controlled rate.
    d. Dextrose inhibits glycogenesis, gluconeogenesis, and lipolysis.

25. When glucagon is administered, what does it do?
    a. Competes for insulin at the receptor sites
    b. Frees glucose from hepatic stores of glycogen
    c. Supplies glycogen directly to the vital tissues
    d. Provides a glucose substitute for rapid replacement

Matching. Match each etiologic factor with its corresponding type of diabetes mellitus. Answers may be used more than once.

Types of DM
a. Type 1
b. Type 2
c. Gestational

Etiologic Factors

_____ 26. Aging process

_____ 27. Autoimmune process

_____ 28. Islet cell antibodies

_____ 29. Obesity

_____ 30. Heredity

_____ 31. Pregnancy

_____ 32. Viral infection

_____ 33. Decreased physical activity

34. Which are preventive measures for diabetes mellitus?
    a. Controlling hypertension
    b. Prenatal care beginning the third trimester of pregnancy
    c. Working in a low-stress environment
    d. Maintaining ideal body weight

35. The diabetic patient is scheduled to have a blood glucose test the next morning. What does the nurse tell the patient to do before coming in for the test?
    a. Eat the usual diet but have nothing after midnight.
    b. Take the usual oral hypoglycemic tablet in the morning.
    c. Eat a clear liquid breakfast in the morning.
    d. Follow the usual diet and medication regimen.

36. The frequency with which the patient should monitor capillary blood glucose levels depends on levels of which element?
    a. Urine glucose
    b. Serum ketones
    c. Serum glucose
    d. Urine ketones

37. Which is considered the earliest sign of diabetic nephropathy?
    a. Positive urine RBCs
    b. Microalbuminuria
    c. Positive urine glucose
    d. Positive urine WBCs

Matching. Match each oral antidiabetic medication with its corresponding nursing intervention.

Medications

a. Chlorpropamide (Diabinese)
b. Metformin (Glucophage)
c. Miglitol (Glyset)
d. Nateglinide (Starlix)

Nursing Interventions

_____ 38. Give drug just before meals.

_____ 39. Hold drug for 48 hours if having x-ray with IV contrast dye (renal).

_____ 40. Hypoglycemic episodes are more likely to occur because of its long duration of action.

_____ 41. Give drug with first bite of each main meal.

42. Which oral agent may cause lactic acidosis?
  a. Nateglinide
  b. Repaglinide
  c. Metformin
  d. Miglitol

43. Which statement about insulin is true?
  a. Exogenous insulin is necessary for management of all cases of type 2 diabetes.
  b. Insulin's effectiveness depends on the individual patient's absorption of the drug.
  c. Insulin doses should be regulated according to self-monitoring urine glucose levels.
  d. Insulin administered in multiple doses per day decreases the flexibility of a patient's lifestyle.

44. Which statement about insulin administration is correct?
  a. Insulin may be given orally, intravenously, or subcutaneously.
  b. Insulin injections should be spaced no closer than one-half inch apart.
  c. Rotating injection sites improves absorption and prevents lipohypertrophy.
  d. In a mixed-dose protocol, the longer-acting insulin should be withdrawn first.

45. The diabetic patient is on a mixed-dose insulin protocol of 8 units regular insulin and 12 units NPH insulin at 7 AM. At 10:30 AM, the patient reports feeling uneasy, shaky, and has a headache. Which is the probable explanation for this?
  a. The NPH insulin's action is peaking, and there is an insufficient blood glucose level.
  b. The regular insulin's action is peaking, and there is an insufficient blood glucose level.
  c. The patient consumed too many calories at breakfast and now has an elevated blood glucose level.
  d. The symptoms are unrelated to the insulin administered in the early morning or diet taken in at lunchtime.

46. The patient will be using an external insulin pump. What does the nurse tell the patient about the pump?
  a. Self-monitoring of blood glucose levels can be done only twice a day.
  b. The insulin supply must be replaced every 2 to 4 weeks.
  c. The pump's battery should be checked on a regular weekly schedule.
  d. The needle site must be changed every 1 to 3 days.

47. The 47-year-old patient with a history of type 2 diabetes mellitus and emphysema who reports smoking three packs of cigarettes per day is admitted to the hospital with a diagnosis of acute pneumonia. The patient is placed on the regular oral antidiabetic agents, sliding scale insulin, and antibiotic medications. On day 2 of hospitalization, the health care provider orders prednisone therapy. What does the nurse expect the blood glucose to do?
    a. Decrease
    b. Stay the same
    c. Increase
    d. Return to normal

48. Which laboratory test is the best indicator of the patient's average blood glucose level and/or compliance with the diabetes mellitus regimen over the last 3 months?
    a. Postprandial test
    b. Oral glucose tolerance test (OGTT)
    c. Casual blood glucose test
    d. Glycosylated hemoglobin (HbA1c)

49. What is the earliest clinical sign of nephropathy?
    a. Proteinuria
    b. Ketonuria
    c. Glucosuria
    d. Microalbuminuria

50. Which insulins are considered to have a rapid onset of action? *(Select all that apply.)*
    a. Novolin 70/30
    b. Glulisine
    c. Humulin N
    d. Aspart
    e. Lispro

51. The diabetic patient has just returned from surgery with stable blood glucose levels between 120 and 180 mg/dL. Which IV solution will promote adequate hydration and stable blood glucose levels?
    a. $D_5$1/2 NS at 125 mL/hr
    b. D_5W at 125 mL/hr
    c. 0.45 % NSS at 100 mL/hr
    d. 0.9% NSS at 100 mL/hr

52. The patient with type 2 diabetes mellitus, usually controlled with a sulfonylurea, develops a urinary tract infection. Due to the stress of the infection, the patient must be treated with insulin. What additional information about this treatment does the nurse relay to the patient?
    a. The sulfonylurea must be discontinued and insulin taken until the infection clears.
    b. Insulin will now be necessary to control the patient's diabetes for life.
    c. The sulfonylurea dose must be reduced until the infection clears.
    d. The insulin is necessary to supplement the sulfonylurea until the infection clears.

Matching. *Match each diabetic complication with its corresponding pathophysiology. Answers may be used more than once.*

Pathophysiology
a. Nephropathy
b. Neuropathy
c. Retinopathy

Complications
_____ 53. Neovascularization
_____ 54. End-stage renal disease
_____ 55. Muscle weakness
_____ 56. Proteinuria
_____ 57. Hemorrhage into the eye
_____ 58. Pain or numbness
_____ 59. Hard exudates on fundus
_____ 60. Permanent blindness

True or False? *Read the statements about sensory alterations in patients with diabetes and write T for true and F for false in the blanks provided. For statements that are false, rewrite the statement to make it true.*

_____ 61. Healing of foot wounds is reduced because of impaired sensation.

_____ 62. Sensory neuropathy, ischemia, and infection are the leading causes of foot disease among diabetics.

_____ 63. Very few patients with diabetic foot ulcers have peripheral sensory neuropathy.

_____ 64. Loss of pain, pressure, and temperature sensation in the foot increases the risk for injury.

65. According to the Diabetes Control and Complication Trial (DCCT) study of type 1 diabetes mellitus patients, intensive therapy with good glucose control resulted in delays in which complications? *(Select all that apply.)*
   a. Macrovascular disease
   b. Cardiovascular disease
   c. Retinopathy
   d. Nephropathy
   e. Neuropathy

Matching. *Match the definition with its corresponding foot condition.*

Foot Conditions
a. Hallux valgus
b. Claw toe deformity
c. Charcot foot

Definitions

_____ 66. Hyperextended toes causing increased pressure on the ball of the foot.

_____ 67. Deformity where the foot is warm, swollen, painful, and walking causes the arch to collapse, giving the foot a "rocker bottom" shape

_____ 68. Turning of the great toe

69. In developing an individualized meal plan for the diabetic patient, which goals are the focus of the plan? *(Select all that apply.)*
   a. Maintaining blood glucose levels at or as close to the normal range as possible
   b. Patient food preferences
   c. Allowing patients to eat as much as they desire
   d. Patient cultural preferences
   e. Limiting food choices only when guided by scientific evidence

70. What is the basic principle of meal planning for the patient with type 1 diabetes mellitus?
   a. Five small meals per day plus a bedtime snack
   b. Taking extra insulin when planning to eat sweet foods
   c. High-protein, low-carbohydrate, and low-fiber foods
   d. Considering the effects and peak action times of the patient's insulin

71. Which statement about dietary concepts for the diabetic patient is true?
    a. Alcoholic beverage consumption is unrestricted.
    b. Carbohydrate counting is emphasized when adjusting dietary intake of nutrients.
    c. Sweeteners should be avoided because of the side effects.
    d. Both soluble and insoluble fiber foods should be limited.

72. What is the recommended protocol for type 2 diabetic patients who must lose weight?
    a. Participate in an aerobic program twice a week for 20 minutes each session.
    b. Slowly increase insulin dosage until mild hypoglycemia occurs.
    c. Reduce calorie intake moderately and increase exercise.
    d. Reduce daily calorie intake to 1000 calories and monitor urine for ketones.

73. What is the recommended calorie reduction for the diabetic patient who must lose weight?
    a. 500 calories/week
    b. 1500 calories/week
    c. 2500 calories/week
    d. 3500 calories/week

74. The diabetic patient who swims for exercise is taught to administer insulin in which area of the body?
    a. Abdomen
    b. Thighs
    c. Arms
    d. Hips

75. The nurse is teaching the diabetic patient about proper foot care. Which instruction does the nurse include?
    a. Use rubbing alcohol to toughen the skin on the soles of the feet.
    b. Wear open-toed shoes or sandals in warm weather to prevent perspiration.
    c. Apply moisturizing cream to the feet after bathing, but not between the toes.
    d. Use cold water for bathing the feet to prevent inadvertent thermal injury.

76. The 25-year-old female patient with type 1 diabetes tells the nurse, "I have two kidneys and I'm still young. I expect to be around for a long time, so why should I worry about my blood sugar?" What is the nurse's best response?
    a. "You have little to worry about as long as your kidneys keep making urine."
    b. "You should discuss this with your physician because you are being unrealistic."
    c. "You would be right if your diabetes was managed with insulin."
    d. "Keeping your blood sugar under control now can help to prevent damage to both kidneys."

77. Self-monitoring of blood glucose levels is most important in which patients? *(Select all that apply.)*
    a. Patients taking multiple daily insulin injections
    b. Patients with mild type 2 diabetes
    c. Patients with hypoglycemic unawareness
    d. Patients using a portable infusion device for insulin administration
    e. Ill patients
    f. Pregnant patients

78. Which statement about sexual intercourse for diabetic patients is true?
    a. The incidence of sexual dysfunction is lower in men than women.
    b. Retrograde ejaculation does not interfere with male fertility.
    c. Impotence is associated with diabetes mellitus in male patients.
    d. Sexual dysfunction in female patients includes inability to achieve pregnancy.

79. The insulin-dependent diabetic patient is planning to travel by air and asks the nurse about preparations for the trip. What does the nurse tell the patient to do?
    a. Pack insulin and syringes in a labeled, crushproof kit in the checked luggage.
    b. Carry all necessary diabetes supplies in a clearly identified pack aboard the plane.
    c. Ask the flight attendant to put the insulin in the galley refrigerator once on the plane.
    d. Take only minimal supplies and get the prescription filled at his or her destination.

80. Which statement by the diabetic patient indicates an understanding of the principles of self-care?
    a. "I don't like the idea of sticking myself so often to measure my sugar."
    b. "I plan to measure the sugar in my urine at least four times a day."
    c. "I plan to get my spouse to exercise with me to keep me company."
    d. "If I get a cold, I can take my regular cough medication until I feel better."

81. After a 2-hour glucose challenge, which result demonstrates impaired glucose tolerance?
    a. Less than 100 mg/dL
    b. Less than 140 mg/dL
    c. Greater than 140 mg/dL
    d. Greater than 250 mg/dL

82. The 50-year-old patient seen in the emergency department (ED) reported nausea, vomiting, and dehydration. When admitted to the hospital, the patient's fasting blood glucose was over 500 mg/dL, and a blood gas showed a pH of 7.38. The patient was diagnosed with diabetes and treated with insulin and fluids. What do these events tell the nurse about the patient?
    a. The diabetes is temporary.
    b. The patient will only require insulin when stressed or ill; the diabetes is temporary.
    c. The pancreas is producing enough insulin to prevent ketoacidosis.
    d. The pancreas is not producing enough insulin to prevent ketoacidosis.

83. The patient with type 2 diabetes often has which laboratory value?
    a. Elevated thyroid studies
    b. Elevated triglycerides
    c. Ketones in the urine
    d. Low hemoglobin

84. The patient has been diagnosed with diabetes. Which aspects does the nurse consider in formulating the teaching plan for this patient? *(Select all that apply.)*
    a. Covering all needed information in one teaching session
    b. Assessing visual impairment regarding insulin labels and markings on syringes
    c. Assessing manual dexterity to determine if the patient is able to draw insulin into a syringe
    d. Assessing patient motivation to learn and comprehend instructions
    e. Assessing the patient's ability to read printed material

85. Which are signs and symptoms of *mild* hypoglycemia? *(Select all that apply.)*
    a. Headache
    b. Weakness
    c. Cold, clammy skin
    d. Irritability
    e. Pallor
    f. Tachycardia

86. The patient with type 1 diabetes is taking a mixture of NPH and regular insulin at home. The patient has been NPO for surgery since midnight. What action does the nurse take regarding the patient's morning dose of insulin?
    a. Administer the dose that is routinely prescribed at home because the patient has type 1 diabetes and needs the insulin.
    b. Administer half the dose because the patient is NPO.
    c. Hold the insulin with all the other medications because the patient is NPO and there is no need for insulin.
    d. Contact the health care provider for an order regarding the insulin.

87. The patient with type 2 diabetes is taking a mixture of NPH and regular insulin at home. The patient has been NPO for surgery since midnight. What action does the nurse take regarding the patient's morning dose of insulin?
    a. Administer the dose that is routinely prescribed at home because the patient has type 2 diabetes and needs the insulin.
    b. Administer half the dose because the patient is NPO.
    c. Hold the insulin with all the other medications because the patient is NPO and there is no need for insulin.
    d. Contact the health care provider for an order regarding the insulin.

88. The patient with diabetes has signs and symptoms of hypoglycemia. The patient is alert and oriented with a blood glucose of 56 mg/dL. What does the nurse do next?
    a. Give a glass of orange juice with two packets of sugar and continue to monitor the patient.
    b. Give a glass of orange or other type of juice and continue to monitor the patient.
    c. Give a complex carbohydrate and continue to monitor the patient.
    d. Administer D50 IV push and give the patient something to eat.

89. The patient with diabetes has signs and symptoms of hypoglycemia. The patient has a blood glucose of 56 mg/dL, is not alert but responds to voice, and is confused and is unable to swallow fluids. What does the nurse do next?
    a. Give a glass of orange juice with two packets of sugar and continue to monitor the patient.
    b. Give a glass of orange or other type of juice and continue to monitor the patient.
    c. Give a complex carbohydrate and continue to monitor the patient.
    d. Administer D50 IV push.

90. The patient has been receiving insulin in the abdomen for 3 days. On day 4, where does the nurse give the insulin injection?
    a. Deltoid
    b. Thigh
    c. Abdomen, near the navel
    d. Abdomen, but in an area different from the previous day's injection
    e. Abdomen, in the same area as the previous day's injection

91. Place the injection sites in order of speed of absorption using the numbers 1 through 4, with 1 having the fastest absorption and 4 having the slowest absorption.
    _____ a. Buttocks
    _____ b. Abdomen
    _____ c. Deltoid
    _____ d. Thigh

Matching. *Match the insulin characteristics with the corresponding types of insulin. Answers may be used more than once.*

Types of Insulin
a. Insulin glargine (Lantus)
b. Regular insulin
c. NPH insulin

Insulin Characteristics
_____ 92. This type of insulin is used in most regimens for basal insulin coverage.
_____ 93. This type of insulin is a long-acting insulin analogue given once daily at bedtime for basal insulin coverage.
_____ 94. When mixing insulins, this type is always drawn up first.
_____ 95. This type of insulin should be given 30 minutes before meals.
_____ 96. This type of insulin should not be diluted or mixed with any other insulin or solution.

CASE STUDY: THE PATIENT WITH DIABETES MELLITUS

Use a separate sheet of paper to answer the questions in this Case Study. Answer guidelines for this Case Study are available on your Evolve website at http://evolve. elsevier.com/Iggy/ in the "Prepare for Class" folder.

The patient is a 48-year-old unconscious woman admitted to the ED. She has a known history of type 1 diabetes mellitus. Her daughter accompanies her and tells the staff that her mother has had the "flu" and has been unable to eat or drink very much. The daughter is uncertain whether her mother has taken her insulin in the past 24 hours. The patient's vital signs are temperature 101.8° F; pulse 120, weak and irregular; respiration 22, deep, and fruity odor; and blood pressure 80/42 mm Hg. Blood specimens and arterial blood gases are drawn and an IV infusion begun.

1. Based on this patient's history, give the probable changes in laboratory results for serum glucose, serum osmolarity, serum acetone, BUN, arterial pH, and arterial Pco_2. What medical emergency do these data indicate?

2. What type of IV solutions should the nurse be prepared to administer to this patient? What drugs should the nurse be prepared to give? Explain your answers.

3. The patient is placed on continuous cardiac monitoring. What is the rationale for this intervention?

4. During the first 24 hours, what complications should the nurse monitor for in this patient? Why?

5. The patient eventually becomes normoglycemic, regains consciousness, and begins a 1500-calorie diabetic diet. Develop a teaching-learning plan for her about this diet.

6. Before this emergency, this patient had been monitoring urine glucose and ketones for self-care and insulin administration. Her physician prescribes blood glucose monitoring instead of urine testing. What is the rationale for this change?

7. Which aspect of diabetic self-care should the nurse discuss with this patient before her discharge?

8. The patient is to be discharged on a mixed-dose regimen for insulin. She is to receive 10 units regular insulin and 18 units NPH insulin before breakfast and another 5 units regular insulin and 12 units NPH at dinnertime. Develop a teaching-learning plan for these medications.

9. Considering the patient's insulin protocol, the patient should keep in mind what principles about the actions of the insulins she is taking?

10. What should the nurse discuss with this patient about diabetes, insulin, and illness? What can this patient do to prevent future emergency episodes? Consider "Instructions for Sick Day" rules.

Assessment of the Renal/Urinary System

CHAPTER 68

STUDY/REVIEW QUESTIONS

Matching. Match the terms with their correct definitions.

Terms

a. Nephron
b. Glomerulus
c. Renin
d. Aldosterone
e. Antidiuretic hormone (ADH)
f. Prostaglandin E_2 (PGE$_2$)
g. Bradykinin
h. Erythropoietin
i. Vitamin D
j. Glomerular filtration

Definitions

_____ 1. Increases kidney reabsorption of sodium and water

_____ 2. "Working" unit of the kidney

_____ 3. Also known as vasopression

_____ 4. Series of specialized capillary loops

_____ 5. First process in urine formation

_____ 6. Hormone helps to regulate blood flow, glomerular filtration rate (GFR), and blood pressure

_____ 7. Acts on distal tubule and collecting duct to increase sodium and water excretion

_____ 8. Needed to absorb calcium in the intestinal tract and to regulate calcium balance

_____ 9. Produced and released in response to decreased oxygen tension in renal blood supply

_____ 10. Small hormone that dilates the afferent arteriole and increases capillary membrane permeability to some solutes

11. The patient has sustained a minor kidney injury. Which structure must remain functional in order for urine to be removed from the blood?
    a. Medulla
    b. Nephron
    c. Calyx
    d. Capsule

12. Based on knowledge of the normal function of the kidney, which large particles are not found in the urine because they are too large to filter through the glomerular capillary walls? *(Select all that apply.)*
    a. Blood cells
    b. Albumin
    c. Other proteins
    d. Electrolytes
    e. Water

13. What is the average urine output of a healthy adult for a 24-hour period?
    a. 500 mL to 1000 mL per day
    b. 1500 mL to 2000 mL per day
    c. 3000 mL to 5000 mL per day
    d. 5000 mL to 7000 mL per day

14. Kidney function, in particular the GFR, is compromised when the systolic blood pressure drops below what reading?
    a. 50 mm Hg
    b. 70 mm Hg
    c. 80 mm Hg
    d. 100 mm Hg

15. Damage to which renal structure or tissues can change the actual production of urine?
    a. Renal parenchyma
    b. Convoluted tubules
    c. Calyces
    d. Ureters

16. The patient has been immobilized for several days after a motor vehicle accident. The nurse encourages ambulation to stimulate the movement of urine through the ureter by what phenomenon?
    a. Peristalsis
    b. Gravity
    c. Pelvic pressure
    d. Backflow

17. Which renal change associated with aging does the nurse expect the older adult patient to report?
    a. Nocturnal polyuria
    b. Micturition
    c. Hematuria
    d. Dysuria

18. The older adult male patient has a history of an enlarged prostate. The patient is most likely to report which symptom associated with this condition?
    a. Inability to sense the urge to void
    b. Difficulty starting the urine stream
    c. Excreting large amounts of very dilute urine
    d. Frequent leakage of small amounts of urine

19. Impairment in the thirst mechanism associated with aging makes the older adult patient more vulnerable to which disorder?
    a. Hypovolemia
    b. Hypocalcemia
    c. Hypokalemia
    d. Hyponatremia

20. The nurse is talking to a group of older women about changes in the urinary system related to aging. What symptom is likely to be the common concern for this group?
    a. Incontinence
    b. Hematuria
    c. Retention
    d. Dysuria

Fill in the blanks.

21. The most important roles of the kidneys are to maintain body fluid _____ and _____, and to filter _____ products for elimination.

22. The kidneys help regulate blood pressure and _____ balance.

23. The kidneys have a rich blood supply and receive _____% to _____% of the total cardiac output.

24. Normal GFR averages _____ mL/min.

25. GFR is controlled by blood _____ and blood _____.

26. _____ increases tubular permeability to water, allowing water to leave the tube and be reabsorbed into the capillaries.

27. Where sodium goes, _____ follows.

28. During water reabsorption, the membrane of the distal convoluted tubule is more permeable to water due to the influence of _____ _____.

29. The primary function of the proximal convoluted tubule is _____ of water and electrolytes.

30. The nurse is taking a history on the 55-year-old patient who denies any serious chronic health problems. Which sudden-onset sign/symptom suggests possible kidney disease in this patient?
    a. Weakness
    b. Hypertension
    c. Confusion
    d. Dysrhythmia

31. Which patient narrative describes the symptom of dysuria?
    a. "I have to pee all the time."
    b. "I have to wait before the pee starts."
    c. "It burns when I pee."
    d. "It feels like I am going to pee in my pants."

32. The nurse and nutritionist are evaluating the diet and nutritional therapies for the patient with kidney problems. Blood urea nitrogen (BUN) levels for this patient are tracked because of the direct relationship to the intake and metabolism of which substance?
    a. Lipids
    b. Carbohydrates
    c. Protein
    d. Fluids

33. The nurse is taking a history on the patient with a change in urinary patterns. In addition to the medical and surgical history, what does the nurse ask the patient about to complete the assessment? *(Select all that apply.)*
    a. Occupational exposure to toxins
    b. Use of illicit substances, such as cocaine
    c. Financial resources for payment of treatments
    d. Religious beliefs about urination
    e. Potential exposure to sexually transmitted disease

34. The nurse is determining whether the patient has a history of hypertension because of the potential for kidney problems. Which question is best to elicit this information?
    a. "Do you have high blood pressure?"
    b. "Do you take any blood pressure medications?"
    c. "Have you ever been told that your blood pressure was high?"
    d. "When was the last time you had your blood pressure checked?"

35. The patient appears very uncomfortable with the nurse's questions about urinary functions and patterns. What is the best technique for the nurse to use to elicit relevant information and decrease the patient's discomfort?
    a. Defer the questions until a later time.
    b. Direct the questions toward a family member.
    c. Use anatomic or medical terminology.
    d. Use the patient's own terminology.

36. The nurse is taking a nutritional history on the patient. The patient states, "I really don't drink as much water as I should." What is the nurse's best response?
    a. "We should probably all drink more water than we do."
    b. "It's an easy thing to forget; just try to remember to drink more."
    c. "What would encourage you to drink the recommended 3 liters per day?"
    d. "I'd like you to read this brochure about kidney health and fluids."

37. When patients have problems with the kidneys or urinary tract, what is the most common symptom that prompts them to seek medical attention?
    a. Change in the frequency or amount of urination
    b. Pain in flank or abdomen or pain when urinating
    c. Noticing a change in the color or odor of the urine
    d. Exposure to a nephrotoxic substance

38. Which ethnic group has the highest risk for end-stage renal disease secondary to diabetes mellitus and hypertension?
    a. Caucasian Americans
    b. African Americans
    c. Asian Americans
    d. Native Americans

39. Which over-the-counter product used by the patient does the nurse explore further for potential impact on renal function?
    a. Peroxide-containing mouthwash
    b. Milk of magnesia laxative
    c. Vitamin C
    d. NSAIDs

40. The nurse is performing an assessment of the renal system. What is the first step in the assessment process?
    a. Percuss the lower abdomen; continue toward the umbilicus
    b. Observe the flank region for asymmetry or discoloration
    c. Listen for a bruit over each renal artery
    d. Lightly palpate the abdomen in all quadrants

41. The nurse is auscultating the renal artery and hears a bruit. What does this finding indicate?
    a. Acute renal failure
    b. Renal artery stenosis
    c. Renal artery aneurysm
    d. Renal tumor

42. The patient has anorexia, nausea and vomiting, muscle cramping, and pruritus. How does the nurse interpret these findings?
    a. Oliguria
    b. Azotemia
    c. Anuria
    d. Uremia

43. The patient is diagnosed with renal artery stenosis. Which sound does the nurse expect to hear by auscultation when a bruit is present in a renal artery?
    a. Quiet, pulsating sound
    b. Swishing sound
    c. Faint wheezing
    d. No sound at all

44. Which volume of urine does the nurse expect to find documented for the patient who is oliguric?
    a. Between 100 and 300 mL in 24 hours
    b. Greater than 2000 mL in 24 hours
    c. Less than 100 mL in 24 hours
    d. Greater than 400 mL during the night

45. The nurse is assessing the patient for bladder distention. What technique does the nurse use?
    a. Gently palpate for the outline of the bladder, percuss the lower abdomen, continue toward the umbilicus until dull sounds are no longer produced.
    b. Gently palpate for the outline of the bladder, auscultate for sounds in the lower abdomen.
    c. Place one hand under the back and palpate with the other hand over the bladder, percuss the lower abdomen until tympanic sounds are no longer produced.
    d. Use the hand to depress the bladder as the patient takes a deep breath, then percuss.

46. The patient reports flank pain or tenderness. What technique does the nurse use to assess for costovertebral tenderness?
    a. Percuss the nontender flank and assess for rebound.
    b. Thump the CVA area with the flat surface of the hand.
    c. Thump the CVA area with a clenched fist.
    d. Place one hand flat over the CVA area, thump with the other fist.

47. The nurse is preparing to assess the female patient's urethra. In addition to gloves, which equipment does the nurse obtain to perform the initial assessment?
    a. Glass slide
    b. Good light source
    c. Speculum
    d. Cotton swab

Matching. Match each urine specimen finding with its corresponding characteristic.

Findings
a. Color
b. Odor
c. Turbidity
d. Specific gravity
e. pH
f. Glucose
g. Ketone bodies
h. Protein
i. Microalbuminuria
j. Sediment
k. Cells
l. Cast
m. Crystals
n. Bacteria

Characteristics
_____ 48. Less than 7 acidic, greater than 7 alkaline
_____ 49. Byproduct of fatty acid metabolism, not seen in urine
_____ 50. Only identified by microscopic examination for protein
_____ 51. Structure found around cell, bacteria, protein, and clumps
_____ 52. Urine is normally sterile; these multiply and grow
_____ 53. Urochrome pigment
_____ 54. 1.000 to 1.35
_____ 55. Not normally in the urine
_____ 56. Cells, casts, crystals, and bacteria
_____ 57. Various salts
_____ 58. Epithelial cells, RBC, WBC, tubular cells
_____ 59. Not seen in urine until blood sugar above 220 mg/dL
_____ 60. Cloudiness or haziness
_____ 61. Faint ammonia

62. The nurse is caring for the patient with dehydration. Which laboratory test results does the nurse anticipate to see for this patient?
a. BUN and creatinine ratio stay the same.
b. BUN rises faster than creatinine level.
c. Creatinine rises faster than BUN.
d. BUN and creatinine have a direct relationship.

63. What does the BUN test measure?
a. Renal excretion of nitrogen
b. GFR
c. Creatinine clearance
d. Urine output

64. Which patient is most likely to have a decreased calcium level?
a. Patient with nephritis
b. Patient with cystitis
c. Patient with a Foley catheter
d. Patient with urinary retention

65. The nurse performs a dipstick urine test for the patient being evaluated for kidney problems. Glucose is present in the urine. How does the nurse interpret this result?
a. Blood glucose level is greater than 220 mg/dL.
b. The kidneys are failing to filter any glucose.
c. The patient is at risk for hypoglycemia.
d. The renal threshold has not been exceeded.

66. In addition to kidney disease, which patient condition causes the BUN to rise above the normal range?
a. Anemia
b. Asthma
c. Infection
d. Malnutrition

67. The community health nurse is talking to a group of African-American adults about renal health. The nurse encourages the participants to have which type of yearly examination to screen for kidney problems?
    a. Renal ultrasound
    b. Serum creatinine and blood urea nitrogen
    c. Urinalysis and microalbuminuria
    d. 24-hour urine collection

68. Which test is the best indicator of kidney function?
    a. Urine osmolarity
    b. Serum creatinine
    c. Urine pH
    d. Color of urine

69. In relation to kidney problems, what does an increase in the ratio of BUN to serum creatinine indicate?
    a. Highly suggestive of renal dysfunction
    b. Definitive for renal dysfunction
    c. Suggests nonrenal factors causing an elevation in BUN
    d. Suggests nonrenal factors causing an elevation in serum creatinine

70. Which urine characteristic listed on a urinalysis report arouses the nurse's suspicion of a problem in the urinary tract?
    a. Cloudiness
    b. Straw color
    c. Ammonia odor
    d. One cast per high-powered field

71. Complete the chart below to indicate abnormal urinalysis findings and the significance of these findings.

Test	Abnormal Findings	Significance of Abnormal Findings
Color		
Odor		
Turbidity		
Specific gravity		
pH		
Glucose		
Ketones		
Protein		
Bilirubin (urobilinogen)		
Red blood cells (RBCs)		
White blood cells (WBCs)		
Casts		
Crystals		
Bacteria		
Parasites		
Leukoesterase		
Nitrites		

72. The patient has a urinalysis ordered. When is the best time for the nurse to collect the specimen?
    a. In the evening
    b. After a meal
    c. In the morning
    d. After a fluid bolus

73. During the day, the nursing student is measuring urine output and observing for urine characteristics in the patient. Which abnormal finding in the urine is the most urgent finding that must be reported to the supervising nurse?
    a. Specific gravity is decreased.
    b. Output is decreased.
    c. pH is decreased.
    d. Color has changed.

74. A 24-hour urine specimen is required from the patient. Which strategy is best to ensure that all the urine is collected for the full 24-hour period?
    a. Instruct the unlicensed assistive personnel (UAP) to collect all the urine.
    b. Put a bedpan or commode next to the bed as a reminder.
    c. Place a sign in the bathroom reminding the patient to save the urine.
    d. Verbally remind the patient about the test.

75. Place the steps of using a bedside bladder scanner in the correct order using the numbers 1 through 8.

    _____ a. Select the male or female icon on the bladder scanner.

    _____ b. Aim the scan head towards the expected location of the bladder.

    _____ c. Place the probe midline about 1.5 inches (4 cm) above the pubic bone.

    _____ d. Explain the purpose and what sensations to expect.

    _____ e. Listen for the sound of a beep and a volume display.

    _____ f. Place an ultrasound gel pad right above the symphysis pubis.

    _____ g. Press and release the scan button.

    _____ h. Repeat for best accuracy.

76. The patient is scheduled for an IV urography. Which medication is discontinued at the time of the procedure and for at least 48 hours until renal function has been re-evaluated?
    a. Glucophage (Metformin)
    b. Diphenhydramine (Benadryl)
    c. Prednisone (Deltasone)
    d. Acetylcysteine (Mucomyst)

77. Several patients are scheduled for testing to diagnose potential kidney problems. Which test requires the patient to have a urinary catheter inserted before the test?
    a. IV urography
    b. Computed tomography
    c. Cystography
    d. Kidney scan

78. The patient has had an IV urography. What is included in the postprocedural care for this patient?
    a. Bowel cleansing with laxatives
    b. IV or oral fluid hydration
    c. Administration of captopril (Capoten)
    d. Insertion of a urinary catheter

79. Which diagnostic test incorporates contrast dye, but does not place the patient at risk for nephrotoxicity?
    a. IV urography
    b. Renal angiography
    c. Voiding cystourethrogram
    d. Computed tomography

80. The nurse is reviewing the results of a patient's ultrasound of the kidney. The report reveals an enlarged kidney which suggests which possible problem?
    a. Polycystic kidney
    b. Kidney infection
    c. Renal carcinoma
    d. Chronic renal disease

81. The patient returns to the unit after a kidney scan. Which instruction about the patient's urine does the nurse give to the UAP caring for the patient?
    a. It is radioactive, so it should be handled with special biohazard precautions.
    b. It does not place anyone at risk because of the small amount of radioactive material.
    c. Its radioactivity is dangerous only to those who are pregnant.
    d. It is potentially dangerous if allowed to sit for prolonged periods in the commode.

82. The nurse is alerted by the radiology department that the patient had a "captopril renal scan." What does the nurse monitor for when the patient returns from the procedure?
    a. Cardiac dysrhythmias
    b. Urine discoloration
    c. Signs of dehydration
    d. Orthostatic hypotension

83. The nurse is teaching the patient scheduled for an ultrasonography. What preprocedural instruction does the nurse give the patient?
    a. Void just before the test begins.
    b. Drink a lot water.
    c. Stop routine medications.
    d. Complete a bowel preparation.

84. The patient had a cystoscopy. After the procedure, what does the nurse expect to see in this patient?
    a. Pink-tinged urine
    b. Bloody urine
    c. Very dilute urine
    d. Decreased urine output

85. The patient is scheduled for retrograde urethrography. Postprocedural care is similar to postprocedural care given for which test?
    a. Ultrasonography
    b. Computed tomography
    c. IV urography
    d. Cystoscopy

86. The patient has had a cystometrography. What is the priority nursing diagnosis for this patient related to this procedure?
    a. Risk for Infection
    b. Knowledge Deficit
    c. Acute Pain
    d. Activity Intolerance

87. The patient has had urine stream testing. What is the primary nursing intervention in the postprocedural care of this patient?
    a. Monitoring vital signs
    b. Cleaning the perineal area
    c. Monitoring for infection
    d. Rehydrating the patient

88. The patient has undergone a renal biopsy. What does the nurse monitor for in the patient related to this procedure?
    a. Nephrotoxicity
    b. Hemorrhage
    c. Urinary retention
    d. Hypertension

89. The patient has undergone a renal biopsy. In the immediate postprocedural period, the nurse notifies the health care provider about which finding?
    a. Hematuria
    b. Localized pain at the site
    c. "Tamponade effect"
    d. Decreasing urine output

CASE STUDY: ASSESSING THE RENAL/URINARY SYSTEM IN THE OLDER ADULT

Use a separate sheet of paper to answer the questions in this Case Study. Answer guidelines for this Case Study are available on your Evolve website at http://evolve. elsevier.com/Iggy/ in the "Prepare for Class" folder.

A 74-year-old man comes to the clinic for changes in urinary patterns. He reports, "I am pretty healthy for my age. I do have some of the typical problems that all old folks have, but nothing serious."

1. What types of questions would the nurse ask using Gordon's functional assessment?

2. Identify changes related to aging and appropriate nursing interventions for older adults with regard to the renal system.

3. The patient is scheduled to have a series of urologic studies for diagnostic purposes. The physician orders the following: urinalysis, urine for culture and sensitivity, BUN, serum creatine, and 24-hour urine for creatinine clearance. The tests will be conducted on an outpatient basis. Describe what the nurse should do to instruct the patient in the collection of these laboratory specimens.

4. Which specimens should be collected first?

5. The patient returns the collection container with a 24-hour urine specimen to the physician's office. As he gives it to the nurse, he comments, "I had a hard time remembering to save it all. Actually, I think I missed some when I forgot and used a bathroom at the shopping mall yesterday." What should the nurse do?

6. Further tests are ordered for the patient, including a renal ultrasound and IV pyelography (IVP). These are scheduled at an outpatient radiology clinic. Design a teaching-learning plan for the patient to prepare him for these studies.

7. Following the ultrasound and IVP, what assessments should be made for the patient?

Care of Patients with Urinary Problems

69 CHAPTER

STUDY/REVIEW QUESTIONS

Matching. Match the terms with their correct definitions.

Terms

a. Cystitis
b. Bacteriuria
c. Colonization
d. *Escherichia coli*
e. Urosepsis
f. Frequency
g. Dysuria
h. Urgency
i. Trabeculation
j. Hunner's ulcers
k. Pyuria
l. Cystocele

Definitions

_____ 1. Bacteria in the urine

_____ 2. Urge to urinate frequently in small amounts

_____ 3. Inflammation of the bladder

_____ 4. Feeling that urination will occur immediately

_____ 5. Bacteriuria is without symptoms of infection

_____ 6. White blood cells (WBCs) in the urine

_____ 7. Causes about 90% of urinary tract infections (UTIs)

_____ 8. Type of bladder lesion

_____ 9. Pain or burning with urination

_____ 10. Abnormal thickening of the bladder wall caused by urinary retention and obstruction

_____ 11. Herniation of the bladder into the vagina

_____ 12. Spread of the infection from the urinary tract to the bloodstream

True or False? Read the statements and write T for true or F for false in the blanks provided. If the statement is false, correct the statement to make it true.

_____ 13. In the hospital, UTIs are the most common nosocomial infection.

_____ 14. Infections of the urinary tract and kidneys are common, especially among men.

_____ 15. Noninfectious cystitis is caused by irritation from chemicals or radiation.

_____ 16. Colonization always progresses to acute infection or renal insufficiency.

_____ 17. About 50% of patients with indwelling catheters become infected within 1 week of catheter insertion.

18. The nurse is caring for the patient with an indwelling catheter. What interventions does the nurse use to minimize catheter-related infections? *(Select all that apply.)*
   a. Consider appropriate alternatives to an indwelling catheter.
   b. Use sterile technique for daily routine handling of equipment.
   c. Select the largest catheter available.
   d. Apply antiseptic solutions or antibiotic ointments to the perineal area.
   e. Maintain a closed system irrigation by ensuring connections are sealed securely.
   f. Irrigate the catheter daily.
   g. Keep urine collection bags below the level of the bladder at all times.

19. The patient reports intense urgency, frequency, and bladder pain. Urinalysis results show WBCs and RBCs and urine culture results are negative for infection. How does the nurse interpret these findings?
   a. Interstitial cystitis
   b. Urethritis
   c. Bacteriuria
   d. Infectious cystitis

20. The nurse is teaching the patient about bladder and urinary health. What information does the nurse include? *(Select all that apply.)*
   a. Have a minimal fluid intake of 3 L daily, unless contraindicated.
   b. Drink more water rather than sugar-containing drinks.
   c. Avoid urinary stasis by urinating every 6 to 8 hours.
   d. Bathe daily or thoroughly wash the perineal and urethral areas.
   e. Avoid straining or pushing when expelling urine.

21. The nurse is performing an initial physical assessment on the patient reporting frequency, urgency, hematuria, low-grade fever, and dysuria. What technique does the nurse use?
   a. Have the patient void and then use a bedside bladder scanner to assess for the amount of residual urine.
   b. Ask the patient to undress from the waist down; drape for privacy and inspect the urethral meatus.
   c. Ask the patient to void; examine the urine and then inspect the lower abdomen and palpate the urinary bladder.
   d. Palpate the bladder to check for distention; have the patient void and then repalpate to check for bladder emptying.

22. The young female patient reports experiencing burning with urination. What question does the nurse ask to differentiate between a vaginal infection and a urinary infection?
   a. "Have you noticed any blood in the urine?"
   b. "Have you had recent sexual intercourse?"
   c. "Have you noticed any vaginal discharge?"
   d. "Have you been voiding less frequently?"

23. The patient reports symptoms indicating a UTI. The nurse obtains an order for which diagnostic test to verify a UTI?
   a. Urine testing for leukocyte esterase and nitrate
   b. Urinalysis for white and red blood cells
   c. Complete blood count
   d. Voiding cystourethrography

24. The patient is diagnosed with a fungal UTI. Which drug does the nurse anticipate the patient will be treated with?
   a. Sulfa drugs
   b. Cephalosporins
   c. Ketoconazole
   d. Quinolones

25. The nurse is teaching the patient about self-care measures to prevent UTIs. Which daily fluid intake does the nurse recommend to the patient to prevent a bladder infection?
   a. 2 to 3 L of water
   b. 3 to 6 glasses of iced tea
   c. 4 to 6 cups of electrolyte fluid
   d. 3 to 4 glasses of juice

26. The nursing student sees an order for a urinalysis for the patient with frequency, urgency, and dysuria. In order to collect the specimen, what does the student do?
    a. Use sterile technique to insert a small-diameter (6 Fr) catheter.
    b. Instruct the patient on how to collect a clean-catch specimen.
    c. Tell the patient to urinate approximately 10 mL into a specimen cup.
    d. Take the urine from a bedpan and transfer it into a specimen cup.

27. The nurse is reviewing the laboratory results for the older adult patient with an indwelling catheter. The urine culture is pending, but the urinalysis shows greater than 10^5 colony-forming units, and the differential WBC count shows a "left shift." How does the nurse interpret these findings?
    a. Interstitial cystitis
    b. Urosepsis
    c. Complicated cystitis
    d. Radiation-induced cystitis

28. The patient has UTI symptoms but there are no bacteria in the urine. The physician suspects interstitial cystitis. The nurse prepares patient teaching material for which diagnostic test?
    a. Urography
    b. Abdominal sonography
    c. Computed tomography (CT)
    d. Cystoscopy

29. The cystoscopy results for the patient include a small-capacity bladder, the presence of Hunner's ulcers, and small hemorrhages after bladder distention. How does the nurse interpret this report?
    a. Urosepsis
    b. Complicated infection cystitis
    c. Interstitial cystitis
    d. Urethritis

30. Several patients at the clinic have been diagnosed with UTIs. Which patients may need to be hospitalized? *(Select all that apply.)*
    a. Postmenopausal patient
    b. Patient with a long-term indwelling catheter
    c. Diabetic patient
    d. Immunosuppressed patient
    e. Pregnant patient

31. The nurse is counseling the patient with recurrent cystitis about dietary therapy. What information does the nurse give to the patient?
    a. Drink 50 mL of concentrated cranberry juice every day.
    b. Limit calorie intake during peaks of infection.
    c. Caffeine, carbonated beverages, and tomato products cause cystitis.
    d. Cranberry tablets are more effective than juice or fluids.

32. The patient received an antibiotic prescription several hours ago and has started the medication, but states needing "some relief from the burning." What comfort measures does the nurse suggest to the patient?
    a. Take over-the-counter acetaminophen.
    b. Sit in a sitz bath and urinate into the warm water.
    c. Place a cold pack over the perineal area.
    d. Rest in a recumbent position with legs elevated.

33. The patient's recurrent cystitis appears to be related to sexual intercourse. The patient seems uncomfortable talking about the situation. What communication technique does the nurse use to assist the patient?
    a. Have a frank and sensitive discussion with the patient.
    b. Give the patient reading material with instructions to call with any questions.
    c. Call the patient's partner and invite the partner to discuss the problem.
    d. Talk about other topics until the patient feels more comfortable disclosing.

34. The male college student comes to the clinic reporting burning or difficulty with urination and a discharge from the urethral meatus. Based on the patient's chief complaint, what is the most logical question for the nurse to ask about the patient's past medical history?
    a. "Do you have a history of a narrow urethra or a stricture?"
    b. "Could you have been exposed to a sexually transmitted disease (STD)?"
    c. "Do you have a history of kidney stones?"
    d. "Have you been drinking an adequate amount of fluids?"

35. The patient is diagnosed with urethral stricture. What findings does the nurse expect to see documented in the patient's chart for this condition?
    a. Pain on urination
    b. Pain on ejaculation
    c. Overflow incontinence
    d. Hematuria and pyuria

36. The patient is diagnosed with a urethral stricture. The nurse prepares the patient for which temporary treatment?
    a. Dilation of the urethra
    b. Antibiotic therapy
    c. Fluid restriction
    d. Urinary diversion

37. The patient reports the loss of small amounts of urine during coughing, sneezing, jogging, or lifting. Which type of incontinence do these symptoms describe?
    a. Urge
    b. Overflow
    c. Functional
    d. Stress

38. The nurse is caring for the obese older adult patient with dementia. The patient is alert and ambulatory, but has functional incontinence. Which nursing intervention is best for this patient?
    a. Help the patient to lose weight.
    b. Help the patient apply an estrogen cream.
    c. Offer assistance with toileting every 2 hours.
    d. Intermittently catheterize the patient.

39. Which patient is mostly likely to have mixed incontinence?
    a. Older woman who had four full-term pregnancies
    b. Patient with a stroke who has neurologic deficits
    c. Patient with benign prostatic hypertrophy
    d. Patient with a pelvic fracture

40. The nurse is caring for the older adult patient with urinary incontinence. The patient is alert and oriented, but refuses to use the call bell and has fallen several times while trying to get to the bathroom. What is the priority nursing diagnosis?
    a. Acute Confusion
    b. Noncompliance
    c. Risk for Falls
    d. Functional Urinary Incontinence

41. The nurse is performing an assessment on the patient with probable stress incontinence. Which assessment technique does the nurse use to validate stress incontinence?
    a. Assess the abdomen to estimate bladder fullness.
    b. Check for residual urine using a portable ultrasound.
    c. Catheterize the patient immediately after voiding.
    d. Ask the patient to cough while wearing a perineal pad.

42. The advanced practice nurse is performing a digital rectal examination (DRE) and notes that the rectal sphincter contracts on digital insertion. How does the nurse interpret this finding?
    a. Nerve supply to the bladder is most likely intact.
    b. Adequate strength in the pelvic floor.
    c. A rectocele is placing pressure on the bladder.
    d. Normal function for the bowel and bladder.

43. The nurse identifies the nursing diagnosis of Stress Urinary Incontinence related to weak pelvic muscles for the middle-aged patient. The patient is highly motivated to participate in self-care. Which interventions does the nurse include in the treatment plan? *(Select all that apply.)*
    a. Keep a detailed diary of urine leakage, activities, and foods eaten.
    b. Wear absorbent pads and undergarments during the assessment process.
    c. Teach pelvic floor (Kegel) exercise therapy.
    d. Teach about vaginal cone therapy.
    e. Drink orange juice every day for 4 to 6 weeks.
    f. Refer to a nutritionist for diet therapy for weight reduction.

44. The patient has been performing Kegel exercises for 2 months. How does the nurse know whether the exercises are working?
    a. Incontinence is still present, but the patient states that it is less.
    b. The patient is able to stop the urinary stream.
    c. There are no complaints of urgency from the patient.
    d. The patient is using absorbent undergarments for protection.

45. The home health nurse is assessing the older adult patient who refuses to leave the house to see friends or participate in usual activities. She reports taking a bath several times a day and becomes very upset when she has an incontinent episode. What is the priority nursing diagnosis for this patient?
    a. Disturbed Body Image
    b. Stress Urinary Incontinence
    c. Social Isolation
    d. Risk for Impaired Skin Integrity

46. The nurse is evaluating outcome criteria for the patient being treated for urge incontinence. Which statement indicates the treatment has been successful?
    a. "I'm following the prescribed therapy, but I think surgery is my best choice."
    b. "I still lose a little urine when I sneeze, but I have been wearing a thin pad."
    c. "I had trouble at first, but now I go to the toilet every 3 hours."
    d. "I have been using the bladder compression technique and it works."

47. The nurse is teaching the patient with urge incontinence about dietary modifications. What is the best information the nurse gives to the patient about fluid intake?
    a. Drink at least 2000 mL per day unless contraindicated.
    b. Drink 120 mL every hour or 240 mL every 2 hours and limit fluids after dinner.
    c. Drink fluid freely in the morning hours, but limit intake before going to bed.
    d. Drinking water is especially good for bladder health.

48. The patient has agreed to try a bladder training program. What is the priority nursing intervention in starting this therapy?
    a. Start a schedule for voiding (e.g., every 30 minutes).
    b. Teach the patient to be alert, aware, and able to resist the urge to urinate.
    c. Convince the patient that he or she controls the bladder; the bladder does not control the patient.
    d. Give a thorough explanation of the problem of urge incontinence.

49. The older adult patient with a cognitive impairment is living in an extended care facility. The patient is incontinent, but as the family points out, "he will urinate in the toilet if somebody helps him." Which type of incontinence does the nurse suspect in this patient?
    a. Urge
    b. Overflow
    c. Functional
    d. Stress

50. The nurse is designing a habit training bladder program for the older adult patient who is alert but mildly confused. What task associated with the training program is delegated to the unlicensed assistive personnel (UAP)?
    a. Tell the patient it is time to go to the toilet and assist him to go on a regular schedule.
    b. Help the patient record the incidents of incontinence in a bladder diary.
    c. Change the patient's incontinence pants (or pad) every 2 hours.
    d. Gradually encourage independence and increase the intervals between voidings.

51. Which patient with incontinence is most likely to benefit from a surgical intervention?
    a. Patient with vaginal atrophy and altered urethral competency
    b. Patient with reflex (overflow) incontinence caused by obstruction
    c. Patient with stress incontinence caused by coughing and sneezing
    d. Patients with urge incontinence or overactive bladder

52. The nurse is teaching the patient a behavioral intervention for bladder compression. In order to correctly perform the Credé method, what does the nurse teach the patient to do?
    a. Insert the fingers into the vagina and gently push against the vaginal wall.
    b. Breathe in deeply and direct the pressure towards the bladder during exhalation.
    c. Empty the bladder, wait a few minutes, and attempt a second bladder emptying.
    d. Apply firm and steady pressure over the bladder area with the palm of the hand.

53. The physician has recommended intermittent self-catheterization for the patient with long-term problems of incomplete bladder emptying. Which information does the nurse give the patient about the procedure?
    a. Perform proper handwashing and cleaning of the catheter to reduce the risk for infection.
    b. Use a large lumen catheter and good lubrication for rapid emptying of the bladder.
    c. Catheterize yourself whenever the bladder gets distended.
    d. Use sterile technique, especially if catheterization is done by a family member.

54. The nurse is reviewing a care plan for the patient who has functional incontinence. There is a note that containment is recommended, especially at night. What is the major concern with this approach?
    a. Skin breakdown
    b. Cost of care and materials
    c. Self-esteem of the patient
    d. Risk for falls

55. The nurse is caring for the patient with functional incontinence. The UAP reports that "the linens have been changed four times within the past 6 hours, but the patient refuses to wear a diaper." What does the nurse do next?
    a. Thank the UAP for the hard work and advise to continue to change the linens.
    b. Call the health care provider to obtain an order for an indwelling catheter.
    c. Instruct the UAP to stop using the word "diaper" and instead use "incontinence pants."
    d. Assess the patient for any new urinary problems and ask about toileting preferences.

56. Which dietary changes does the nurse suggest to the patient with stress incontinence?
    a. Limit fluid intake to no more than 2 L/day.
    b. Peel all fruit before consuming.
    c. Avoid alcohol and caffeine.
    d. Avoid smoked or salted foods.

57. The patient is considering vaginal cone therapy, but is a little hesitant because she does not understand how it works. What does the nurse tell her about how vaginal cone therapy improves incontinence?
    a. It mechanically obstructs urine loss from the urethra.
    b. It repositions the bladder to reduce compression.
    c. It increases the normal flora of the perineum.
    d. It strengthens pelvic floor muscles.

58. The patient with urinary incontinence is prescribed oxybutynin (Ditropan). What precautions or instructions does the nurse provide related to this therapy?
    a. Avoid aspirin or aspirin-containing products.
    b. Increase fluids and dietary fiber intake
    c. Report any unusual vaginal bleeding.
    d. Change positions slowly, especially in the morning.

59. Teaching intermittent self-catheterization for incontinence is appropriate for which patients? *(Select all that apply.)*
    a. 90-year-old female patient with hypertension
    b. 25-year-old male patient with paraplegia
    c. 35-year-old female patient with stress incontinence
    d. 70-year-old patient who wears absorbent briefs
    e. 18-year-old patient with a severe head injury

True or False? *Read each statement and write T for true or F for false in the blanks provided. If the statement is false, rewrite the statement to make it true.*

_____ 60. Habit training is not appropriate for the patient who is confused or cognitively impaired.

_____ 61. Limiting fluid intake decreases the risk for incontinence.

_____ 62. Use of penile clamps requires vigilance and manual dexterity.

_____ 63. Drug therapy has no role as an intervention for reflex urinary incontinence.

64. The patient is admitted for an elective orthopedic surgical procedure. The patient also has a personal and family history for urolithiasis. Which circumstance creates the greatest risk for recurrent urolithiasis?
    a. Giving the patient milk with every meal tray
    b. Keeping the patient NPO for extended periods
    c. Giving the patient an opioid narcotic for pain
    d. Inserting an indwelling catheter for the procedure

65. The patient reports severe flank pain. The report indicates that urine is turbid, malodorous, and rust colored; RBCs, WBCs, and bacteria are present; and microscopic analysis shows crystals. What does this data suggest?
    a. Pyuria and cystitis
    b. Staghorn calculus with infection
    c. Urolithiasis and infection
    d. Dysuria and urinary retention

66. The patient reports severe flank pain, bladder distention, and nausea and vomiting with increasingly smaller amounts of urine with frank blood. The patient states, "I have kidney stones and I just need some pain medication." What is the nurse's priority concern?
    a. Controlling the patient's pain
    b. Checking the quantity of blood in the urine
    c. Flushing the kidneys with oral fluids
    d. Determining if there is an obstruction

67. The nurse is caring for the patient with a urolithiasis. Which medication is likely given in the acute phase to relieve the patient's severe pain?
    a. Ketorolac (Toradol)
    b. Oxybutynin chloride (Ditropan)
    c. Propantheline bromide (Pro-Banthine)
    d. Morphine sulfate

68. The patient returns to the medical-surgical unit after having extracorporeal shock wave lithotripsy (ESWL). What is an appropriate nursing intervention for the postprocedural care of this patient?
    a. Strain the urine to monitor the passage of stone fragments.
    b. Report bruising that occurs on the flank of the affected side.
    c. Continuously monitor ECG for dysrhythmias.
    d. Apply a local anesthetic cream to the skin of the affected side.

69. The nurse is teaching self-care measures to the patient who had lithotripsy for kidney stones. What information does the nurse include? *(Select all that apply.)*
    a. Finish the entire prescription of antibiotics to prevent UTIs.
    b. Balance regular exercise with sleep and rest.
    c. Dink at least 3 L of fluid a day.
    d. Watch for and immediately report bruising after lithotripsy.
    e. Urine may be bloody for several days.
    f. Pain in the region of the kidneys or bladder is expected.
    g. Report pain, fever, chills, or difficulty with urination to the health care provider.

70. The patient with a history of kidney stones presents with severe flank pain, nausea, vomiting, pallor, and diaphoresis. He reports freely passing urine, but it is bloody. What is the priority nursing diagnosis?
    a. Risk for Deficient Fluid Volume
    b. Risk for Ineffective Tissue Perfusion
    c. Impaired Urinary Elimination
    d. Acute Pain

71. Which clinical manifestation indicates to the nurse that the management intervention for the patient with a kidney stone is effective?
    a. Urine is blood-tinged.
    b. Pulse rate is 75 beats/min.
    c. Urine output is 50 mL/min.
    d. Pulse oximeter reading is 94%.

72. The urine output of the patient with a kidney stone has decreased from 40 mL/hr to 5 mL/hr. What is the nurse's priority action?
    a. Ensure IV access and notify the physician.
    b. Perform the Credé maneuver on the patient's bladder.
    c. Test the urine for ketone bodies.
    d. Document the finding and continue monitoring.

Matching. Indicate which intervention is most appropriate for each type of stone.

Interventions
a. Captopril
b. Thiazide diuretic
c. Sodium bicarbonate
d. Pyridoxine

Types of Stones

_____ 73. Calcium-containing stone

_____ 74. Uric acid-containing stone

_____ 75. Oxalate-containing stone

_____ 76. Cystine-containing stone

77. Which patient has the highest risk for bladder cancer?
    a. 60-year-old male patient with chronic alcoholism
    b. 25-year-old male patient with type 1 diabetes mellitus
    c. 60-year-old female patient who smokes two packs of cigarettes per day and works in a chemical factory
    d. 25-year-old female patient who has had three episodes of bacterial (*Escherichia coli*) cystitis in the past year

78. The employee health nurse is conducting a presentation for employees who work in a paint manufacturing plant. In order to protect against bladder cancer, the nurse advises that everyone who works with chemicals should do what?
    a. Shower with mild soap and rinse well before they come to work.
    b. Use personal protective equipment such as gloves and masks.
    c. Limit their exposure to chemicals and fumes at all times.
    d. Avoid hobbies such as furniture refinishing that further expose to chemicals.

79. The nurse is talking to a 68-year-old male patient who is a smoker and has a long history of occupational exposure to toxic chemicals. Because this patient has a high risk for bladder cancer, the nurse is concerned about which urinary complaint?
    a. Frequency
    b. Nocturia
    c. Painless hematuria
    d. Incontinence

80. The patient has had surgery for bladder cancer. To prevent recurrence of superficial bladder cancer, the nurse anticipates that the physician is likely to recommend which treatment?
    a. No treatment is needed for this benign condition.
    b. Intravesical instillation of a single-agent chemotherapy.
    c. Radiation therapy to the bladder, ureters, and urethra.
    d. Intravesical instillation of bacille Calmette-Guérin.

81. Which statement by the patient indicates effective coping with a Kock's pouch?
    a. "I don't have any discomfort, but the pouch frequently overflows."
    b. "My wife has been irrigating the pouch daily. She likes to do it."
    c. "I check the pouch every 2 to 3 hours depending on my fluid and diet."
    d. "I wash the pouch every day, just like they told me to do in the hospital."

82. The patient has had a bladder suspension and a suprapubic catheter is in place. The patient wants to know how long the catheter will remain in place. What is the nurse's best response?
    a. "Typically it remains for 24 hours postoperatively."
    b. "It will be removed at your first clinic visit."
    c. "When you can void on your own, it will be removed."
    d. "When you can void and the residual urine is less than 50 mL."

83. The patient is returning from the postanesthesia care unit after surgery for bladder cancer resulting in a cutaneous ureterostomy. Where does the nurse expect the stoma to be located?
    a. On the perineum
    b. At the beltline
    c. On the posterior flank
    d. In the midabdominal area

CASE STUDY: THE PATIENT WITH URINARY INCONTINENCE

Use a separate sheet of paper to answer the questions in this Case Study. Answer guidelines for this Case Study are available on your Evolve website at http://evolve. elsevier.com/Iggy/ in the "Prepare for Class" folder.

The patient is a 45-year-old female who has had several full-term pregnancies. She is active and generally healthy, saying, "I take good care of myself." She comes to the clinic for advice about "losing a little urine when I laugh." She reports voiding between 6 and 10 times a day depending on fluid intake. She denies dysuria, back pain, hematuria, fever, or vaginal discharge.

1. What should be included in the assessment of a patient with incontinence?

2. What are the most common types of urinary incontinence? Which type is the patient most likely to have?

3. Identify at least three nursing diagnoses specific to the patient who also has a diagnosis of urinary incontinence.

4. Why is this patient a good candidate for Kegel exercises? What information should the nurse give about performing the exercises?

5. What topics would the nurse include in the teaching plan for this patient?

CHAPTER 70
Care of Patients with Renal Disorders

STUDY/REVIEW QUESTIONS

Matching. *Match each characteristic of patients with polycystic disease to its corresponding gene trait. Answers may be used more than once.*

Gene Traits

a.   Autosomal recessive

b.   Autosomal dominant

Characteristics

_____ 1.   This is the most common form of polycystic kidney disease (PKD).

_____ 2.   Both parents must carry a mutated allele; both mutated alleles must be inherited.

_____ 3.   Nearly 100% who inherit a PKD gene will develop renal cysts by age 30.

_____ 4.   Half develop renal failure by age 50.

_____ 5.   Most die in early childhood.

_____ 6.   Child has a 1 in 4 chance of inheriting autosomal polycystic disease.

7.   The patient's parent has the autosomal dominant form of PKD. Which abnormal vital sign is the greatest concern for the nurse to follow up with because of the family history of PKD?
   a.   Pulse of 100 beats/min
   b.   Temperature of 100.6° F
   c.   Blood pressure of 130/86 mm Hg
   d.   Respiratory rate of 22/min

8.   The nurse is interviewing the patient with suspected PKD. What questions does the nurse ask the patient? *(Select all that apply.)*
   a.   "Is there any family history of PKD or kidney disease?"
   b.   "At what age was your parent diagnosed with PKD?"
   c.   "Have you had any constipation or abdominal discomfort?"
   d.   "Have you noticed a change in urine color or frequency?"
   e.   "Do you have a history of sexually transmitted disease?"
   f.   "Is there a family history of sudden death from a myocardial infarction?"
   g.   "Have you had any problems with headaches?"

9. The patient has a family history of autosomal dominant form of PKD and has therefore been advised to monitor for and report symptoms. What is an early symptom of PKD?
   a. Headache
   b. Pruritus
   c. Edema
   d. Nocturia

10. The patient reports dull, aching pain and the urinalysis is negative for infection. The nurse identifies the nursing diagnosis of Chronic Pain related to enlarging kidneys compressing abdominal contents. What nursing intervention is best for this patient?
    a. Administer trimethoprim/sulfamethoxazole (Bactrim).
    b. Apply dry heat to the abdomen or flank.
    c. Teach methods of relaxation such as deep breathing.
    d. Administer around-the-clock NSAIDs.

11. Why may the patient with PKD experience constipation?
    a. Polycystic kidneys enlarge and put pressure on the large intestine.
    b. Patient becomes dehydrated because the kidneys are dysfunctional.
    c. Constipation is a side effect from the medications given to treat PKD.
    d. Patients with PKD have special dietary restrictions that cause constipation.

12. The nurse is developing a teaching plan for the patient with PKD. Which topics does the nurse include? *(Select all that apply.)*
    a. Teach how to measure and record blood pressure.
    b. Assist to develop a schedule for self-administering drugs.
    c. Instruct to take and record weight twice a month.
    d. Teach to keep blood pressure records.
    e. Explain the potential side effects of the drugs.
    f. Review high-protein, low-fat diet plan.

13. The patient with PKD reports sharp flank pain followed by blood in the urine. How does the nurse interpret these signs/symptoms?
    a. Infection
    b. Ruptured cyst
    c. Increased kidney size
    d. Ruptured renal artery aneurysm

14. The patient with PKD reports a severe headache and is at risk for a berry aneurysm. What is the nurse's priority action?
    a. Assess the pain and give a PRN pain medication.
    b. Reassure the patient that this is an expected aspect of the disease.
    c. Assess for neurologic changes and check vital signs.
    d. Monitor for hematuria and decreased urinary output.

15. The patient with PKD reports nocturia. What is the nocturia caused by?
    a. Increased fluid intake in the evening
    b. Increased hypertension
    c. Decreased renal concentrating ability
    d. Detrusor irritability

16. The nurse is reviewing the patient's laboratory results. Which laboratory abnormality in the patient with PKD indicates disease progression?
    a. Hypercalcemia
    b. Hypokalemia
    c. Proteinuria
    d. Homocystinuria

17. The patient is suspected of having PKD. Which diagnostic study has minimal risks and can reveal PKD?
    a. Kidneys-ureters-bladder (KUB) x-ray
    b. Urography
    c. Renal sonography
    d. MRI with contrast

18. Which pain management strategy does the nurse teach the patient who has pain from infected renal cysts of PKD?
    a. Take nothing by mouth.
    b. Increase the dose of NSAIDs.
    c. Assume a high Fowler's position.
    d. Apply dry heat to the abdomen or flank.

19. The patient with PKD usually experiences constipation. What does the nurse recommend?
    a. Stool softeners and increased fluids
    b. Decreased dietary fiber and laxatives
    c. Laxatives and decreased fluids
    d. Daily tap water enemas and fiber supplements

20. The patient with PKD has nocturia. What does the nurse encourage the patient to do?
    a. Drink 2 liters of fluid daily.
    b. Restrict fluid in the evening.
    c. Only drink 1000 mL/24 hr.
    d. Take diuretics as ordered.

21. Which type of medication is the best choice to control hypertension in the patient with PKD?
    a. ACE inhibitors
    b. Beta blockers
    c. Calcium channel blockers
    d. Potassium-sparing diuretics

22. After the nurse instructs the patient with PKD on home care, the patient knows to contact the physician immediately when what sign/symptom occurs?
    a. Urine is blood-tinged.
    b. Weight has increased by 3 pounds in 3 days.
    c. Two days have passed since the last bowel movement.
    d. Morning systolic blood pressure has decreased by 5 mm Hg.

23. The older adult male patient calls the clinic because he has "not passed any urine all day long." What is the nurse's best response?
    a. "Try drinking several large glasses of water and waiting a few more hours."
    b. "Are you having any other symptoms such as flank pain or fever?"
    c. "You could have an obstruction, so you should come in to be checked."
    d. "I am sorry, but I really can't comment about your problem over the phone."

24. The patient reports straining to pass very small amounts of urine today, despite a normal fluid intake, and reports having the urge to urinate. The nurse palpates the bladder and finds that it is distended. How does the nurse interpret these findings?
    a. Urethral stricture
    b. Hydroureter
    c. Hydronephrosis
    d. PKD

25. The patient is diagnosed with hydronephrosis. What is a complication that could result from this condition?
    a. Damage to the nephrons
    b. Kidney cancer
    c. Kidney stone
    d. Structural defects

26. Which clinical manifestation in the patient with an obstruction in the urinary system is associated specifically with a hydronephrosis?
    a. Flank asymmetry
    b. Chills and fever
    c. Urge incontinence
    d. Decreased urine volume

27. The older adult male patient reports an acute problem with urine retention. The nurse advises the patient to seek medical attention because permanent kidney damage can occur in what time frame?
    a. In less than 6 hours
    b. In less than 48 hours
    c. Within several weeks
    d. Within several years

28. The nurse is reviewing the laboratory results for the patient being evaluated for trouble with passing urine. The urinalysis shows tubular epithelial cells on microscopic examination. How does the nurse interpret this finding?
    a. The obstruction is resolving.
    b. The obstruction is prolonged.
    c. Glomerular filtration rate (GFR) is reduced.
    d. GFR is adequate.

29. The patient had a nephrostomy and a nephrostomy tube is in place. What is included in the postoperative care of this patient?
   a. Assess the amount of drainage in the collection bag.
   b. Irrigate the tube to ensure patency.
   c. Keep the patient NPO for 6 to 8 hours.
   d. Review the results of the clotting studies.

30. The nurse is caring for the patient with a nephrostomy. The nurse notifies the physician about which assessment finding?
   a. Urine drainage is red-tinged 4 hours post-surgery.
   b. Amount of drainage decreases and the patient has back pain.
   c. There is a small steady drainage for the first 4 hours postsurgery.
   d. The nephrostomy site looks dry.

Matching. *Match the factors or manifestations to the renal disorders they are primarily associated with. Answers may be used more than once.*

Renal Disorders
a. Associated with acute pyelonephritis
b. Associated with chronic pyelonephritis
c. Common to both acute and chronic pyelonephritis
d. Common to neither acute nor chronic pyelonephritis

Factors and Manifestations

_____ 31. Obstruction with reflex

_____ 32. Abscess formation

_____ 33. Alcohol abuse

_____ 34. Active bacterial infection

_____ 35. Decreased urine specific gravity

_____ 36. CVA tenderness/pain

_____ 37. Structural deformities

_____ 38. Neurogenic impairment of voiding

_____ 39. Undergone manipulation of the urinary tract

40. The nurse is assessing the patient who reports chills, high fever, and flank pain with urinary urgency and frequency. On physical examination, the patient has costovertebral angle (CVA) tenderness, pulse is 110 beats/min, and respirations are 28/min. How does the nurse interpret these findings?
   a. Complicated cystitis
   b. Acute pyelonephritis
   c. Chronic pyelonephritis
   d. Acute glomerulonephritis

41. The physician informs the patient with acute pyelonephritis that abscess formation is common and recommends diagnostic testing to identify the presence of an abscess. Which test does the nurse prepare the patient for?
   a. Renal arteriography
   b. Cystourethrogram
   c. Radionuclide scintillation
   d. Urodynamic flow studies

42. The patient with chronic pyelonephritis returns to the clinic for follow-up. Which behavior indicates the patient is meeting the expected outcomes to conserve existing renal function?
    a. Drinks a liter of fluid every day
    b. Considers buying a home blood pressure cuff
    c. Reports self-administration of antibiotics as prescribed
    d. Takes pain medication on a regular basis

43. Which patient is at greatest risk for the development of chronic pyelonephritis?
    a. 80-year-old woman who takes diuretics for mild heart failure
    b. 80-year-old man who drinks four cans of beer per day
    c. 36-year-old woman with diabetes mellitus who is pregnant
    d. 36-year-old man with diabetes insipidus

44. The patient is diagnosed with acute pyelonephritis. What is the priority nursing diagnosis for this patient?
    a. Deficient Knowledge
    b. Excess Fluid Volume
    c. Acute/Chronic Pain
    d. Activity Intolerance

45. The nurse is giving discharge instructions to the patient who had pyelolithotomy. What topics does the nurse include in the teaching plan? *(Select all that apply.)*
    a. Controlling blood pressure
    b. Restricting fluids
    c. Eating properly to promote healing
    d. Completing oral antibiotics
    e. Monitoring changes in urine output

46. The patient has come to the clinic for follow-up of acute pyelonephritis. Which action does the nurse reinforce to the patient?
    a. Complete all antibiotic regimens.
    b. Report episodes of nocturia.
    c. Stop taking the antibiotic when pain is relieved.
    d. Notify the physician of any over-the-counter drug use.

True or False? Read each statement and write T for true or F for false in the blanks provided. If the statement is false, correct the statement to make it true.

_____ 47. In PKD, the kidney tissue is eventually replaced by nonfunctioning cysts which look like clusters of grapes.

_____ 48. The kidneys are the only organs that are affected by PKD.

_____ 49. The effect on the renin-angiotensin system in the kidney in PKD results in decreased blood pressure.

_____ 50. Hydronephrosis, hydroureter, and urethral stricture have much in common because they are all forms of congenital anomalies.

_____ 51. Renal tissue changes in chronic glomerulonephritis are caused by trauma and elevated body temperature.

_____ 52. Rapidly progressive glomerulonephritis is related to previous multisystem disease.

_____ 53. The underlying pathology of nephrosclerosis is abscess formation, inflammation, and narrowing of the renal tubules.

_____ 54. A renal cell carcinoma that has metastasized to the lungs would be considered Stage I.

55. The patient is admitted for acute glomerulonephritis. In reviewing the patient's past medical history, which systemic conditions does the nurse suspect may have caused acute glomerulonephritis and will include in the overall treatment plan?
    a. Systemic lupus erythematosus and diabetic nephropathy
    b. Myocardial infarction and atrial fibrillation
    c. Ischemic stroke and hemiparesis
    d. Blunt trauma to the kidney with hematuria

56. The nurse is assessing the patient with possible acute glomerulonephritis. During the inspection of the hands, face, and eyelids, the nurse is primarily observing for evidence of which factors?
    a. Redness
    b. Edema
    c. Rashes
    d. Dryness

57. The nurse is assessing the patient with glomerulonephritis and notes crackles in the lung fields and neck vein distention. The patient reports mild shortness of breath. Based on these findings, what does the nurse do next?
    a. Check for CVA tenderness or flank pain.
    b. Obtain a urine sample to check for proteinuria.
    c. Assess for additional signs of fluid overload.
    d. Alert the physician about the respiratory symptoms.

58. The GFR of the patient with acute glomerulonephritis is 50 mL/min. What is the nurse's interpretation of this finding?
    a. GFR is normal; therapy is effective.
    b. GFR is high; the patient is at risk for dehydration.
    c. GFR is low; the patient is at risk for infection.
    d. GFR is low; the patient is at risk for fluid overload.

59. The patient is very ill and is admitted to the intensive care unit with rapidly progressive glomerulonephritis. The nurse monitors the patient for manifestations of which organ system failure?
    a. Immune system
    b. Cardiac
    c. Liver
    d. Renal

60. The patient is diagnosed with chronic glomerulonephritis. The patient's spouse reports that the patient is irritable, forgetful, and has trouble concentrating. Which assessment finding does the nurse expect further examination will reveal?
    a. Low oxygen saturation
    b. Elevated blood urea nitrogen
    c. High white count with a left shift
    d. Low blood pressure and bradycardia

61. The nurse is reviewing the laboratory results for the patient with chronic glomerulonephritis. The serum albumin level is low. What else does the nurse expect to see?
    a. Proteinuria
    b. Elevated hematocrit
    c. Very low urine specific gravity
    d. Low white blood cell count

62. The patient has chronic glomerulonephritis. In order to assess for uremic symptoms, what does the nurse do?
    a. Evaluate the blood urea nitrogen (BUN).
    b. Ask the patient to extend the arms and hyperextend the wrists.
    c. Gently palpate the flank for asymmetry and tenderness.
    d. Auscultate for the presence of an S_3 heart sound.

63. The nurse is reviewing the laboratory results for the patient with chronic glomerulonephritis. The phosphorus level is 5.3 mg/dL. What else does the nurse expect to see?
    a. Serum calcium level below the normal range
    b. Serum potassium level below the normal range
    c. Falsely elevated serum sodium level
    d. Elevated serum levels for all other electrolytes

64. The nurse is reviewing arterial blood gas results of the patient with acute glomerulonephritis. The pH of the sample is 7.35. As acidosis is likely to be present because of hydrogen ion retention and loss of bicarbonate, how does the nurse interpret this data?
    a. Normal pH with respiratory compensation
    b. Acidosis with failure of respiratory compensation
    c. Alkalosis with failure of metabolic compensation
    d. Normal pH with metabolic compensation

65. The nurse is taking a history on the patient with chronic glomerulonephritis. What is the patient most likely to report?
    a. History of antibiotic allergy
    b. Intense flank pain
    c. Malnutrition and weight loss
    d. Mild edema and hypertension

66. Which patient history factor is considered a causative factor for acute glomerulonephritis?
    a. Cystitis 6 months ago
    b. Strep throat 3 weeks ago
    c. Kidney stones 2 years ago
    d. Mild hypertension diagnosed 1 year ago

67. The patient with acute glomerulonephritis has edema of the face. The blood pressure is moderately elevated and the patient has gained 2 pounds within the past 24 hours. The patient reports fatigue and refuses to eat. What is the priority nursing diagnosis?
    a. Fatigue
    b. Imbalanced Nutrition: Less Than Body Requirements
    c. Impaired Urinary Elimination
    d. Excess Fluid Volume

68. The patient with acute glomerulonephritis is required to provide a 24-hour urine specimen. What does the nurse expect to see with the specimen?
    a. Smoky or cola-colored urine
    b. Clear and very dilute urine
    c. Urine that is full of pus and very thick
    d. Bright orange-colored urine

69. Which nursing intervention is applicable for the patient with acute glomerulonephritis?
    a. Restricting visitors to adults only
    b. Using a lift sheet to turn the patient
    c. Inspecting the vascular access
    d. Measuring abdominal girth daily

70. Which diagnostic tests and results does the nurse expect to see with acute glomerulonephritis? *(Select all that apply.)*
    a. Urinalysis revealing hematuria
    b. Urinalysis revealing proteinuria
    c. Microscopic red blood cell casts
    d. Normal urine sedimentation assay
    e. 24-hour urine for creatinine clearance decreased
    f. Serum nitrogen level decreased
    g. Serum albumin levels decreased
    h. Antistreptolysin-O titers increased

71. The patient has late-stage chronic glomerulonephritis. Which treatment does the nurse discuss and educate the patient about?
    a. Appropriate anti-infective medications
    b. Dialysis or transplantation
    c. Radiation therapy
    d. Immunosuppressive agents

72. The nurse is caring for the patient with nephrotic syndrome. What interventions are included in the plan of care for this patient? *(Select all that apply.)*
    a. Dietary protein must be increased.
    b. Administer mild diuretics.
    c. Assess for edema.
    d. Administer antihypertensive medications.
    e. Assess the patient's hydration status.

73. The nurse is reviewing laboratory results for the patient with suspected kidney problems. Which manifestation is a hallmark for nephrotic syndrome?
    a. Flank asymmetry
    b. Proteinuria greater than 3.5 g of protein in 24 hours
    c. Serum sodium 148 mmol/L
    d. Serum cholesterol (total) 190 mg/dL

74. The patient is newly admitted with nephrotic syndrome and has proteinuria, edema, hyperlipidemia, and hypertension. What is the priority nursing diagnosis for this patient?
    a. Imbalanced Nutrition: More Than Body Requirements
    b. Risk for Urinary Retention
    c. Risk for Imbalanced Fluid Volume
    d. Deficient Knowledge

75. The patient is diagnosed with chronic interstitial nephritis. Which nursing action is relevant and specific for this patient's medical condition?
    a. Avoid analgesic use.
    b. Use disposable gloves.
    c. Monitor for fever.
    d. Place the patient in isolation.

76. Which ethnic group is mostly likely to develop end-stage renal disease related to hypertension?
    a. Caucasian Americans
    b. Asian Americans
    c. Native Americans
    d. African Americans

77. The patient with diabetic nephropathy reports having frequent hypoglycemic episodes "so my doctor reduced my insulin which means my diabetes is improving." What is the nurse's best response?
    a. "Congratulations! You must be following the diet and lifestyle instructions very carefully."
    b. "When kidney function is reduced, the insulin is available for a longer time and thus less of it is needed."
    c. "You should probably talk to your doctor again. You have been diagnosed with nephropathy and that changes the situation."
    d. "Let me get you a brochure about the relationship of diabetes and kidney disease. It is a complex topic and hard to understand."

78. The student nurse is assisting in the postoperative care of the patient who had a recent nephrectomy. The student demonstrates a reluctance to change the linens because "the patient seems so tired." The nurse reminds the student that a priority assessment for this patient is to assess for which factor?
    a. Skin breakdown on the patient's back
    b. Blood on the linens beneath the patient
    c. Urinary incontinence and moisture
    d. The patient's ability to move self in bed

79. After a nephrectomy, the patient has a large urine output because of adrenal insufficiency. What does the nurse anticipate the priority intervention for this patient will be?
    a. ACE inhibitor to control the hypertension and decrease protein loss in urine
    b. Straight catheterization or bedside bladder scan to measure residual urine
    c. IV fluid replacement because of subsequent hypotension and oliguria
    d. IV infusion of Temsirolimus to inhibit cell division and prevent metastasis

80. The patient with a renal abscess who is receiving antibiotics is ordered an additional treatment by the physician. The nurse prepares patient education material for which procedure?
    a. Surgical incision or needle aspiration
    b. Hemodialysis
    c. Insertion of a suprapubic catheter
    d. Cystostomy

81. The 53-year-old patient is newly diagnosed with renal artery stenosis. What clinical manifestation does the nurse observe when the patient first seeks health care?
    a. Sudden onset of hypertension
    b. Urinary frequency and dysuria
    c. Nausea and vomiting
    d. Flank pain and hematuria

82. The patient has been informed by the physician that treatment will be needed for renal artery stenosis. The nurse prepares to teach about a variety of treatment options. What treatments will the nurse include in the teaching plan? *(Select all that apply.)*
    a. Renal transplant
    b. Hypertension control
    c. Percutaneous transluminal balloon angioplasty
    d. Renal bypass surgery
    e. Synthetic blood vessel graft
    f. Percutaneous ultrasonic pyelolithotomy

83. What change in diabetic therapy may be needed for the patient who has diabetic nephropathy?
    a. Fluid restriction
    b. Decreased activity level
    c. Decreased insulin dosages
    d. Increased caloric intake

84. The patient has had one kidney removed as a treatment for renal cancer. The patient's spouse asks, "Does the good kidney take over immediately? I know a person can live with just one kidney." What is the nurse's best response?
    a. "The other kidney will provide adequate function, but this may take days or weeks."
    b. "The other kidney alone isn't able to provide adequate function, so supplemental therapies will be needed."
    c. "That's a good question. Remember to ask your doctor next time he or she comes in."
    d. "It varies a lot, but within a few days we expect everything to normalize."

85. After a nephrectomy, one adrenal gland remains. Based on this knowledge, which type of medication replacement therapy does the nurse expect the patient who had a nephrectomy to receive?
    a. Potassium
    b. Steroid
    c. Calcium
    d. Estrogen

86. The nurse is caring for the patient with renal cell carcinoma. What symptoms and findings does the nurse expect to see in this patient? *(Select all that apply.)*
    a. Urinary tract infection
    b. Erythrocytosis
    c. Hypercalcemia
    d. Liver dysfunction
    e. Decreased sedimentation rate
    f. Hypertension
    g. Hematuria

87. The nurse is caring for the patient with renal cell carcinoma. What does the nurse expect to find documented about the patient's initial assessment?
    a. Flank pain, gross hematuria, palpable renal mass, and renal bruit
    b. Gross hematuria, hypertension, diabetes, and oliguria
    c. Dysuria, polyuria, dehydration, and palpable renal mass
    d. Nocturia and urinary retention with difficulty starting stream

88. The patient is diagnosed with renal cancer and the physician recommends the best therapy. Which treatment does the nurse anticipate teaching the patient about?
    a. Chemotherapy
    b. Surgical removal
    c. Hormonal therapy
    d. Radiation therapy

89. The patient returning to the unit after a left radical nephrectomy for renal cell carcinoma is concerned about severe pain on the right side. What does the nurse tell the patient?
    a. "The right kidney was repositioned to take over the function of both kidneys."
    b. "I'll call your doctor for an order to increase your pain medication."
    c. "The pain is likely to be from being positioned on your right side during surgery."
    d. "Would you like to talk with someone who had this surgery last year and now is fully recovered?"

90. The nurse is caring for the postoperative nephrectomy patient. The nurse notes during the first several hours of the shift a marked and steady downward trend in blood pressure. How does the nurse interpret this finding?
    a. Hypertension has been corrected.
    b. Internal hemorrhage is possible.
    c. The other kidney is failing.
    d. This is an expected response to medication.

91. The nurse is caring for the patient after a nephrectomy. The nurse notes that the urine flow was 50 mL/hr at the beginning of the shift, but several hours later has dropped to 30 mL. What is the nurse's priority action?
    a. Notify the physician for an order for an IV fluid bolus.
    b. Document the finding and continue to monitor for downward trend.
    c. Troubleshoot the drainage system to make sure there are no obstructions.
    d. Obtain the patient's weight and compare it to baseline.

92. The nurse is caring for the patient who had a nephrectomy yesterday. To manage the patient's pain, what is the best plan for analgesia therapy?
    a. Limit narcotics because of respiratory depression.
    b. Give an oral analgesic when the patient can eat.
    c. Alternate parenteral and oral medications.
    d. Give parenteral medications on a schedule.

93. The patient is brought to the emergency department (ED) after being involved in a fight in which the patient was kicked and punched repeatedly in the back. What does the nurse include in the initial physical assessment? (Select all that apply.)
    a. Take complete vital signs.
    b. Check apical and peripheral pulses.
    c. Inspect both flanks for asymmetry or penetrating injuries of the lower chest or back.
    d. Inspect the abdomen for bruising or penetrating wounds.
    e. Deeply palpate the abdomen for signs of rigidity.
    f. Percuss the abdomen for distention.
    g. Inspect the urethra for gross bleeding.

94. The ED nurse is preparing the patient with renal trauma for emergency surgery. What is the best task to delegate to the unlicensed assistive personnel (UAP)?
    a. Set the automated blood pressure machine to cycle every 30 minutes.
    b. Inform the family about surgery and assist them to the surgery waiting area.
    c. Go to the blood bank and pick up the units of packed red cells.
    d. Insert a Foley catheter if there is no gross bleeding at the urethra.

95. The patient has sustained renal injury. In order to assist the patient to undergo the best diagnostic test to determine the extent of injury, what does the nurse do?
    a. Obtain a clean catch urine specimen for urinalysis.
    b. Give an IV fluid bolus before renal arteriography.
    c. Give an explanation of computed tomography.
    d. Obtain a blood sample for hemoglobin and hematocrit.

CASE STUDY: THE PATIENT WITH PKD

Use a separate sheet of paper to answer the questions in this Case Study. Answer guidelines for this Case Study are available on your Evolve website at http://evolve. elsevier.com/Iggy/ in the "Prepare for Class" folder.

A 30-year-old white male patient comes to the clinic reporting dull, aching abdominal and flank pain. He reports nocturia and a family history of autosomal dominant PKD. He reports no known personal health problems, although he was instructed to monitor his blood pressure at home and he admits to "not doing so well with that." Today his blood pressure is 130/90 mm Hg; pulse is 72 and regular; respirations 12/min, and temperature is 98.8° F.

1. What additional information should the nurse elicit during the interview?
2. What are the key features of PKD?
3. Describe the causes of pain for patients with PKD.
4. What are typical findings of a urinalysis in a patient with PKD?
5. What are the causes of hypertension and renal ischemia in a patient with PKD?
6. What is the risk involved with other organs and tissues in the progression of PKD?
7. Patients with PKD often have other tissue involvement. List several of the complications that can be present.
8. List reasons that patients diagnosed with PKD may need a nursing diagnosis of Impaired Coping.
9. Identify priority nursing care needs for the patient with PKD.
10. What would the nurse include in the teaching plan for this patient?

71 CHAPTER

Care of Patients with Acute Renal Failure and Chronic Kidney Disease

STUDY/REVIEW QUESTIONS

True or False? Read each statement and write T for true or F for false in the blanks provided. If the statement is false, correct the statement to make it true.

_____ 1. When kidney function declines gradually, as occurs most often with chronic kidney disease (CKD) also known as chronic renal failure (CRF), 90% to 95% of the nephrons must be destroyed before renal failure is obvious.

_____ 2. The problems that occur with renal failure are related to fluid volume excess, electrolyte- and acid-base abnormalities, buildup of nitrogen-based wastes, and loss of kidney hormone function.

_____ 3. With shock or other problems causing an acute reduction in renal blood flow, the kidney compensates by constricting renal blood vessels, activating the renin-angiotensin-aldosterone pathway, and releasing antidiuretic hormone.

_____ 4. When pressure in the renal tubules exceeds glomerular pressure, glomerular filtration stops.

_____ 5. Acute renal failure (ARF) may occur with no loss of nephrons.

Matching. Match each cause to its corresponding urologic change. Answers may be used more than once.

Urologic Changes
a. Prerenal
b. Intrarenal
c. Postrenal

Causes

_____ 6. Urethral cancer

_____ 7. Heart failure

_____ 8. Vasculitis

_____ 9. Sepsis

_____ 10. Exposure to nephrotoxins

_____ 11. Renal calculi

_____ 12. Atony of bladder

_____ 13. Renal artery stenosis or thrombosis

_____ 14. Shock

15. The community health nurse is designing programs to reduce kidney problems and renal failure among the general public. In order to do so, the nurse targets health promotion and compliance with therapy for people with which conditions?
    a. Diabetes mellitus and hypertension
    b. Frequent episodes of sexually transmitted disease
    c. Osteoporosis and other bone diseases
    d. Gastroenteritis and poor eating habits

16. The nurse is caring for the patient who had hypovolemic shock secondary to trauma in the emergency department (ED) 2 days ago. Based on the pathophysiology of hypovolemia and prerenal azotemia, what does the student nurse assess every hour?
    a. Urinary output
    b. Presence of edema
    c. Urine color
    d. Presence of pain

17. The nurse is talking to the older adult male patient who is reasonably healthy for his age, but has benign prostatic hypertrophy (BPH). Which condition does the BPH potentially place him at risk for?
    a. Prerenal azotemia
    b. Postrenal azotemia
    c. Acute tubular necrosis
    d. Acute glomerulonephritis

18. Which patient is taking a combination of drugs that are the most nephrotoxic?
    a. Angiotensin-converting enzyme (ACE) inhibitors and aspirin
    b. Angiotensin II receptor blockers and antacids
    c. Aminoglycoside antibiotics and NSAIDs
    d. Calcium channel blockers and antihistamines

19. The nurse is caring for the patient with the nonoliguric form of ARF. Which factor contributes to the prognosis for this patient?
    a. The clinical manifestations are more readily and easily observed.
    b. Attentive nursing care has resulted in the patient having the nonoliguric form.
    c. The urine output remains nearly normal and the treatment is less complicated.
    d. The nonoliguric form occurs in younger people who have better baseline health.

20. The patient with ARF secondary to which factor has the worst prognosis and the lowest chance for recovery?
    a. Radiographic contrast dye
    b. Glomerulonephritis
    c. Kidney stone
    d. Dehydration

21. The nurse has obtained a urine specimen from the patient and has used a dipstick to test the urine. Which abnormal finding is the earliest sign of renal tubular damage?
    a. Presence of blood
    b. Presence of leukocytes
    c. Presence of glucose
    d. Decreased urine specific gravity

22. The nurse is caring for the patient receiving gentamycin. Because this drug has potential for nephrotoxicity, which laboratory results does the nurse monitor? *(Select all that apply.)*
    a. Blood urea nitrogen (BUN)
    b. Creatinine
    c. Drug peak and trough levels
    d. Prothrombin time (PT)
    e. Platelet count
    f. Hemoglobin and hematocrit

23. The nurse is assessing the patient with ARF. The nurse notes bladder distention and the patient reports "feeling the urge to urinate." Urine sodium level is 40 mEq/L; specific gravity of 1.010. How does the nurse interpret these findings?
    a. Prerenal azotemia
    b. Intrarenal failure
    c. Postrenal failure
    d. Oliguric phase

24. The patient has been diagnosed with ARF, but the cause is uncertain. The nurse prepares patient education material about which diagnostic test?
    a. Flat plate of the abdomen
    b. Renal ultrasonography
    c. Computed tomography
    d. Renal biopsy

25. The patient is in the diuretic phase of ARF. During this phase, what is the nurse mainly concerned about?
    a. Assessing for hypertension and fluid overload
    b. Monitoring for hypovolemia and electrolyte loss
    c. Adjusting the dosage of diuretic medications
    d. Balancing diuretic therapy with intake

26. The patient with prerenal azotemia is administered a fluid challenge. In evaluating response to the therapy, which outcome indicates that the goal was met?
    a. Patient reports feeling better and indicates an eagerness to go home.
    b. Patient produces urine soon after the initial bolus.
    c. The therapy is completed without adverse effects.
    d. The physician orders a diuretic when the challenge is completed.

27. The nurse is caring for the patient with ARF and notes a trend of increasing elevated BUN levels. How does the nurse interpret this information?
    a. Breakdown of muscle for protein which leads to an increase in azotemia
    b. Sign of urinary retention and decreased urinary output
    c. Expected trend that can be reversed by increasing dietary protein
    d. Ominous sign of impending irreversible kidney failure

28. The nurse is caring for the patient with prerenal azotemia. What are the primary treatment goals in the initial phase that prevents permanent kidney damage for this patient? *(Select all that apply.)*
    a. Correct blood volume.
    b. Increase blood pressure.
    c. Manage kidney infections.
    d. Relieve the obstruction.
    e. Improve cardiac output.

29. The patient sustained extensive burns and depletion of vascular volume. The nurse expects which changes in vital signs and urinary function?
    a. Decreased urine output, postural hypotension, tachycardia
    b. Increased urine output, bounding pulses, tachycardia
    c. Bradycardia, hypertension, polyuria
    d. Dysrhythmias, hypertension, oliguria

30. The nurse is taking a history of the patient at risk for renal failure. What does the nurse ask the patient about during the interview? *(Select all that apply.)*
    a. Exposure to nephrotoxic chemicals
    b. Recent weight loss
    c. History of diabetes mellitus, hypertension, systemic lupus erythematosus
    d. Recent surgery, trauma, or transfusions
    e. Leakage of urine when coughing or laughing
    f. Use of antibiotics, NSAIDs, or ACE inhibitors

31. Which disorder may mimic the presentation of prerenal azotemia?
    a. Heart failure
    b. Diabetes mellitus
    c. Pneumonia
    d. Compartment syndrome

32. The patient with ARF is anorexic and refuses to eat. The nurse notifies the health care provider to obtain an order for which intervention?
    a. Normal saline to prevent dehydration
    b. Nutritional consult for a calculated diet
    c. Total parenteral nutrition (TPN) with appropriate laboratory monitoring
    d. Nasogastric tube for enteral feedings

33. Which symptoms does the nurse expect to see in the patient with intrarenal ARF? *(Select all that apply.)*
    a. Oliguria/anuria
    b. Hypotension
    c. Shortness of breath
    d. Jugular vein distention
    e. Decreased central pressure
    f. Weight loss
    g. Rales and crackles
    h. Nausea and anorexia

34. The nurse is caring for the patient with signs and symptoms of prerenal azotemia. A fluid challenge is performed to promote renal perfusion by doing what?
    a. Administering normal saline 500 to 1000 mL infused over 1 hour
    b. Administering drugs to suppress aldosterone release
    c. Instilling warm, sterile normal saline into the bladder
    d. Having the patient drink several large glasses of water

35. The patient has ARF related to nephrotoxic acute tubular necrosis (ATN). In order to maintain cell integrity, improve glomerular filtration rate (GFR), and improve renal blood flow, which medication does the nurse anticipate the health care provider will prescribe?
    a. Digoxin
    b. Alpha-adrenergic blockers
    c. Beta blockers
    d. Calcium channel blockers

36. The patient with ARF has a high rate of catabolism. What is this related to?
    a. Increased levels of catecholamines, cortisol, and glucagon
    b. Inability to excrete excess electrolytes
    c. Conversion of body fat into glucose
    d. Presence of retained nitrogenous wastes

37. The nurse is caring for the patient in the ICU who sustained blood loss during a traumatic accident. In order to assess for prerenal azotemia, which signs and symptoms does the nurse observe for? *(Select all that apply.)*
    a. Hypotension
    b. Bradycardia
    c. Decreased urine output
    d. Decreased cardiac output
    e. Increased central venous pressure
    f. Lethargy

38. The patient with ARF is receiving total parenteral nutrition (TPN). What is the goal of TPN?
    a. Preserve lean body mass
    b. Promote tubular reabsorption
    c. Create a negative nitrogen balance
    d. Prevent infection

Matching. *Match each characteristic with its corresponding device. Answers may be used more than once, and there may be more than one answer for a characteristic.*

Devices

a. Continuous arteriovenous hemofiltration (CAVH)
b. Continuous arteriovenous hemodialysis and filtration (CAVHD)
c. Continuous venovenous hemofiltration (CVVH)

Characteristics

_____ 39. Requires placement of arterial and venous catheter

_____ 40. Requires a double-lumen venous catheter

_____ 41. Uses pump

_____ 42. Arterial pressure of at least 60 mm Hg

_____ 43. Removes water and electrolytes

_____ 44. Risk of air embolus

_____ 45. Uses dialysate to remove nitrogenous waste

Matching. *Match each characteristic with its corresponding stage of renal failure. Answers may be used more than once, and there may be more than one answer for a characteristic.*

Stages

a. Reduced renal reserve
b. Renal insufficiency
c. End-stage renal disease (ESRD)

Characteristics

_____ 46. Excessive waste products

_____ 47. Increased BUN and creatinine

_____ 48. Dialysis

_____ 49. Primary reduction in function

_____ 50. Nephrons compensate

_____ 51. Hypertension

_____ 52. Stress of illness can rapidly compromise this stage

_____ 53. Therapy slows, but does not halt progression

_____ 54. Severe fluid overload

_____ 55. Severe electrolyte and acid-base imbalances

_____ 56. Renal osteodystrophy

57. The nurse is taking a history on the patient with diabetes and hypertension. Because of the patient's high risk for developing kidney problems, which early sign of CRF does the nurse assess for?
    a. Decreased output with subjective thirst
    b. Urinary frequency of very small amounts
    c. Pink or blood-tinged urine
    d. Increased output of very dilute urine

58. The patient's laboratory results show an elevated creatinine level. The patient's history reveals no risk factors for kidney disease. Which question does the nurse ask the patient to shed further light on the laboratory result?
    a. "How many hours of sleep did you get the night before the test?"
    b. "How much fluid did you drink before the test?"
    c. "Did you take any type of antibiotics before taking the test?"
    d. "When and how much did you last urinate before having the test?"

59. The nurse is reviewing the patient's laboratory results. In the early phase of CRF, what does the nurse expect to see?
    a. Higher than normal potassium
    b. Lower than normal sodium
    c. Higher than normal calcium
    d. Lower than normal phosphorus

60. The patient with CRF has a potassium level of 8 mEq/L. The nurse notifies the health care provider after assessing for which sign/symptom?
    a. Cardiac dysrhythmias
    b. Respiratory depression
    c. Tremors or seizures
    d. Decreased urine output

61. The nurse is assessing the patient with renal failure and notes a marked increase in the rate and depth of breathing. The nurse recognizes this as Kussmaul respiration, which is the body's attempt to compensate for which condition?
    a. Hypoxia
    b. Alkalosis
    c. Acidosis
    d. Hypoxemia

62. The patient is diagnosed with renal osteo-dystrophy. What does the nurse instruct the unlicensed assistive personnel (UAP) to do in relation to this patient's diagnosis?
    a. Assist the patient with toileting every 2 hours.
    b. Gently wash the patient's skin with a mild soap and rinse well.
    c. Handle the patient gently because of risk for fractures.
    d. Assist the patient with eating because of loss of coordination.

63. The patient with CKD develops severe chest pain, an increased pulse, low-grade fever, and a pericardial friction rub with a cardiac dysrhythmia and muffled heart tones. The nurse immediately alerts the physician and prepares for which emergency procedure?
    a. Pericardiocentesis
    b. Continuous venovenous hemofiltration
    c. Renal dialysis
    d. Cardiopulmonary resuscitation

64. All patients with hypertension or diabetes should have yearly screenings for which factor?
    a. Creatinine
    b. BUN
    c. Glycosuria
    d. Microalbuminuria

65. The nurse is assessing the patient with renal failure. What is an early neurologic manifestation of renal failure that could potentially be resolved with dialysis?
    a. Lethargy
    b. Unequal pupils
    c. Severe motor impairment
    d. Unilateral weakness

66. The night shift nurse sees the patient with renal failure sitting up in bed. The patient states, "I feel a little short of breath at night or when I get up to walk to the bathroom." What assessment does the nurse do?
    a. Check for orthostatic hypertension because of potential volume depletion.
    b. Auscultate the lungs for crackles which indicate fluid overload.
    c. Check the pulse and blood pressure for possible decreased cardiac output.
    d. Assess for normal sleep pattern and need for a PRN sedative.

67. What does the breath often smell like in the patient with CRF?
    a. Fruit
    b. Feces
    c. Urine
    d. Blood

68. The patient with CRF reports chronic fatigue and lethargy with weakness and mild shortness of breath with dizziness when rising to a standing position. In addition, the nurse notes pale mucous membranes. Based on the patient's illness and the presenting symptoms, which laboratory result does the nurse expect to see?
    a. Low hemoglobin and hematocrit
    b. Low white cell count
    c. Low blood glucose
    d. Low oxygen saturation

69. The nurse is assessing the skin of the patient with ESRD. Which clinical manifestation is considered a sign of very advanced disease?
    a. Ecchymoses
    b. Sallowness
    c. Pallor
    d. Uremic frost

70. The nurse notes an abnormal laboratory test finding for the patient with CRF and alerts the health care provider. The nurse also consults with the nutritionist because an excessive dietary protein intake is directly related to which factor?
    a. Elevated serum creatinine level
    b. Protein presence in the urine
    c. Elevated BUN level
    d. Elevated serum potassium level

71. In collaboration with the nutritionist, the nurse teaches the patient about which diet recommendations for management of CRF? *(Select all that apply.)*
    a. Controlling protein intake
    b. Limiting fluid intake
    c. Restricting potassium
    d. Increasing sodium
    e. Restricting phosphorus
    f. Eating enough calories to meet metabolic need
    g. Avoiding vitamin supplements

72. The patient receives dialysis therapy and the health care provider has ordered sodium restriction to 4 g daily. What does the nurse teach the patient?
    a. Add only small amounts of salt at the table or during cooking.
    b. Foods high in sodium (e.g., processed foods, fast foods) should be strictly avoided.
    c. Herbs and spices can be used in place of salt to enhance food flavor.
    d. Bland foods with very minimal amounts of spicing are the best choice.

73. In order to assist the patient in the prevention of osteodystrophy, which intervention does the nurse perform?
    a. Administer phosphate binders at mealtimes.
    b. Encourage the patient to eat high-quality protein foods.
    c. Assist the patient to ambulate and exercise several times a day.
    d. Encourage the patient to drink extra milk at mealtimes.

74. The nurse prepares to administer medications to the patient with CRF. The nurse calls the health care provider as a reminder that the patient might need which nutritional supplements? *(Select all that apply.)*
    a. Iron
    b. Magnesium
    c. Phosphorus
    d. Calcium
    e. Vitamin D
    f. Water-soluble vitamins

75. The nurse is caring for the patient with ESRD and dialysis has been initiated. Which drug order does the nurse question?
    a. Erythropoietin
    b. Diuretic
    c. ACE inhibitor
    d. Calcium channel blocker

76. The nurse monitors the CRF patient's daily weights because of the risk for fluid retention. What instructions does the nurse give to the UAP?
    a. Weigh the patient daily at the same time each day, same scale, with the same amount of clothing.
    b. Weigh the patient daily and add 1 kilogram of weight for the intake of each liter of fluid.
    c. Weigh the patient in the morning before breakfast and weigh the patient at night just before bedtime.
    d. Ask the patient what his or her normal weight is and then weigh the patient before and after each voiding.

77. The patient with CKD is taking digoxin. Which signs of digoxin toxicity does the nurse vigilantly monitor for? *(Select all that apply.)*
    a. Nausea and vomiting
    b. Visual changes
    c. Respiratory depression
    d. Restlessness or confusion
    e. Headache or fatigue
    f. Atrial fibrillation

78. The nurse is caring for the patient with CKD. The nurse anticipates that dosage adjustments will be made for which drugs? *(Select all that apply.)*
    a. Antibiotics
    b. Opioids
    c. Insulin
    d. NSAIDs
    e. Oral antidiabetics

79. The nurse is evaluating the patient's treatment response to erythropoietin (Epogen). Which hematocrit reading indicates that the goal is being met?
    a. 10%
    b. 30%
    c. 50%
    d. At baseline

80. The patient has been receiving erythropoietin (Epogen). Which statement by the patient indicates that the therapy is producing the desired effect?
    a. "I can do my housework with less fatigue."
    b. "I have been passing more urine than I was before."
    c. "I have less pain and discomfort now."
    d. "I can swallow and eat much better than before."

81. Which behavior is the strongest indicator that the patient with ESRD is not coping well with the illness and may need a referral for psychological counseling?
    a. Displays irritability when the meal tray arrives
    b. Refuses to take one of the drugs because it causes nausea
    c. Repeatedly misses dialysis appointments
    d. Seems distracted when the physician talks about the prognosis

82. The patient with CKD is restless, anxious, and short of breath. The nurse hears crackles that begin at the base of the lungs. The pulse rate is increased and the patient has frothy, blood-tinged sputum. What does the nurse do next?
    a. Facilitate transfer to the ICU for aggressive treatment.
    b. Place the patient in a high Fowler's position.
    c. Monitor vital signs and assess breath sounds.
    d. Administer a loop diuretic such as furosemide (Lasix).

83. Which patients are candidates for CAVH? *(Select all that apply.)*
    a. Patient with fluid volume overload
    b. Patient who needs long-term management
    c. Hemodynamically unstable patient
    d. Patient who is ready for discharge to home
    e. Patient who is resistant to diuretics

84. As the patient with ESRD experiences isosthenuria, what must the nurse be alert for?
    a. The diuretic stage
    b. Fluid volume overload
    c. Dehydration
    d. Alkalosis

85. The nurse is caring for the patient with CRF. The family asks about when renal replacement therapy will begin. What is the nurse's best response?
    a. "As early as possible to prevent further damage in stage I."
    b. "When there is renal insufficiency and metabolic wastes accumulate."
    c. "When the kidneys are unable to maintain a balance in body functions."
    d. "It will be started with diuretic therapy to enhance the remaining function."

86. Which are the most accurate ways to monitor kidney function in the patient with CRF? *(Select all that apply.)*
    a. Monitoring intake and output
    b. Checking urine specific gravity
    c. Reviewing BUN and serum creatinine levels
    d. Reviewing x-ray reports
    e. Consulting the nutritionist's notes

87. As a result of kidney failure, excessive hydrogen ions cannot be excreted. With acid retention, the nurse is most likely to observe what type of respiratory compensation?
    a. Cheyne-Stokes respiratory pattern
    b. Increased depth of breathing
    c. Decreased respiratory rate and depth
    d. Increased arterial carbon dioxide levels

88. The nurse is assessing the patient with uremia. Which gastrointestinal changes does the nurse expect to find? *(Select all that apply.)*
    a. Halitosis
    b. Hiccups
    c. Anorexia
    d. Nausea
    e. Vomiting
    f. Salivation
    g. Stomatitis

89. Which chronic renal patients are candidates for hemodialysis? *(Select all that apply.)*
    a. Patient with fluid overload who does not respond to diuretics
    b. Patient with medication-controlled hypertension
    c. Patient with severe neurologic problems
    d. Patient with a decreased attention span and decreased cognition
    e. Patient with worsening anemia and pruritus

90. The home health nurse is evaluating the home setting for the patient who wishes to have in-home hemodialysis. What is important to have in the home setting to support this therapy?
    a. Specialized water treatment system to provide a safe, clean water supply
    b. Large dust-free space to accommodate and store the dialysis equipment
    c. Modified electrical system to provide high voltage to power the equipment
    d. Specialized cooling system to maintain strict temperature control

91. The nursing student is explaining principles of hemodialysis to the nursing instructor. Which statement by the student indicates a need for additional study and research on the topic?
    a. "Dialysis works as molecules from an area of higher concentration move to an area of lower concentration."
    b. "Blood and dialyzing solution flow in opposite directions across an enclosed semipermeable membrane."
    c. "Excess water, waste products, and excess electrolytes are removed from the blood."
    d. "Bacteria and other organisms can also pass through the membrane."

92. The patient and family are trying to plan a schedule that coordinates with the patient's dialysis regimen. The patient asks, "How often will I have to go and how long does it take?" What is the nurse's best response?
    a. "If you are compliant with the diet and fluid restrictions, you spend less time in dialysis, about 12 hours a week."
    b. "Most patients require about 12 hours per week; this is usually divided into three 4-hour treatments."
    c. "It varies from patient to patient. You will have to call your health care provider for specific instructions."
    d. "If you gain a large amount of fluid weight, a longer treatment time may be needed to prevent severe side effects."

93. The patient is undergoing a dialysis treatment and exhibits a progression of symptoms which include headache, nausea, and vomiting; decreased level of consciousness; and seizure activity. How does the nurse interpret these symptoms?
    a. Dialysis disequilibrium syndrome
    b. Expected manifestations in ESRD
    c. Transient symptoms in a new dialysis patient
    d. Adverse reaction to the dialysate

94. The nurse is caring for the patient with an arteriovenous shunt. What instructions are given to the UAP regarding the care of this patient?
    a. Palpate for thrills and auscultate for bruits every 4 hours.
    b. Check for bleeding at needle insertion sites.
    c. Assess the patient's distal pulses and circulation.
    d. Do not take blood pressure readings in the arm with the shunt.

95. The nurse is assessing the patient's extremity with an arteriovenous graft. The nurse notes a thrill and a bruit, and the patient reports numbness and a cool feeling in the fingers. How does the nurse interpret this information in regards to the shunt?
    a. It is functional and symptoms are expected.
    b. It is functional but the patient has "steal syndrome."
    c. It is directing the blood flow in the wrong direction.
    d. It is not functional and therefore causing numbness.

96. The nurse is providing postdialysis care for the patient. In comparing vital signs and weight measurements to the predialysis data, what does the nurse expect to find?
    a. Blood pressure and weight are reduced.
    b. Blood pressure is increased and weight is reduced.
    c. Blood pressure and weight are similar to predialysis measurements.
    d. Blood pressure is low and weight is the same.

97. The nurse is assessing the patient who has just returned from hemodialysis. What is an unexpected finding that warrants notification of the health care provider?
    a. Feeling of malaise
    b. Nausea and anorexia
    c. Muscle cramps in the legs
    d. Bleeding at the access site

98. The nurse is caring for the patient with an arteriovenous fistula. What is included in the nursing care for this patient? *(Select all that apply.)*
    a. Keep small clamps handy by the bedside.
    b. Encourage routine range-of-motion exercises.
    c. Avoid venipuncture or IV administration on the arm with the access device.
    d. Instruct the patient to carry heavy objects to build muscular strength.
    e. Assess for manifestations of infection at needle sites.
    f. Instruct the patient to sleep on the side with the affected arm in the dependent position.

99. The patient has returned to the medical-surgical unit after having a dialysis treatment. The nurse notes that the patient is also scheduled for an invasive procedure on the same day. What is the primary rationale for delaying the procedure for 4 to 6 hours?
    a. The patient was heparinized during dialysis.
    b. The patient will have cardiac dysrhythmias after dialysis.
    c. The patient will be incoherent and unable to give consent.
    d. The patient needs routine medications that were delayed.

100. The nurse alerts the physician about changes in the patient's condition and the patient is diagnosed with dialysis disequilibrium syndrome. The nurse prepares to assist in the administration of which treatment?
    a. IV normal saline fluid bolus
    b. Diuretics and antihypertensives
    c. Barbiturates and anticonvulsants
    d. Morphine and anticoagulants

101. Which renal patient is the best candidate for peritoneal dialysis (PD)?
    a. Patient with peritoneal adhesions
    b. Patient with a history of extensive abdominal surgery
    c. Patient with peritoneal membrane fibrosis
    d. Patient with a history of difficulty with anticoagulants

102. Place the sequence of steps of PD in the correct order using the numbers 1 through 3.
    _____ a. Fluid stays in the cavity for a specified time prescribed by the physician.
    _____ b. 1 to 2 L of dialysate is infused by gravity over a 10- to 20-minute period.
    _____ c. Fluid flows out of the body by gravity into a drainage bag.

103. The physician has ordered intraperitoneal heparin for the patient with a new PD catheter to prevent clotting of the catheter. What does the nurse advise the patient to do?
    a. Watch for signs of bleeding such as bruising or bleeding from the gums.
    b. Make a follow-up appointment for coagulation studies.
    c. Be aware that intraperitoneal heparin does not affect clotting times.
    d. Be aware that heparin will be given with a small subcutaneous needle.

Matching. Match the terms with their correct descriptions.

Terms
a. Continuous ambulatory peritoneal dialysis (CAPD)
b. Continuous connect system
c. Disconnect system
d. Automated peritoneal dialysis (APD)
e. Intermittent peritoneal dialysis (IPD)
f. Continuous-cycle peritoneal dialysis (CCPD)

Descriptions

_____ 104. Combines osmotic pressure gradients with true dialysis

_____ 105. Infusion of four 2 L exchanges of dialysate; exchanges occur 7 days a week

_____ 106. The extra opening of the system increases the risk for infection

_____ 107. Empty bag and tubing are folded beneath clothing until they are used for outflow

_____ 108. Permits in-home dialysis during sleep, allowing dialysis-free waking hours

_____ 109. Uses an automated cycling machine

110. The home health nurse is visiting the patient who independently performs PD. Which question does the nurse ask the patient to assess for the most common problem associated with PD?
    a. "Have you noticed any signs or symptoms of infection?"
    b. "Are you having any pain during the dialysis treatments?"
    c. "Is the dialysate fluid slow or sluggish?"
    d. "Have you noticed any leakage around the catheter?"

111. The nurse is teaching the patient about performing PD at home. In order to identify the earliest manifestation of infection, what does the nurse instruct the patient to do?
    a. Monitor temperature routinely.
    b. Check the effluent for cloudiness.
    c. Be aware of feelings of malaise.
    d. Monitor for abdominal pain.

112. During PD, the nurse notes slowed dialysate flow. What does the nurse do to troubleshoot the system? *(Select all that apply.)*
    a. Ensure that the drainage bag is elevated.
    b. Inspect the tubing for kinking or twisting.
    c. Ensure that clamps are open.
    d. Turn the patient to the other side.
    e. Make sure the patient is in good body alignment
    f. Instruct the patient to stand or cough.
    g. Milk the tubing for particulate matter.

113. The patient has just started PD therapy and reports some mild pain when the dialysate is flowing in. What does the nurse do next?
    a. Immediately report the pain to the health care provider.
    b. Try warming the dialysate in the microwave oven.
    c. Reassure the patient that some pain is expected for the first week or two.
    d. Assess the connection tubing for kinking or twisting.

114. The nurse is caring for the patient requiring PD. In order to monitor the patient's weight, what does the nurse do?
    a. Check the weight after a drain and before the next fill to monitor the patient's "dry weight."
    b. Calculate the "dry weight" by weighing the patient every day and comparing the measurements to baseline.
    c. Determine "dry weight" by comparing the patient's weight to a standard weight chart based on height and age.
    d. Weigh the patient each day and count fluid intake and dialysate volume to determine the patient's "dry weight."

115. The nurse is monitoring the patient's PD treatment. The total outflow is less than the inflow. What does the nurse do next?
    a. Instruct the patient to ambulate.
    b. Notify the health care provider.
    c. Record the difference as intake.
    d. Put the patient on fluid restriction.

116. Which patients are likely to be excluded from receiving a transplant? *(Select all that apply.)*
    a. Patient who had breast cancer 6 years ago
    b. HIV-positive patient
    c. Patient with a chemical dependency
    d. 70-year-old patient
    e. Patient with diabetes mellitus

117. A daughter is considering donating a kidney to her mother for organ transplant. What information does the nurse give to the daughter about the criteria for donation? *(Select all that apply.)*
    a. Age limit is at least 21 years old.
    b. Systemic disease and infection must be absent.
    c. There must be no history of cancer.
    d. Hypertension or renal disease must be absent.
    e. There must be adequate renal function as determined by diagnostic studies.
    f. The donor must understand the surgery and be willing to give up the organ.
    g. There must be no allergies to medications.

118. The nurse is caring for the renal transplant patient in the immediate postoperative period. During this initial period, for what time frame does the nurse assess the urine output at least hourly?
    a. First 8 hours
    b. First 12 hours
    c. First 24 hours
    d. First 48 hours

119. The intensive care nurse is caring for the renal transplant patient who was just transferred from the recovery unit. Which finding is the most serious within the first 12 hours after surgery and warrants immediate notification of the transplant surgeon?
    a. Diuresis with increased output
    b. Pink and bloody urine
    c. Abrupt decrease in urine
    d. Low-grade fever

120. The nurse is caring for the transplant patient who is 3 days postsurgery. The nurse notes a sudden and abrupt decrease in urine. The nurse alerts the health care provider because this is a sign of which anomaly?
    a. Rejection
    b. Thrombosis
    c. Stenosis
    d. Infection

CASE STUDY: THE PATIENT WITH CONTINUOUS AMBULATORY PERITONEAL DIALYSIS (CAPD)

Use a separate sheet of paper to answer the questions in this Case Study. Answer guidelines for this Case Study are available on your Evolve website at http://evolve. elsevier.com/Iggy/ in the "Prepare for Class" folder.

A 36-year-old woman is married and has two adopted children. She is diagnosed with polycystic kidney disease (PKD), and she will soon have to go on dialysis or consent to a renal transplant.

1. What additional data should the nurse collect to help the patient make the best decision for herself?

2. How would the nurse briefly describe the process of dialysis to the patient? Include information about the following questions:
    a. In peritoneal dialysis, what is the membrane through which the process occurs?
    b. Identify the types of peritoneal dialysis.
    c. What is used to prevent fibrin clot formation in peritoneal dialysis?
    d. How is peritonitis identified and diagnosed in the patient receiving dialysis?
    e. List three advantages of using peritoneal dialysis instead of hemodialysis.

3. Identify the source of possible problems with the flow of dialysate in patients with peritoneal dialysis.

4. What are the protein needs of the patient receiving peritoneal dialysis?

5. Due to the long distance the patient lives from the medical center, she elects to begin CAPD. What would be included in a plan of hospital care for the patient for this procedure?

6. What could the nurse explain and demonstrate about the steps of caring for the dialysis catheter?

7. The patient has been performing PD at home. She calls the nurse to report about outflow from the first peritoneal dialysis. What does the nurse tell the patient about the appearance of the outflow?

72
CHAPTER

Assessment of the Reproductive System

STUDY/REVIEW QUESTIONS

True or False? *Read the statements about reproductive physiology and write T for true or F for false in the blanks provided. If the statement is false, correct the statement to make it true.*

_____ 1. The ovaries produce the sex steroid hormones, estrogen, progesterone, androgen, and relaxin.

_____ 2. Artificial menopause can be surgically induced.

_____ 3. The vas deferens of the internal reproductive system of the male aids in maturation of the sperm.

_____ 4. The first menstrual cycles are typically ovulatory and regular.

5. The advanced practice nurse is performing a genitourinary reproductive examination of the male patient. Which technique does the practitioner use?
   a. Examine the left and right side of the scrotal sac for symmetry.
   b. Obtain a sample of penile discharge by gently milking or squeezing the penis.
   c. Palpate the prostate gland on the posterior surface of the testis.
   d. Transilluminate swollen areas of the scrotum in a dark room with a penlight.

6. The nurse is interviewing a 52-year-old woman reporting irregular and decreased flow of menses for several months. Suspecting that the patient has entered the life phase of the "climacteric," which question does the nurse ask?
   a. "Is there any chance you could be pregnant?"
   b. "Are you having any discomfort during intercourse?"
   c. "Do your breasts feel tender or swollen?"
   d. "Are you having any unusual vaginal discharge?"

7. The 45-year-old woman is being prepared for diagnostic testing to confirm the presence of the climacteric. What does the nurse do to prepare the patient?
   a. Place the patient in the lithotomy position for a Papanicolaou (Pap) test.
   b. Obtain a clean catch urine specimen for a pregnanediol level.
   c. Draw a blood sample for follicle-stimulating hormone and luteinizing hormone levels.
   d. Obtain the equipment and position the patient for a vaginal wet smear.

8. Which woman may experience artificial menopause?
   a. 65-year-old with osteoporosis
   b. 35-year-old who had radiation to the ovaries
   c. 42-year-old who had a laparoscopy
   d. 53-year-old who has hot flashes

9. The nurse is talking with the female patient about what to expect after a pelvic examination. What does the nurse tell the patient?
   a. "You may have some mild abdominal pain."
   b. "You may have dizziness because of orthostatic hypotension."
   c. "You can expect some light red bleeding for 1 to 2 hours."
   d. "You should eat crackers and light meals for nausea or anorexia."

10. The patient is undergoing an infertility workup. Which test best evaluates the presence of a tubal dysfunction?
    a. Hysterosalpingography
    b. Computed tomography
    c. Urologic studies
    d. Radioimmunoassay

11. The nurse is conducting a sex education class for a group of sixth-grade boys and their parents. One of the parents asks the nurse to explain the signs of puberty to the boys. Which statements does the nurse include? *(Select all that apply.)*
    a. "Your scrotum and testes will enlarge, usually between 11 and 13 1/2 years of age."
    b. "You will see growth of hair in your armpits."
    c. "Your skin may feel dry, tight, or seem flaky because of increased testosterone levels."
    d. "Your voice will deepen and may 'crack' because of thickening of the vocal cords."
    e. "You might have pimples on your face or back because of sebaceous gland activity."
    f. "You will have a delay in reaching full muscle mass and body size until age 14 or 15."

12. The nurse is conducting health education for a group of men who are at high risk for prostate cancer. For which age group does the nurse recommend annual digital rectal examinations (DRE) and prostate-specific antigen (PSA) blood tests?
    a. Over 35 years of age
    b. Over 40 years of age
    c. Over 50 years of age
    d. Over 60 years of age

13. A couple is trying to conceive a child. Based on the physiology of normal spermatogenesis, the nurse suggests that the husband avoid which activity before intercourse?
    a. Practicing karate
    b. Kicking a soccer ball
    c. Surfing in the ocean
    d. Sitting in a hot tub

14. A mother is very concerned that her 13-year-old son is not showing any physical signs of puberty because her daughter was fully developed and menstruating by age 13. What is the nurse's best response to the mother?
    a. "Your son will start his growth spurt by his 14th birthday, so I wouldn't worry at this time."
    b. "Boys usually mature physically before girls, so your son needs to see your family doctor."
    c. "Girls usually mature physically about 2 years before boys, so I wouldn't be concerned at this time."
    d. "Boys and girls mature at about the same age; let's review some factors that may be delaying his development."

15. The patient is 13 1/2 years of age and experienced menarche 4 months ago. Her mother is very concerned that her daughter has had very irregular menstrual cycles since then. What is the nurse's best response to the mother?
    a. Her daughter must see a doctor for a pelvic examination.
    b. A pregnancy test must be done.
    c. Her daughter's cycles will adjust themselves within the next 2 years.
    d. The irregularity is normal after the onset of menstruation.

16. Which statement about the function of the female breasts is correct?
    a. They produce hormones that moderate the menstrual cycle.
    b. Their function is to provide milk for the mother's baby.
    c. They provide milk for the mother's baby and are a source of sexual sensation.
    d. Their main function is to allow for passive transfer of antibodies to the baby after birth.

Fill in the blanks.

17. The normal pH of the vagina is _____ to _____, which is necessary to decrease the vagina's susceptibility to infection.

18. Failure of ovulation is associated with a greater risk for _____ cancer.

19. It is not unusual for the breast on the woman's _____ side to appear larger because of the more developed pectoral muscle base.

20. Most girls begin to menstruate between _____ and _____ years of age.

21. Women with a greater percentage of _____ _____ have higher estrone levels after menopause.

22. Estrogen is needed by bone tissue for _____ _____ uptake.

23. The first visible sign of puberty in males is enlargement of the scrotum and testes, which typically occurs between _____ and _____ years of age.

24. Penile erection can result from _____ stimulation and _____ mechanisms.

25. The prostate gland secretes a milky alkaline fluid that enhances sperm _____ and neutralizes acidic _____ secretions.

26. In many women, the breasts become slightly larger and tender during the _____ period.

27. The nurse is teaching a women's health education class and advising participants about the pelvic exam procedure. Which point does the nurse make about pelvic exams?
    a. The patient must douche before the exam to allow for better visualization of the cervix.
    b. The patient must have a full bladder so it is easier to identify on palpation.
    c. The pelvic exam is indicated every 3 years if a patient is sexually active.
    d. The pelvic exam can be used to assess for infection or menstrual irregularities.

28. The nurse is taking a history on the 27-year-old man and his wife who are having trouble conceiving. Which disease does the nurse asks the husband if he had after puberty?
    a. Chicken pox
    b. Rubella
    c. Mumps
    d. Influenza

29. The adult patient tells the nurse practitioner that she has been performing breast self-examination as directed, but was wondering when to have her first mammogram. The nurse tells the patient that a baseline mammogram is to be performed at what age?
    a. 25
    b. 30
    c. 40
    d. 50

30. The adult patient is scheduled to have an endometrial biopsy. What does the nurse teach this patient about the test?
    a. Abdominal cramping will last 1 to 2 weeks.
    b. Vaginal discharge will be heavy at times but will last only 10 to 14 days.
    c. Sexual activity should be postponed until the vaginal discharge stops.
    d. General anesthesia will be used for the procedure.

31. Which common cancer in young adult men can be treated effectively if found early?
    a. Prostate
    b. Colon
    c. Penile
    d. Testicular

32. A mother is very concerned that her 17-year-old daughter has not started menstruating. The nurse assesses the patient for what factors related to delayed puberty?
    a. Low percentage of body fat
    b. Family history of genital cancer
    c. Use of illicit substances
    d. Inadequate iron and calcium intake

33. During a sex education class, the nurse explains about menstruation. What information does the nurse include?
    a. A female's first menstruation is one sign of puberty.
    b. Consult a doctor if the menstrual period does not start by age 14.
    c. For 1 to 2 years after the first menstruation, pregnancy is impossible.
    d. The ideal menstrual cycle is every 30 days.

34. The 40-year-old patient has an enlarged prostate gland. The nurse designs interventions to assist the patient with which issue?
    a. Infertility
    b. Nocturia and incontinence
    c. Sexual dysfunction
    d. Swelling and discharge

35. Which gynecologic procedure requires local or general anesthesia for the patient?
    a. Colposcopy
    b. Laparoscopy
    c. Transvaginal scan
    d. Mammography

36. The nurse is scheduling several patients for an endometrial biopsy with aspiration. Which patient has the most flexibility for scheduling the procedure?
    a. 35-year-old who has been trying to get pregnant for 3 years
    b. 23-year-old with very heavy menstrual periods for 2 years
    c. 57-year-old who has been postmenopausal for 3 years
    d. 45-year-old with unusually long time lapses between menses

37. The nurse is giving discharge instructions to the patient who had an endometrial biopsy and aspiration. What does the nurse include in the discharge instructions?
    a. Heavy bleeding and cramping are expected for 1 to 2 days.
    b. Avoid intercourse or douching for at least 1 month.
    c. Results of the biopsy are usually available within 72 hours.
    d. Bedrest with bathroom privileges is advised for 24 hours.

38. The nurse is assisting the physician with fluid aspiration from a breast mass. Which type of fluid suggests the patient may have cancer?
    a. Bloody
    b. Clear
    c. Light yellow
    d. Dark green

Matching. Match each diagnostic test with its corresponding definition.

Diagnostic Tests

a. Culture
b. DNA HPV
c. Serologic test
d. VDRL
e. Pap smear
f. FTA-ABS
g. Wet preparation
h. ELISA
i. PSA
j. Follicle-stimulating hormone (FSH)

Descriptions

_____ 39. Detects cancerous and precancerous cells of the cervix

_____ 40. Screens for prostate cancer

_____ 41. Detects the causative agent of syphilis

_____ 42. Identifies 13 high-risk types of human papillomavirus (HPV) associated with the development of cervical cancer

_____ 43. Test used to screen for syphilis

_____ 44. Involves the use of a spray on preparation and a glass slide

_____ 45. Decreased levels indicate possible infertility, anorexia nervosa, or neoplasm

_____ 46. Detects antigen-antibody reactions

_____ 47. Detects the presence of a chlamydial infection

_____ 48. Determines appropriate antibiotic therapy

49. Which female patient does the nurse alert about the need to have a rubella titer?
    a. 63-year-old whose last gynecologic exam was 3 years ago
    b. 26-year-old who plans to get pregnant within the next 3 years
    c. 35-year-old who gave birth 2 months ago
    d. 40-year-old recently diagnosed with uterine cancer

50. The patient is diagnosed with a chlamydial infection but is reluctant to spend the money for treatment because she is asymptomatic and does not have a job or health insurance. The nurse advises her that chlamydial infections can result in which condition?
    a. Female infertility
    b. Male partner infertility
    c. Amenorrhea
    d. Teratogenic effects

51. In recalling dietary intake for a recent 24-hour period, the female patient describes eating eggs, whole milk, and bacon for breakfast; fried chicken and French fries for lunch; three-cheese pizza and ice cream for dinner. This type of diet places her at increased risk for which disorder?
    a. Osteoporosis
    b. Fatigue and low libido
    c. Early menopause
    d. Cancer of the breast and ovaries

52. Which female patient must be advised to eat foods that contain folic acid and vitamins B_6 and B_{12}?
    a. Patient who uses oral contraceptives
    b. Patient with heavy menstrual periods
    c. Patient who is perimenopausal
    d. Patient with salpingitis

53. The nurse is taking a history from the female patient whose mother was given diethylstilbestrol (DES) during pregnancy. What must the nurse advise this patient about?
    a. Probability of heavy and irregular periods and the likelihood of premature menopause
    b. Need for regular gynecologic examinations because of the increased risk for reproductive tract cancer
    c. Need for genetic counseling before conceiving because of the increased risk for teratogenic effects
    d. Reduced estrogen levels that will contribute to thinning of the vaginal walls and sensation of dryness

54. Which is a risk factor for prostate cancer?
    a. Never being circumcised
    b. History of difficulty sustaining an erection
    c. First-degree relatives with prostate cancer
    d. Patient's current age

55. The 40-year-old woman has heavy vaginal bleeding. Which question is the priority in evaluating the patient's chief complaint?
    a. "Is the bleeding related to the menstrual cycle or intercourse?"
    b. "Are you having any sensations of pain or cramping?"
    c. "Are you sexually active and do you use oral contraceptives?"
    d. "Are you feeling weak, dizzy, or lightheaded?"

56. The young woman reports that she has a genital discharge causing irritation and odor. She feels embarrassed, but insists that she has not had recent sexual relations. What does the nurse assess for? *(Select all that apply.)*
    a. Current use of antibiotic medications
    b. Type of clothing and undergarments
    c. Age of onset of menses
    d. Presence of genital or orifice lesions
    e. Recent change of diet
    f. Chronic presence of the discharge

57. The 18-year-old patient who has recently become sexually active will be undergoing her first pelvic examination. What does the nurse do to prepare the patient for this new experience? *(Select all that apply.)*
    a. Show the equipment to be used and demonstrate the assessment procedures.
    b. Teach relaxation and breathing techniques to enhance a sense of control.
    c. Inform about what will be done and what she will feel as the examination proceeds.
    d. Ask if she has ever been sexually abused; prepare her for being touched in the genital area.
    e. Call the mother into the examination room for support.

58. The patient calls to make an appointment for a routine pelvic exam. What type of instructions does the nurse give the patient about preparing for the exam?
    a. Do not douche for at least 24 hours before the exam.
    b. Do not eat or drink anything after midnight to decrease bowel and bladder discomfort.
    c. The genital area must be cleaned with mild soap and water before the exam.
    d. If you are having your period, do not wear a tampon; use a menstrual pad.

59. The nurse is teaching the patient about the contraindications for hysteroscopy. What does the nurse tell the patient?
    a. During the procedure, normal or abnormal cells can be pushed through the fallopian tubes and into your pelvic cavity; therefore pregnancy is contraindicated.
    b. The procedure causes irritation and can be very painful if your vaginal tissue is dry or fragile; therefore, the procedure is not recommended for postmenopausal women.
    c. The procedure can cause a lot of bleeding so a recent prescription of an anticoagulant is contraindicated.
    d. During the procedure, an iodine-based dye is used, so allergies to shellfish or iodine are contraindications.

60. The nurse is preparing the equipment and supplies needed to prepare a cervical biopsy specimen. Which item does the nurse obtain?
    a. Container with formalin solution
    b. Several glass slides with KOH solution
    c. Several culture tubes with growth medium
    d. Sterile container for aspirate fluid

Matching. Match each dysfunction with its etiology.

Dysfunctions
a. Teratogenic effects
b. Vaginal dryness, increased yeast infections, impotence
c. Failure of ovulation
d. Ovarian dysfunction
e. Decreased spermatogenesis, libido, or impotence
f. Increased risk of endometrial cancer
g. Pelvic scarring and adhesions or infertility
h. Altered sexual response
i. Orchitis, sterility

Etiology
_____ 61. Low levels of body fat or poor nutrition
_____ 62. Infertility in women
_____ 63. Substance abuse
_____ 64. Rubella in pregnant women
_____ 65. Mumps in postpubertal males
_____ 66. Endocrine disorders
_____ 67. Chronic disorders of nervous, respiratory, or cardiovascular system
_____ 68. Associated with a greater risk for endometrial cancer
_____ 69. Pelvic inflammatory disease (PID), salpingitis

70. The nurse is preparing the patient for a pelvic exam. Which task does the nurse delegate to the unlicensed assistive personnel (UAP)?
    a. Clarify the purpose of the exam and instruct the patient to wait for the doctor.
    b. Explain to the patient that a mirror can be used for teaching if the patient so desires.
    c. Have the patient undress completely and drape her adequately to protect modesty.
    d. Obtain a three-dimensional model and demonstrate the assessment procedures to the patient.

71. The nurse is moving the patient into the lithotomy position for a pelvic exam. Which statement describes the lithotomy position?
    a. Patient lies supine on the table with knees in flexion and thighs adducted.
    b. Patient's buttocks extend slightly beyond the edge of the table; thighs are abducted.
    c. Patient's hips are slightly elevated and legs abducted.
    d. Patient lies in a modified recovery position with upper knees in full flexion.

72. The nurse is teaching the patient about the pelvic exam process. The nurse explains that the examiner will ask her to squeeze the vaginal opening closed after two fingers are inserted. What is the purpose of this exercise?
    a. To assess perineal support and strength of vaginal walls
    b. To assess for urinary and bowel incontinence
    c. To determine if there is a vaginal fistula
    d. To check the size of the birth passage

73. Which phrase describes a rectocele?
    a. Bulge in the anterior vaginal wall
    b. Bulge in the posterior vaginal wall
    c. Passage between the rectum and vagina
    d. Lump of hard feces in the rectum

74. The nurse is preparing the equipment for a pelvic exam. What does the nurse do?
    a. Obtain the smallest speculum available.
    b. Lubricate the speculum with water-soluble gel.
    c. Position the speculum with the blades open.
    d. Adjust the water faucet to obtain warm water.

75. Before a gynecologic exam, the nurse explains the bimanual exam to the patient. What does the nurse tell the patient about this part of the exam?
    a. A warmed speculum is inserted into the vagina to visualize the cervix for color, shape, erosions, or lesions.
    b. Two fingers are inserted into the vagina; the opposite hand is placed on the abdomen and is pressed downwards.
    c. Two hands are used to gently examine the external genitalia by separating the labia folds and vaginal opening.
    d. The palmar surface of one hand is used to deeply palpate the abdomen, and the fingertips of the other hand are used to gently palpate.

76. The nurse is assisting the patient after completion of a pelvic exam. To ensure safety, what does the nurse do?
    a. Provide the patient with tissues or disposable towelettes to clean the perineum.
    b. Give the patient a perineal pad to absorb any dye or discharge.
    c. Give instruction for additional follow-up care, especially if wet smears were obtained.
    d. Evaluate for signs of dizziness before letting the patient get off the examining table.

77. The nurse is caring for the patient who had a laparoscopy. What does postoperative care for this patient include? *(Select all that apply.)*
    a. Administer oral analgesics for incisional pain.
    b. Notify the physician of complaints of referred shoulder pain.
    c. Reassure the patient that most painful sensations disappear within 4 to 6 weeks.
    d. Instruct the patient to change the small adhesive bandage as needed.
    e. Teach the patient to observe the incision for signs of infection or hematoma.
    f. Remind the patient to avoid strenuous activity for 4 to 6 weeks after the procedure.

78. The nurse is helping the patient schedule an appointment for a hysteroscopy. When does the nurse advise the patient that the procedure should be done?
    a. 5 days after menses have ceased
    b. 5 days before the beginning of menses
    c. During the menstrual period
    d. Whenever she can take 3 to 4 days off of work

79. In which patients is a hysteroscopy contraindicated? *(Select all that apply.)*
    a. Patient with suspected cervical cancer
    b. Infertile patient
    c. Patient with an infection of the reproductive tract
    d. Menopausal patient
    e. Pregnant patient
    f. Patient with suspected endometrial cancer

80. The nurse is giving discharge instructions to the patient who had a breast biopsy and aspiration. What does the nurse include in the discharge instructions? *(Select all that apply.)*
    a. Inform that discomfort is usually mild and is controlled with analgesics or the use of ice or heat.
    b. Advise to check the area or incision for bleeding and edema.
    c. Instruct to wear a properly supportive bra continuously for 2 days after surgery.
    d. Advise that numbness around the biopsy site may last 2 to 3 days.
    e. Include instructions for breast self-examination.

81. Place the steps of vulvar self-examination in the correct order using the numbers 1 through 5.
    _____ a. Feel and visually inspect the area.
    _____ b. Examine the area around the vaginal opening from the mons pubis to the perianal area.
    _____ c. Report new nodes, warts, growths of any type, ulcers, sores, blisters, change in skin color, painful areas, areas of itching or inflammation, or any change in vaginal discharge.
    _____ d. Use a handheld mirror to see your external genitalia.
    _____ e. Sit in a well-lighted area on a soft surface (bed or carpeted floor).

CASE STUDY: THE PERIMENOPAUSAL PATIENT

Use a separate sheet of paper to answer the questions in this Case Study. Answer guidelines for this Case Study are available on your Evolve website at http://evolve. elsevier.com/Iggy/ in the "Prepare for Class" folder.

A 52-year-old woman comes to the clinic for a routine gynecologic exam. She reports noticing irregular and lighter periods for the past 4 months. She suspects she is perimenopausal. She is requesting health and self-care information related to "the change of life."

1. Identify the different areas to be included in a genitoreproductive nursing history.
2. Discuss the difference between the terms *menopause* and *climacteric*.
3. Describe six of the physical changes that occur in a woman's body during climacteric and include the etiology of the physical change.
4. Identify appropriate nursing interventions to address the changes related to aging for this patient.

Care of Patients with Breast Disorders

73

CHAPTER

STUDY/REVIEW QUESTIONS

Matching. *Match the terms with their correct definitions.*

Terms

a. Fibroadenoma
b. Microcysts
c. Macrocysts
d. Ductal ectasia
e. Gynecomastia
f. Lymphedema of the affected limb
g. Breast augmentation
h. Papilloma
i. Ductal carcinoma in situ (DCIS)
j. Peau d'orange

Definitions

_____ 1. Most common benign tumor in women during the reproductive years

_____ 2. Dimpling, orange-peel appearance of the skin

_____ 3. Surgery to enhance the size, shape, or symmetry of breasts

_____ 4. Small, nonpalpable cysts inside the breast glands

_____ 5. Easily felt and can reach up to two inches across

_____ 6. Benign breast problem usually seen in women approaching menopause

_____ 7. Pedunculated outgrowth of tissue

_____ 8. Early noninvasive form of breast cancer

_____ 9. Usually a benign condition of breast enlargement in men

_____ 10. Abnormal accumulation of protein fluid in the subcutaneous tissue

11. Which patient group is most likely to present with fibroadenoma as a common breast problem?
    a. Women in their reproductive years
    b. Older women who have never had children
    c. Very young women who have had multiple children
    d. Women in their postmenopausal years

12. The nurse is preparing an information packet about reconstructive breast surgery. What information does the nurse include about health risks for large-breasted women?
    a. Increased risk for fungal infections and backaches
    b. Decreased difficulty in nursing a baby
    c. Likelihood of foul discharge from the nipples
    d. Increased risk for fibrocystic disease

13. A pregnant woman discovers an oval-shaped, freely mobile, rubbery mass in her breast. The physician recommends diagnostic testing for probable fibroadenoma. The nurse anticipates and prepares patient information for which diagnostic test?
    a. Breast ultrasound examination
    b. Chest x-ray
    c. Mammography
    d. Wet preparation

14. The patient with fibrocystic breast condition (FBC) has just undergone fine needle aspiration to drain the cyst fluid and reduce pressure and pain. At what points does the nurse prepare patient education material about breast biopsy? *(Select all that apply.)*
    a. If hormonal replacement therapy is prescribed
    b. If fluid is not aspirated
    c. If the mammogram shows suspicious findings
    d. If fluid buildup recurs
    e. If the mass remains palpable after aspiration
    f. If aspirated fluid reveals cancer cells

15. The patient with FBC is prescribed drug therapy to manage symptoms. The nurse prepares teaching materials for which group of medications?
    a. Anti-androgen agents, calcium supplements, opioids
    b. Monoclonal antibody agents, corticosteroids
    c. Aromatase inhibitors, potassium supplements, NSAIDs
    d. Oral contraceptives, vitamin therapy, diuretics

16. The nurse recommends which self-care measures to help the patient reduce pain and manage symptoms associated with FBC? *(Select all that apply.)*
    a. Temporarily discontinue drug therapy just before menses.
    b. Take mild analgesics as needed.
    c. Limit salt intake before menses to help decrease swelling.
    d. Wear a supportive bra.
    e. Locally apply ice or heat to provide temporary relief of pain.
    f. Massage breasts frequently during peak episodes of pain.

17. The 54-year-old woman has identified a hard breast mass with irregular borders, redness, and edema. She reports a greenish-brown nipple discharge and enlarged axillary nodes. Based on the patient's age and description of the symptoms, what does the nurse suspect?
    a. Fibroadenoma
    b. Fibrocystic breast condition
    c. Ductal ectasia
    d. Intraductal papilloma

18. The nurse notes in the documentation that the patient has a round, firm, nontender, mobile breast mass not attached to breast tissue or the chest wall. What does this describe?
    a. Fibroadenoma
    b. Fibrocystic disease
    c. Breast cysts
    d. Ductal ectasia

19. The nurse is reviewing discharge instructions for the patient who had breast augmentation surgery. What does the nurse include in these instructions? *(Select all that apply.)*
    a. Expect soreness in chest and arms for several months.
    b. Breasts will feel tight and sensitive; the breast skin may feel warm or itchy.
    c. Anticipate having difficulty raising the arms over the head.
    d. Perform lifting, pushing, and pulling exercises several times a day.
    e. Walk every few hours to prevent deep vein thrombi.
    f. Expect some swelling for 3 to 4 weeks after surgery.

20. What is the most common breast dysfunction found in the male breast?
    a. Nipple discharge
    b. Nipple retraction
    c. Gynecomastia
    d. Disseminated breast cancer

Fill in the blanks.

21. The two main features of FBC are _____ _____ and _____.

22. The 5-year survival rate for women with localized breast cancer is 98%, whereas the rate drops to 81% when the breast cancer has spread to the _____ _____ nodes.

23. The most common sites of metastatic disease from breast cancer are _____, _____, _____, and _____.

24. Fibroadenoma of the breast is more likely to enlarge during _____.

25. FBC is thought to be caused by an imbalance in the normal _____ to progesterone ratio.

26. The nurse is preparing an information packet about cancer screening based on the American Cancer Society recommendations. What information does the nurse include in the packet?
    a. A baseline screening mammogram is recommended at 25 years of age for those with high risk, and biannual screenings are recommended beginning at age 25.
    b. A baseline screening mammogram is recommended at 30 years of age, and yearly screening for women is recommended beginning at age 40.
    c. A baseline screening mammogram is recommended at 40 years of age, and yearly screening for women is recommended beginning at age 40.
    d. A baseline screening mammogram is recommended at 50 years of age, and yearly screening for women is recommended beginning at age 50.

27. The female patient has been told her breast tumor is 3 cm, nonfixed, with axillary metastasis. Based on this information, what stage of breast cancer is most likely present?
    a. I
    b. II
    c. III
    d. IV

28. According to the latest studies, which woman has the greatest risk of developing breast cancer?
    a. Physician, age 56, who had her first child at age 38
    b. Ballet dancer, age 20, who has a 5-year-old son
    c. Radiation technician, age 24, who had her menarche at age 13
    d. Postmenopausal woman, age 52, who had breast reduction surgery at age 26

29. The nurse is counseling the woman recently diagnosed with breast cancer. Which factor has the most influence on the patient's choice for treatment?
    a. Age at the time of diagnosis
    b. Overall health status
    c. Personal choice and type of insurance
    d. Extent and location of metastasis of the breast mass

30. The young patient is suspected of having invasive breast cancer. Based on the types and frequencies of breast cancer, what is the patient most likely to be diagnosed with?
    a. FBC
    b. Infiltrating ductal carcinoma
    c. Lobular carcinoma in situ
    d. DCIS

31. Which factor is the incidence of breast disease most closely related to?
    a. Weight
    b. Aging
    c. Ethnic background
    d. Socioeconomic status

32. Cancer surveillance in high-risk women involves breast self-examination (BSE), clinical breast examination (CBE), and mammography. Cancer surveillance is used to detect cancer in its early stages and is referred to as what kind of prevention?
    a. Primary
    b. Secondary
    c. Tertiary
    d. Prophylactic

33. How is the three-pronged approach to early detection of breast cancer defined as?
    a. BSE, annual CBE, and ultrasound
    b. CBE, mammogram, and ultrasound
    c. Mammogram, BSE, and CBE
    d. BSE, mammogram, and ultrasound

34. Which factor makes the mammogram a more sensitive screening tool than other tests?
    a. Higher compliance rate than BSE because it is less painful
    b. Less expensive than other tests that identify tumor markers
    c. Able to reveal masses too small to be palpated manually
    d. Able to differentiate between fluid and solid masses

35. The nurse is teaching the 24-year-old patient about BSE. When does the nurse tell her to perform BSE?
    a. The day before her menstrual flow is due
    b. On the third day after her menstrual flow starts
    c. When ovulation occurs
    d. One week after her menstrual flow starts

36. The nurse is teaching the thin, small-breasted woman how to perform BSE. The patient keeps palpating her ribs and reporting lumps. What technique does the nurse use to help her identify the ribs?
    a. Have her stand in front of a mirror and look at the rib contour.
    b. Reassure her that because she is thin, she is feeling her ribs.
    c. Demonstrate how to follow the rib to the sternum.
    d. Put her in a supine position so that breast tissue falls to the sides.

37. The patient stopped having menses about a year ago. When does the nurse advise the patient to perform BSE?
    a. The first day of every other month
    b. Continue on schedule even though menses have ceased
    c. The last day of each month
    d. Any day as long as the schedule is consistent

38. The student nurse is preparing to teach the Navajo patient about breast cancer and BSE. After reading culturally relevant material, which teaching method does the student decide is best for this patient?
    a. Show the patient a video.
    b. Have the patient attend a lecture.
    c. Supply reading material for the patient.
    d. Practice on a manikin.

39. The nurse is teaching the young patient about BSE. Which statement by the patient indicates a need for further instruction?
    a. "I should perform BSE on a monthly basis from now on."
    b. "I see my health care provider annually, but I should perform BSE."
    c. "BSE is a self-care measure that I can use to prevent breast cancer."
    d. "The best time to perform BSE is 1 week after my menstrual period."

40. What type of teaching increases the likelihood that a woman will be more compliant with the performance of regular monthly BSE?
    a. Learning from a pamphlet at home
    b. Learning at a clinic or office
    c. Seeing a television program about the risks for developing breast cancer
    d. Reading magazine articles

41. The advanced practice nurse is performing a CBE. The practitioner places the patient in which position to begin the examination?
    a. Supine position with a pillow under the shoulder and the arm raised above the head
    b. The arms raised over the head to expose the surface underneath the breast for inspection
    c. Standing position with the hands on the hips
    d. Sitting or standing with the arms down at the sides

42. During a CBE, the examiner observes a discharge from the nipple. What is most important to include in the documentation of this finding?
    a. Area of "the clock" that was compressed when the discharge was released
    b. Amount of pressure required for the discharge to be released
    c. Frequency and technique the patient uses for BSE
    d. History of difficulty or pain when attempting to breast-feed

43. Upon performing a CBE, which patient has a symptom that suggests advanced disease?
    a. Patient with gynecomastia
    b. Patient with an oval-shaped, mobile, rubbery mass
    c. Patient with a thin, milky discharge from the nipple
    d. Patient with a skin change of peau d'orange

True or False? Read each statement and write T for true or F for false in the blanks provided. If the statement is false, correct the statement to make it true.

_____ 44. Ninety percent of women will have fibrocystic changes sometime during their lives.

_____ 45. Fibroadenomas are the most common benign tumor in women during the menopausal years.

_____ 46. Many symptoms of breast cancer are the same as those seen in benign disorders.

_____ 47. Having cysts or fibrosis increases a woman's chance of developing breast cancer.

_____ 48. Ductal ectasia is a precursor to breast cancer risk, especially in postmenopausal women.

_____ 49. DCIS should be treated to prevent development of an invasive breast cancer, but it is not harmful at this stage.

_____ 50. Most men who present with nipple discharge are diagnosed with breast cancer.

_____ 51. Having two first-degree relatives with breast cancer doubles the risk for breast cancer.

_____ 52. Characteristics of patients at high risk for breast cancer include early menarche, late menopause, first pregnancy after 30 years of age, or nullipara.

53. The patient has returned from breast reconstruction surgery with a Jackson-Pratt drain in place that is patent and draining serosanguineous fluid. The nurse notices that at 8:00 AM, the drainage container is full. It was last emptied at 6:00 AM. The total drainage for the last 2 hours is measured at 145 mL. What is the priority nursing intervention?
    a. Notify the health care provider about the amount and type of drainage for last 2 hours.
    b. Empty the drain every 2 hours so the suction will be more effective.
    c. Chart the type and amount of drainage and continue to monitor.
    d. Reinforce the drain site with a sterile bulky dressing.

54. The patient had a partial mastectomy yesterday and the nurse writes on the nursing care plan "Anxiety related to removal of breast tissue." What is the nurse's priority intervention?
    a. Use distraction until the patient improves and is able to think more clearly.
    b. Encourage the patient to have a positive attitude so she will heal faster.
    c. Ensure that the patient takes PRN anxiolytic medication every 4 to 6 hours.
    d. Encourage the patient to discuss her fears and ask questions about her concerns.

55. The patient had a partial mastectomy. When teaching about care of the arm on the affected side, what does the nurse tell the patient?
    a. Start arm exercises as soon as the drains are removed from the incision.
    b. Keep the arm elevated so the elbow is above the shoulder and the wrist is above the elbow.
    c. Do not take blood pressure in the arm on the affected side for the first 6 months after surgery.
    d. Do push-ups and arm circles on a routine basis for a full recovery.

56. The patient has recently been diagnosed with breast cancer. What is the most likely priority preoperative nursing diagnosis for this patient?
    a. Deficient Knowledge
    b. Readiness for Enhanced Decision Making
    c. Fear
    d. Anxiety

57. Which intervention is priority in the nursing care plan for the patient after a modified radical mastectomy?
    a. Position the patient on the affected side to aid with gravity flow of drainage from the incision site.
    b. Immobilize the arm on the affected side for the first 24 hours postoperatively.
    c. Assess the patient for anxiety because it can impede the healing process.
    d. Teach the patient signs and symptoms of infection and how to monitor for altered wound healing.

58. The patient who had surgery for breast cancer appears in need of continued community support. The nurse refers the patient to which organization?
    a. Reach to Recovery
    b. Empty Arms
    c. Resolve
    d. NAMI

59. The nurse is counseling the woman who has had several discussions with the health care provider about her risk for breast cancer. The nurse reinforces that prophylactic mastectomy would have what effect on her risk for developing breast cancer?
    a. Increases the risk
    b. Eliminates the risk
    c. Decreases the risk
    d. Doubles the risk

60. Which woman has the highest risk for developing breast cancer?
    a. 68-year-old who has taken hormone replacement therapy
    b. 35-year-old with three children
    c. 23-year-old who started menstruating at age 12
    d. 40-year-old who has two cousins who have had breast cancer

61. Which interventions incorporate research findings related to higher breast cancer mortality rates among African-American women? *(Select all that apply.)*
    a. Ask high-end retail stores to do promotional campaigns encouraging mammograms.
    b. Make a list of facilities that do diagnostic screenings in low-income neighborhoods.
    c. Identify bus routes that serve hospitals and clinics and advocate for increased service.
    d. Encourage women to have breast cancer screening because insurance pays for it.
    e. Take all opportunities to teach patients to do BSE.

62. The patient found a mass in her breast 6 months ago. What question does the nurse ask related to possible metastases of a potential cancer?
    a. "Why did you wait 6 months before seeking medical attention?"
    b. "Have you noticed any joint or bone pain or other changes in your body?"
    c. "Have you ever had any exposure to radiation or toxic chemicals?"
    d. "Has your sister or mother ever been diagnosed with breast cancer?"

63. The patient has just been diagnosed with advanced breast cancer. Which behavior by the patient is the strongest indicator of readiness for additional patient teaching and information?
    a. Cheerfully talking about her family and the vacation they will take to Europe
    b. Being active and angrily throwing her belongings into her suitcase
    c. Crying and being upset, asking the nurse to call a spiritual counselor
    d. Being quiet and thoughtfully fingering the lace on her new bra

64. The patient in the medical-surgical unit says to the nursing student, "My doctor told me I have advanced breast cancer and I want to give you this bracelet, because you have been so sweet to me today." What does the student nurse do next?
    a. Contact the charge nurse because the patient may be signaling intentions of suicide.
    b. Sit with the patient and allow her to take the lead in the conversation.
    c. Contact the nursing instructor because the news is overwhelming.
    d. Explain to the patient that it is unethical for students to accept expensive gifts.

65. The nurse is reviewing the laboratory results from the postmenopausal woman being evaluated for a breast mass. What type of metastases does the increased serum calcium and alkaline phosphatase levels suggest?
    a. Brain
    b. Bone
    c. Lung
    d. Liver

66. The nurse is talking to the woman recently diagnosed with breast cancer who confides, "I am going to use nutritional and herbal therapy instead of taking drugs and radiation that would make my hair fall out." What is the nurse's best response?
    a. "Some research shows benefits when complementary therapy is combined with conventional medicine."
    b. "What did your physician tell you about all of your possible treatment options?"
    c. "You really shouldn't use alternative nutritional therapies as a replacement for conventional therapies."
    d. "Where did you hear about this nutritional and herbal treatment?"

67. The nurse is caring for the patient who had a right-sided modified radical mastectomy. Which task does the nurse delegate to the UAP?
    a. Observe the drainage in the Jackson-Pratt drain.
    b. Take blood pressure on the right arm only.
    c. Assist the patient to ambulate the day after surgery.
    d. Instruct the patient about arm positioning.

68. The patient is lying in bed after a mastectomy. How does the nurse position the patient?
    a. Head of the bed up at least 30 degrees with the affected arm elevated on a pillow
    b. Supine body position with the affected arm positioned straight by the side
    c. Any position that is the most comfortable to the patient
    d. Side-lying position with the unaffected side down towards mattress

69. The patient is one day postsurgery after a mastectomy and is anxious to begin the prescribed exercises. Which exercise is appropriate for the patient's first efforts?
    a. Flex the fingers so that the hands slowly "walk" up the wall.
    b. Squeeze the affected hand around a soft, round object.
    c. Swing the rope in small circles and gradually increase to larger circles.
    d. Grab the ends of the rope, and extend the arms until they are straight.

70. The patient is being discharged with a prescription for tamoxifen to decrease the chance of breast cancer recurrence. Because of the common side effect, what does the nurse suggest to the patient in taking this drug?
    a. Have soda crackers and ginger ale on hand.
    b. Install a handrail around the bathtub.
    c. Purchase a scale to monitor body weight.
    d. Buy a soft-bristle toothbrush.

71. The patient is prescribed trastuzumab (Herceptin) for breast cancer. What is the priority nursing intervention for this patient?
    a. Obtain an order for baseline ECG.
    b. Assess for signs of bleeding.
    c. Premedicate with an antiemetic.
    d. Rotate injection sites.

72. The nurse is designing a teaching plan for the patient who had surgery for breast cancer. What information does the nurse include in the plan? *(Select all that apply.)*
    a. Do not use lotions or ointments on the area.
    b. Delay using deodorant under the affected arm until healing is complete.
    c. Swelling and redness of the scar itself are considered normal and permanent.
    d. Report any increased heat and tenderness of the area to the surgeon.
    e. Wear loose pajamas at home for 6 to 8 weeks.
    f. Begin active range-of-motion exercises 1 week after surgery.

CASE STUDY: THE PATIENT WITH FIBROCYSTIC BREAST DISEASE

Use a separate sheet of paper to answer the questions in this Case Study. Answer guidelines for this Case Study are available on your Evolve website at http://evolve. elsevier.com/Iggy/ in the "Prepare for Class" folder.

A 26-year-old woman reports during her annual gynecologic examination that she has been feeling fullness and soreness before her menstrual period and that she has felt some "marbles" in her breast. She is using contraceptive gel for prevention of pregnancy. The nurse palpates numerous nodules in both breasts and tells the patient that this is most likely fibrocystic change in the breast tissue.

1. What should the nurse tell the patient about diagnostic testing that will be done?

2. What kinds of treatments might the nurse instruct the patient about after the diagnosis of fibrocystic breast disease (FBD) is confirmed?

3. What teaching should the nurse do to prepare the patient to care for her symptoms?

4. Identify six instructions necessary for the nurse to teach a woman before having her demonstrate a BSE.

74
CHAPTER

Care of Patients with Gynecologic Problems

STUDY/REVIEW QUESTIONS

Matching. *Match each term to its corresponding definition.*

Terms
a. Uterine prolapse
b. Myometrium
c. Cystocele
d. Leiomyomas
e. Urethrovaginal
f. Vulvovaginitis
g. Fibroid
h. Rectocele
i. Dysmenorrhea
j. Polyp
k. Chocolate cyst
l. Bartholin cyst

Descriptions
_____ 1. Area of endometriosis inside of an ovary
_____ 2. Protrusion of the bladder through the vaginal wall
_____ 3. Results in leakage of urine into the vagina
_____ 4. Painful menstrual flow
_____ 5. Protrusion of the rectum through the vaginal wall
_____ 6. Inflammation of the lower genital tract
_____ 7. A common disorder of the vulva
_____ 8. Weakened pelvic floor muscles and a full feeling in the vagina
_____ 9. Uterine muscle
_____ 10. Also called fibroids
_____ 11. Most common slow-growing pelvic tumor
_____ 12. Most common benign neoplastic growth of the cervix

Fill in the blank.

13. The cause of primary dysmenorrhea is thought to be increased production and release of uterine _____, which peak at the onset of menses.

14. Secondary dysmenorrhea begins with an _____ disease condition.

15. Hormone replacement therapy increases the menopausal patient's risk for _____ _____.

16. In endometriosis, the monthly cyclic bleeding occurs at an _____ site of implantation, which irritates and scars the surrounding tissue.

17. Without _____, prolonged estrogen stimulation causes the endometrium to grow, causing disordered shedding of the uterine lining.

18. The 22-year-old patient reports pain associated with her menstrual periods. What questions does the nurse ask when taking the patient's history? *(Select all that apply.)*
    a. "How old were you when you started menstruation?"
    b. "When did you first start having pain?"
    c. "What is a typical menstrual period for you?"
    d. "Have you ever been pregnant?"
    e. "What kind of contraceptives do you use?"
    f. "Do you have a history of frequent urinary tract infections?"

19. The health care provider recommends use of antiprostaglandin therapy for the patient with dysmenorrhea. How does the nurse instruct the patient to take the medication for maximum effectiveness?
    a. Start at the onset of symptoms.
    b. Take on a regular daily basis.
    c. Take on an empty stomach.
    d. Start at the end of each menstrual cycle.

20. What nonpharmacologic therapy may be recommended to the patient to relieve the pain and discomfort associated with dysmenorrhea?
    a. Dietary supplements
    b. Increased level of activity, such as walking, during pain episodes
    c. Wearable cold pack on the lower abdomen
    d. Relaxation techniques such as acupressure or acupuncture

21. A current treatment of primary dysmenorrhea includes which medication?
    a. Serotonin-reuptake inhibitors (SSRIs)
    b. Beta blockers
    c. Nonsteroidal anti-inflammatory drugs (NSAIDs)
    d. Prostaglandin stimulators

22. Which physiologic factor is thought to be the etiologic cause of dysmenorrhea?
    a. Increased production of gonadotropin-releasing hormone
    b. Increased production of prostaglandins
    c. Decreased production of progesterone
    d. Decreased production of estradiol

23. What does the nurse do to assist the health care provider in verifying a diagnosis of premenstrual syndrome (PMS)?
    a. Teach the patient to record two menstrual cycles to include pattern of symptoms.
    b. Obtain blood and urine specimens to test hormone levels.
    c. Prepare the patient for a pelvic and bimanual examination.
    c. Schedule an appointment for magnetic resonance-guided focused ultrasound.

24. Which woman is at greatest risk for having PMS?
    a. 26-year-old caring for her first child
    b. 15-year-old who recently started smoking
    c. 46-year-old who had a death in the family 6 months ago
    d. 34-year-old mother of four who is recently divorced

25. Which dietary therapy does the nurse recommend to the patient with PMS as being the most beneficial?
    a. Limit intake of calcium, magnesium, and sodium.
    b. Limit intake of sugar, red meat, and alcohol.
    c. Lose at least 10 pounds over a period of 6 months.
    d. Eat three balanced meals a day with increased fiber.

26. The patient has PMS. What is the nurse's role in the therapy that the health care provider is likely to first suggest for this patient?
    a. Advise not to abruptly discontinue SSRIs.
    b. Teach about the side effects associated with oral contraceptives.
    c. Instruct to monitor for bleeding signs, such as bruising or bleeding from the gums.
    d. Teach how to prepare for a magnetic resonance-guided focused ultrasound.

27. The obese 54-year-old patient describes excessive menstrual bleeding that occurs approximately every 10 days. The nurse prepares the patient for which diagnostic test that is used to evaluate for endometrial cancer?
    a. Bimanual pelvic examination
    b. Transvaginal ultrasound
    c. Sonohysterography
    d. Endometrial biopsy

28. The patient is diagnosed with dysfunctional uterine bleeding. During the pelvic exam, the health care provider determines that the bleeding is acute and heavy. What is the nurse's priority action?
    a. Prepare the patient for immediate transport to the operating room.
    b. Establish a peripheral IV site for hormonal therapy.
    c. Obtain and administer a hormonal contraceptive patch.
    d. Administer injectable medroxyprogesterone acetate (Depo-Provera).

29. The patient who is very upset asks the nurse, "My doctor says I have endometriosis. That sounds so horrible. What does it mean?" What is the nurse's best response?
    a. "It is an early warning sign of endometrial cancer, but you still need more testing."
    b. "A special type of tissue, called endometrial tissue, is outside of your uterus."
    c. "It's the growth of a special tissue which grows rapidly, but it is not dangerous."
    d. "It is a type of infection and inflammation of the endometrial tissue."

30. The patient is a 53-year-old woman who reports distressing perimenopausal symptoms. She asks the nurse about the possibility of taking hormone replacement therapy (HRT). What is the nurse's best response?
    a. "The cautious consensus is to offer HRT for the shortest period of time at the lowest possible dose to relieve symptoms."
    b. "Since 2002, HRT is not recommended because of unexpected increased risk for coronary heart disease and breast cancer."
    c. "HRT is not recommended because estrogen given alone can cause endometrial cancer, gallbladder disease, deep vein thrombosis, and stroke."
    d. "HRT is currently offered to selective patients as a one-time dose, but the dose is very high and there are side effects."

31. The 36-year-old patient has been having hot flashes, crying spells, and mood swings. Her physician wants to prescribe HRT for her perimenopausal symptoms. In consideration of her age, what is this patient experiencing?
    a. Early-onset menopause
    b. Late-onset menarche
    c. Normal menopause
    d. Signs of ovarian cancer

32. What is the primary treatment for dysfunctional uterine bleeding in perimenopausal women?
    a. Hysterectomy
    b. HRT
    c. Radiation
    d. Chemotherapy

33. The patient has been diagnosed with atrophic vaginitis. The nurse prepares teaching information about which type of treatment?
    a. A 25 mg infusion of conjugated estrogens
    b. Dilation and curettage (D&C)
    c. Vaginal estrogen therapy (ET) as a ring, tablet, or cream
    d. Endometrial ablation

34. What is the major reason for the onset of menopause and resulting atrophy of the vulvar organs?
    a. Decrease in levels of follicle-stimulating hormone
    b. Increase in levels of prostaglandin
    c. Decrease in levels of estrogen
    d. Increase in levels of luteinizing hormone

35. The patient is suffering from postmenopausal vaginal dryness. The nurse advises her to use which over-the-counter product to decrease sexual discomfort related to intercourse?
    a. Hydrocortisone cream
    b. Water-soluble gel
    c. Petroleum jelly
    d. Vitamin A and D ointment

36. The patient with which reproductive condition is most likely prescribed raloxifene (Evista) or alendronate (Fosamax) as an additional therapy to prevent associated complications?
    a. Dysfunctional uterine bleeding
    b. Premenstrual syndrome
    c. Dysmenorrhea
    d. Menopause

37. Which is a common cause of vaginitis?
    a. Taking antibiotics
    b. Swimming in lakes
    c. Wiping from front to back
    d. Wearing inappropriate clothing

38. The nurse is advising the patient about self-care for vulvitis, which is caused by a non-pathologic condition. What information does the nurse provide? *(Select all that apply.)*
    a. Wash the area daily with hydrogen peroxide.
    b. Take a sitz bath for 30 minutes several times a day.
    c. Apply prescribed topical drugs, such as hydrocortisone.
    d. Remove any irritants or allergens (e.g., change detergents).
    e. Apply a topical lindane cream or lotion.
    f. Apply wet compresses.

39. The patient with a high fever, headache, flu-like symptoms, and fainting is admitted with the diagnosis of toxic shock syndrome. What additional clinical manifestations does the nurse assess for?
    a. Sunburn-like rash with peeling of palms
    b. Sore throat and swollen lymph nodes
    c. Severe hypertension and confusion
    d. Polyuria and diaphoresis

40. The nurse is teaching a group of women about preventing toxic shock syndrome. What information does the nurse provide to the group? *(Select all that apply.)*
    a. "Do not use tampons under any circumstances."
    b. "Use sanitary napkins at night."
    c. "Do not use a vaginal sponge for more than 30 hours at a time."
    d. "If you use a diaphragm, remove it within 24 hours after intercourse."
    e. "Do not use a diaphragm during your menstrual period."

41. The patient is admitted with toxic shock syndrome. What organism is frequently associated with this syndrome when it occurs as a menstrually related infection?
    a. *Escherichia coli*
    b. *Staphylococcus aureus*
    c. *Haemophilus influenzae*
    d. Beta-hemolytic streptococcus

42. The patient reports the sensation of feeling as if "something is falling out" along with painful intercourse, backache, and a feeling of heaviness or pressure in the pelvis, with urinary frequency. Which question does the nurse ask to assess for a cystocele?
    a. "Are you having urinary frequency or urgency?"
    b. "Do you feel constipated?"
    c. "Have you had problems with hemorrhoids?"
    d. "Have you had any heavy vaginal bleeding?"

43. The patient is recovering from repair of a cystocele. What postprocedure intervention does the nurse teach the patient?
    a. Perform perineal floor exercises.
    b. Take sitz baths three times a day.
    c. Perform povidone-iodine douches every other day.
    d. Maintain bedrest for the first 6 weeks.

44. The patient has had a posterior colporrhaphy. What is included in the nursing care of this patient? *(Select all that apply.)*
    a. Administer pain medication before having a bowel movement.
    b. Instruct to avoid straining during a bowel movement.
    c. Resume regular activities after discharge from the hospital.
    d. Provide sitz baths.
    e. Promote a low-residue (low-fiber) diet.

45. The patient is diagnosed with a fistula. The nurse identifies the nursing diagnosis Risk for Impaired Skin Integrity related to leakage of feces into the vagina. What nursing interventions best address this issue? *(Select all that apply.)*
    a. Assist with frequent perineal hygiene.
    b. Offer sitz baths and perineal cleaning with mild, unscented soap and water.
    c. Douche frequently with high-flow pressure and deodorizing solutions.
    d. Suggest sanitary napkins or disposable undergarments.
    e. Design a bladder and bowel training program.
    f. Apply vitamin A and D ointment to excoriated tissues.
    g. Evaluate for depression or other emotional response.

Matching. *Match the terms with their correct definitions.*

Terms
a. Intramural leiomyomas
b. Submucosal leiomyomas
c. Subserosal leiomyomas
d. Pedunculated leiomyomas
e. Parasitic fibroid

Definitions
_____ 46. May extend to the broad ligament, pressing other organs
_____ 47. Contained in the uterine wall within the myometrium
_____ 48. Occasionally breaks off and attaches to other tissues
_____ 49. Can cause bleeding and disrupt pregnancy
_____ 50. Attached by a stalk to the outside of the uterus

51. The patient is diagnosed with uterine leiomyomas. What does the nurse expect to see in the documentation for this patient as the chief presenting complaint?
    a. Vaginal pressure and fullness
    b. Abnormal vaginal bleeding
    c. Intermittent pain
    d. Urinary dysfunction

52. The patient with uterine leiomyomas reports a feeling of pelvic pressure, constipation, urinary frequency, and says "I can't button my pants anymore." What does the nurse assess for to further evaluate the patient's symptoms?
    a. Fluid imbalance
    b. Abdominal distention or enlargement
    c. Bowel and bladder incontinence
    d. Vaginal bleeding or discharge

53. The patient has had a pelvic examination and needs an additional diagnostic test for possible uterine leiomyomas. The nurse prepares the patient for which first-choice diagnostic test?
    a. Transvaginal ultrasound
    b. Laparoscopy
    c. Hysteroscopy
    d. Magnetic resonance imaging (MRI)

54. What is the priority nursing diagnosis most commonly seen preoperatively and postoperatively in the patient with leiomyomas?
    a. Risk for Infection
    b. Acute Pain
    c. Risk for Altered Tissue Perfusion
    d. Anxiety

55. The patient has undergone uterine artery embolization for treatment of uterine leiomyomas. What does the nurse include in the discharge teaching for this patient?
    a. Expect cramping to continue for 2 to 4 weeks.
    b. Pain or bleeding are not expected and should be reported.
    c. A flu-like illness may develop.
    d. Return to work or daily routine in 24 hours.

56. The patient has had a myomectomy. For what reason does the nurse remind the patient to record this procedure in personal health records and to inform current and future health care providers?
    a. There will be difficulty in carrying a pregnancy to full-term.
    b. Menstrual periods are more likely to be heavy and prolonged.
    c. There is an increased risk for uterine cancer.
    d. Future deliveries must be via cesarean section.

57. The patient has just undergone a transcervical endometrial resection (TCER) performed via hysteroscopy. What is the priority assessment for this patient in postoperative care?
    a. Pain
    b. Bleeding
    c. Confusion
    d. Urinary symptoms

58. The patient with cancer has also been diagnosed with uterine leiomyomas. Which procedure does the nurse prepare the patient for?
    a. Myomectomy
    b. Hysterectomy
    c. HRT
    d. Magnetic resonance-guided focused ultrasound

59. The patient who had a total abdominal hysterectomy is anxious to resume her activities because she has young children at home. What postprocedure information does the nurse provide to the patient? *(Select all that apply.)*
    a. Climb stairs to build strength and endurance.
    b. Avoid sitting for prolonged periods.
    c. Do not lift anything heavier than 5 lbs.
    d. Walk 2 to 3 miles per day.
    e. Do not drive for at least 4 weeks or until the surgeon approves.

60. The patient who had a total abdominal hysterectomy comes to the clinic for a 6-week follow-up appointment. Which patient demeanor is the strongest indicator that there is a need for psychological referral?
    a. Quiet and withdrawn but able to correctly answer questions
    b. Tense and impatient but answers questions correctly
    c. Disheveled and lackluster but answers correctly with repeated prompting
    d. Cheerful and distractible but answers correctly with excessive detail

61. What does discharge teaching for the woman who had a total abdominal hysterectomy include?
    a. Sexual activity may be resumed usually in 2 to 3 weeks if the incision has healed.
    b. Pain will decrease in about 2 to 3 days but may last for up to 6 weeks.
    c. Daily exercise such as walking is encouraged after the first 6 weeks.
    d. Wound care includes showering but no tub baths.

62. The patient reporting swelling in the perineal area is diagnosed with a Bartholin cyst. Non-surgical management is recommended. What does the nurse instruct the patient to do?
    a. Apply moist heat (e.g., sitz baths or hot wet packs) to the vulva.
    b. Return immediately to the clinic if the cyst ruptures.
    c. Contact all sexual partners about the need for treatment.
    d. Change the dressing at least three times a day.

63. The older adult patient is being treated for endometrial cancer. Which common symptoms does the nurse expect to find in the patient's record that was reported before the patient was diagnosed?
    a. Pelvic pain
    b. Nausea and anorexia
    c. Dysfunctional uterine bleeding
    d. Vaginal discharge

64. The nurse is giving instructions to the patient scheduled for intracavity radiation therapy (IRT). What do the nurse's postprocedure instructions include?
    a. Ambulate with assistance.
    b. Maintain high Fowler's position.
    c. Restrict visitors for 2 weeks.
    d. Provide a low-residue diet.

65. The nurse is caring for the patient with a radioactive sealed implant. Which task can be delegated to unlicensed assistive personnel (UAP)?
    a. Save linens until radioactive source is removed, then dispose of linens as usual.
    b. Wear a dosimeter film badge while caring for the patient for protection.
    c. Use a long-handled forceps to dispose of the radioactive source in the toilet.
    d. Arrange beds so that two patients undergoing the treatment can share the room.

66. The patient is receiving external radiation therapy for treatment of endometrial cancer. What task does the nurse delegate to the UAP?
    a. Gently wash the markings outlining the treatment site.
    b. Monitor for signs of skin breakdown, especially in the perineal area.
    c. Assist the patient to ambulate if she feels fatigue or tiredness.
    d. Clean the Foley catheter and meatus with mild soap and water.

67. The patient receiving external radiation therapy treatments reports fatigue, loss of energy, and experiencing an "emotional crisis every day and my hair is falling out." What does the nurse do first to help the patient adapt to body changes?
    a. Suggest participation in self-management.
    b. Encourage the patient to ventilate feelings.
    c. Help the patient to select a wig or scarf.
    d. Encourage the patient to talk to her family.

68. The nurse encourages the teenage patient to receive the human papillomavirus (HPV) vaccine (Gardasil) because it protects against which type of cancer?
    a. Endometrial cancer
    b. Cervical cancer
    c. Ovarian cancer
    d. Uterine cancer

69. Which statement about pelvic examinations and Pap smears is correct?
    a. Begin screening precautions within 3 years after having sexual intercourse or by the age of 21.
    b. Sexually active women should have annual screening regardless of underlying health problems or history.
    c. Postmenopausal women should have a final pelvic examination 1 to 2 years after the onset of menopause.
    d. Screening precautions every 2 to 3 years are sufficient for adult women who are sexually active.

70. Which classic symptom is indicative of invasive gynecologic cancer in the older patient?
    a. Swelling of one leg
    b. Dark and foul-smelling discharge
    c. Painless vaginal bleeding
    d. Flank pain

71. The nurse is taking a history on the patient with probable gynecologic cancer. Which clinical manifestation is a sign of metastasis?
    a. Watery, blood-tinged vaginal discharge
    b. Painless vaginal bleeding
    c. Dark and foul-smelling discharge
    d. Dysuria and hematuria

72. The patient had loop electrosurgical excision procedure (LEEP) for treatment and diagnosis of cervical cancer. In the discharge instructions, what does the nurse tell the patient to expect after the procedure?
    a. Spotting
    b. Vaginal bleeding similar to menses
    c. Clotting and cramps lasting 24 hours
    d. Heavy watery discharge

73. The nurse is teaching several patients being discharged after treatment of gynecologic cancer. Which patient is most likely to need a home health care nurse and the assistance of a UAP?
    a. Patient who had a hysterectomy
    b. Patient who had a conization
    c. Patient who had a pelvic exenteration
    d. Patient who had cryotherapy

74. The nurse has identified the nursing diagnosis of Disturbed Body Image for the patient who had pelvic exenteration. Which patient behavior is the best indicator that the patient is coping and adapting successfully?
    a. Refusing to look at the wound site, but encouraging the nursing students to look
    b. Withdrawn and quiet, sitting passively when the nurse performs wound care
    c. Asking questions about the wound care, but reluctant to do self-care
    d. Frequently staring at the wound site, but appearing afraid to touch the area

75. The patient has undergone a skinning vulvectomy for cancer of the vulva. What is the major focus of nursing care for this patient?
    a. Sexual dysfunction and dyspareunia
    b. Wound healing and pain relief
    c. Hemorrhage and potential for shock
    d. Bowel and bladder function

76. The nurse is giving discharge instructions to the patient with a vulvectomy. What information does the nurse include? *(Select all that apply.)*
    a. Use a sitz bath, tub, or whirlpool bath once or twice a day for wound care.
    b. Thoroughly clean the tub before each use.
    c. Use a squeeze bottle with a saline solution and squirt over the wound area.
    d. Wear incontinence pants or absorbent pads for 7 to 10 days.
    e. Antiperistaltic drugs are usually given for 7 to 10 days to prevent defecation.
    f. Perineal care after voidings or bowel movements may prevent contamination.

77. The patient undergoing which procedure has the greatest need for referral to sexual counseling because of the nature of the surgery?
    a. Vulvectomy
    b. Myomectomy
    c. Vaginectomy
    d. Hysterectomy

CASE STUDY: THE PATIENT WITH ENDOMETRIOSIS

Use a separate sheet of paper to answer the questions in this Case Study. Answer guidelines for this Case Study are available on your Evolve website at http://evolve. elsevier.com/Iggy/ in the "Prepare for Class" folder.

A 28-year-old woman comes to the gynecologist's office reporting persistent lower abdominal pain that peaks just before menstrual flow, and she has had difficulty getting pregnant. She is very frustrated and wants to know "what's wrong" with her.

1. What will the nurse focus on during the history-taking?

2. What will the nurse tell the patient about usual testing procedures for endometriosis?

3. What interventions will the nurse describe to the patient as usual treatment for endometriosis?

4. What type of complementary and alternative therapies could the nurse discuss with the patient?

5. What are the goals of nursing management for the patient with endometriosis?

75
CHAPTER

Care of Male Patients with Reproductive Problems

STUDY/REVIEW QUESTIONS

Fill in the blanks.

1. Of all malignancies, prostate cancer is one of the _____ growing, and it metastasizes in a _____ pattern.

2. Men over _____ years old have the greatest risk for prostate cancer.

3. Testicular cancer is the most common malignancy in men _____ to _____ years of age.

4. Patients with early stage seminomas have a _____-year survival rate of 96% with orchiectomy and radiation therapy.

5. _____ cancer usually occurs as a painless, wart-like growth or ulcer on the glans under the prepuce.

6. Prostate-specific antigen (PSA) is a glycoprotein produced solely by the prostate. After treatment for prostate cancer, what does an elevated PSA level indicate?
   a. Recurrence of the prostate cancer
   b. Intolerance of cancer therapy
   c. Presence of a malignancy elsewhere in the body
   d. Reduction of the prostate gland tissue

7. The nurse is interviewing the patient with advanced prostatic cancer. Based on the most common site for the metastasis of prostate cancer, which question does the nurse ask?
   a. "Are you having pain in your back or pelvis?"
   b. "Do you feel short of breath after minor exertion?"
   c. "Have you had headaches or blurred vision?"
   d. "Are you having nausea or stomach cramps?"

8. The nurse is reviewing the laboratory results for the patient with metastasis of prostate cancer to the bone. Which elevated level does the nurse expect to see?
   a. Alpha fetoprotein
   b. Blood urea nitrogen
   c. Serum alkaline phosphatase
   d. Serum creatinine

9. The nurse is counseling a 25-year-old man recently exposed to mumps. He reports never having the mumps during childhood. What does the nurse advise the patient to do?
   a. Contact the health care provider for gamma globulin.
   b. Use scrupulous hand hygiene and avoid crowds.
   c. Go to the health department for a mumps vaccination.
   d. Watch for the signs and symptoms of urethritis.

10. The patient reports scrotal pain, edema, a heavy feeling in the testicle, dysuria, and discharge from the penis. These clinical manifestations are common to which two disorders?
    a. Orchitis and epididymitis
    b. Priapism and scrotal torsion
    c. Benign prostatic hyperplasia (BPH) and prostate cancer
    d. Hydrocele and varicocele

11. The adult male patient who had a prostatectomy earlier this morning has a Foley catheter with continuous bladder irrigation. What type of urinary drainage does the nurse expect to see in this patient?
    a. Light pink with small clots
    b. Bright red with small clots
    c. Dark burgundy with no clots
    d. Minimal for the first 12 hours

12. The nurse is teaching the patient diagnosed with erectile dysfunction about the common treatments and therapies. Which topics does the nurse include? *(Select all that apply.)*
    a. Phosphodiesterace-5 (PDE-5) inhibitors
    b. Transurethral suppositories
    c. Vacuum devices
    d. Anticholinergics
    e. Penile injections
    f. Penectomy

13. Which statement about testicular cancer is true?
    a. Testicular cancer typically occurs bilaterally.
    b. Testicular cancer occurs most often in older African-American men.
    c. Elevated alpha-fetoprotein level is used as a tumor marker for testicular cancer.
    d. Elevated alpha-fetoprotein level indicates metastasis of testicular cancer.

14. During the first 24 hours after prostatectomy, what is the priority assessment in the nursing care plan?
    a. Hemorrhage
    b. Infection
    c. Hydronephrosis
    d. Confusion

15. Which type of surgery is used to treat BPH while leaving no incision?
    a. Suprapubic prostatectomy
    b. Perineal prostatectomy
    c. Retropubic prostatectomy
    d. Transurethral resection

16. The patient is diagnosed with prostatitis. Which intervention does the nurse use to alleviate the discomfort associated with this condition?
    a. Stool softeners to prevent straining
    b. Nonsteroidal anti-inflammatory drugs (NSAIDs) to prevent pain
    c. Comfort measures such as sitz baths for pain
    d. Antispasmodics to relieve bladder pain

Matching. Match each term with its corresponding fact.

Terms

a.   Spermatocele
b.   Organic erectile dysfunction
c.   Hydrocele
d.   Phimosis
e.   Varicocele
f.   Cryptorchidism
g.   Penectomy
h.   Circumcision
i.   Testicular torsion
j.   Scrotal support
k.   Priapism
l.   Prostatitis
m.   Azoospermia

Facts

_____ 17.   Results from a disorder in the lymphatic drainage of the scrotum, causing a mass around the testis

_____ 18.   Uncontrolled, very painful penile erection without sexual desire

_____ 19.   Gradual deterioration of function

_____ 20.   Increased risk of suicide after this procedure

_____ 21.   Inflammation can result from a viral or bacterial infection, sexually transmitted disease (STD), or a psychosexual problem

_____ 22.   If not done at birth, requires strict personal hygiene to clean the prepuce

_____ 23.   Very painful; a medical emergency

_____ 24.   Palpation reveals a "wormlike" mass

_____ 25.   Usually requires no intervention unless the patient reports discomfort

_____ 26.   Promotes drainage and comfort after surgery

_____ 27.   Undescended testis with increased risk for testicular cancer

_____ 28.   Prepuce is constricted so that it cannot be retracted over the glans

_____ 29.   Absence of living sperm is common in patients with testicular cancer

30.   The patient has BPH. Based on this medical diagnosis, with what does the nurse prepare to assist the patient?
a.   PRN pain medications
b.   Urinary stasis or retention
c.   Erectile dysfunction
d.   Constipation

31.   The nurse is interviewing the patient to determine the presence of lower urinary tract symptoms (LUTS) associated with BPH. What does the nurse question the patient about? *(Select all that apply.)*
a.   Difficulty in starting and continuing urination
b.   Urinary urgency
c.   Reduced force and size of the urinary stream
d.   Postvoid dribbling
e.   Nocturia
f.   Pain with urination
g.   Sensation of incomplete bladder emptying

32. The nurse is preparing to assess the obese patient who reports subjective symptoms and urinary patterns associated with BPH. Which technique does the nurse use to perform the physical assessment?
    a. Instruct the patient to undress from the waist down, then inspect and palpate the bladder.
    b. Have the patient drink several large glasses of water and percuss the bladder.
    c. Apply gentle pressure to the bladder to elicit urgency; then instruct the patient to void.
    d. Instruct the patient to void and then use the bedside ultrasound bladder scanner.

33. The advanced practice nurse is preparing to examine the patient's prostate gland. Before the exam, what does the nurse tell the patient?
    a. He may feel the urge to defecate or faint as the prostate is palpated.
    b. He should lie supine with knees bent in a fully flexed position.
    c. The examination is very painful, but it lasts just a few seconds.
    d. The gland will be massaged to obtain a fluid sample for possible prostatitis.

34. The nurse is reviewing the laboratory results from the patient being evaluated for LUTS. What does an elevated PSA level and serum acid phosphatase level in this patient indicate?
    a. Infection
    b. Prostate cancer
    c. Renal involvement
    d. Infertility

35. The patient has an enlarged prostate. What is the gold standard test for bladder obstruction?
    a. Urodynamic pressure-flow study
    b. Bladder scan
    c. Transrectal ultrasound
    d. Cystoscopy

36. The patient is being treated for both BPH and hypertension. Which alpha blocker does the nurse anticipate will be prescribed for the patient?
    a. Doxazosin (Cardura)
    b. Finasteride (Proscar)
    c. Dutasteride (Avodart)
    d. Sildenafil (Viagra)

37. The nurse is designing a teaching plan for the patient with an enlarged prostate and obstructive symptoms. What does the nurse teach the patient to avoid?
    a. Sexual intercourse
    b. Diuretics
    c. Straining to urinate
    d. Citrus fruits

Matching. *Match the definitions of treatment options for BPH with the correct terminology.*

Terms
a. Thermotherapy
b. Transurethral needle ablation (TUNA)
c. Transurethral microwave therapy (TUMT)
d. Interstitial laser coagulation (ILC)
e. Electrovaporization

Definitions
_____ 38. Low radio frequency energy shrinks the prostate.

_____ 39. Several noninvasive techniques to destroy excess prostate tissue using heat methods.

_____ 40. High-frequency electrical current cuts and vaporizes excess tissue.

_____ 41. Laser energy coagulates excess tissue.

_____ 42. High temperatures heat and destroy excess tissue.

43. Which patients meet the criteria for a having a transurethral resection of the prostate (TURP)? *(Select all that apply.)*
   a. Patient with acute urinary retention and hematuria
   b. Patient with hydronephrosis
   c. Patient with an acute urinary tract infection
   d. Patient with a kidney stone
   e. Patient with chronic urinary tract infections

44. The patient is undergoing large volume bladder irrigation. During and after the procedure, the nurse observes the patient for confusion, muscle weakness, and increased gastrointestinal motility related to which potentially adverse effect of large volume irrigation?
   a. Hyponatremia
   b. Hypovolemia
   c. Hypoactivity
   d. Hypotension

45. The patient has had a TURP with a three-way urinary catheter taped to the left thigh. Which position does the nurse instruct the patient to maintain for the left leg?
   a. Abducted
   b. Hip slightly flexed
   c. Elevated
   d. Straight

46. The older adult patient had a TURP at 8:00 AM. At 3:00 PM the nurse assesses the patient. Which finding does the nurse report to the physician?
   a. Patient reports a continuous urge to void.
   b. Patient has painful spasms after trying to void around catheter.
   c. Patient is restless and picks at tubes.
   d. Patient keeps moving and burgundy-colored output is noted.

47. The nurse notes bright red blood with numerous clots on the patient who has had a TURP with continuous bladder irrigation (CBI). After notifying the surgeon, what does the nurse do next?
   a. Increases the CBI rate or irrigates the catheter with saline.
   b. Discontinues the CBI and removes the three-way catheter.
   c. Starts an IV infusion and draws blood for type and cross.
   d. Gives oxygen via nasal cannula and stays with the patient.

48. The nurse is giving discharge instructions to the patient who had a TURP. What does the nurse include in the instructions?
   a. Reassurance that loss of control of urination or dribbling of urine is temporary
   b. Instructions about how to apply a condom catheter and monitor for skin breakdown
   c. Advice about how to control bleeding and passage of blood clots
   d. Information about the side effects related to aminocaproic acid (Amicar)

49. Based on American Cancer Society (ACS) recommendations, what does the nurse teach the patient about screening for prostate cancer?
   a. Beginning at age 30, all men should have an annual digital rectal examination.
   b. All African-American men should start screening at 45 years of age.
   c. Men with multiple first-degree young relatives with prostate cancer at an early age should begin screening at age 40.
   d. Asian-American men should start screening at 55 years of age.

50. The nurse is teaching the patient at risk for prostate cancer about food sources of lycopene, a powerful anticancer antioxidant. Which food does the nurse suggest?
   a. Red meat
   b. Fish
   c. Watermelon
   d. Oatmeal

51. Which sign or symptom is considered a late sign of prostate cancer?
    a. Difficulty starting urination
    b. Hematuria
    c. Frequent bladder infections
    d. Urinary retention

52. The older male patient is scheduled for an annual physical including a PSA and a digital rectal examination (DRE). How are these two tests scheduled for the patient?
    a. PSA is drawn before the DRE.
    b. DRE is done several weeks before the PSA.
    c. PSA is reviewed first because DRE may be unnecessary.
    d. Both tests can be done at the convenience of the patient.

53. The nurse is reviewing PSA results for the patient who had a prostatectomy for prostate cancer several weeks ago. The PSA level is 40 ng/mL. How does the nurse interprets this data?
    a. This is an expected PSA level during this stage of the treatment.
    b. The cancer was completely removed during the surgery.
    c. The cancer is most likely recurring.
    d. There is prostate irritation and infection occurring.

54. The patient had a transrectal ultrasound with biopsy. After this procedure, what does the nurse instruct the patient to do? *(Select all that apply.)*
    a. Report fever, chills, bloody urine, and any difficulty voiding.
    b. Avoid strenuous physical activity.
    c. Limit fluid intake, especially in the first 24 hours after the procedure.
    d. Expect a small amount of bleeding that makes the urine turn pink.
    e. Expect some mild perineal and abdominal pain.

55. The older adult patient's wife is very upset because "my husband was just told that he had prostate cancer. He feels fine now, but the doctor told him to watch and wait. Why are we just watching? What are we watching for?" What is the nurse's best response?
    a. "Prostate cancer is very slow-growing. Your husband will be scheduled for regular DRE and PSA testing and I will make you a list of symptoms to watch for."
    b. "This is very upsetting news. Let's sit down and talk about how you feel and then I will have the doctor talk to you again."
    c. "It's okay, don't be upset. This is a very common way to handle prostate cancer for men that are your husband's age."
    d. "I can get you some information about prostate cancer. This will help you to understand why the doctor said this to your husband."

56. The nurse is caring for the patient who had an open radical prostatectomy. During the assessment, the nurse notes that the penis and scrotum are swollen. What does the nurse do next?
    a. Notify the physician and monitor for an inability to void or increasing pain.
    b. Elevate the scrotum and penis; apply ice to the area, 20 minutes on and 20 minutes off.
    c. Assist the patient to increase mobility, especially early ambulation.
    d. Observe the urethral meatus for redness and discharge and monitor urine output.

57. The nurse is teaching the patient who had an open radical prostatectomy about how to manage the common potential long-term complications. What does the nurse teach the patient?
    a. How to perform testicular self-examination
    b. How to manage a permanent suprapubic catheter
    c. How to perform Kegel perineal exercises
    d. Dietary modifications to acidify the urine

58. The patient has undergone external beam radiation therapy (EBRT) for palliative treatment of prostate cancer. What suggestions does the nurse make to help the patient manage acute radiation cystitis secondary to EBRT?
    a. Limit intake of water and other fluids.
    b. Avoid intake of coffee, colas, and teas.
    c. Increase consumption of dairy products.
    d. Wash genitals with mild soap and water.

59. The patient is receiving internal radiation therapy (brachytherapy) and has had a low-dose radiation seed implanted directly into the prostate gland. What nursing implication is related to this therapy?
    a. Ensure that any staff member or visitor who is pregnant is not exposed to the patient.
    b. Organize the nursing care so that exposure to the patient is limited to a few minutes.
    c. Instruct UAP that all urine specimens should be immediately discarded.
    d. Teach the patient that fatigue is common, but should pass after several months.

60. The patient is prescribed the LHRH agonist leuprolide (Lupron) for treatment of a prostate tumor. What possible side effect of this medication does the nurse advise the patient about?
    a. Nipple discharge
    b. Scrotal enlargement
    c. Fragility of the skin
    d. Erectile dysfunction

61. The patient reports having uncomfortable and unsettling episodes of "hot flashes" after receiving hormonal therapy for a prostate tumor. To alleviate this symptom, which prescription medication does the nurse assist the patient in obtaining?
    a. Biphosphonate drug such as pamidronate (Aredia)
    b. Anti-androgen drug such as bicalutamide (Casodex)
    c. Hormonal inhibitor drug such as megestrol acetate (Megace)
    d. Antimuscarinic agents such as tolterodine (Detrol)

62. The nurse is teaching the patient about self-care following a radical prostatectomy. What does the nurse include in the health teaching? *(Select all that apply.)*
    a. Teach how to care for the indwelling catheter and manifestations of infection.
    b. Walk short distances.
    c. Restrict lifting to no more than 25 lbs. for up to 3 weeks.
    d. Maintain an upright position and do not walk bent or flexed.
    e. Avoid vigorous exercise for at least 4 weeks.
    f. Shower rather than soak in a bathtub for the first 2 to 3 weeks.
    g. PSA blood tests are taken 12 weeks after surgery and then once a year.

63. The patient reports having erectile dysfunction and is seeking a prescription for sildenafil (Viagra). Because of the potential for dangerous drug-drug interactions, the nurse asks the patient specifically if he takes which type of drug?
    a. NSAIDs
    b. Nitrates
    c. Opioids
    d. Antilipemics

64. The advanced practice nurse is performing a testicular exam on the young white male patient. The practitioner finds a lump, which the patient reports is painless. This finding is considered the most common manifestation of which disease or disorder?
    a. Testicular cancer
    b. Erectile dysfunction
    c. Prostate cancer
    d. Epididymitis

65. Which statement about diagnostic biomarkers for testicular cancer is true?
    a. Presence of alpha-fetoprotein in adults is abnormal.
    b. Beta human chorionic gonadotropin (hCG) is found only in pregnant women.
    c. Lactate dehydrogenase (LDH) increases when there is tumor cell destruction.
    d. There are no true biomarkers for testicular cancer.

66. The young male patient has been diagnosed with testicular cancer. He and his wife had been trying to conceive a child for several months. What information does the nurse give the couple about sperm storage?
    a. Arrangements for sperm storage should be made as soon as possible after diagnosis.
    b. Sperm collection should be completed after radiation therapy or chemotherapy.
    c. Two or three samples should be collected 6 days apart.
    d. Saving sperm prevents fears related to erectile dysfunction.

67. The nurse is caring for the patient who had minimally invasive surgery (MIS) for testicular cancer. The nurse is also caring for the patient who had an open radical retroperitoneal lymph node dissection for testicular cancer. The nurse anticipates that the second patient has more of a risk for which condition?
    a. Paralytic ileus
    b. Urinary incontinence
    c. Metastatic disease
    d. Fluid overload

68. The nurse is teaching the patient who had an open retroperitoneal lymph node dissection. What instructions does the nurse give to the patient? *(Select all that apply.)*
    a. Do not lift anything over 5 lbs.
    b. Limit intake of fluids to 1000 mL per day.
    c. Do not drive a car for several weeks.
    d. Notify the surgeon if chills, fever, or increasing tenderness or pain around the incision site occur.
    e. Resume usual activities within 1 week after discharge, except for lifting.
    f. Perform monthly testicular self-examination on the remaining testis.
    g. Have follow-up diagnostic testing for at least 3 years after the surgery.

69. Yesterday the patient underwent the surgical removal of a hydrocele with a drain inserted. He calls the clinic for advice because he is unable to remember the discharge instructions. The nurse advises him to come into the clinic if he experiences which sign/symptom?
    a. Some serosanguineous drainage
    b. Malodorous and purulent drainage
    c. Moderate incision pain
    d. Scrotal swelling and edema

70. The advanced practice nurse is examining the testicles and scrotum of the patient. The practitioner notes that the scrotum feels "wormlike" when palpated. What is the significance of this finding?
    a. A varicocele can cause infertility.
    b. A spermatocele can cause infection.
    c. A hydrocele can become very enlarged.
    d. A varicocelectomy is advisable.

71. The nurse is caring for the middle-aged male patient who had a total penectomy. Which behavior by the patient is the strongest indicator that he needs referral for psychological assistance?
    a. He is looking at pictures of his wife and children.
    b. He is embarrassed because he has to sit down to urinate.
    c. He gets angry at the nurse for leaving the door open.
    d. He starts planning a hunting trip in a remote area.

72. The nurse is giving instructions to the UAP about hygienic care for the older adult patient who is uncircumcised. What does the nurse instruct the UAP to do?
    a. Defer cleaning the penis because of patient embarrassment.
    b. Replace the foreskin over the penis after bathing.
    c. Observe the penis and the foreskin for redness or odor.
    d. Avoid touching the foreskin because of hypersensitivity.

73. Which medical conditions can be associated with priapism? *(Select all that apply.)*
    a. Leukemia
    b. Sickle cell disease
    c. Diabetes mellitus
    d. Myocardial infarction
    e. Renal failure
    f. Malignancies

74. The patient comes to the emergency department reporting fever, chills, dysuria, urethral discharge, and a boggy, tender prostate. On exam there is a urethral discharge which shows WBCs. What does the nurse suspect in this patient?
    a. Acute bacterial prostatitis
    b. Chronic bacterial prostatitis
    c. Chronic pelvic pain syndrome
    d. Asymptomatic inflammatory prostatitis

75. The nurse is teaching the patient with chronic prostatitis. What information does the nurse include?
    a. The importance of increasing fluid intake and long-term antibiotic therapy.
    b. Avoid sexual intercourse or masturbation until symptoms subside.
    c. Prostatitis is infectious and contagious so condoms should always be used.
    d. Avoid tub baths, hot tubs, sitz baths, or swimming in heated swimming pools.

76. The nurse is talking to the 25-year-old male patient who was diagnosed and successfully treated for epididymitis. What is an important topic for the nurse to discuss with this patient?
    a. His desire to have children.
    b. The likelihood of urinary symptoms.
    c. The notification of his sexual partners.
    d. Current self-image of his sexuality.

CASE STUDY: THE PATIENT WITH URINARY RETENTION SECONDARY TO PROSTATE ENLARGEMENT

Use a separate sheet of paper to answer the questions in this Case Study. Answer guidelines for this Case Study are available on your Evolve website at http://evolve. elsevier.com/Iggy/ in the "Prepare for Class" folder.

A 73-year-old man comes to the ambulatory urgent care center reporting burning on urination, urgency, dribbling of urine, and a feeling of bladder fullness. He states that he has noticed a gradual change in his urinary pattern over the past few months but attributes it to "old age." He adds that he would not have come in at all except that he noticed some burning when he urinated today. He also says his back has been hurting, but he attributes that to yard work and gardening.

1. When interviewing this patient, what questions should the nurse ask?
2. What are the symptoms of LUTS?
3. What symptoms differentiate an obstructive problem from a nonobstructive problem?
4. What nursing diagnoses would be appropriate for this patient?
5. What laboratory tests and/or procedures can be expected for this patient?
6. The patient is diagnosed with BPH. State four effects of BPH on urinary elimination.

76
CHAPTER

Care of Patients with Sexually Transmitted Disease

STUDY/REVIEW QUESTIONS

1. Which symptom is the first sign of primary syphilis?
   a. Small painless, indurated, smooth, weeping lesion
   b. There are no symptoms, so a history of potential exposure is essential
   c. Malaise, low-grade fever, and general muscular aches and pains
   d. Rash that tends to change from papules to squamous papules to pustules

2. The patient calls the nurse suspecting a one-time exposure to syphilis that occurred about 4 weeks ago. The patient reports being asymptomatic and abstinent since the incident. What is the nurse's best response?
   a. "The first sign is a chancre which will usually develop by the third week."
   b. "Continue abstinence for up to 90 days and observe the genitalia for painless sores."
   c. "Use a latex or polyurethane condom for genital and anal intercourse."
   d. "The chancre can appear anywhere and then disappear, so you must come in for testing."

3. The patient is admitted for emergency surgery after an accident. In addition, the patient has a pustular rash related to secondary syphilis. What instructions does the nurse give to the unlicensed assistive personnel (UAP)?
   a. Gloves should be worn at all times when touching the patient.
   b. The lesions are highly contagious, so the patient should do his or her own hygienic care.
   c. No instructions are given to the UAP because patient confidentiality is essential.
   d. If the skin is open and draining pus or fluid, use gloves during patient care.

4. The patient is being tested for *T. pallidum*, and the first slide is negative. The patient's health care provider is relatively inexperienced. What is the nurse's primary concern?
   a. The patient must be told that he did not have syphilis.
   b. The patient must be directed to return in 3 days for a repeat test.
   c. The patient must be treated prophylactically with penicillin.
   d. The patient must be educated about preventing sexually transmitted diseases (STDs).

5. The patient is diagnosed with primary syphilis. The nurse prepares to administer and educate the patient about which treatment regimen?
   a. Benzathine penicillin G given intramuscularly as a single 2.4 million units dose, and follow-up evaluation at 6, 12, and 24 months
   b. Benzathine penicillin G given intramuscularly for 7 days, and follow-up evaluation at 6, 12, and 24 months
   c. Ceftriaxone (Rocephin) 125 mg intramuscularly in a single dose, plus azithromycin (Zithromax) 1 g orally in a single dose, and follow-up evaluation at 6, 12, and 24 months
   d. Metronidazole (Flagyl) 500 mg orally twice daily for 14 days, and follow-up evaluation at 6, 12, and 24 months

6. How is a Jarisch-Herxheimer reaction treated?
   a. Oxygen, epinephrine, and antihistamines
   b. Emergency IV fluid resuscitation
   c. Analgesics and antipyretics
   d. Monitoring for symptom resolution

7. The patient is diagnosed with late tertiary syphilis. In addition to central nervous system involvement, what findings does the nurse see documented in the patient's record?
   a. Chancres on the genitalia, lips, or nipples
   b. Rash on the palms and soles of the feet
   c. Benign lesions of the skin, mucous membranes, and bone
   d. Contagious wart-like lesions and mucous patches

8. The patient is diagnosed with early latent syphilis. Which medication is prescribed for the patient?
   a. Penicillin-G
   b. Doxycycline
   c. Amoxicillin
   d. Tetracycline

9. The patient reports a possible exposure to syphilis. The nurse informs the patient about which screening test?
   a. ELISA serum
   b. VDRL serum
   c. FTA antibody
   d. MHA assay

True or False? *Read each statement and write T for true or F for false in the blanks provided. If the statement is false, correct the statement to make it true.*

_____ 10. Chlamydia, gonorrhea, syphilis, chancroid, HIV infection, and AIDS are reportable to local health authorities in every state.

_____ 11. The causative organism of gonorrhea is *Treponema pallidum*, a spirochete with a slender, spiral shape that resembles a corkscrew.

_____ 12. There are no laboratory or physical examination techniques that alone are both sensitive and specific for the diagnosis of acute pelvic inflammatory disease (PID).

_____ 13. Syphilis is one of the leading causes of infertility and is related to the increase in the number of ectopic pregnancies reported in the United States.

_____ 14. Less common diseases in the United States that are transmitted by sexual contact are lymphogranuloma venereum, chancroid, and granuloma inguinale.

_____ 15. The number-one causative agent associated with PID is *Escherichia coli*.

_____ 16. Standards of care and treatment for STDs are developed by the Food and Drug Administration.

_____ 17. For genital herpes, the goal of medication is to reduce symptoms and discomfort.

_____ 18. Nonoxynol-9 may decrease risk for transmission of HIV during vaginal intercourse and anal intercourse.

19. The patient has had genital herpes–HSV-2 for several years. She is at the clinic for her annual Papanicolaou (Pap) smear and asks about long-term problems. What is the nurse's best response?
    a. "There is an increased risk for PID."
    b. "You are likely to have frequent episodes of vaginitis."
    c. "You have a greater risk for developing cervical cancer."
    d. "When you are pregnant, the fetus will be closely monitored for infection."

20. The nurse is teaching the patient being discharged after treatment for genital herpes. Which patient statement indicates a need for further teaching?
    a. "I can be contagious even when I do not have any lesions."
    b. "If I get pregnant, I need to tell my nurse midwife that I have genital herpes."
    c. "After taking all of my acyclovir, I will not have genital herpes anymore."
    d. "I need to have an annual Pap smear because of my increased risk for cervical cancer."

21. The patient is prescribed doxycycline for the treatment of lymphogranuloma venereum. What additional information does the nurse give the patient about treatment issues?
    a. All sexual partners for 60 days before the patient's symptom onset should be treated.
    b. Even with treatment, expect long-term complications of carditis and arthritis.
    c. The treatment will cure the infection, but lymph nodes will drain chronically.
    d. Watch for and report headache, malaise, arthralgia, and anorexia.

22. Why do women develop complications more often than men when being treated for gonorrhea?
    a. Treatment for the disease can leave women infertile.
    b. The disease is asymptomatic in the early stages.
    c. Estrogen leaves the woman more resistant to antibiotic therapy.
    d. The disease is much more difficult to cure in women.

23. How long is the usual incubation period for gonorrhea?
    a. 3 to 10 days
    b. 10 to 14 days
    c. 2 to 3 weeks
    d. 2 to 3 months

24. The nurse is performing a history and physical on the male patient who reports an STD. Which symptom is the most common in the male with Chlamydia?
    a. Painful intercourse
    b. Urethritis
    c. Dark yellow urine
    d. Thick green discharge

25. When obtaining a complete obstetric-gynecologic history, the nurse also takes a sexual history from the patient. Which approach is the most therapeutic to elicit information from the patient?
    a. Use a checklist to ask "yes" and "no" questions.
    b. Ask the patient to explain his or her sexual history.
    c. Ask directly if the patient has ever had an STD.
    d. Ask open-ended questions.

26. For the nurse to be an effective clinician when working with patients concerning sexuality, STDs, or other sexual concerns, what must the nurse do first?
    a. Take a course on sexual relations and counseling.
    b. Know all about his or her patient's concerns, problems, or needs.
    c. Be aware of his or her own sexual values, attitudes, and sexuality.
    d. Set up a meeting with the patient's sexual partner.

27. The female patient reporting a troublesome vaginal discharge is diagnosed with trichomoniasis and is given medication to treat the infection. What does the nurse teach the patient about the diagnosis?
    a. *Trichomonas vaginalis* is self-limiting, but medicine is needed to treat the vaginal itching.
    b. The patient's sexual partner must be treated if the problem is to be resolved.
    c. The medication should be applied liberally to the external genitalia once a day.
    d. The vaginal infection can cause infertility in childbearing women.

28. Women with PID are at an increased risk for which condition?
    a. Ovarian rupture
    b. Appendicitis
    c. Infertility
    d. STDs

29. What is the most common chief complaint that leads the patient with PID to seek medical health care?
    a. Vaginal itching
    b. Lower abdominal pain
    c. Malaise with fever
    d. Abnormal menstrual flow

30. The patient with PID is on bedrest with bathroom privileges. What position is best for the patient while on bedrest?
    a. Prone
    b. Supine
    c. Side-lying
    d. Semi-Fowler's

31. The patient with PID is discharged home on oral antibiotics. What does the nurse tell the patient regarding her monthly menstrual flow?
    a. "Use tampons only when your menstrual flow is heavy."
    b. "Follow your normal routine for using tampons unless the pain increases."
    c. "Use perineal pads until you are fully recovered."
    d. "Use tampons in the day and perineal pads at night."

32. When performing discharge teaching about resuming sexual relations to the female patient diagnosed with an STD, what does the nurse teach the patient?
    a. Douche within 24 hours after vaginal intercourse.
    b. Sexual relations are prohibited for 3 months.
    c. Intercourse should be postponed until the treatment regimen is completed.
    d. Intercourse is permitted unless there is an increase in abdominal pain.

33. What does the nurse tell the patient with PID about the practice of vaginal douching?
    a. It increases a woman's risk for developing PID.
    b. It should be done daily during the course of the illness.
    c. Vinegar is the only safe solution to use.
    d. Use only disposable equipment.

Matching. Match each STD with its corresponding definition.

Sexually Transmitted Diseases

a. Herpes simplex type 2
b. Secondary syphilis
c. Lymphogranuloma venereum
d. Herpes genitalis
e. Genital warts
f. Primary syphilis
g. Granuloma inguinale
h. Gonorrhea
i. Chancroid
j. Chlamydia
k. Human papillomavirus (HPV)
l. Candida

Definitions

_____ 34. Highly infectious state with the presence of a chancre

_____ 35. An infection limited to the vagina; very irritating, but has no long-term sequelae

_____ 36. Recurrences are not caused by re-infection

_____ 37. Transmitted by direct sexual contact with mucosal surfaces and can be transmitted to the vaginally delivered neonate

_____ 38. Transient painless lesion that gives rise to secondary signs of infection as headache, malaise, or anorexia

_____ 39. In 2006, the U.S. Food and Drug Administration approved a vaccine which provides almost 100% immunity

_____ 40. Most common sexually transmitted viral disease caused by the human papillomavirus (HPV)

_____ 41. Flu-like symptoms and a generalized rash

_____ 42. Nodules that ulcerate, grow together, and become a spreading ulcer, which can become mutilating

_____ 43. Often responsible for causing PID

_____ 44. Genital lesions that are painful and bleed easily caused by *Haemophilus ducreyi*, a gram-negative bacteria

_____ 45. Initial infection that causes blisters which rupture and cause painful lesions

46. The nurse is preparing an information packet about women's health considerations for STDs. What information does the nurse include? *(Select all that apply.)*
   a. Young women generally have excellent knowledge about the risk of STDs.
   b. Young women frequently believe that they are vulnerable to STDs.
   c. Young women mistakenly believe that contraceptives protect them from STDs.
   d. Mucosal tears in postmenopausal women may also place them at greater risk for STDs.
   e. Women have more asymptomatic infections that may delay diagnosis and treatment.

47. The young female patient requires hospitalization for a severe case of genital herpes. What information is given to the patient regarding the long-term consequences?
   a. There is an increased risk of recurrence with an increased susceptibility to re-infection.
   b. There is a risk of neonatal transmission and an increased risk for acquiring HIV infection.
   c. There is an increased risk of recurrence with greater severity of symptoms with each episode.
   d. There is an increased risk for multiple types of reproductive cancers at a young age.

48. The nurse is counseling the patient experiencing recurrent outbreaks of genital herpes. What suggestions for symptomatic treatment does the nurse include?
    a. Oral analgesics, sitz baths, and increased oral fluid intake
    b. Topical anesthetics, nutritional therapy, and warm compresses
    c. Abstinence, frequent bathing, and fluid restriction
    d. Bedrest and application of podofilox (Condylox) 0.5% solution

49. The patient is diagnosed with condylomata acuminata. What are the desired outcomes of management for this patient?
    a. Reduce pain and prevent recurrence
    b. Prevent long-term complications to the cardiac system
    c. Remove the warts and treat the symptoms
    d. Prevent infertility and systemic infection

50. The patient requires treatment for genital warts. Which treatment is done by the patient at home if given the proper instructions?
    a. Imiquimod (Aldara) 5% cream
    b. Cryotherapy with liquid nitrogen
    c. Podophyllin resin 10% in a compound of tincture of benzoin
    d. Trichloroacetic acid (TCA) or bichloroacetic acid (BCA)

51. What is the incubation period for genital warts?
    a. 3 to 7 days
    b. 2 to 20 days
    c. 10 to 90 days
    d. 2 to 3 months

52. The patient has had podophyllin treatment for condylomata acuminata. For which sign/symptom does the nurse tell the patient to return for further treatment?
    a. Discomfort at the site
    b. Bleeding from the site
    c. Infection at the site
    d. Sloughing of parts of warts

53. The male patient reports that a female sexual partner just told him that she was treated for gonorrhea. What symptoms does the nurse ask him about, because they are the most likely to occur with gonorrhea in a male?
    a. Small, painless lump that occurred on the penis, but spontaneously disappeared
    b. Numerous small, painless papillary growths in the genital area
    c. Painful intercourse because of scrotal swelling and epididymitis
    d. Dysuria and a profuse yellowish green or scant clear penile discharge

54. The patient is being treated for gonorrhea. Which single-dose medication order does the nurse question?
    a. Ceftriaxone (Rocephin) 125 mg
    b. Cefixime (Suprax) 400 mg
    c. Azithromycin (Zithromax) 1 g orally
    d. Ciprofloxacin (Cipro) 250 mg

55. The patient is tested for and diagnosed with gonorrhea. The nurse advocates that the choice of drug therapy include medications that concurrently treat which condition?
    a. Genital herpes
    b. Chlamydia
    c. Syphilis
    d. Genital warts

56. The young woman discovers she has Chlamydia after going to her doctor for a routine Pap smear and pelvic exam. She is reluctant to accept the diagnosis, because she is asymptomatic and "does not have any money for unnecessary treatment right now." What is the nurse's best response?
    a. Explain that there is a single-dose of medication which has a one-time cost.
    b. Talk to the woman about her financial situation and help her find resources.
    c. Encourage the patient to express her reluctance and disbelief.
    d. Tell her that it is possible to have Chlamydia without having any symptoms.

57. The patient with an STD freely admits to being a commercial sex worker. In talking to this patient, the nurse recognizes that she has not disclosed a true name, address, or partner contact information. What is the best treatment strategy to use with this patient?
    a. Reassure her that all health data is confidential and will be handled with discretion.
    b. Spend extra time with the patient to enlist trust so that she will give correct information.
    c. Administer a one-dose course of treatment and dispense a box of condoms.
    d. Give her all the medications for a 7-day treatment and convey a nonjudgmental attitude.

58. Which factors increase the risk for PID? *(Select all that apply.)*
    a. Age younger than 26 years
    b. Multiple sexual partners
    c. Intrauterine device (IUD) in place
    d. Caffeine use
    e. History of Chlamydia or gonococcal infection
    f. History of gastrointestinal infections

59. The young female patient with a history of previous STDs has a hunched-over gait and has difficulty getting on the examination table. On observing this behavior, what does the nurse first assess for?
    a. Lower abdominal pain
    b. Lower back pain
    c. Musculoskeletal weakness
    d. Vaginal bleeding

60. The nurse is reviewing laboratory results for the patient with PID. Which lab results does the nurse expect to see? *(Select all that apply.)*
    a. Elevation in white blood cell (WBC) count
    b. Elevation in erythrocyte sedimentation rate (ESR)
    c. Decreased level of C-reactive protein
    d. Presence of human chorionic gonadotropin (hCG) in urine
    e. Presence of more than 10 WBCs per high-power field for vaginal discharge

61. In the emergency department, the patient is diagnosed with PID and there is an order to discharge the patient home with a prescription for antibiotics. What circumstance causes the nurse to question the order for discharge to home?
    a. The patient is several months postpartum, but had very mild symptoms.
    b. The patient is nauseated, but able to tolerate small amounts of oral fluids.
    c. The patient is pregnant, but willing to attempt self-care if properly instructed.
    d. The patient is afraid to go home, but the sister and husband are available to help.

62. The nurse is caring for the patient admitted for PID. Which task does the nurse delegate to the UAP?
    a. Apply a heating pad to the lower abdomen or back.
    b. Place the patient in a semi-Fowler's position.
    c. Ask the patient if the pain is a 2 to 3 on a pain scale of 0 to –10.
    d. Report to the nurse if the patient is anxious about infertility.

63. The patient reports an itching or tingling sensation felt in the skin 1 to 2 days followed by a blister on the penis which ruptured spontaneously with painful erosion. What are these symptoms consistent with?
    a. Syphilis
    b. Genital warts
    c. Genital herpes
    d. Gonorrhea

64. The nurse is teaching a group of high-school students about the use of condoms. What information does the nurse include? *(Select all that apply.)*
    a. Condoms are primarily effective for vaginal intercourse.
    b. Female condoms are too difficult to use for inexperienced partners.
    c. Keep condoms (especially latex) in a cool, dry place out of direct sunlight.
    d. Do not use condoms that are in damaged packages or that are brittle or discolored.
    e. Avoid damaging the condom with fingernails, teeth, or other sharp objects.
    f. Put condoms on the penis before foreplay or arousal.
    g. If you use a lubricant, make sure that the lubricant is water-based.

65. Which STD is associated with an increased risk for cervical cancer?
    a. Syphilis
    b. Condylomata acuminata: HPV type 16
    c. Condylomata acuminata: HPV type 6
    d. PID

66. In performing a genital exam on a teenage patient, the examiner sees multiple large cauliflower-like growths in the perineal area. The patient reports these appeared about 3 months after her first sexual experience. What does the examiner suspect?
    a. Condylomata acuminata
    b. Genital herpes
    c. Salpingitis
    d. Gonorrhea

CASE STUDY: THE PATIENT WITH A SEXUALLY TRANSMITTED DISEASE

Use a separate sheet of paper to answer the questions in this Case Study. Answer guidelines for this Case Study are available on your Evolve website at http://evolve. elsevier.com/Iggy/ in the "Prepare for Class" folder.

A young woman comes to the STD clinic. She is defensive and seems disgusted as she explains to the nurse that she believes she was exposed to an STD. She bases her belief on something a friend told her, but she is reluctant to be more forthcoming about the details. She currently denies symptoms. She is also very angry about "false accusations" that people are making. The nurse validates her decision to come in for examination and diagnosis.

1. The nurse explains that women have more health problems associated with STDs than men. What should the nurse tell the patient?

2. Explain why the patient could present with this angry and defensive behavior. What can the nurse do?

3. What should be included in a nursing assessment of the patient with symptoms of an STD?

4. What are six nursing responsibilities associated with the management of a patient who is newly diagnosed with an STD?

5. The patient is reluctant to disclose the names of sexual partners or talk about partners. What could the nurse do?

6. The patient is diagnosed with Chlamydia. What should be included in the patient education material?

7. What should the nurse include in the patient teaching for a patient who was prescribed oral antibiotics?

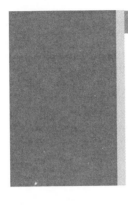

Answer Key for Study/Review Questions

CHAPTER 1

1. d
2. b
3. a
4. c
5. c
6. b
7. d
8. b
9. b
10. b
11. c

CHAPTER 2

1. *Across*
   4. Journaling
   6. Touch
   7. Massage
   10. Aromatherapy

   Down
   1. Imagery
   2. Tai Chi
   3. Acupuncture
   5. Acupressure
   8. AAT
   9. Herbal
2. d
3. (Refer to Table 2-1 in the text.)
4. d
5. a
6. b
7. e
8. c
9. d
10. a, c
11. b
12. a, b, c, e
13. a. Relaxation
    b. Decrease pain
    c. Decrease anxiety
14. c
15. a, b, e, f
16. a. Herbal preparations may cause liver toxicity, potentiate other drugs, alter blood pressure, and cause bleeding.

b. There is potential for serious interactions with prescription drugs such as anticoagulants, hypoglycemics, antidepressants, sedative-hypnotics, and medications with therapeutic ranges such as digoxin/theophylline.

c. Just because herbal preparations are "natural" does not mean they are safe; even if they are safe, it does not mean they are effective.

d. Labels may not accurately describe contents.

e. Never ingest herbs while pregnant or nursing.

f. Herbal preparations are regulated as food and nutritional supplements in the United States by the Food and Drug Administration (FDA) and do not receive the same oversight in preparation and use as medications do.

g. Self-treatment with herbal preparations may delay conventional treatments that may be more effective.

17. a
18. d
19. b

CHAPTER 3

1. a, b, c,
2. Identify any four of the following:
   a. Reorient the patient frequently to his or her location.
   b. Explain all procedures and routines to the patient before they occur.
   c. Provide opportunities for the patient to assist in decision-making.
   d. Encourage the patient's family and friends to visit often.
   e. Establish a trusting relationship with the patient as soon as possible.
   f. Arrange for familiar or special keepsakes to keep at the patient's beside. (See Chart 3-1.)

3. a, c, d, e
4. c
5. a, c, d
6. b, c, e
7. b
8. a, d
9. b
10. a
11. d
12. b
13. c
14. T
15. F
16. F
17. T
18. a
19. a, b, e
20. c
21. a, c
22. c
23. d
24. b
25. a
26. b
27. a
28. a
29. b
30. b
31. d
32. c
33. a
34. b

CHAPTER 4

1. c
2. d
3. a
4. i
5. h
6. f
7. g
8. j
9. b
10. e
11. d
12. T
13. T

14. F; 18% in 2000, estimated by 2050 to be 43.8%
15. T
16. F; people have diverse needs
17. T
18. F; manifestations of pain vary greatly among and within cultures
19. a
20. d
21. a. 3
    b. 1
    c. 2
22. c

CHAPTER 5

1. F; pain is "complex and subjective"
2. T
3. F; there have been only slight improvements
4. T
5. F; to advocate for the patient by *believing* reports of pain
6. a. Age
   b. Gender
   c. Sociocultural environment
7. b
8. c
9. a. Pain confined to the site of origin
   b. Pain along a specific nerve or nerves
   c. Diffuse pain around the site of origin that is not well-localized
   d. Pain perceived in an area away from the site of painful stimulation
10. c
11. a, e, g, j
12. c, d, f
13. b, d, h
14. a
15. a. Skin, subcutaneous tissues, and musculoskeletal structures
    b. Organs and the linings of the body cavities
    c. Nerve fibers, spinal cord, and central nervous system
16. d
17. a
18. CP
19. B
20. AP
21. CP
22. CP
23. B
24. AP
25. a, b
26. b

27. a. 3
    b. 1
    c. 2
    d. 4
28. a, c
29. a, b, e
30. F; IM route is no longer acceptable because of its many disadvantages
31. T
32. T
33. F; plasma concentration increases gradually
34. c, e
35. b, c, e
36. b, c, e, g
37. b
38. c
39. a, c
40. a
41. b
42. c
43. b
44. c
45. c
46. b
47. F; morphine is most commonly used
48. T
49. F; no drug is administered during the lockout interval
50. T
51. F; provides more consistent analgesia
52. T
53. b, c, d, f
54. a, d, e
55. b
56. d
57. d
58. e
59. c
60. b
61. a
62. a
63. a
64. b
65. d
66. d
67. a
68. c
69. a
70. c
71. b
72. T
73. T
74. T

75. F; not easily titrated and only certain patients are able to use this method
76. T
77. F; effective for 72 hours before it has to be changed
78. F; a fever can increase absorption and cause side effects such as sedation
79. c

CHAPTER 6

1. *Across*
   3. RNA
   4. Centromere
   6. Autosomes
   8. Genome
   9. Dizygotic
   10. Transcription
   11. Diploid

   Down
   1. Chromosome
   2. Phenotype
   5. Haploid
   7. Monozygotic
2. 46; 23
3. a
4. same
5. different
6. same
7. a. AR
   b. AD
   c. B
   d. AD
   e. AR
   f. AD
   g. AR
   h. AR
8. T
9. F; the trait cannot be transmitted from father to son
10. T
11. F; female carriers have a 50% risk (with each pregnancy) of transmitting the gene to their children
12. d
13. a, c, d
14. a, c, e, f
15. a. SLR
    b. FC
    c. FC
    d. SLR
    e. SLR
    f. FC

CHAPTER 7

1.

Categories	Action of Substance and Overall Effects on the Body	Examples
Stimulants	Increase alertness, relieve fatigue, euphoria. Effects include increased blood pressure, heart rate, respiration, dilated pupils, decreased appetite.	Caffeine, nicotine, amphetamines, methamphetamines, cocaine
Hallucinogens	Produce behavioral changes that are often multiple and dramatic. Effects include rapidly changing feelings that sometimes incorporate violent and erratic behavior.	Lysergic acid (LSD), phencyclidine (PCP), marijuana
Depressants	Drugs used medically to relieve anxiety, irritability, and tension. Effects include calmness, relaxation, slurred speech, impaired judgment.	Barbiturates, benzodiazepines (such as Rohypnol, gamma hydroxybutyrate, or GHB), alcohol
Narcotics	Drugs used medically to relieve pain. Effects include euphoria, drowsiness, respiratory depression, pinpoint pupils.	Opioids and morphine derivatives, including codeine, morphine, heroin, methadone, oxycodone
Inhalants	Drugs that are inexpensive and easy to obtain legally. Effects include slurred speech, loss of muscle control, impaired judgment, irritation of the eyes, rhinitis, brain and lung damage.	Solvents, nitrites, gases
Steroids	Increased muscle mass. Males: acne, baldness, breast enlargement, shrinkage of penis and testicles. For females: breast reduction and hair growth. Psychological effects may include outbursts of anger ("roid rage"). Life-threatening effects include an acute myocardial infarction and liver cancer.	Anabolic steroids

2. F; are susceptible
3. F; state boards of nursing have peer-assistance programs available
4. F; and the patient's culture
5. F; alcohol, steroids, nicotine, and prescription drugs are also included
6. F; substance abuse can occur at any age
7. T
8. T
9. T
10. T
11. a, c
12. a. Amphetamines
    b. Methamphetamine
13. b
14. b
15. a
16. b
17. b
18. Nicotine; the drug stimulates the body to release epinephrine, causing a sudden release of glucose and other substances. Then after recovery from the stimulant effect, nicotine causes sedation and feelings of depression and fatigue.
19. T
20. T
21. F
22. T
23. F
24. d

25. d
26. b
27. Flushing, increased perspiration, aggression, incoherence; the user is unaware of his or her surroundings and may experience feelings of superior physical strength
28. b
29. c, d, e
30. c
31. T
32. F; dependence can occur in a very short time
33. T
34. T
35. F; exists when a person does not have a strong craving for alcohol or physical dependence, but does have problems related to alcohol use
36. a
37. c
38. a. Minor alcohol withdrawal is characterized by restlessness, anxiety, insomnia, tachycardia, agitation and tremors, diaphoresis, and increased blood pressure.
    b. Major withdrawal includes the above findings, plus hallucinations, vomiting, pronounced diaphoresis, and tremors of the entire body (delirium tremens, or DTs).

    c. Life-threatening withdrawal can include any of the above, plus global confusion, DTs, and the inability to recognize familiar objects or people.
39. c
40. b
41. b
42. d, e
43. a
44. b
45. c
46. d
47. a, b
48. c
49. T
50. T
51. a
52. b
53. e
54. d
55. f
56. b
57. a
58. c

CHAPTER 8

1. e
2. j
3. c or d
4. d

5. a
6. h, i
7. h
8. b
9. c
10. k
11. g
12. f
13. b
14. e
15. b
16. b, h
17. l
18. c
19. d
20. c
21. T
22. T
23. F; constipation, not diarrhea, can be a problem related to decreased motility and mobility
24. T
25. T
26. F; turning the patient every 2 hours may not be sufficient for people who are frail and have thin skin
27. F; fluid restriction is necessary
28. a
29. c
30. a
31. a, c, e
32. a, c, d, e, f
33. a
34. b
35. a
36. a
37. b
38. b
39. a
40. b
41. a
42. b
43. d
44. a, b
45. a
46. a, b, e
47. c
48. c
49. c
50. b
51. b
52. c
53. b
54. a
55. a, b, but can use for checking of residual with c
56. a, b
57. c
58. b
59. c

60. a, b, c
61. a, b, c
62. b
63. b, d, e
64. c
65. d
66. c
67. a
68. a
69. c
70. d
71. c
72. a
73. e
74. c
75. e
76. b

CHAPTER 9

1. c
2. a
3. d
4. b
5. d
6. c
7. c
8. a, c, d, e
9. a. 2
   b. 3
   c. 1
10. c
11. d
12. b, c, d, e
13. b
14. d
15. a
16. c
17. b
18. F; giving food or fluids may actually lead to more discomfort
19. T
20. T
21. F; the most feared is pain
22. T
23. T
24. F; dyspnea is a subjective experience in which the patient experiences an uncomfortable awareness of breathing
25. T
26. T
27. T
28. F; nausea and vomiting commonly occur as death nears, and are not limited to patients with cancer
29. T
30. a
31. c
32. c

CHAPTER 10

1. d
2. b
3. c
4. a
5. e
6. a, b, d, f, g
7. c
8. b
9. d
10. b
11. c
12. b, d
13. d
14. d
15. b
16. c
17. a
18. d
19. b, c, e
20. d
21. b
22. a. U
    b. E
    c. E
    d. U
    e. N
    f. U
    g. E
    h. N
23. a, c, e, f
24. c
25. a
26. c
27. b
28. c
29. a
30. d
31. c
32. b
33. a
34. e
35. c
36. c
37. a
38. a
39. a
40. b
41. c
42. b
43. d
44. a, b, e
45. a. 2
    b. 1
    c. 3
    d. 4
46. b
47. F; there is no universal triage system
48. T

49. F; the nurse is responsible for reassessment
50. F; the nurse may search the patient for protection of the patient, staff, and others
51. T
52. T
53. F; unintentional injury is the leading cause
54. F; to enable recovery and return to patients to productive roles in society

CHAPTER 11

1. a, c, e, f, g
2. b
3. c
4. b
5. a, c, d
6. a, c, f
7. c
8. a
9. d
10. b, c, e
11. a
12. c
13. a, c, d, e
14. c
15. d
16. c
17. a
18. b
19. a
20. d
21. b
22. a
23. a
24. a
25. b
26. a, b, d, g
27. c
28. b
29. a
30. a
31. b
32. c
33. a
34. b
35. a
36. c
37. *Across*
    1. Urticating
    3. Brown recluse
    4. Honeybee
    6. Black widow

    Down
    2. Tarantula
    5. Bark

38. a, b
39. a
40. b
41. b
42. a
43. b
44. b
45. b
46. a
47. c
48. c
49. c
50. a
51. a
52. b
53. a, b, c, e
54. c
55. d
56. d
57. c
58. b
59. b
60. c
61. a
62. c
63. F
64. T
65. T
66. F
67. F
68. T
69. T
70. b
71. c
72. b
73. c
74. d
75. c
76. d
77. a, c, d, e, f
78. c
79. c
80. d
81. d
82. a
83. a, b, d, e
84. a
85. a
86. c
87. b
88. b
89. b, e, g, h
90. a
91. b
92. d
93. b
94. b
95. a

96. c
97. c
98. b
99. c
100. d
101. d
102. a

CHAPTER 12

1. d
2. f
3. k
4. b
5. l
6. m
7. h
8. c
9. i
10. j
11. g
12. a
13. e
14. d
15. a, c, d, g
16. b
17. d
18. b
19. a
20. b
21. c
22. d
23. c
24. d
25. b
26. c
27. c
28. a
29. a
30. d
31. c
32. b
33. d
34. c
35. a
36. b
37. a
38. a, c, d, f
39. d
40. b
41. a
42. b
43. b
44. b
45. a
46. b
47. a

CHAPTER 13

1. c
2. a
3. f
4. d
5. e
6. b
7. a, b, d, f, h
8. a
9. b
10. d
11. b
12. d
13. d
14. b
15. c
16. b
17. c
18. a, b, c, e, f
19. a
20. d
21. c
22. b
23. c
24. a
25. a
26. b
27. b, d, e
28. c
29. a
30. d
31. c
32. c
33. b
34. a
35. c
36. b
37. b
38. f
39. f
40. a
41. d
42. a
43. e
44. b
45. b
46. c
47. d
48. d
49. c
50. e
51. c
52. a
53. a
54. d
55. a, c, d, f
56. b
57. b
58. b
59. d

60. b
61. a
62. c
63. b
64. a
65. a
66. a
67. c
68. a
69. b
70. b
71. d
72. d
73. d
74. a, c, d, e
75. d
76. c
77. a
78. d
79. a, d, e, g
80. b
81. b
82. b
83. a
84. a
85. a
86. b
87. b
88. a
89. a
90. b
91. a
92. a
93. b
94. d
95. c
96. b
97. a
98. b
99. b
100. d
101. b, c, d
102. d
103. b
104. b, c, d
105. a
106. c
107. b
108. b
109. a
110. a
111. a
112. b
113. b
114. b
115. b
116. a
117. b
118. a, e, f, g, h
119. a, c, e, g

120. b
121. a
122. a, b, c, d
123. c
124. c
125. b
126. c
127. a
128. a
129. a
130. a
131. d
132. b
133. c
134. a
135. a
136. b, c, d
137. c
138. a
139. b
140. b
141. a
142. a
143. b
144. b
145. a
146. b
147. a
148. b
149. a
150. b
151. d
152. a
153. a
154. d
155. a
156. c
157. a, b, c
158.

Electrolyte	Reference Range
Sodium (Na^+)	136–145 mEq/L
Potassium (K^+)	3.5–5.0 mEq/L
Calcium (Ca^{2+})	9.0–10.5 mg/dL
Chloride (Cl^-)	98–106 mEq/L
Magnesium (Mg^{2+})	1.3–2.1 mEq/L
Phosphorus (Pi)	3.0–4.5 mg/dL

CHAPTER 14

1. F; acid-base balance occurs through control of hydrogen ion (H^+) production and elimination
2. F; occurs in the red blood cell
3. F; are stronger, but slower to respond
4. T

5. F; main cause is renal reabsorption
6. F; bicarbonate is major buffer
7. F; component is carbon dioxide
8. T
9. F; results in carbon dioxide retention and acidemia
10. F; is more severe
11. acidic
12. 1:20
13. bicarbonate; CO_2
14. b
15. a
16. a
17. c
18. d
19. a
20. d
21. b
22. c
23. $CO_2 + H_2O \rightarrow H_2CO_3 \rightarrow H^+ + HCO_3^-$
24. a. D
    b. D
    c. D
    d. I
    e. I
25. b
26. c
27. c
28. a
29. d
30. b
31. b
32. a, b, e
33. c
34. c
35. a
36. b
37. d
38. c
39. a
40. b, d
41. d
42. a
43. d
44. c
45. c
46. b
47. a
48. d
49. c
50. b
51. a
52. b
53. b
54. b
55. d
56. a
57. c
58. b
59. c

60. c
61. b, d, f
62. b
63. a
64. c
65. a
66. b
67. a
68. b
69. b
70. a
71. a, b, c, e, f
72. c
73. b
74. c
75. d
76. d
77. d
78. b
79. c
80. b
81. a
82. d
83. b
84. b
85. d
86. c, d
87. a
88. b
89. d
90. (Refer to Chart 14-1 in the text.)
91. b
92. c
93. d
94. a
95. a
96. c
97. e
98. b
99. b
100. c
101. c
102. a. Acid
     b. Acid
     c. Alkaline
     d. Acid

CHAPTER 15

1. b
2. a
3. a, b, c, e, g
4. a, b, c
5. c
6. b, d, e, g
7. a
8. d
9. b
10. a
11. d
12. a

13. d
14.

Grade	Criteria
0	No symptoms
1	Erythema with or without pain
2	Pain at access site with erythema and/or edema
3	Pain at access site with erythema and/or edema; streak formation; palpable cord
4	Pain at access site with erythema and/or edema; streak formation; palpable venous cord >1 inch long; purulent drainage

15. b
16. c
17. b
18. c
19. c
20. d
21. a, d, e
22. d
23. a
24. c
25. c
26. a
27. b
28. c
29. a
30. b
31. d
32. d
33. b
34. d
35. b, c, d
36. b
37. c
38. a. P
    b. CID
    c. P
    d. P
    e. CID
39. a, b, c, e
40. c
41. c
42. d
43. a, b, e
44. d
45. a, b, c, d
46. a
47. a. 5
    b. 4
    c. 6
    d. 3
    e. 1
    f. 7
    g. 2

48. c
49. b
50. d
51. c
52. c
53. c
54. a
55. d
56. d
57. c
58. d
59. c
60. a
61. d
62. a
63. *Across*
   1. Infection
   3. Infiltration
   4. Vesicant
   8. Thrombosis

   Down
   2. Extravasation
   5. Phlebitis
   6. Ecchymosis
   7. Allergic
   9. Speed shock

CHAPTER 16

1. d
2. d
3. c
4. e
5. b
6. a
7. a
8. a. EM
   b. EL
   c. U
9. a
10. T
11. F; the nurse performs a comprehensive head-to-toe physical assessment
12. T
13. T
14. F; all baseline laboratory values should be recorded and reported
15. F; all patients, regardless of how minor the procedure or how often they have had surgery, should have discharge planning
16. b, d, e
17. a
18. c
19. b
20. c

21.

Procedure/Exercise	Purpose
Breathing exercises and incentive spirometry	Help to expand lungs, loosen secretions, and maintain adequate air exchange
Coughing and splinting	Performed along with deep breathing. Help to expel secretions, keep the lungs clear, promote full aeration of the lungs, and prevent pneumonia and atelectasis
Antiembolism stockings and elastic wraps	Promote venous return from lower extremities and prevent venous stasis and deep vein thrombosis
Pneumatic compression devices	Devices that provide intermittent periods of compression to the lower leg, thus preventing venous stasis and enhancing venous flow
Early ambulation	Stimulates intestinal motility, enhances lung expansion, mobilizes secretions, promotes venous return, prevents joint rigidity, and relieves pressure
Range-of-motion exercises	Passive or active, these help prevent joint rigidity and muscle contracture

CHAPTER 17

1. a
2. d
3. a
4. b
5. f
6. e
7. c
8. a, b, c, d
9. d
10. b
11. a
12. c
13. b
14. a, b, c, e, g
15. d
16. c
17. b, c, d
18. b
19. e
20. d
21. a
22. c
23. d
24. h
25. d
26. e
27. g
28. f
29. a
30. c
31. b
32. c
33. c
34. e
35. c
36. a
37. b
38. d
39. a, c, d, g

CHAPTER 18

1. d
2. b
3. c, d, e
4. c
5. b
6. c
7. d
8. d
9. a
10. c, e
11. b
12. a, b, d
13. g
14. b
15. c
16. d
17. f
18. a
19. b, c, e
20. g
21. b, c
22. c, d, f
23. d
24. a
25. f
26. g
27. e
28. c, g
29. b, c
30. g
31. f

32. a, b, c
33. d
34. b
35. g
36. a
37. a
38. a. 7
    b. 3
    c. 4
    d. 5
    e. 6
    f. 2
    g. 1
39. b
40. a. 2
    b. 3
    c. 4
    d. 5
    e. 1
41. An evisceration is a surgical emergency. First, call for help and stay with the patient. The person who responds should notify the surgeon immediately and ensure that supplies are brought to the room. Immediately cover the wound with nonadherent dressing premoistened in warm sterile normal saline. If premoistened dressings are not available, moisten the sterile gauze or sterile towels in a sterile irrigation tray with sterile saline, then cover the wound. Do not allow the dressings to dry. Do not attempt to reinsert the protruding organ or viscera. While one nurse is dressing the wound, another should be taking the patient's vital signs, and ensuring that the patient is in a supine position with the hips and knees bent. (See Figure 18-2 in the text for more details.)
42. d
43. b
44. c

CHAPTER 19

1. a, b, c, d, e
2. a, b, c, d, e
3. T
4. T
5. T
6. F
7. F
8. d
9. b
10. a, b, c, d, e
11. b
12. c
13. a
14. d
15. c
16. b

17. a
18. a
19. b
20. c
21. d
22. a, b, c
23. a, b, c, d, e
24. a
25. b
26. a, b, c, d, e
27. b
28. a
29. b
30. a
31. c
32. c
33. a, b, d
34. a
35. b
36. b
37. c
38. a
39. e
40. d
41. a, c
42. d
43. c

44. b
45. e
46. a
47. a, b, c
48. c
49. a
50. d
51. c
52. b
53. c
54. T
55. c, d
56. a
57. b
58. a
59. b
60. c
61. b
62. c
63. a
64. c
65. c
66. a
67. a
68. d
69. b
70. a
71. c

72.

Drug	Use
Cyclosporine	Routine immunosuppression after solid organ transplantation
Tacrolimus FK506 (Prograf)	Maintenance and rescue therapy (to combat acute rejection)
Corticosteroids	Induce general immunosuppression
Daclizumab (Zenapax)	Given before transplant surgery and a few days after surgery to bind to antibodies and reduce T-cell growth and activation
Muromonab-CD3 (Orthoclone OKT3)	An antibody used to prevent T-cell activities

73. e
74. c
75. d
76. b
77. a
78. a

CHAPTER 20

1. a. Connective tissue disease
   b. Degenerative joint disease
   c. Osteoarthritis
   d. Hormone replacement therapy
   e. Erythrocyte sedimentation rate
   f. Total joint replacement
   g. Total joint arthroplasty
   h. Deep vein (venous) thrombosis
   i. Continuous passive motion
   j. Rheumatoid arthritis
   k. Temporomandibular joint
   l. Progressive systemic sclerosis
   m. Systemic lupus erythematosus
2. d
3. a, c, d
4. a
5. d
6. c
7. a
8. c
9. a
10. c
11. b
12. d

13. b, c, d
14. b
15. c
16. a, c, d
17. c
18. a, b, c, e
19. T
20. F
21. a, c, d
22. a
23. c
24. a
25. T
26. T
27. F
28. a
29. d
30. a, c, d, e
31. b
32. a
33. c
34. a
35. a, c d
36. b, d, e
37. d
38. c, e
39. b, c, d
40. b, c, e, f
41. a
42. c
43. b
44. b
45. a, b, c
46. b
47. d
48. a
49. a. L
    b. E
    c. L
    d. L
    e. L
    f. E
    g. E
    h. L
50. a
51. a
52. c
53. a, b, c
54. c
55. b
56. a
57. a
58. a, b, c, d
59. d
60. a, c
61. a. Low
    b. Low
    c. Low
    d. High
    e. High

62. b
63. c
64. g
65. c
66. a, b
67. e
68. i
69. h
70. d
71. f
72. j
73. b
74. a, c
75. a
76. b
77. d
78. c
79. c
80. b
81. d
82. d
83. b
84. d
85. a, c, e
86. a, b, c, d
87. b, d
88. c
89. T
90. T
91. b
92. a, b, c
93. a
94. a
95. d
96. a, b
97. T
98. F; is a disease that mimics the clinical manifestations of gout, but the crystals deposited in the joints are calcium pyrophosphate, not sodium urate
99. a, c, d
100. c
101. g
102. e
103. b
104. d
105. a
106. c
107. f

CHAPTER 21

1. c
2. d
3. a
4. c
5. b
6. e
7. F
8. a. B
   b. C

   c. C
   d. A
   e. B
   f. B
   g. B
   h. C
   i. B
9. b
10. b
11. c
12. a, b, d
13. a, c, d
14. d
15. b
16. b, c, e
17. b
18. a
19. a
20. a, c, d, e
21. a, b, c, d
22. a
23. a, c, d, e
24. d
25. a, b, c
26. T
27. F
28. T
29. a, c, d
30. b, c, d
31. c
32. a, b, d, e
33. d
34. b, c, d, e
35. b, c, d
36. a, b, c
37. a, b, d
38. a, b, d
39. b, d, e
40. a, c, d
41. T
42. T
43. F; lesions resulting from Kaposi's sarcoma are small, purplish brown, raised, and usually not painful or itchy
44. T
45. T
46. F; patients with HIV should know that as CD4+ counts lower, clinical manifestations increase, not decrease
47. T
48. T
49. F; antiretroviral therapy only inhibits viral replication and does not kill the virus.
50. F; HIV is more easily transmitted from infected male to uninfected female than infected female to uninfected male
51. a, c
52. b
53. a. 2

   b. 4
   c. 1
   d. 3
54. a. D
   b. NC
   c. D
   d. D
55.

Drug	Classification	Therapeutic Use	Nursing Intervention
Pentamidine isethionate	Antiprotozoal (anti-infective)	*Pneumocystis carinii* pneumonia	Monitor blood pressure during IM and IV administration. Instruct to lie supine during drug administration. Monitor blood glucose levels for hypoglycemia and hyperglycemia. Evaluate IM sites for pain, redness, induration, and IV sites for phlebitis. Monitor renal, hepatic, and hematology lab values.
Metronidazole (Flagyl)	Antiprotozoal (anti-infective)	Cryptosporidiosis Giardiasis	Monitor for neurologic symptoms, especially for numbness and paresthesia of extremities. Monitor I & O. Fluid intake must be enough to maintain urinary output of 2000 mL. Monitor urinalysis results.
Zidovudine (Retrovir)	Nucleoside-analog-reverse transcriptase inhibitor	Inhibits viral DNA synthesis and replication	Monitor CBC, Hgb, MCV, reticulocyte count, CD4 cell count, HIV RNA plasma levels. Instruct about common adverse effects including headache, nausea, insomnia, and myalgia.
Ritonavir (Norvir)	Protease inhibitor	Prevents viral replication	Monitor CBC with differential and platelet count, hepatic and kidney function tests, lipid profile, electrolytes, blood glucose, CD4 cell count, plasma levels of HIV RNA.
Enfuvirtide (Fuzeon)	Fusion inhibitor	Blocks fusion of HIV with a host cell; prevents infection of new cells	Monitor hepatic function tests, lipid profile, and CBC with differential.
Nevirapine (Viramune)	Non-nucleoside-analog reverse transcriptase inhibitor	Protects uninfected cells, suppresses viral replication, does not kill the virus	Monitor hepatic and kidney function tests, electrolytes, and CBC.
Fluconazole (Diflucan)	Antifungal (anti-infective)	Candidiasis, cryptococcal meningitis	Monitor hepatic and kidney function tests, electrolytes, and CBC.

56. d

CHAPTER 22

1. b
2. a, b, c
3. a
4. b
5. d
6. a
7. e
8. c
9. a
10. b
11. d
12. a
13. c
14. d
15. c
16. a
17. d
18. b
19. a, b
20. b, d
21. b
22. a
23. c
24. d
25. e
26. a, b, e
27. a, b, e, f
28. b
29. T
30. T
31. F; after the proper dose of epinephrine is administered to a patient having an anaphylactic reaction, the same dose may be repeated every 15 to 20 minutes if needed
32. T
33. T
34. F; latex allergens may enter the body through inhalation, direct contact with blood vessels during surgery, or via direct contact with the skin
35. T
36. T
37. F; corticosteroids or other anti-inflammatory agents work faster than Benadryl in type IV delayed hypersensitivity reactions
38. F; patients with bee sting allergies should carry a kit that contains injectable epinephrine for immediate treatment as needed
39. a
40. a
41. a
42. a, d, e
43. b

44. c
45. a, b, d, e
46. c
47. c
48. b
49. a, b, c, d
50. a, b
51. c
52. a
53. b
54. a
55. b
56. a
57. d
58. c
59. a, d, f
60. d
61. a
62. c
63. a
64. d
65. a
66. a

CHAPTER 23

1. b, c
2. b
3. a, c, e, f
4. a, b, c, f
5. T
6. T
7. F; blood cells do not produce fibronectin
8. T
9. F; G0 state
10. F; euploid
11. T
12. T
13. F, to lose the specific appearance of the parent cell
14. c
15. a, b, c, d, f
16. b, c, d, f
17. a, b, c, d
18. a, b, e
19. T
20. T
21. T
22. F; if promotion occurs and the cancer cell is able to divide
23. T
24. a, b, e
25. a, b, c, e
26. c
27. a
28. a, b, c, d, e
29. T
30. T
31. F
32. a, c, e

33. c
34. a
35. a, c, d, e
36. a. R
    b. C
    c. C
    d. R
    e. C
    f. C
    g. R
37. a, b, c, d
38. a, b, c, e
39. a, b, e
40. b, c, d
41. a, b, d, e
42. a, b, c, d, e
43. a, b, c, e
44. a, b, c
45. c
46. a
47. b, c
48. a, b, c, d, e
49. a, b, c, e
50. a, c, f

CHAPTER 24

1. b
2. b, c, e
3. c
4. d
5. b, d
6. F; pain does not always accompany cancer
7. T
8. F; the purpose of cancer treatment is to prolong survival time or improve quality of life
9. T
10. a
11. a, b, c, d
12. c
13. b
14. a, b
15. a, b, c
16. b
17. T
18. F; the total dose of radiation needed depends on the size and location of the tumor and on the radiation sensitivity of the tumor and surrounding normal tissues
19. F; some damage to normal tissues cannot be avoided during radiation therapy
20. T
21. F; the optimum dose of radiation is one that can kill the cancer cells with an acceptable level of damage to normal tissues

22. T
23. T
24. F; with needles and seed implants, the patient emits radiation while the implant is in place, but the excreta are not radioactive
25. T
26. a
27. a, b, c
28. b
29. a
30. a
31. a, b, c, e
32. c
33. c
34. c
35. b
36. d
37. a
38. b
39. b
40. b
41. b, c
42. c
43. c
44. a
45. a. V
    b. V
    c. I
    d. V
    e. I
46. a, b
47. a, b
48. d
49. c
50. a, c, f
51. a, c, d
52. b, c, f
53. T
54. F
55. a
56. c
57. a
58. b
59. a
60. a, b, c, e
61. b
62. a
63. d
64. b
65. c
66. d
67. a
68. c
69. b
70. c
71. d
72. c

CHAPTER 25

1. c
2. f
3. d
4. g
5. h
6. e
7. b
8. a
9. a
10. b
11. c
12. a
13. a, b, c, d, g
14. a
15. e
16. d
17. a
18. a
19. c
20. b
21. d
22. b, e
23. a, e
24. b, e
25. c
26. T
27. T
28. F; phagocytosis is an essential mechanism in host defense
29. F; gloves are not impervious barriers, and hands should be washed with soap and water or rubbed with an alcohol-based cleanser after removing the gloves
30. F; artificial nails have been linked to a number of outbreaks due to poor fingernail health and hygiene
31. F; *nosocomial infection* means that the infection occurred while receiving health care, not that it was caused by health care
32. a. 2
    b. 1
    c. 3
    d. 4
33. d
34. c
35. d
36. b
37. a
38. a, b, c, d
39. d, e, f, g
40. g
41. h
42. f
43. e
44. d
45. c
46. b
47. a
48. d
49. T
50. F; a fever, generally a temperature greater than 101° F, is one of the indicators of a systemic infection
51. T
52. F; a *superinfection* is either a reinfection or a second infection with the same kind of microorganism
53. a, b, c, d
54. a. Erythromycin, tetracycline, gentamicin
    b. Antifungal agents
    c. Actinomycin
    d. Penicillins and cephalosporins
55. b
56. g
57. i
58. f
59. h
60. b
61. a
62. c
63. d
64. e
65. b
66. b, c, e
67. a
68. c
69. b
70. d

CHAPTER 26

1. b
2. a
3. b
4. b
5. c
6. a
7. a
8. b
9. c
10. c
11. b
12. c
13. a
14. c
15. a
16. c
17. d
18. e
19. h
20. c
21. b
22. i
23. j
24. f
25. g
26. a
27. a
28. b
29. b, c, e, f, g
30. d
31. b
32. b
33. Y
34. N
35. N
36. Y
37. Y
38. Y
39. N
40. Y
41. a, b, d, f
42. a
43. c
44. c
45. b
46. c
47. d
48. d
49. a
50. b
51. e
52. c
53. a
54. c
55. a
56. b
57. c
58. d
59. a
60. b
61. b
62. c
63. a
64. a, b, c, d, f, g
65. d
66. a
67. a
68. i
69. h
70. e
71. d
72. f
73. g
74. c
75. b
76. c
77. d
78. c
79. a, c, e, f
80. a
81. F; Langerhans cells engulf any foreign substances (antigens) that invade the body when the skin is injured
82. T
83. T

84. F; epidermis has no blood supply
85. F; baldness is related to hereditary factors
86. T
87. F; evaluate all skin areas on a monthly basis
88. F; use standard precautions; some may be placed in contact isolation
89. T

CHAPTER 27

1. m
2. k
3. i
4. d
5. b
6. f
7. l
8. j
9. c
10. a
11. e
12. h
13. g
14. a
15. b, c, d, f
16. d
17. b
18. b
19. c
20. c
21. b
22. d
23. T
24. F; in dry climates
25. F; the chronic wound is allowed to heal from the inside out
26. T
27. T
28. F; skin graft must have adequate blood supply, be free of infection, and be completely immobilized
29. F; herpes zoster manifests with pain, itching, and tenderness
30. F; pediculosis capitis is usually treated with chemical agents
31. T
32. a, b, d, e
33. a
34. a
35. d
36. a
37. a, b, c, e
38. b
39. a, d, e, g
40. d
41. b
42. c
43. a
44. e

45. a
46. b
47. b
48. c
49. c
50. a
51. a
52. a, c, d
53. a
54. a
55. c
56. c
57. e
58. b
59. h
60. g
61. a
62. d
63. e
64. f
65. i
66. j
67. k
68. l
69. c
70. d
71. c
72. b
73. b
74. a
75. a. 1
    b. 8
    c. 7
    d. 4
    e. 6
    f. 5
    g. 3
    h. 2
76. c
77. a, c, d
78. b
79. c
80. a
81. c
82. c
83. d
84. b
85. b
86. b
87. c
88. a, b, c, e, f
89. b
90. d
91. a
92. c
93. d
94. a
95. a
96. b
97. d

98. c
99. a
100. c

CHAPTER 28

1. i
2. e
3. g
4. a
5. d
6. h
7. c
8. f
9. b
10. k
11. j
12. a
13. c
14. b, c, d, e
15. d
16. a
17. c
18. d
19. c
20. b
21. b
22. b
23. b
24. a, c, d, e
25. b
26. a
27. b
28. c
29. b
30. F
31. T
32. T
33. T
34. T
35. T
36. F
37. T
38. F
39. T
40. d
41. b
42. b
43. a, b, c, e
44. c
45. b
46. a
47. c
48. b
49. a
50. c
51. a
52. 40 mL/hr
53. c
54. b
55. c

56. b
57. F
58. T
59. F
60. T
61. T
62. T
63. d
64. a, c, e
65. a
66. b
67. a, b, c, e
68. a
69. b
70. c
71. d
72. (Refer to Table 28-1 in the text)
73. a, b, d, e
74. b
75. a, d
76. b
77. a, b, d, f
78. c
79. a
80. a
81. a
82. b, c, d
83. T
84. T
85. F
86. F
87. T
88. a
89. a
90. a
91. a
92. a
93. c
94. c
95. c
96. b
97. f
98. e
99. a
100. d
101. g
102. b
103. b
104. b, c, d
105. c
106. c
107. d
108. b, d, f
109. a
110. a
111. d
112. *Across*
    2. Desquamation
    3. Eschar
    5. Shock

    7. Superficial
    8. Partial
    9. Blanch
    11. Emergent
    13. Third spacing

Down
    1. Pigskin
    4. Remobilization
    6. Full
    10. Contact
    12. Moist
    14. Dry

CHAPTER 29

1. a
2. a
3. b
4. b
5. b
6. a
7. b
8. a
9. a
10. a
11. b
12. b
13. c
14. a
15. b
16. a
17. b
18. c
19. a
20. c
21. e
22. b
23. a
24. d
25. g
26. f
27. b
28. b
29. c
30. a
31. b
32. d
33. c
34. b
35. b
36. b
37. a
38. d
39. b
40. c
41. b
42. c
43. a
44. (Refer to Figure 29-10 in the text)
45. a

46. a, b, c, d
47. d
48. c
49. a
50. c
51. c
52. c
53. a
54. b
55. c
56. b
57. b
58. b
59. g
60. f
61. e
62. a
63. c
64. b
65. c
66. d
67. b
68. c
69. a
70. a
71. c
72. a. Y; vasoconstriction causes decreased peripheral blood flow
    b. Y; low hemoglobin count results in reduced oxygen-carrying abilities of RBCs
    c. Y; abnormal-shaped red blood cell interferes with blood flow
    d. N; hypothermia causes vasoconstriction
    e. N; oxygen administration route has no direct effect on the device itself
    f. Y; peripheral vasoconstriction occurs when peripheral vascular system shuts down
    g. N; this can affect respirations but not the pulse oximetry device directly
    h. Y; deeper coloration of the nail bed than those of whites can cause artificially low results by 3% to 5%
    i. N; it makes no difference in the ability to read the saturation, even though women have larger airways than men
    j. N; the pulse oximetry can be low because of respiratory diseases affecting the ability to oxygenate but not affect the device itself, causing an artificially low result
    k. N; this is part of a respiratory assessment and can affect the patient's ability to breathe but not cause artificially low results

73. d
74. d
75. b
76. b
77. d
78. c
79. d
80. d
81. a
82. b
83. a
84. a

CHAPTER 30

1. T
2. T
3. T
4. F; the amount of oxygen should be regulated by parameters such as pulse oximetry/blood gas/respiratory assessment to administer the lowest level possible with least harmful side effects, not just symptom management
5. T
6. F; oxygen does not itself burn but is needed for something to burn
7. b, c, e
8. b, d, e
9. b
10. b
11. c
12. c
13. c
14. d
15. c
16. a, b, c, d, e
17. b
18. c
19. c
20. a, c, d, e
21. a
22. d
23. d
24. c
25. (Refer to Tables 30-1 and 30-2 in the text)
26. c
27. c
28. a
29. a, b, d, e, f, g
30. b
31. a
32. a
33. c
34. d
35. c
36. c
37. b
38. d
39. a

40. a
41. b
42. a
43. b
44. a. 1
    b. 2
    c. 6
    d. 9
    e. 3
    f. 4
    g. 8
    h. 7
    i. 5
45. a. 2
    b. 10
    c. 1
    d. 4
    e. 7
    f. 3
    g. 8
    h. 6
    i. 5
    j. 9
46. d
47. a
48. d
49. d
50. d
51. c
52. h
53. c
54. d
55. a
56. g
57. f
58. b
59. e
60. d
61. b
62. c
63. b
64. c
65. b
66. c
67. c

CHAPTER 31

1. c
2. a, b, c, f
3. c
4. a
5. a
6. c
7. c
8. d
9. c
10. c
11. b
12. c
13. c

14. a
15. b
16. b
17. c
18. c
19. a
20. d
21. a
22. a
23. c
24. b
25. b
26. d
27. a
28. a
29. c
30. b
31. c
32. d
33. d
34. T
35. T
36. T
37. F; erythroplasia; white lesions are leukoplakia
38. T
39. F; specific locations and small tumors
40. T
41. F; partial laryngectomy
42. T
43. T
44. d
45. a, c, e, f
46. a
47. c
48. b
49. a
50. a
51. d
52. c
53. c
54. a
55. d
56. a
57. a
58. b
59. c
60. d
61. d
62. b
63. c
64. a
65. c
66. a
67. b
68. d
69. a, d, e, f
70. c

71.

Procedure	Description	Resulting Voice Quality
Laser surgery	Tumor reduced or destroyed by laser beam through laryngoscope	Normal/hoarse
Transoral cordectomy	Tumor (early lesion) resected through laryngoscope	Normal/hoarse (high cure rate)
Laryngofissure	No cord removed (early lesion)	Normal (high cure rate)
Supraglottic partial laryngectomy	Hyoid bone, false cords, and epiglottis removed Neck dissection on affected side performed if nodes involved	Normal/hoarse
Hemilaryngectomy or vertical laryngectomy	One true cord, one false cord, and one-half of thyroid cartilage removed	Hoarse voice
Total laryngectomy	Entire larynx, hyoid bone, strap muscles, one or two tracheal rings removed Nodal neck dissection if nodes involved	No natural voice

CHAPTER 32

1. a, b
2. b
3. c
4. c
5. b, c
6. b
7. b, c
8. a
9. b
10. a, b, c
11. a
12. a
13. a
14. c
15. a
16. c
17. a
18. b, c
19. a
20. a
21. a
22. a, c, d, f
23. c
24. b
25. c
26. a
27. d
28. b
29. c
30. d
31. b, c, d, e
32. c
33. b
34. b
35. b
36. c
37. c
38. b
39. d
40. c
41. d
42. b
43. b
44. c
45. a
46. b
47. d
48. b
49. a
50. b
51. b
52. c
53. a
54. a
55. b
56. c
57. d
58. b
59. c
60. (See Chart 32-5.)
61. c
62. c
63. a. 2
    b. 6
    c. 5
    d. 3
    e. 4
    f. 7
    g. 1
64. c
65. c
66. a
67. a
68. a, c, d, f
69. d
70. b
71. c
72. a
73. T
74. T
75. T
76. T
77. T
78. F; risk decreases after 15 years
79. F; all factors contribute
80. F; the reverse is true
81. T
82. T
83. F; a missing gene in women can make those who smoke at a higher risk
84. F; symptoms are a late sign
85. F; there are no screening tools for lung cancer; x-rays may indicate advanced disease
86. F; cancer cells are not always in the sputum; various methods are used for diagnostic testing (see text)
87. T
88. T
89. a
90. c
91. d
92. a
93. d
94. c
95. c
96. b
97. b
98. c
99. c
100. d
101. b
102. b
103. a
104. T
105. T
106. T
107. a
108. c
109. a
110. c
111. a

CHAPTER 33

1. c
2. d

3. b
4. d
5. b
6. c
7. b
8. b
9. d
10. c
11. c
12. a
13. c
14. c
15. a
16. b
17. b
18. a
19. c
20. a
21. b
22. c
23. a, b, c, e
24. a. 8
    b. 5
    c. 7
    d. 11
    e. 2
    f. 12
    g. 3
    h. 6
    i. 10
    j. 4
    k. 9
    l. 1
25. b
26. b
27. d
28. d
29. a
30. c
31. d
32. a
33. c
34. a
35. c
36. c
37. d
38. d
39. a
40. b
41. b
42. c
43. a
44. b
45. b
46. a
47. a, b, d, e
48. a, b, d, e
49. b
50. c
51. b, c, d, f

52. c
53. b
54. b
55. c
56. d
57. a
58. a
59. d
60. c
61. d
62. d
63. d
64. b
65. a
66. b
67. b
68. b
69. d
70. a
71. a, b, c, d
72. a
73. a
74. a
75. c
76. d
77. b
78. c
79. c
80. b
81. a
82. a, b, d, e, f
83. b

CHAPTER 34

1. F; blood clots are the most common
2. T
3. T
4. T
5. T
6. T
7. F; most common sites are thrombi in deep veins in the legs or pelvis
8. c
9. a, b, c, g
10. a
11. b
12. d
13. b
14. a
15. d
16. a, d, e
17. Y; postoperative immobility; decreased fluids; usually older than 50 years of age
18. Y; hypercoagulability and immobility
19. N; out of bed; home; no risk
20. Y; damage to veins; increases risk
21. Y; increase viscosity of blood; older than 60 years of age; hospitalized

22. Y; abnormal red blood cells
23. N; no causes
24. Y; obesity—large abdomen causes decreased venous return and increases risk for DVT
25. N; no causes
26. Y; risk for amniotic fluid PE
27. N; no causes
28. Y; decreased mobility; surgical patient
29. Y; clot to brain, lung, intestine
30. Y; no muscle pumping; stagnation of blood in legs; risk for DVT
31. N; not all patients; however, this is a consideration in determining risk
32. b
33. c
34. d
35. b
36. d
37. b, c, d, f
38. c
39. c
40. b
41. a
42. c
43. F; perfusion normal, but ventilation is inadequate
44. T
45. F; perfusion is decreased
46. T
47. T
48. T
49. F; lung is normally dry, but in ARDS lung fluid increases
50. F; lung volume decreases and compliance decreases
51. T
52. T
53. b
54. a, c, d, f
55. c
56. a
57. b
58. d
59. b, c, e, g
60. a
61. c
62. b
63. a. Low oxygen; give oxygen
    b. Metabolic acidosis with respiratory compensation; correct metabolic cause
    c. Respiratory acidosis; increase ventilation, encourage pursed-lip breathing
    d. Respiratory alkalosis; decrease ventilation, have patient rebreathe ventilations

e. Normal ABG result; no treatment needed

f. Respiratory acidosis; give oxygen, patient likely to be intubated

64. d
65. b
66. b
67. d
68. b
69. d
70. b
71. c
72. b
73. a
74. c
75. b
76. a
77. a
78. b
79. c
80. b
81. a
82. a
83. b
84. a
85. a
86. c
87. b
88. a
89. a
90. b
91. a, b, c, e, g
92. b
93. c
94. a, c, e
95. c
96. c
97. c
98. a
99. b
100. d
101. a
102. c
103. b, c, d, e, f
104. c
105. c
106. a
107. a
108. b
109. b
110. a
111. a
112. a, b, c, e, g
113. a, b, c
114. c
115. b
116. a
117. a, b, c
118. a
119. f

120. c
121. b
122. h
123. a
124. g
125. e
126. d
127. i
128. j
129. c
130. b
131. a
132. d
133. d
134. a. 3
   b. 5
   c. 7
   d. 4
   e. 8
   f. 1
   g. 2
   h. 6
135. a, b, d
136. b, d, e, f
137. c
138. d
139. b
140. a
141. a

CHAPTER 35

1. g
2. b
3. i
4. h
5. f
6. e
7. c
8. d
9. a
10. a. SA node rate is 60 to 100 beats/min
    b. AV node rate is 40 to 60 beats/min
    c. Purkinje fibers rate is 20 to 40 beats/min
11. c
12. e
13. a
14. d
15. b
16. a, c, d
17. a, d, e, f
18. a
19. c
20. a
21. a, b, d, f
22. a, b, e
23. b
24. F; diastolic blood pressure

25. F; systolic blood pressure
26. T
27. T
28. T
29. T
30. F; the left ventricle
31. T
32. a. 3
    b. 1
    c. 2
    d. 5
    e. 4
33. c
34. b
35. b
36. d
37. c
38. a
39. c
40. d
41. One-half pack/day × 2 years = 1 pack-year
42. a
43. a
44. a
45. b
46. a
47. a
48. c
49. d
50. b, d
51. c
52. a
53. (Refer to Figure 35-7 in the text.)
54. F; begins with inspection
55. T
56. T
57. F; detected by auscultation
58. T
59. F; best heard at the lower left sternal border or the apex
60. F; to listen for high-frequency sounds
61. T
62. a, b, c
63. f
64. d
65. c
66. a, b, c
67. a
68. f
69. b
70. e
71. b
72. e
73. a, c
74. d
75. b
76. a, c, d, e, f
77. b

78. c
79. c
80. T
81. T
82. F
83. F
84. T
85. a
86. b
87. a
88. c
89. d
90. b
91. a
92. d
93. b
94. a
95. e
96. c
97. a
98. a
99. a, b, d
100. c
101. a, b, d
102. a
103. b
104. a
105. c
106. d
107. T
108. F; do not require informed consent
109. T
110. F; effective for detecting an acute MI and define its location and size
111. F; is not placed in isolation
112. T
113. T
114. T
115. T
116. T
117. F; multigated blood pool scanning is a noninvasive test that evaluates cardiac motion and calculates ejection fraction
118. T
119. T
120. F; is useful
121. c
122. d
123. a
124. d
125. c, d, e, f, g
126. b
127. b

CHAPTER 36

1. sinoatrial (SA) node
2. Bundle of His; Purkinje fibers
3. delay
4. automaticity
5. Contractility

6. conductivity
7. excitability
8. Atrial kick
9. b
10. b
11. c
12. c
13. d
14. a
15. c
16. f
17. e
18. b
19. (Refer to Figure 36-5 in the text.)
20. a
21. c
22. a
23. a
24. d
25. a
26. c
27. d
28. d
29. c
30. a
31. c
32. d
33. a. 6
    b. 3
    c. 1
    d. 5
    e. 4
    f. 2
34. a
35. b
36. a, b, e, f
37. d
38. b, c, e
39. T
40. T
41. F; the QRS complex is formed
42. T
43. T
44. F; of ventricles to occur
45. F; reflects electrical activity
46. b
47. a
48. d
49. 60 (1500 divided by 25)
50. 50; bradycardia
51. b
52. b
53. c
54. g
55. d
56. e
57. f
58. h
59. c
60. a

61. b
62. f
63. b
64. c
65. a, b, c, d
66. d
67. c
68. d
69. a
70. a
71. b
72. b
73. a
74. d
75. a
76. b
77. c
78. a
79. a
80. T
81. F; there is a delay in the AV node conduction, but all impulses reach the ventricles
82. T
83. T
84. T
85. F; first-degree block may not need intervention
86. c
87. b
88. c
89. d
90. a
91. b
92. b
93. b
94. d
95. b
96. c
97. b
98. c
99. a
100. a, b, d, f
101. c
102. b
103. d
104. c
105. d
106. e
107. a
108. b
109. f
110. c
111. a
112. c
113. a. 1
     b. 3
     c. 6
     d. 4
     e. 5

f. 7

g. 2

114. c

115. a

116. a, b, d

117. F; treats spontaneous sustained ventricular tachycardia (VT) or ventricular fibrillation (VF) unrelated to a myocardial infarction or other causes amenable to correction

118. T

119. T

120. F; in cardioversion shock, the defibrillator is set in the synchronized mode to avoid discharging the shock during the T wave

121. T

122. T

123. a

124. c

125. b, c, d, f

126. a. 4

b. 1

c. 3

d. 5

e. 2

127. b, c, e

128. c

129. a, c, d, f

130. atrial flutter

131. bradycardia with premature atrial contraction (PAC)

132. atrial tachycardia

133. atrial fibrillation

134. sinus arrest

135. sinus tachycardia

136. ventricular fibrillation

137. normal sinus rhythm with PVC

138. ventricular fibrillation

139. ventricular tachycardia

140. asystole

141. atrial fibrillation

142. atrial flutter

143. normal sinus rhythm with PJC

144. PVCs (bigeminy)

CHAPTER 37

1. b

2. e

3. c

4. d

5. f

6. a

7. left ventricle

8. diminishes; pulmonary

9. fluid overload

10. increase

11. sympathetic stimulation

12. c

13. c

14. a, c, e

15. a, b, c, e, f

16. d

17. d

18. d

19. b

20. c

21. c

22. d

23. d

24. b

25. b

26. a

27. a

28. a, b, c, e

29. a, d, e

30. a

31. d

32. c

33. b

34. c

35. a

36. d

37. c

38. a

39. d

40. a

41. b

42. a

43. c

44. b

45. a, b, c, e

46. b

47. c, d, e, f

48. b

49. a

50. T

51. T

52. F; mitral valve prolapse and aortic insufficiency are associated

53. F; urgent surgery is indicated

54. T

55. T

56. T

57. T

58. T

59. b

60. d

61. a

62. e

63. a, b

64. c

65. a

66. e

67. b

68. a

69. a, b

70. c

71. c

72. d

73. d

74. b

75. d

76. b

77. a

78. a

79. c

80. c

81. a

82. a

83. b

84. b

85. c

86. b

87. a

88. c

89. a

90. b, c, e, f, g, h

91. d

92. c

93. b

94. e

95. a

96. f

97. g

98. b

99. a

100. a

101. c

102. a

103. b

104. a

105. c

106. a, d, e, f

107. b

108. c

109. a

110. b

111. b

112. F; is surgical excision of the pericardium (pericardiectomy)

113. T

114. F; 2 to 6 weeks

115. T

116. T

117. T

118. b

119. c

120. b

121. a

122. c

123. b

124. a

125. b

126. a, b, c, e

127. T

128. T

129. T

130. F

131. T

132. F
133. a
134. b
135. a, e, f, g

CHAPTER 38

1.   T
2.   T
3.   T
4.   F; increases the systemic arterial pressure
5.   T
6.   F; effects of hyperglycemia
7.   T
8.   T
9.   T
10. F; a modifiable factor
11. d
12. b
13. a
14. d
15. b
16. d
17. b
18. a
19.

Cholesterol Test	Target Levels
Total serum cholesterol	Below 200 mg/dL
LDL-C level (for healthy people)	Below 100 mg/dL
LDL-C level (for people with CVD or diabetes)	Less than 70 mg/dL
HDL-C level	40 mg/dL or above

20. b, c, d
21. b, c, d
22. a
23. b
24. b
25. b, c, d, e, g
26. b
27. a
28. d
29. a
30. b, c, d, e
31. c
32. (Refer to Table 38-3 in the text.)
33. a
34. b
35. d
36. a
37. c

38. a
39. b
40. a, b, c, f
41. b
42. d
43. b
44. b
45. a. A
     b. A
     c. V
     d. V
     e. A
     f. A
     g. A
     h. A
     i. V
     j. A
     k. A
     l. A
     m. V
     n. A
     o. V
46. a, b, c, f
47. a
48. b
49. c
50. d
51. b
52. b
53. a
54. c
55. a, b, d, f
56. c
57. c
58. a, c, d, e
59. a, c, d
60. F; one or more arteries are dilated with a balloon catheter advanced through a cannula, which is inserted into or above an occluded/stenosed artery
61. F; the purpose of improving circulation to a given area; it is not a cure
62. T
63. T
64. T
65. F; reocclusion may occur within a year of treatment in some patients; others may be occlusion-free for 3 to 5 years
66. b
67. a, b, c, e
68. b
69. a
70. d
71. a
72. b
73. d
74. a
75. a
76. b
77. c

78. b
79. a
80. a
81. c
82. a
83. b, c
84. a, b
85. a
86. b, d, e, f, g, h
87. a
88. c
89. b
90. b
91. d
92. b
93. a
94. b
95. a, b, c, e, f
96. a
97. c
98. c
99. d
100. a
101. a
102. c
103. a, b, c, d
104. b
105. a
106. d
107. b
108. a. BD
     b. RD
     c. RD
     d. BD
     e. BD
     f. RD
109. b
110. a
111. c
112. a
113. d
114. a
115. c
116. a
117. c
118. F; may be absent; therefore, monitor patients who are known to be at risk
119. F; positive Homans' sign appears in only a small percentage of patients with DVT, and false-positive findings are common
120. T
121. T
122. F; within 5 days
123. T
124. F; associated with stasis of blood flow, endothelial injury, and/or hypercoagulability, known as *Virchow's triad*
125. T
126. T

127. T
128. F; venograms are not performed frequently today for DVT due to complications from the contrast medium, including sensitivity and acute renal failure
129. F; UFH inhibits fibrin formation; the drug does nothing to the existing clot
130. d
131. b
132. c
133. c
134. c
135. a, b, c
136. a
137. a, b, c, d, f, g
138. b
139. c
140. d
141. a
142. a, b, c, e
143. a
144. c
145. c
146. F; changed weekly
147. F; moistened with zinc oxide
148. T
149. T
150. F; applied from the toes to the knee
151. T
152. T
153. b
154. a
155. a, b, d, e
156. a
157. a, b, c, d, e, f
158. a
159. c
160. a, b, d, e
161. c
162. c
163. b
164. b
165. a. 6
    b. 3
    c. 2
    d. 5
    e. 4
    f. 1
166. c

CHAPTER 39

1. e
2. a
3. f
4. b
5. h
6. c
7. d
8. i
9. g

10. j
11. oxygen
12. predictable
13. sympathetic; endocrine
14. cardiac
15. skin; skeletal muscles
16. b, c, d, e
17. a
18. d
19. b, c, d, f
20. a, b, d, e
21. d
22. b
23. c
24. d
25. d
26. b
27. c
28. d
29. c
30. a
31. b
32. a
33. b
34. a
35. a
36. b
37. a
38. a. Cry
    b. Col
    c. Col
    d. Cry
    e. Col
39. c
40. a
41. c
42. d
43. c
44. a, b, e, f, g
45. b
46. a
47. c
48. a
49. b
50. b
51. d
52. b
53. d
54. c
55. a
56. b
57. b
58. (Refer to Table 39-5 in the text.)
59. b
60. c
61. c
62. a
63. c
64. d
65. d

66. c
67. d
68. b
69. c
70. a
71. a
72. d
73. c
74. c
75. a, c, d, f
76. d
77. a, b, c, e, f
78. b
79. d
80. b
81. a
82. T
83. F; shock progresses in a predictable, orderly fashion, but death is not inevitable
84. F; in the early stages of shock, the blood pressure is within normal limits or slightly decreased because of adequate compensatory mechanisms
85. T
86. T
87. T
88. T
89. T
90. F; cause an increase in cardiac output
91. T
92. d
93. f
94. e
95. b
96. a
97. d
98. e
99. a
100. f
101. d
102. a
103. c
104. a
105. a
106. f
107. a
108. f
109. a

CHAPTER 40

1. f
2. b
3. g
4. d
5. c
6. h
7. k
8. i

9. e
10. j
11. a
12. ruptures; aggregation; formation
13. 40
14. myocardial infarction; 5
15. 64.5; 70.4
16. hours
17. collateral circulation; anaerobic metabolism
18. a
19. a
20. b
21. d
22. b, c, f
23. c
24. a
25. c
26. a
27. a. 4
    b. 5
    c. 1
    d. 2
    e. 3
28. a. A
    b. MI
    c. MI
    d. A
    e. MI
    f. A
    g. A
    h. MI
    i. MI
29. T
30. T
31. T
32. F; leading cause of death for both men and women in the most prevalent ethnic groups
33. T
34. F; have an incidence of MI that equals that of men
35. T
36. T
37. F; which may increase the heart contractility and afterload
38. T
39. a, c
40. b
41. a. 3
    b. 1
    c. 5
    d. 2
    e. 4
42. b
43. d
44. c
45. a
46. a

47. d
48. a, b, d, e
49. a
50. c
51. F; accounts for over one-third of deaths
52. T
53. F; does not reduce the risk of CAD
54. T
55. T
56. F; intense exercise may be associated with plaque rupture and increase the number of cardiac episodes
57. F; does not increase
58. T
59. (Refer to Table 40-3 in the text.)
60. b
61. a, b, c, e, g
62. a, c, d, f, g
63. a
64. b
65. c
66. d
67. b
68. c
69. d
70. c
71. c
72. b
73. b
74. a, b, c, e, g
75. b
76. T
77. T
78. F; streptokinase is not fibrin-specific, and not commonly used
79. F; greater than 30 minutes
80. T
81. b
82. a, b, c, e, f
83. a, b, d, e, f
84. b, c, d
85. a
86. b
87. a
88. b
89. b
90. a
91. b
92. c
93. a
94. a
95. c
96. a
97. a, b, d, e, f
98. c
99. b
100. a
101. c

102. a
103. c
104. a
105. b
106. a
107. a, c, d, f
108. a
109. b
110. b, c, d, e
111. a, b, d, e, f
112. b
113. b
114. d
115. a
116. b
117. d
118. b
119. a
120. c
121. a, b, c, e
122. b
123. b, c, d
124. c
125. a
126. b
127. a
128. a, b, c, d, e, f
129. b
130. c
131. e
132. b
133. a
134. c
135. d
136. f

CHAPTER 41

1. T
2. T
3. T
4. F
5. F
6. T
7. T
8. T
9. F
10. T
11. F
12. T
13. F
14. F
15. T
16. T
17. F
18. T
19. T
20. T
21. T

22. T
23. F
24. F
25. T
26. a, b, c, d
27. d
28. a, b, c, d
29. b

30. F
31. T
32. T
33. T
34. F
35. F
36. a
37. d, e
38. b

6. c
7. a
8. c
9. b
10. b
11. a
12. a, b, c, d, e
13. d
14. a, b, c, d, e
15. a, b, d
16. a
17. a
18. c
19. a, b, d, e, f
20. a
21. a, b
22. a, b, c, d, e
23. a
24. c
25. b
26. c
27. a, b, c, e, f
28. a
29. c
30. b
31. a, b, c, d, e
32. c
33. a, c, d, e
34. a
35. a
36. a
37. a
38. b
39. a
40. a
41. b
42. a
43. ATP
44. TTP
45. ATP
46. TTP
47. ATP
48. ATP
49. TTP
50. ATP
51. ATP
52. b
53. c, e
54. c
55. b
56. d
57. a
58. b
59. c

39.

Test	Significance of Abnormal Findings
Red blood cell (RBC) count	Decreased levels—possible anemia or hemorrhage; Increased levels—possible chronic hypoxia or polycythemia vera
Hemoglobin (Hgb)	(Same as for RBC)
Hematocrit (Hct)	(Same as for RBC)
Mean cell volume (MCV)	Increased levels—macrocytic cells, possible anemia; Decreased levels—microcytic cells, possible iron deficiency anemia
Mean cell hemoglobin (MCH)	(Same as for MCV)
Mean cell hemoglobin concentration (MCHC)	Increased levels—spherocytosis or anemia; Decreased levels—iron deficiency anemia or a hemoglobinopathy
White blood cell (WBC) count	Increased levels—associated with infection, inflammation, autoimmune disorders, and leukemia; Decreased levels—prolonged infection or bone marrow suppression
Total iron binding capacity (TIBC)	Increased levels—iron deficiency; Decreased levels—anemia, hemorrhage, hemolysis
Iron (Fe)	Increased levels—iron excess, hemochromocytosis, liver disorders, megablastic anemia; Decreased levels—possible iron deficiency anemia, hemorrhage
Serum ferritin	(Same as for iron)
Platelet count	Increased levels—polycythemia vera or malignancy; Decreased levels—bone marrow suppression, autoimmune disease, hypersplenism
Hemoglobin electrophoresis	Variations indicate hemiglobinopathies
Direct Coombs' and indirect Coombs' test	Positive findings indicate antibodies to RBCs
Prothrombin time (PT)	Increased time—possible deficiency of clotting factors V and VII; Decreased time—vitamin K excess
Bleeding time	Increased time—inadequate platelet function or number, clotting factor deficiencies
Fibrin degradation products	Increased levels—disseminated intravascular coagulation of fibrinolysis

40. d
41. T
42. T
43. F
44. F
45. T

CHAPTER 42

1. a, b, c, d, e, f
2. a, b, c, d, e
3. d
4. a
5. a, d, f

60.

Transfusion Reactions	Associated Characteristics and Symptoms
Febrile transfusion reactions	Occur most often in patients with anti-WBC antibodies, a situation that can develop after multiple transfusions. The patient develops chills, tachycardia, fever, hypotension, and tachypnea. WBC filters may be used to trap WBCs and prevent their infusion into the patient.
Hemolytic transfusion reactions	Caused by blood type or Rh incompatibility. When blood containing antigens different from the patient's own is infused, antigen-antibody complexes are formed in the patient's blood. The reaction may be mild with fever and chills, or life-threatening with disseminated intravascular coagulation and circulatory collapse. Other manifestations include apprehension, headache, chest pain, low back pain, tachycardia, tachypnea, hypotension, hemoglobinuria, and a sense of impending doom. Onset may be immediate or may not occur until subsequent units have been transfused.
Allergic transfusion reactions	Most often seen in patients with a history of allergy. They may have urticaria, itching, bronchospasm, or anaphylaxis. Onset usually occurs during or up to 24 hours after the transfusion. Patients with a history of allergy can be given leukocyte-reduced or washed RBCs in which WBCs and plasma have been removed.
Bacterial transfusion reactions	Occur as a result of contaminated blood products. Usually a gram-negative organism is the source because these bacteria grow rapidly in blood stored under refrigeration. Symptoms include tachycardia, hypotension, fever, chills, and shock. Onset is rapid.
Circulatory overload	Can occur when a blood product is infused too quickly. Most common with whole-blood transfusions or when the patient receives multiple transfusions. Older adults are most at risk. Symptoms include hypertension, bounding pulse, distended jugular veins, dyspnea, restlessness, and confusion. Management and prevention strategies include monitoring intake and output, infusing blood products more slowly, and giving diuretics.
Transfusion-associated graft-versus-host disease (TA-GVHD)	Rare but life-threatening problem that can occur in both immunosuppressed and immunocompetent patients. Its cause in immunosuppressed patients is similar to that of GVHD in which donor T-cell lymphocytes attack host tissue. Manifestations usually occur within 1 to 2 weeks and include thrombocytopenia, anorexia, nausea, vomiting, chronic hepatitis, weight loss, and recurrent infection. TA-GVHD has an 80% to 90% mortality rate but can be prevented by using irradiated blood products; irradiation destroys T-cells and their cytokine products.

CHAPTER 43

1. b
2. c
3. a
4. f
5. d
6. g
7. e
8. d
9. a
10. d
11. b

12. a. P
    b. B
    c. B
    d. P
    e. P
    f. P
    g. B
    h. P
13. b
14. d
15. a
16. c
17. PNS

18. SNS
19. PNS
20. PNS
21. SNS
22. SNS
23. d
24. a
25. a
26. d
27. c
28. a
29. c
30. c

31. (See Table 43-4.)

Cranial Nerve	Function
I: Olfactory	Smell
II: Optic	Vision
III: Oculomotor	Eye movement via medial and lateral rectus and inferior oblique and superior rectus muscles; lid elevation via the levator muscle; pupil constriction; ciliary muscles
IV: Trochlear	Eye movement via superior oblique muscles
V: Trigeminal	Sensation from skin of face and scalp and mucous membranes of mouth and nose; muscles of mastication (chewing)
VI: Abducens	Eye movement via lateral rectus muscles
VII: Facial	Pain and temperature from ear area; deep sensations from the face; taste from anterior two-thirds of the tongue; muscles of the face and scalp; lacrimal, submandibular, and sublingual salivary glands
VIII: Vestibulocochlear	Hearing; equilibrium
IX: Glossopharyngeal	Pain and temperature from ear; taste and sensations from posterior one-third of tongue and pharynx; skeletal muscles of the throat; parotid glands
X: Vagus	Pain and temperature from ear; sensations from pharynx, larynx, thoracic and abdominal viscera; muscles of the soft palate, larynx, and pharynx; thoracic and abdominal viscera; cells of secretory glands; cardiac and smooth muscle innervation to the level of the splenic flexure
XI: Accessory	Skeletal muscles of the pharynx and larynx and sternocleidomastoid and trapezius muscles
XII: Hypoglossal	Skeletal muscles of the tongue

32. d
33. c
34. a
35. a
36. d
37. c
38. e
39. b
40. a
41. f
42. a
43. a
44. d
45. e
46. a
47. c
48. b
49. b
50. b
51. a
52. b
53. b
54. c
55. d
56. b
57. c
58. d
59. a
60. d
61. c
62. a
63. d
64. a, b, c, d, f
65. a

CHAPTER 44

1. a
2. b
3. b
4. a
5. a
6. a
7. b
8. a
9. a
10. a
11. b

12. b
13. b
14. a
15. b
16. a
17. b
18. b
19. a
20. a, b, e, f
21. d
22. d
23. a

24.

Stages of Migraine Headache	Associated Characteristics and Symptoms
Prodrome (or prodromal) phase	Specific symptoms such as food cravings or mood changes
Aura phase (if present)	Visual changes, flashing lights, or diplopia (double vision)
Headache phase	Pain may last a few hours to a few days
Termination phase	Intensity of the headache decreases
Postprodrome phase	Patient is often fatigued, may be irritable, and has muscle pain

25. a
26. c
27. c
28. b
29. a
30. d
31. c
32. a

33. b
34. d
35. b
36. d
37. b
38. c
39. a
40. b

41. a
42. c
43. b
44. c

45. b
46. c
47. d
48. b
49. c

50.

Stages of Parkinson Disease	Associated Characteristics and Symptoms
Stage 1: Initial	Unilateral limb involvement Minimal weakness Hand and arm trembling
Stage 2: Mild	Bilateral limb involvement Masklike facies Slow, shuffling gait
Stage 3: Moderate	Postural instability Increased gait disturbances
Stage 4: Severe disability	Akinesia Rigidity
Stage 5: Complete ADLS dependence	

51. b
52. c
53. a
54. b
55. a, b, c, e
56. a
57. c
58. d
59. b
60. b
61. c
62. b

CHAPTER 45

1. b
2. b
3. a
4. d
5. c
6. a, b, c, e
7. b
8. c
9. a
10. a
11. d
12. c
13. d
14. c
15. b
16. a
17. c
18. (See Chart 45-8.)
19. b
20. a
21. a
22. b
23. a
24. b

25. c
26. a
27. b
28. a
29. d
30. c
31. a
32. b
33. b
34. d
35. a
36. c
37. e
38. b
39. a
40. d
41. a, b, c, e, f
42. c
43. b
44. d
45. a
46. b
47. c
48. d
49. a
50. b
51. T
52. F
53. T
54. F
55. T
56. F

CHAPTER 46

1. j
2. d
3. a

4. c
5. m
6. h
7. g
8. f
9. i
10. b
11. k
12. l
13. e
14. b
15. c
16. c
17. d
18. d
19. a
20. c
21. a
22. T
23. T
24. F; GBS is self-limiting and paralysis is temporary
25. F; combination shows no additional benefit
26. T
27. T
28. b
29. a
30. a
31. T
32. T
33. F; women are affected three times more than men
34. T
35. T
36. F; deficient in acetylcholine
37. a
38. d
39. c
40. b
41. a
42. c
43. a
44. c
45. b
46. c
47. b
48. d
49. b
50. (See Table 46-3.)
51. b
52. d
53. b
54. c
55. a
56. b
57. d
58. d
59. b

60. c
61. a
62. c
63. c
64. d
65. b
66. a, b, e, f
67. ulnar; radial; femoral; sciatic
68. 24
69. urge to move
70. trigger zone
71. trauma; infection
72. 48; 5
73. inflammatory
74. c
75. c
76. c
77. b
78. b
79. d
80. a
81. a, b, c, f
82. c
83. a
84. a
85. b
86. a
87. b
88. b
89. b
90. a
91. b
92. b
93. b
94. a
95. b, c, d, f
96. c

CHAPTER 47

1. b
2. a
3. b
4. b
5. b
6. a
7. b
8. a
9. b
10. b
11. a, b, d, e
12. d
13. c
14. a
15. b
16. b
17. b
18. b
19. d
20. g
21. e

22. b
23. c
24. f
25. a
26. c
27. b
28. a
29. a
30. c
31. (See Table 47-1.)
32. b
33. c
34. c
35. a, b, d, e, f
36. a, b, c, e
37. a, b, d, f
38. a
39. a
40. b
41. a
42. b
43. a
44. b
45. a
46. b
47. a
48. a
49. c
50. b
51. a
52. c
53. a
54. b
55. a
56. d
57. b
58. a
59. h
60. d
61. a
62. b
63. g
64. e
65. i
66. f
67. c
68. c
69. c
70. a
71. b
72. c
73. a
74. d
75. c
76. a
77. c
78. c
79. c
80. b
81. a, b, d, e

82. a
83. b
84. a
85. a
86. a
87. b
88. b
89. a
90. a
91. b
92. a
93. b
94. b
95. a
96. b
97. c
98. d
99. a, c, d, f
100. b
101. a
102. d
103. c
104. b
105. d
106. c
107. d
108. d
109. b
110. a
111. c

CHAPTER 48

1. c
2. a. 4
   b. 2
   c. 3
   d. 1
   e. 5
3. b, d
4. a
5. c
6. a
7. d
8. b
9. d
10. d
11. e
12. a
13. c
14. b
15. a, b, c, e
16. a, b, c, d

17.

Health History	Reason for Obtaining Information
Family history and genetic risk	Some eye conditions have familial tendencies or genetic predisposition
Current medical systemic diseases	Systemic medical conditions may cause vision complications; previous surgery or trauma may cause current difficulties; specifically ask about laser surgeries
Types of sports activities in which patient participates	Discuss the use of eye protection when playing specific sports
All medications	Medications may cause ocular changes or complications with vision

18. d
19. b, c
20. c
21. a
22. d
23. b
24. c
25. e
26. a, e, f
27. a, c, d
28. b
29. b, d, f
30. d, e
31. c
32. a
33. d
34. b
35. e
36. c
37. d, e
38. c
39. F; does not affect vision
40. T
41. F; located in the upper outer part of the orbit
42. F; protrusion of the eye
43. F; the patient is able to see at 20 feet what a "healthy eye" can see at 70 feet
44. a, c, d, f, g
45. b
46. f
47. e
48. a
49. d
50. c

CHAPTER 49

1. b
2. c
3. d
4. e
5. a
6. a, b, c
7. a, b, c, d, e
8. c
9. c
10. a, e, f
11. b, c, d, e
12. a, b, e
13. c
14. F; no pain or eye redness is associated with age-related cataract formation
15. T
16. T
17. F; rate of progression in each eye is usually different
18. T
19. (Refer to Table 49-1.)
20. a, b, c, d, e,

21.

	Primary Open-Angle Glaucoma	Angle-Closure Glaucoma
Prevalence	Most common	Rare
Symptoms	Asymptomatic: gradual loss of vision fields may go unnoticed. Foggy vision; reduced accommodation; mild aching in eyes or headaches	Severe pain around eyes; vomiting; headache; halos around lights; sudden blurred vision with decreased light perception.
Onset	Gradual	Sudden
Physical examination	Visual fields initially show a small crescent-shaped defect that gradually progresses to a larger field defect	Sclera may appear reddened, and cornea foggy. Anterior chamber is shallow; aqueous humor is cloudy; pupil is moderately dilated and nonreactive.
Tonometry reading	Between 22 and 21 mm Hg	May be 30 mm Hg or higher

22. a. Physically constricting the pupil so that the ciliary muscle is contracted, which allows better circulation of the aqueous humor to the site of absorption
b. Reducing the production of aqueous humor

23.

Drug	Classification	Action	Nursing Implication
Timolol	Beta blocker	Reduce aqueous humor production	Monitor the patient's heart rate and blood pressure. (See Chart 50-2, "Drug Therapy for Eye Problems," for others.)
Pilocarpine	Direct-acting miotic	Constricts the pupil and contracts the ciliary muscle, thus enhancing aqueous outflow	May cause blurred vision for 1 to 2 hours after use; vision in low light environments is difficult because of pupillary constriction. (See Chart 50-2, "Drug Therapy for Eye Problems," for others.)
Latanoprost	Prostaglandin agonist	Improves the outflow of aqueous humor	May cause a permanent color change in the iris that does not affect vision. (See Chart 50-2, "Drug Therapy for Eye Problems," for others.)

24. a, b, e
25. d
26. a, b, e
27. c
28. a, b, c, e
29. a
30. b
31. c
32. c
33. b, c
34. c
35. reading, writing, close work, activities which increase IOP
36. b
37. d
38. b
39. a
40. c

41.

	Radial Keratotomy (RK)	Photorefractive Keratotomy (PRK)	Laser-in-situ Keratomileusis (LASIK)
Indication	Outpatient treatment for mild to moderate myopia.	Outpatient procedure for treatment of mild to moderate stable myopia and low astigmatism, and for some corneal conditions. One eye is treated at a time, with a wait of 3 months between treatments.	Outpatient procedure for correction of near-sightedness, far-sightedness, and astigmatism. Both eyes are usually treated at the same time.
Procedure	Surgical incisions are made through 90% of the peripheral cornea; as a result, the cornea is flattened, and the image is focused closer to the retina.	An excimer laser pulses a beam onto the outer surface of the central cornea, removing small portions of the tissue surface. The cornea is reshaped so that the image is focused on the retina.	The superficial layers of the cornea are lifted temporarily, and brief but powerful laser pulses reshape the deeper corneal layers. The corneal flap is then replaced into its original position.
Postoperative Recovery	May have several days of moderate discomfort after surgery. Patient may still need some visual correction after surgery because slight overcorrection or undercorrection of the refractive error is possible.	Eye is patched after surgery; complete healing to best vision may take 6 months. Usually corrects distance vision problems, but reading glasses may still be needed.	Most patients report improved vision within an hour; complete healing to best vision may take up to 4 weeks. Procedure has less pain than PRK and less time to best vision. Overcorrection or undercorrection is possible, requiring a mild prescription for a continued refractive error.

42. c
43. c
44. d
45. Melanoma
46. d
47. a, b, c, d
48. d
49. b
50. c

CHAPTER 50

1. a
2. c
3. a
4. b
5. b
6. c
7. a
8. c
9. b
10. a. 2
    b. 3
    c. 4
    d. 5
    e. 1
    f. 6
11. a, d
12. c
13. a
14. d
15. b
16. e
17. d
18. a, c, e, f

19. b
20. c, d, e
21. c
22. Air conduction
23. d
24. e
25. f
26. b
27. c
28. a
29. b
30. a, b, c
31. b
32. c
33. a
34. d
35. b
36. a
37. a
38. c
39. c
40. a
41. b

CHAPTER 51

1. a, b, c, e
2. b, c, d, e
3. d
4. a
5. c
6. c
7. b
8. a
9. a
10. b
11. b, c, e, f
12. a
13. a
14. a, b, e
15. b
16. a, b, c, d, e
17. b, c, d, e
18. vertigo
19. a, b, c, e
20. a, b, c, e
21. c
22. a, c, d
23. a
24. T
25. c
26. b
27. a, b, c, d, e
28. a, b, e
29. a, c, e
30. a, b, c, e
31. c, d
32. c
33. e
34. d
35. i

36. h
37. f
38. b
39. g
40. a
41. b, d, e
42. T
43. T
44. F; do not irrigate an ear that has an eardrum perforation or otitis media
45. F; insects are killed before removal unless they can be coaxed out with a light or humming noise
46. F; only trained health care providers should use this method of earwax removal
47. T
48. F; a myringotomy drains middle ear fluid and immediately removes pain in cases of otitis media
49. F; tinnitus is a common problem of patients with ear disorders, but it can be mild or it can be so severe that it interferes with thinking and attention span

CHAPTER 52

1.

Type of Bone	Example
1. Long bones	Femur
2. Short bones	Phalanges
3. Flat bones	Scapula
4. Irregular bones	Inner ear or carpal bones
5. Sesamoid bones	Patella

2. a
3. b
4. h
5. c
6. b
7. e
8. d
9. a
10. k
11. f
12. j
13. i
14. g
15. c
16. b
17. c
18. a
19. F; the knee is a synovial-type joint; shoulder and hip joints are "ball-and-socket" joints
20. T

21. F; rotation only
22. T
23. F; and slight rotation
24. d
25. c
26. a
27. g
28. a
29. b
30. i
31. e
32. h
33. f
34. d
35. c
36. F; bone density decreases
37. F; synovial joint cartilage degenerates with age
38. T
39. b
40. d
41. c
42. d
43. c
44. d
45. a
46. b
47. d
48. (See Table 52-2 in the text.)
49. b, c, e
50. a
51. b
52. c
53. d
54. a
55. a, b, d, e
56. a, b
57. a
58. c
59. e
60. b
61. a
62. d
63. F; African-American men have denser bones than African-American women
64. T
65. F; such as dark green leafy vegetables
66. *Across*
   1. Varum
   3. Gait
   4. Mobility

   Down
   1. Valgum
   2. Scoliosis
67. k
68. e
69. a

70. f
71. b
72. c
73. g
74. i
75. j
76. m
77. l
78. d
79. h

CHAPTER 53

1. b
2. c
3. a
4. c
5. a
6. b
7. a
8. a
9. c
10. b
11. a
12. b
13. a
14. c
15. b
16. a
17. b
18. c
19. c
20. a
21. b
22. a
23. b, c
24. a
25. c
26. b
27. a
28. a, b, c, f
29. b
30. a
31. c
32. a
33. c
34. d
35. f
36. d
37. c
38. a
39. e
40. b
41. b
42. c
43. a
44. b
45. a
46. b
47. a
48. b

49. d
50. a
51. b
52. d
53. a
54. c
55. a
56. b
57. a, c, d
58. d
59. T
60. T
61. F; often extends into the soft tissue
62. F; dull pain and swelling occur over a long period
63. T
64. b
65. a
66. b
67. b
68. a
69. b
70. a
71. c
72. a, b, f
73. a
74. a
75. a
76. c
77. c
78. e
79. a
80. b
81. d
82. a
83. c
84. b
85. c
86. d
87. a
88. b
89. b
90. a
91. c
92. b
93. a
94. b
95. b
96. a
97. b
98. b
99. a
100. b
101. b
102. a
103. b
104. c
105. a
106. c
107. d

108. e
109. a
110. b
111. b
112. d
113. e
114. e
115. a
116. c
117. d
118. T
119. T
120. T
121. F; screened for scoliosis during their middle-school years
122. F; nonstructural scoliosis results
123. F; methods of treatment for adults differ

CHAPTER 54

1. c
2. d
3. b
4. a
5. a, b, d, f
6. d
7. b
8. a
9. b
10. c
11. a
12. c
13. a
14. a. 4
    b. 5
    c. 1
    d. 3
    e. 2
15. d
16. b, c, d
17. d
18. a
19. b
20. b
21. d
22. c
23. b
24. c
25. b
26. a
27. a
28. c
29. a
30. b
31. d
32. c
33. b
34. e
35. d
36. b

37. a
38. c
39. f
40. d
41. c
42. a
43. d
44. a
45. c
46. d
47. a
48. d
49. b
50. (See Chart 54-3.)
51. a. 6
    b. 4
    c. 1
    d. 2
    e. 5
    f. 3
52. b
53. b
54. c
55. a
56. c
57. b
58. c
59. d
60. c
61. b
62. d
63. c
64. e
65. a
66. b
67. d
68. c
69. d
70. c

71. b
72. c
73. c
74. a, b, c, e
75. b
76. a, b, e
77. F; medial meniscus is more likely to tear
78. T
79. F; 6 to 9 months or longer
80. F; athletes who participate in strenuous sports
81. T
82. F; a strain is excessive stretching of a muscle or tendon
83. T
84. T
85. F; cannot maintain abduction
86. a, c, d
87. b
88. c
89. d
90. c
91. d
92. d
93. b
94. a
95. c
96. d
97. a. 5
    b. 1
    c. 2
    d. 4
    e. 3
    f. 6
98. b, c, e, g
99. b
100. a

CHAPTER 55

1. n
2. i
3. t
4. p
5. b
6. r
7. q
8. s
9. d
10. h
11. o
12. e
13. c
14. m
15. k
16. a
17. j
18. f
19. g
20. l
21. a, b, c
22. T
23. F
24. T
25. T
26. a, b, c, d, e
27. a. 4
    b. 3
    c. 2
    d. 1
28. a. 1
    b. 3
    c. 4
    d. 2
29. d
30. d
31. c
32. b
33. a

34.

Assessment Finding	Significance
Fruity-smelling breath	Could be indication the patient has an elevated blood sugar
Asymmetry in the upper quadrants of the abdomen	Right upper quadrant—could indicate changes in the liver, gallbladder, duodenum, head of the pancreas, hepatic flexion of the colon or part of the ascending and transverse colon
	Left upper quadrant—could indicate changes in the left lobe of the liver, stomach, spleen, body and tail of the pancreas, splenic flexure of the colon or part of the transverse and descending colon
Asymmetry in the lower quadrants of the abdomen	Left lower quadrant—could indicate changes in the descending colon, sigmoid colon, left ureter, left ovary and fallopian tube, or the left spermatic cord
	Right lower quadrant—could indicate changes in the cecum, appendix, right ureter, right ovary and fallopian tube, or right spermatic cord
Cullen's sign	Indication of intra-abdominal bleeding
Bruit heard over the abdominal aorta	Usually indicates presence of an aneurysm
Diminished or absent bowel sounds	Often diminished or absent after abdominal surgery or in the patient with peritonitis or paralytic ileus
Loud, gurgling bowel sounds	Result from hypermotility of the bowel (borborygmus); usually heard in the patient with diarrhea or gastroenteritis, or above a complete intestinal obstruction

35. a, b, e
36. a
37. i
38. g
39. a
40. h
41. d
42. f
43. e
44. b
45. c
46. d
47. c
48. b
49. a

CHAPTER 56

1. d
2. a
3. d
4. b
5. c
6. a
7. a
8. e
9. c
10. a
11. d
12. b
13. c
14. d
15. d
16. d
17. b
18. c
19. a

20. c
21. b
22. T
23. T
24. F
25. T
26. T
27. a
28. c
29. c
30. a

CHAPTER 57

1. b
2. a
3. T
4. T
5. F
6. a
7. d
8. b
9. e
10. c
11. f
12. h
13. g
14. i
15. b
16. d
17. a
18. a
19. d
20. d
21. b
22. T
23. T

24. F
25. T
26. a, b, c, d, e
27. b
28. a
29. F
30. T
31. T
32. F
33. T
34. F
35. a
36. b
37. T
38. T
39. T
40. T
41. a, b, c, d, e

CHAPTER 58

1. T
2. F
3. T
4. T
5. F
6. T
7. a, c, d
8. a
9. b
10. d
11. a
12. b
13. d
14. a
15. d

16. T
17. T
18. F
19. T
20. F
21. T
22. c
23. a
24. d
25. b
26. d
27. a, b, c, d, e
28. b
29. c
30. a, b, c, d, e
31. a, b, c, d, e
32. a
33. a
34. c
35. T
36. T
37. F
38. F
39. T
40. T
41. a, c
42. b, c, d, e
43. c
44. T
45. T
46. T
47. F
48. T
49. a
50. a

CHAPTER 59

1. T
2. T
3. F
4. T
5. T
6. F
7. F
8. T
9. a
10. a, b, c, d, e
11. d
12. a
13. f
14. c
15. b
16. e
17. g
18. c
19. d
20. c
21. b
22. T
23. T

24. T
25. T
26. F
27. F
28. T
29. T
30. b
31. a
32. a
33. d
34. a
35. c
36. d
37. b
38. a
39. T
40. T
41. T
42. F
43. F
44. F
45. T
46. T
47. a
48. a, b, c, d, e
49. b
50. b
51. d
52. c
53. a
54. T
55. T
56. T
57. T
58. F
59. T
60. a
61. b, c, d, e
62. c
63. T
64. T
65. T
66. T
67. F
68. T
69. T
70. a
71. c
72. T
73. T
74. T
75. F
76. T
77. d

CHAPTER 60

1. T
2. T
3. T
4. F

5. F
6. T
7. a, b
8. b
9. b, c
10. T
11. T
12. F
13. T
14. c
15. a
16. b
17. c
18. c
19. T
20. T
21. F
22. T
23. d
24. b
25. c, d, e
26. a
27. a. UC
    b. CD
    c. UC
    d. CD
    e. UC
    f. UC
    g. CD
28. a
29. b
30. a
31. b
32. a, b, e
33. c
34. e
35. d
36. f
37. a
38. b
39. c
40. d
41. d
42. T
43. T
44. F
45. T
46. T
47. F
48. d
49. a
50. c
51. c
52. c
53. a
54. b
55. b
56. c
57. a
58. b

59. a, b, c, d
60. c
61. a
62. b
63. d
64. F
65. F
66. T
67. T
68. T
69. T

CHAPTER 61

1. T
2. T
3. F
4. T
5. F
6. T
7. T
8. T
9. T
10. F
11. a, b, c, d, e
12. d
13. b
14. j
15. a
16. f
17. i
18. c
19. g
20. e
21. h
22. d
23. b
24. a, b, c, d, e, f
25. b
26. c
27. b
28. a, c, d, e, f
29. a
30. a
31. d
32. T
33. T
34. T
35. T
36. T
37. a
38. d
39. F
40. T
41. T
42. F
43. F
44. T
45. T
46. a, b, c, d, e
47. a, b, c, d, e

48. T
49. F
50. F
51. T
52. T
53. T
54. F
55. T
56. T
57. a
58. d
59. b, c, d, e
60. a, b, c
61. T
62. T
63. T
64. F
65. T
66. T
67. F
68. T
69. T
70. T

CHAPTER 62

1. a
2. c
3. c
4. a
5. f
6. c
7. a
8. d
9. b
10. e
11. g
12. h
13. b
14. d
15. a
16. b
17. b
18. T
19. T
20. T
21. T
22. F
23. d
24. e
25. c
26. a
27. d
28. b
29. b
30. c
31. a
32. d
33. b
34. F
35. T

36. T
37. T
38. F
39. T
40. F
41. T
42. T
43. d
44. a
45. c
46. d
47. c
48. c
49. T
50. T
51. F
52. T
53. F
54. T

CHAPTER 63

1. T
2. T
3. T
4. F
5. F
6. a, b, c, d, e
7. a, c, d, e
8. a
9. b
10. a, b, c, d, e
11. b
12. f
13. g
14. b
15. a
16. d
17. e
18. c
19. h
20. i
21. F
22. T
23. F
24. T
25. T
26. F
27. T
28. T
29. F
30. T
31. F
32. F
33. T
34. T
35. a, c, d, e
36. e
37. f
38. c
39. d

40. a
41. b
42. b
43. d
44. b
45. c
46. a
47. T
48. F
49. T
50. F
51. F
52. T
53. b
54. a
55. d
56. d
57. a, b, c, d, e
58. c
59. b
60. c
61. a
62. b
63. T
64. T
65. T
66. T
67. F
68. b, c, d, e
69. a, c, d, e
70. d
71. d
72. d

CHAPTER 64

1. a, c, d, e
2. c
3. b
4. h
5. e
6. c
7. d
8. l
9. a
10. f
11. i
12. c
13. e
14. j
15. g
16. k
17. b
18. b
19. e
20. a
21. a
22. d
23. T
24. F; duration of effect is short
25. F; must be free to bind

26. F; except for two hormones that are not stored and must be continuously produced
27. T
28. F; hormone clearance occurs through cellular uptake, enzymatic breakdown, and GI or urinary excretion
29. T
30. T
31. T
32. T
33. F; the pituitary gland also has these factors
34. a
35. b

36.

Endocrine Gland	Principal Hormones Secreted
a. Hypothalamus	CRH, TRH, GnRH, GHRH, GHIH, PIH, MIH
b. Anterior pituitary	TSH, ACTH, LH, FSH, PRL, GH, MSH
c. Posterior pituitary	ADH, oxytocin
d. Thyroid	T_3, T_4, calcitonin
e. Parathyroid	Parathyroid hormone
f. Adrenal cortex	Cortisol, aldosterone
g. Pancreas	Insulin, glucagon, somatostatin
h. Ovary	Estrogen, progesterone
i. Testes	Testosterone

37. b
38. a
39. b
40. a
41. a
42. b
43. F; affects carbohydrate, protein, and fat metabolism
44. T
45. F; ACTH from the anterior pituitary
46. F; peaks occur in the morning
47. T
48. T
49. a, b, c, e
50. F; located anteriorly
51. F; iodine and protein intake
52. F; two distinct lobes
53. F; increases in response
54. a
55. d
56. a, b, c, e
57. b, c, d

58. d
59. d
60. c
61. b
62. d
63. b
64. b, c, d, e
65. b
66. c
67. b
68. d
69. a
70. a
71. b
72. b
73. a, b, c, d
74. b
75. c, d, e, f
76. a, b, d, e
77. b
78. d
79. b

CHAPTER 65

1.

Dysfunction	Cause	Result
Primary pituitary dysfunction	Problem within the pituitary gland: shock with hypotension causing pituitary infarction, rapid loss of body fat, tumor, radiation of the head or brain, trauma, infection, AIDS	Undersecretion of hormones (hypofunction) or oversecretion of hormones (hyperfunction)
Secondary pituitary dysfunction	Dysfunction of hypothalamus: infection, trauma, tumor	Undersecretion of hormones (hypofunction) or oversecretion of hormones (hyperfunction)

2. a, b, c, e
3. c, e
4. a, b, d, e
5. c
6. a
7. a
8. d
9. b
10. c
11. a
12. a, b, c, d, e
13. d, e
14. d
15. c
16. d
17. c
18. c, d, e
19. a, b, c, d
20. b, c, d, e, f
21. b
22. b
23. a
24. c
25. b
26. F; massive diuresis increases plasma osmolality
27. F; excessive output of dilute urine even with decreased intake and thirst
28. T
29. F; less than 1.005
30. T
31. b
32. a, b
33. a, c, d, e
34. c
35. c

36.

	Cause	Evidence
Diabetes insipidus	ADH deficiency or inability of the kidney to respond to ADH, resulting in excretion of large volumes of dilute urine	Frequent urination, excessive thirst, poor skin turgor, dry mucous membranes, excretion of large volumes of dilute urine, low specific gravity and osmolarity
SIADH	ADH excess resulting in water retention, increased ECF volume, and dilutional hyponatremia	Water retention, weight gain, increased ECF volume, dilutional hyponatremia

37. b
38. b
39. c
40. a, c, d
41. a
42. c
43. a. Decreases
    b. Increases
    c. Increases
44. b
45. b
46. d
47. b
48. b
49. d
50. d
51. d
52. d
53. a, d, f, h
54. c
55. b, c, e
56. a
57. a
58. d
59. b
60. b
61. d
62. b
63. a, b, c, d, e
64. a
65. a
66. a, c, d
67. b
68. d

69.

Clinical Finding	Adrenal Insufficiency	Cushing's Syndrome
a. Serum sodium level	Decrease	Increase
b. Serum potassium level	Increase	Decrease
c. ECF volume	Decrease	Increase
d. Blood pressure	Decrease	Increase
e. Serum glucose level	Decrease	Increase
f. Cortisol level	Decrease	Increase

70. d
71. c

CHAPTER 66

1. d
2. a
3. b
4. a
5. a
6. a
7. b
8. a
9. a
10. b
11. a
12. a
13. b
14. a
15. b
16. a
17. b
18. a
19. a
20. b
21. b
22. a
23. a
24. c
25. b
26. b
27. d
28. b
29. a
30. b
31. c
32. e
33. b
34. d
35. c
36. a
37. T

38. F; not hereditary; however, there is a genetic susceptibility to the antibodies
39. T
40. T
41. T
42. T
43. T
44. T
45. F; hyperthyroidism, particularly Graves' disease, causes these cardiac problems
46. T
47. T
48. F; no radiation precautions are necessary because the dose is low
49. T
50. d
51. c
52. a
53. b
54. d
55. e
56. a
57. b
58. c
59. a, c, d
60. a
61. b
62. a, c, d, e
63. a, b, c, e
64. a
65. a, b
66. a, b, c, g
67. e
68. f, h
69. d
70. c, d, e
71. f

72. f
73. b
74. f
75. c
76. f
77. h
78. i
79. f
80. b, c, d, e, g, h
81. a, b, c, d, e
82. d
83. c, d
84. b
85. a
86. b
87. b
88. d
89. c
90. b
91. c
92. b
93. b
94. d
95. a
96. b
97. a
98. c
99. b
100. d
101. c
102. b
103. b
104. a
105. b
106. b
107. a

108.

Laboratory Test	Hyperparathyroidism	Hypoparathyroidism
a. Serum calcium	Increase	Decrease
b. Serum phosphate	Decrease	Increase
c. Serum PTH	Increase	Decrease

109. a
110. a, b, c
111. a, b, c, d, e
112. a, c
113. b
114. a, c, d

CHAPTER 67

1. c
2. b
3. a
4. c
5. b

6. a
7. c
8. b
9. c
10. a
11. b
12. c
13. d
14. d
15. c
16. c
17. a, b, d
18. b, c, d, e
19. a, b

20. a
21. c
22. d
23. c
24. c
25. b
26. b
27. a
28. a
29. b
30. b
31. c
32. a
33. b

34. d
35. a
36. c
37. b
38. d
39. b
40. a
41. c
42. c
43. b
44. c
45. b
46. d
47. c
48. d
49. d
50. b, d, e
51. a
52. d
53. c
54. a
55. b
56. a
57. c
58. b
59. c
60. c
61. F; because of impaired circulation
62. T
63. F; 60% to 90% have peripheral sensory neuropathy
64. T
65. a, b, c, d, e
66. b
67. c
68. a
69. a, b, d, e
70. d
71. b
72. c
73. d
74. a
75. c
76. d
77. a, c, d, e, f
78. c
79. b

80. c
81. c
82. c
83. b
84. b, c, d, e
85. a, b d
86. d
87. d
88. b
89. d
90. d
91. a. 4
    b. 1
    c. 2
    d. 3
92. c
93. a
94. b
95. b
96. a

CHAPTER 68

1. d
2. a
3. e
4. b
5. j
6. c
7. f
8. i
9. h
10. g
11. b
12. a, b, c
13. b
14. b
15. b
16. a
17. a
18. b
19. a
20. a
21. volume; composition; waste
22. acid-base
23. 20; 25
24. 125

25. pressure; flow
26. Antidiuretic hormone (ADH)
27. water
28. antidiuretic hormone (ADH)
29. reabsorption
30. b
31. c
32. c
33. a, b, e
34. c
35. d
36. c
37. b
38. b
39. d
40. b
41. b
42. d
43. b
44. a
45. a
46. d
47. b
48. e
49. g
50. i
51. l
52. n
53. a
54. d
55. h
56. j
57. m
58. k
59. f
60. c
61. b
62. b
63. a
64. a
65. a
66. c
67. c
68. b
69. c
70. a

71.

Test	Abnormal Findings	Significance of Abnormal Findings
Color	Dark amber Very pale yellow Dark red or brown Other	Concentrated urine Diluted urine Blood in the urine; brown also may indicate increased urinary bilirubin level, red may also indicate the presence of myoglobin Other color changes may result from diet or medications
Odor	Foul smell	Possible infection, dehydration, or ingestion of certain foods or drugs
Turbidity	Cloudy urine	Infection, sediment, or high levels of urinary protein
Specific gravity	Increased level above 1.030 Decreased level below 1.000	Decreased renal perfusion, inappropriate antidiuretic hormone secretion, or congestive heart failure Chronic renal insufficiency, diabetes insipidus, malignant hypertension, diuretic administration, and lithium toxicity
pH	Changes in level	Change in diet, administration of medications, infection, freshness of the specimen, acid-base imbalance, altered renal function
Glucose	Presence of glucose	Hyperglycemia or a decrease in the renal threshold for glucose
Ketones	Presence of ketones	Incomplete metabolism of fatty acids as in diabetic ketoacidosis, prolonged fasting, anorexia nervosa
Protein	Increased amount above 0.8 mg/dL	Stress, infection, recent strenuous exercise, glomerular disorders
Bilirubin (urobilinogen)	Presence of bilirubin	Hepatic or biliary disease or obstruction
Red blood cells (RBCs)	Increased amount of 0-2 per high-power field	Normal with indwelling or intermittent catheterization or menses but may reflect tumor, stones, trauma, glomerular disorders, cystitis, or bleeding disorders
White blood cells (WBCs)	Increased amount above 0-3 per high-power field (males) and 0-5 per high-power field (females)	Infectious or inflammatory process anywhere in the renal/urinary tract, renal transplant rejection, fever, exercise
Casts	Increased amounts	Presence of bacteria or protein, which is seen in severe renal disease and could also indicate urinary calculi
Crystals	Presence of crystals	Presence of normal or abnormal crystals may indicate that the specimen has been allowed to stand
Bacteria	Increased amounts above 1000 colonies/mL	Need for urine culture to determine the presence of urinary tract infection
Parasites	Presence of parasites	Presence of *Trichomonas vaginalis* indicates infection, usually of the urethra, prostate, or vagina
Leukoesterase	Presence of leukoesterase	Urinary tract infection
Nitrites	Presence of nitrites	Urinary *Escherichia coli*

72. c
73. b
74. c
75. a. 2
   b. 5
   c. 4
   d. 1
   e. 7
   f. 3
   g. 6
   h. 8
76. a
77. c
78. b
79. c

80. a
81. b
82. d
83. b
84. a
85. c
86. a
87. b
88. b
89. d

CHAPTER 69

1. b
2. f

3. a
4. h
5. c
6. k
7. d
8. j
9. g
10. i
11. l
12. e
13. T
14. F; especially among women
15. T

16. F; colonization usually does not progress unless the patient has other pathologic problems
17. T
18. a, e, g
19. a
20. a, b, d
21. c
22. c
23. a
24. c
25. a
26. b
27. b
28. d
29. c
30. b, c, d, e
31. a
32. b
33. a
34. b
35. c
36. a
37. d
38. c
39. a
40. c
41. d
42. a
43. a, b, c, d, f
44. b
45. a
46. c
47. b
48. d
49. c
50. a
51. b
52. d
53. a
54. a
55. d
56. c
57. d
58. b
59. a, b, d
60. F; is appropriate, if caregivers are conscientious in the scheduled toileting routine
61. F; increases the osmolarity and concentration of urine, making it more irritating and stimulating the urge to urinate
62. T
63. F; cholinergic agents may be used as short-term therapy for patients with reflex incontinence, particularly after surgery
64. b
65. c
66. d

67. d
68. a
69. a, b, c, e, g
70. d
71. b
72. a
73. b
74. c
75. d
76. a
77. c
78. b
79. c
80. d
81. c
82. d
83. d

CHAPTER 70

1. b
2. a
3. b
4. b
5. a
6. a
7. c
8. a, b, c, d, g
9. d
10. c
11. a
12. a, b, d, e
13. b
14. c
15. c
16. c
17. c
18. d
19. a
20. a
21. a
22. b
23. c
24. a
25. a
26. a
27. b
28. b
29. a
30. b
31. b
32. a
33. d
34. a
35. d
36. c
37. b
38. b
39. c
40. b
41. c

42. c
43. c
44. c
45. a, c, d, e
46. a
47. T
48. F; cysts can form in the other tissues such as the vessels and liver. Other organs can be displaced.
49. F; results in increased blood pressure
50. F; the commonality for the three is obstruction
51. F; caused by ischemia, fluid and electrolyte imbalance, and hypertension
52. T
53. F; is related to decreased renal blood flow, ischemia, and renal fibrosis
54. F; Stage IV
55. a
56. b
57. c
58. d
59. d
60. b
61. a
62. b
63. a
64. a
65. d
66. b
67. d
68. a
69. d
70. a, b, c, e, g, h
71. b
72. b, c, d, e
73. b
74. c
75. c
76. d
77. b
78. b
79. c
80. a
81. a
82. b, c, d, e
83. c
84. a
85. b
86. b, c, d, f, g
87. a
88. b
89. c
90. b
91. c
92. d
93. a, b, c, d, f, g
94. c
95. c

CHAPTER 71

1. T
2. T
3. T
4. T
5. F; may occur with the loss of 50% of nephrons as opposed to CRF which may not occur until 90% to 95% are lost
6. c
7. a
8. b
9. a
10. b
11. c
12. c
13. b
14. a
15. a
16. a
17. b
18. c
19. c
20. a
21. d
22. a, b, c
23. c
24. d
25. b
26. b
27. a
28. a, b, e
29. a
30. a, c, d, f
31. a
32. c
33. a, c, d, g, h
34. a
35. d
36. a
37. a, c, d, f
38. a
39. a
40. b, c
41. c
42. a
43. a
44. c
45. b
46. c
47. b, c
48. c
49. a
50. a
51. a, b, c
52. a
53. b
54. c
55. c
56. c
57. d
58. c
59. b
60. a
61. c
62. c
63. a
64. d
65. a
66. b
67. c
68. a
69. d
70. c
71. a, b, c, e, f
72. c
73. a
74. a, d, e, f
75. b
76. a
77. a, b, d, e, f
78. a, c, e
79. b
80. a
81. c
82. b
83. a, c, e
84. b
85. c
86. a, b, c
87. b
88. a, b, c, d, e, g
89. a, c, d, e
90. a
91. d
92. b
93. a
94. d
95. b
96. a
97. d
98. a, b, c, e
99. a
100. c
101. d
102. a. 2
    b. 1
    c. 3
103. c
104. e
105. a
106. c
107. b
108. d
109. f
110. a
111. b
112. b, c, d, e, g
113. c
114. a
115. c
116. b, c
117. b, c, d, e, f
118. d
119. c
120. b

CHAPTER 72

1. T
2. T
3. F; the epididymis
4. F; are anovulatory and irregular
5. d
6. b
7. c
8. b
9. b
10. a
11. a, b, d, e
12. b
13. d
14. c
15. d
16. c
17. 4; 5
18. endometrial
19. dominant
20. 10; 16
21. body fat
22. calcium
23. 11; 13 1/2
24. tactile; psychogenic
25. motility; vaginal
26. premenstrual
27. d
28. c
29. c
30. c
31. d
32. a
33. a
34. b
35. b
36. c
37. c
38. a
39. e
40. i
41. f
42. b
43. d
44. g
45. j
46. c
47. h
48. a
49. b
50. a
51. d
52. a
53. b

54. c
55. d
56. a, b, d, f
57. a, b, c
58. a
59. a
60. a
61. d
62. f
63. e
64. a
65. i
66. b
67. h
68. c
69. g
70. c
71. b
72. a
73. b
74. d
75. b
76. d
77. a, d, e
78. a
79. a, c, e, f
80. a, b, e
81. a. 4
     b. 3
     c. 5
     d. 2
     e. 1

CHAPTER 73

1. a
2. j
3. g
4. b
5. c
6. d
7. h
8. i
9. e
10. f
11. a
12. a
13. a
14. b, c, e, f
15. d
16. b, c, d, e
17. c
18. a
19. b, c, e, f
20. c
21. fibrosis; cysts
22. regional lymph
23. bone; lungs; brain; liver
24. pregnancy
25. estrogen
26. c

27. b
28. a
29. d
30. b
31. b
32. b
33. c
34. c
35. d
36. c
37. d
38. a
39. c
40. b
41. d
42. a
43. d
44. F; over half will have changes
45. F; during the reproductive years
46. T
47. F; does not increase
48. F; ductal ectasia does not affect risk
49. T
50. T
51. F; increase is five-fold
52. T
53. a
54. d
55. b
56. d
57. d
58. a
59. c
60. a
61. b, c, e
62. b
63. d
64. b
65. b
66. b
67. c
68. a
69. b
70. c
71. a
72. a, b, d, f

CHAPTER 74

1. k
2. c
3. e
4. i
5. h
6. f
7. l
8. a
9. b
10. d

11. g
12. j
13. prostaglandins
14. underlying
15. breast cancer
16. ectopic
17. progesterone
18. a, b, c, d, e
19. a
20. d
21. c
22. b
23. a
24. d
25. b
26. b
27. d
28. b
29. b
30. a
31. a
32. b
33. c
34. c
35. b
36. d
37. a
38. b, c, d, f
39. a
40. b, c, d, e
41. b
42. a
43. a
44. a, b, d, e
45. a, b, d, e, f
46. c
47. a
48. e
49. b
50. d
51. b
52. b
53. a
54. c
55. c
56. d
57. b
58. b
59. b, c, e
60. c
61. d
62. a
63. c
64. d
65. a
66. c
67. d
68. b
69. a

70. c
71. d
72. a
73. c
74. c
75. b
76. a, b, c, e, f
77. c

CHAPTER 75

1. slowest; predictable
2. 65
3. 15; 34
4. 5
5. Penile
6. a
7. a
8. c
9. a
10. a
11. a
12. a, b, c, e
13. c
14. a
15. d
16. c
17. c
18. k
19. b
20. g
21. l
22. h
23. i
24. e
25. a
26. j
27. f
28. d
29. m
30. b
31. a, c, d, e, g
32. d
33. d
34. b
35. a
36. a
37. b
38. b
39. a
40. e
41. d
42. c
43. a, b, e
44. a

45. d
46. d
47. a
48. a
49. c
50. c
51. b
52. a
53. c
54. a, b, d
55. a
56. b
57. c
58. b
59. d
60. d
61. c
62. a, b, d, f
63. b
64. a
65. a
66. a
67. a
68. c, d, e, f, g
69. b
70. a
71. d
72. b
73. a, b, c, f
74. a
75. a
76. c

CHAPTER 76

1. a
2. d
3. a
4. b
5. a
6. c
7. c
8. a
9. b
10. T
11. F; causative organism of syphilis
12. T
13. F; pelvic inflammatory disease is one of the leading causes
14. T
15. F; is *Neisseria gonorrhoeae*
16. F; are developed by the Centers for Disease Control and Prevention

17. T
18. F; nonoxynol-9 may increase risk
19. c
20. c
21. a
22. b
23. a
24. b
25. d
26. c
27. b
28. c
29. b
30. d
31. c
32. c
33. a
34. f
35. l
36. a
37. h
38. c
39. k
40. e
41. b
42. g
43. j
44. i
45. d
46. c, d, e
47. b
48. a
49. c
50. a
51. d
52. c
53. d
54. d
55. b
56. b
57. c
58. a, b, c, e
59. a
60. a, b, e
61. c
62. b
63. c
64. c, d, e, g
65. b
66. a